Handbook of

WOMEN'S HEALTH

An evidence-based approach

This practical handbook provides a clear and comprehensive evidence-based primary-care guide to the care of women in ambulatory practice, intended for general and family practitioners, nurses, physicians assistants and all those who practice primary care of women. It emphasizes preventive care and well-woman care throughout the life cycle of a woman, including sexuality, contraception, medical care in pregnancy, and psychological and important medical concerns. It stresses the strength of evidence underlying common practices of care of women.

- It recognizes and pays heed to the cultural, social and psychological differences that impact on women's health
- It conveys a consistently positive message in terms of seeking solutions to women's health care problems and emphasizes preventive health care
- It provides insightful tips and checklists to highlight women's common health problems and effective evidence-based treatment
- Suitable for health care workers of all levels and specialties who practice primary care of women

Dr. Rosenfeld is a family physician, fellow of the American Academy of Family Physicians, and Assistant Professor of General Internal Medicine at Johns Hopkins School of Medicine. She graduated from Johns Hopkins School of Medicine and completed a residency in Family Practice at Case Western University Hospitals, Cleveland, Ohio. She practiced on the Eastern Shore of Maryland and then became Associate Program Director of the St. Francis Family Practice Residency in Wilmington, Delaware. She was Professor of Family Medicine, then, at East Tennessee State University and Program Director of the Family Practice Residency in Bristol, Tennessee. She is author and editor of *Women's Health in Primary Care* (1997) and coauthor of the American Academy of Family Physicians' *Quick Guide to Women's Health* (2000). She has authored over 50 articles and research articles on women's health.

Handbook of

WOMEN'S HEALTH

An evidence-based approach

Edited by **Jo Ann Rosenfeld**

Johns Hopkins School of Medicine

LIVERPOOL
JOHN MOORES UNIVERSITY
AVRIL ROBARTS LRC
TEL. 0151 231 4022

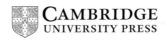

CAMBRIDGE
UNIVERSITY PRESS

PUBLISHED BY THE PRESS SYNDICATE OF THE UNIVERSITY OF CAMBRIDGE
The Pitt Building, Trumpington Street, Cambridge, United Kingdom

CAMBRIDGE UNIVERSITY PRESS
The Edinburgh Building, Cambridge CB2 2RU, UK
40 West 20th Street, New York NY10011-4211, USA
10 Stamford Road, Oakleigh, VIC 3166, Australia
Ruiz de Alarcón 13, 28014 Madrid, Spain
Dock House, The Waterfront, Cape Town 8001, South Africa

http://www.cambridge.org

© Cambridge University Press 2001

This book is in copyright. Subject to statutory exception
and to the provisions of relevant collective licensing agreements,
no reproduction of any part may take place without
the written permission of Cambridge University Press.

First published 2001

Printed in the United Kingdom at the University Press, Cambridge

Typeface Utopia 10/14pt   *System* Poltype ® [v n]

A catalogue record for this book is available from the British Library

Library of Congress Cataloguing in Publication data

Handbook of women's health: an evidence-based approach / edited by Jo Ann Rosenfeld.
   p.   cm.
Includes bibliographical references and index.
ISBN 0 521 78833 1
1. Women – Health and hygiene – Handbooks, manuals, etc.   2. Evidence-based medicine –
Handbooks, manuals, etc.   I. Rosenfeld, Jo Ann.
[DNLM: 1. Womens Health – Handbooks.   2. Evidence-Based Medicine – Handbooks.
3. Primary Health Care – Handbooks. WA 39 H2366 2001]
RA778.H225   2001
613'.04244 – dc21   00-068873

ISBN 0 521 78833 1

Every effort has been made in preparing this book to provide accurate and up-to-date
information which is in accord with accepted standards and practice at the time of publication.
Nevertheless, the authors, editors and publisher can make no warranties that the information
contained herein is totally free from error, not least because clinical standards are constantly
changing through research and regulation. The authors, editors and publisher therefore
disclaim all liability for direct or consequential damages resulting from the use of material
contained in this book. Readers are strongly advised to pay careful attention to information
provided by the manufacturer of any drugs or equipment that they plan to use.

Contents

Common medical problems   481

Contributors

Kathyrn Andolsek, MD
Duke University Medical Center
PO Box 2914
Durham, NC 27710
USA

Barbara S. Apgar, MD, MS
883 Sciomeadow Drive
Ann Arbor, MI 4810
USA

Kay Bauman, MD. MPH
University of Hawaii
Wahiawa Hospital
95–390 Kuahelani Avenue
Mililani, HI 96789
USA

Deborah Bostock, MD
Uniformed Services University
Dept of Family Practice
4301 Jones Bridge Rd
Bethesda, MD 20814-4799
USA

Abenaa Brewster, MD
Johns Hopkins Oncology Center
422 North Bond Street
Baltimore, MD 21231
USA

Ann Brown, MD
Box 3611
Duke University Medical Center
Durham, NC 27710
USA

Sandra Burge, PhD
University of Texas Health Science Center,
Department of Family Practice
7703 Floyd Curl Drive
San Antonio, TX 78284-7701
USA

Pamela Connor, PhD
1127 Union Avenue
Memphis, TN 38104
USA

Nancy Davidson, MD
Johns Hopkins Oncology Center
422 North Bond Street
Baltimore, MD 21231
USA

Mari Egan, MD
Northwestern University Medical School
Morton Bldg
303 East Chicago Avenue
Chicago, IL 61611
USA

Amy Ellwood, MSW
Dept of Family Medicine and Community
Medicine
6375 Charleston Boulevard
Las Vegas, NV 89146
USA

William Hueston, MD
Medical University of South Carolina
Department of Family Medicine
295 Calhoun Street
Charleston, SC 29403-8702
USA

Rebecca Jaffe, MD
3105 Limestone Road
Suite 200
Wilmington, DE 19808-2151
USA

Janet Lair, MD
Box 3886
Duke University Medical Center
Durham, NC 27710
USA

Patricia Lenahan, PhD
Dept of Family Medicine and Community
Medicine
6375 Charleston Boulevard
Las Vegas, NV 89146
USA

Diane Madlon-Kay, MD
Regions Hospital
640 Jackson Street, Suite 8
St Paul, MN 55101
USA

Cathy Morrow, MD
Maine-Dartmouth Family Practice
4 Sheridan Road
Fairfield, ME 04937
USA

Kris Pena, MD
9101 Franklin Square Drive
Suite 205
Baltimore, MD 21237
USA

Kathy Reilly, MD
900 Northeast 10th Street
Oklahoma City, OK 73104
USA

Jo Ann Rosenfeld, MD
1112 Nicodemus Road
Reisterstown, MD 21136
USA

Rebecca Saenz, MD
University of Mississippi Medical Center
2500 North State Street
Jackson, MS 39216
USA

Ellen Sakornbut, MD
University of Tennessee at Memphis
Department of Family Practice
1121 Union Avenue
Memphis, TN 38104-6646
USA

Jeannette South-Paul, MD
Uniformed Services University
Dept of Family Practice
4301 Jones Bridge Rd
Bethesda, MD 20814-4799
USA

Laura Tavernier, MD
1127 Union Avenue
Memphis, TN 38104
USA

Valerie Ulstad, MD
10551 Morgan Ave South
Bloomington, MN 55431
USA

Cheryl Woodson, MD
Uniformed Services University
Dept of Family Practice
4301 Jones Bridge Road
Bethesda, MD 20814-4799
USA

Common abbreviations used in the text

AIDS	acquired immune deficiency syndrome
b.i.d.	twice daily
BMI	body mass index
CDC	Centers for Disease Control and Prevention
CHD	coronary heart disease
CT	computed tomography
FDA	US Food and Drug Administration
HDL	high density lipoprotein
HIV	human immunodeficiency virus
HRT	hormone replacement therapy
i.m.	intramuscular
IU	international unit
i.v.	intravenous
IUD	intrauterine device
LDL	low density lipoprotein
MPA	medroxyprogesterone acetate
MRI	magnetic resonance imaging
NSAIDs	nonsteroidal antiinflammatory drugs
OCPs	oral contraceptive pills
OR	odds ratio
p.o.	by mouth
Pap smear	Papanicolaou smear
PCOS	polycystic ovary syndrome
PID	pelvic inflammatory disease
q.d.	daily
q.h.s.	before sleep
q.i.d.	four times daily
RCT	randomized controlled trial
RR	relative risk
STD	sexually transmitted disease
t.i.d.	three times daily
UTI	urinary tract infection

Normal blood values in women and during pregnancy

Laboratory value	Physiological change during pregnancy	Prepregnancy value	Pregnancy value, third trimester
Hematology			
ESR	No change	Westegren 0–20 mm/h	Same
Hematocrit	Decreased	39.8%	33.5%
MCV	No change	80–96 μm^3	Same
Platelet count	No change	150 000–300 000/mm^2	Same
Platelet concentration	Unchanged or slightly decreased	150 000–300 000/μL	< 100 000/μL abnormal
RBC count	Reduced	4.2–5.4 million/mm^2	4.0 million/mm^2
Red cell volume	Increased 30%	1400 ml	1600 mL
Total blood volume	Increased	4000 ml	5430 mL
WBC count	Increased	6000–9000 cells/mm^2	Variable
Chemistry			
Albumin	Decreased	3.3–5.2 g/dL	2.5–4.5 g/dL
Alkaline phosphatase	Increased	35–150 IU/L	2–4 × normal: 60–200 IU/L
ALT, AST	Unchanged	1–40 IU/L	Same
Amylase	Unchanged	25–125 IU/L	90–350 IU/L
Blood urea nitrogen	Decreased	13 mg/dL	9 mg/dL
Chloride, serum	Slightly decreased	96–106 mEq/L	93–100 mEq/L
Cholesterol	Increased	100–199 mg/dL	180–280 mg/dL
HDL		35–150 mg/dL	
VLDL		5–40 mg/dL	
LDL		0–125 mg/dL	
Triglycerides		0–199 mg/dL	
Creatinine, serum	Decreased	0.8 mg/dL	0.4–0.6 mg/dL
Ferritin	Slightly increased	20–200 ng/mL	50–200 ng/mL
Glucose, fasting	Decreased	70–115 mg/dL	60–105 mg/dL
Hemoglobin A1c	Unchanged	3–5% of total hemoglobin	Same
Lipase	Decreased		
Total serum protein concentration	Decreased 20%		
Uric acid	Decreased	4–6 mg/100 mL	3.5 mg/100 mL
Hormone levels			
Prolactin	Increased	1–20 ng/mL	50–400 ng/mL
Testosterone	Increased	20–75 ng/dL	40–200 ng/dL
Thyroid hormones			
Serum T4	Increased	7–12 μg/100 mL	10–16 μg/100 mL
T3RU	Decreased	24–36%	22%
Coagulation factors			
Factor XI, XII, antithrombin III	Decreased 50–70%		
Fibrinogen	Increased	170–410 mg/dL	450 mg/dL
All other coagulation factors	Increased		

WBC, white blood cell; RBC, red blood cell; ESR, erythrocyte sedimentation rate; MCV, mean corpuscular volume; ALT, alanine aminotransferase; AST, aspartate aminotransferase; HDL, high density lipoprotein; LDL, low density lipoprotein; VLDL, very low density lipoprotein.

Introduction

Jo Ann Rosenfeld, MD

The purpose of this book is to consider the woman and her health needs in her position in her life cycle, her family, and society. Women have historically been "the other" in medical care. Sigmund Freud and Erik Erikson considered women's development to be deviant from the normal, which was men's. Although the Greeks Hippocrates and Soranus wrote about women's medical needs, women's health concerns have either been considered abnormal, or, traditionally, been condensed to their gynecological functions and disorders, perhaps because these were their only valued functions. Since the 1860s and the organization of medicine, women's health and those who provided for it were usually considered one of the least important parts of medicine. In the past 20 to 40 years, women's health concerns have begun to take their place as topics worthy of discussion.

Recognizing that combining "all women" into any classification is fraught with difficulties, this book attempts to distinguish and point out the differences and individualities of women. Women are more likely to be different than all alike, and must be treated as individuals.

Because much of clinical experience and research does not separate or study women independently, this book examines the strength and depth of evidence, using clinical experience and data discovered on studies on women, when available, and on men, when research on women is lacking. Thus, at times, deciding on the best way to help the woman manage health concerns may be difficult.

Finally, realizing that women seek physicians' care for a variety of purposes, only some of which are medical diseases, this book emphasizes collaborative care between the woman and her physician. Women's health concerns are not all diseases, nor should all women be considered patients. Contraception, fertility, infertility, cigarette, alcohol and drug abuse, sexuality, life changes, and family problems need collaboration and cooperative care, not disease management. Emphasizing prevention, this book will help practitioners' daily work with women to promote health.

1 Singular health care of women

Jo Ann Rosenfeld, MD

The way women's health concerns have been handled, examined, and researched by the medical establishment may be different from that of men. Women's health concerns have been considered different and abnormal when compared with that of men. Yet differences between men and women, noted in medicine and by physicians, may be more creations of society and its expectations than of nature;[1] women are more similar to men than they are different.

Research

Exclusion and extension

1. Researchers have historically assumed that data collected and extended from male subjects, often middle-aged white men, applied to women of all ages (and the elderly) as well.[2] The American Medical Association (AMA) has said "Medical treatments for women are based on a male model, regardless of the fact that women may react differently to treatments than men or that some diseases manifest themselves differently in women than men. The results of medical research on men are generalized to women without sufficient evidence of applicability to women."[3]

2. Exclusion: Women, children, ethnic minorities and the elderly have been excluded from research protocols. The justification given for this "is lack of data, but there is also a belief that health iniquities are a smaller problem for women than men."[4]

   For example, research into the acquired immune deficiency syndrome (AIDS) is almost completely androcentric. Until 1993 the US Centers for Disease Control (CDC) failed to recognize different manifestations of human immunodeficiency virus (HIV) infection in women, such as pelvic inflammatory disease (PID), vaginal infections and cervical cancer. AIDS vaccine trials and mandatory screening of pregnant women continue the different treatment of women in research.

Yet, the percentage of women with AIDS is increasing and women are at least twice as susceptible to HIV infection compared with men. The first large AIDS study on women started only in 1994 and is following 2500 women with AIDS.[5]

3. Marginalization: What research that has been done on women's problems has emphasized female childbearing concerns. For example, there is extensive research on female contraception while comparable research on men has been neglected.[2] Research in this area ignored women, unless it considered increasing, improving or controlling fertility, in which case women shared an unequal and almost exclusive burden.

> Medical treatments for women are based on a male model, regardless of the fact that women may react differently to treatments than men.

New guidelines for research

In 1994, realizing these disparities, the National Institutes of Health (NIH) issued new guidelines for research funding. In addition to continuing inclusion of women and members of minority groups in research, the NIH has been tasked with:

1. Ensuring that women and members of minorities are included in all human subject research. "Women of childbearing potential should not be routinely excluded from participation in clinical research."[6]

2. For phase III trials, ensuring that women and minorities "must be included such that valid analyses of differences in intervention effect can be accomplished".[6]

3. Cost is not an acceptable reason for excluding these groups.

4. The NIH must "initiate programs and support for outreach efforts to recruit these groups into clinical studies."[6]

5. "Over the past decade [the 1990s], there has been growing concern that the drug development process does not produce adequate information about the effect of drugs in women . . .. Analyses of published clinical trials in certain therapeutic areas (notably cardiovascular disease) have indicated that there has been little or no participation of women in many of the studies."[7]

6. The FDA may even have a requirement that women are included in early studies if disease is serious and affects women.[7]

Women in population studies

1. Except for the Framingham study, in which 2200 women were included to act as a control group for the study of the development of heart disease in men, most early, large, prospective population studies excluded or did not actively recruit women. In the past two decades, there have been several important long-term women-only studies.

2. The Nurses' Health Study (NHS) enrolled 120 000 women aged between age 30 and 55 years; participants, now aged 50 to 75, have been followed for more than 20 years. Every two years, this cohort fills out extensive questionnaires about their health and lifestyles and the questions are periodically changed, allowing examination of the relationship between different lifestyle factors and medical outcomes.[8]

3. Other large population studies that involved women are listed in Table 1.1. Realizing some of these research deficits, recently the Women's Health Initiative (WHI) was started. It is a large-scale multicenter randomized trial, evaluating 163 000 postmenopausal women, and examining preventative therapies including hormone replacement treatment (HRT), heart disease, osteoporosis and breast cancer, and the first results cannot be expected until approximately 2006.[9]

Societal differences between men and women that affect health

Men and women may live different lives within society and the way they live affects their health.

Caregiving

1. Women are more likely to be caregivers to children, spouses, and the elderly family members, putting themselves at risk of increased stress and role stresses. Women are more likely to perform duties at home and work. Twenty five percent of women working full time also care for a relative.

2. Long-term care for relatives is a familial responsibility that usually devolves upon women. Lower income women bear a disproportionate burden in caring for elderly relatives.[10]

3. Caregivers are more likely to suffer anxiety, depression and role stress, and accompanying medical problems.

Insurance

Women are more likely to be uninsured and underinsured. They may work parttime or in professions or jobs that do not provide insurance, and, if

Table 1.1. Population studies that examined the health of many women

Author(s)	Title	Comments
Colditz, Stampf and others	Nurses' Health Study	Prospective cohort of 121 701 female registered nurses (98% white) 30–55 years old when started in 1976. Followed 12 or more years
Buring	Women's Health Study	1992: > 38 000 health care professional women, looking at effect of aspirin on heart attacks
	Women's Health Initiative	Prospective study of more than 163 000 postmenopausal women testing impact of low fat diets, estrogen, and calcium and vitamin D on breast cancer, osteoporosis, hip fractures and cardiovascular disease
	Framingham Study	2200 women used to study cardiovascular disease
	PEPI Trial	Postmenopausal Estrogen/Progestin Intervention Trial 1987 from National Heart Lung and Blood Institute found that orally administered estrogen alone or in combination with progesterone increased levels of HDL cholesterol in 875 postmenopausal women over 3 years of follow-up
Clay	Royal College of General Practitioners Oral Contraception Study	1400 general practitioners looking at 46 000 women half of whom used OCPs
	1993 NIAID Women's Interagency HIV study	2500 women with AIDS

HDL, high density lipoprotein.

divorced or single, may not be eligible for spouse's or family insurance. By 2025, only 37 percent of women in the USA aged 65 to 69 years will still be in their first marriage.[11] This makes it less likely for these women to receive preventive and continuing health services.

Living circumstances

Within each disease process, the circumstances for women may be different from those of men and these circumstances must be taken into account in the care of women with health problems.

1. For example, men with chronic obstructive lung disease (COPD) are very likely to be in their 60s, be insured (at least by Medicare in the USA) be married, and have a wife to help with their care and activities of daily living (ADLs). Women with COPD are more likely to be in their 50s, living alone, and uninsured. If they need help, family members or community groups may be needed.

2. Similarly, women with severe drug abuse problems (see Chapter 27) are more likely than men to be multiply addicted, homeless, and with children. In caring for the woman with addiction, dealing with her individual circumstances is very important.

Elderly women

1. Among the elderly, more men are married, and many more women are living alone (two-thirds of women versus one-half of men). Dietary recommendations may be easier to suggest to, and will be followed by, a married man whose wife does the cooking, than to a single woman.

2. Women are more likely to be widowed and live widowed a longer time than men. As well, many men are less prepared to experience loss, and women have more years to adapt to their loss. Men are less accepting of relocation.

3. Many more elderly men have an adequate income and perceive their health status as excellent. Fewer men have activity restrictions and very few men have impairments in ADLs. Women are more likely to be disabled.[12] Older women, in the USA are two times more likely to be living below the poverty level. Women may be less likely to follow exercise recommendations or obtain prescription medications that are not covered by Medicare.

4. Women are more likely to smoke at home, while men smoke during breaks at work. Women are less likely to use smoking cessation programs, especially work-related programs, and are less likely to quit.

5. More women are elderly, and the older the population the greater the percentage who are women. More women (38 percent) live to 85 years than men (18 percent). From age 65 to 69 years there are 81 men per 100 women, but over age 85 there are only 39 men per 100 women.[12]

6. Drug use: The average elderly woman takes eight drugs daily.[13] Women and the elderly are more likely to have comorbid disease processes and to be taking more medications that affect the drug investigated. Other drug use may affect a particular drug's pharmacokinetics.

7. Pharmacokinetics: Older women have a lower blood volume, decreased gastric acid and reduced intestinal motility. Older women are more likely to suffer central nervous system (CNS) side effects such as confusion, disorientation, delirium, and hallucinations.

Table 1.2. Percentage of participants in drug studies by gender

Drug type	1983 Men	1983 Women	1989 Men	1989 Women	GAO 1992 Men	GAO 1992 Women
Antiinflammatory	32–36	60–68	31	69	35–40	60–65
Cardiovascular	64–72	27–36	36–59	33–64	31–85	15–70
Antibiotic	48–57	43–52	67	33	33–89	11–67
Antiulcer	77	23	69–72	28–31	40–67	33–60

GAO, General Accounting Office figures.

8. Older women are more likely to use outpatient services and less likely to be hospitalized than older men.[14]

The average elderly woman takes eight drugs daily.

Inherent physical and medical differences between women and men

Immunology

Women are immunologically stronger – less susceptible to infection and more likely to contract autoimmune diseases.

Drug use and metabolism

1. Drug studies, especially phase III trials, historically were performed on white middle-aged and adult men (Table 1.2). Some drug studies, such as those of heart disease and antibiotic medications, used primarily men, although these problems are just as important in women. On the other hand, antiarthritis and antiinflammation drugs were tested primarily in women. The percentages given in Table 1.2 have not changed much in the past 20 years.
2. Recent requirements have added ethnic minorities, children, the elderly, and women as populations on which all drugs must be studied. Many of the elderly are women. Drug use, distribution, and toxicity may be fundamentally different in women and the elderly than in men.
3. Women are more likely to receive prescriptions during a physician's visit, receive a prescription for psychotropic medications, and spend more money on prescription and nonprescription drugs.[15]
4. Variations in drug pharmacokinetics can arise from many factors.

Women are more likely to receive prescriptions during a physician's visit.

a. Women have longer gastric emptying time and less gastric acid. They have slower intestinal transit time and these differences are independent of hormone use and menstrual status. Women metabolize some common substances, such as alcohol, differently from men, and women have an increased and quicker bioavailability with the same amount of alcohol ingested.

b. Women have a larger percentage of fat and a lower total body water value, except when they are pregnant. Antidepressant levels are dependent on body size and fat levels; side effects and therapeutic levels may occur at lower doses than they do in men.

c. Age affects pharmacokinetics. Older people have decreased renal function. For example, younger people metabolize theophylline more quickly.

d. Men have different renal function with higher serum urinary creatinine levels and higher creatinine clearance values, affecting the clearance of drugs, such as antibiotics, metabolized and eliminated by the kidneys. Nonpregnant women may need lower doses of renally eliminated drugs than men.

e. Individual differences, such as size or muscle mass, may affect pharmacokinetics or health. While not all women are the same size, more women are likely to be smaller and have smaller muscle mass than most men. For example, women were found to have a greater mortality with coronary artery angioplasty. When studies compared body size and size of coronary arteries, it was found that the variable was not "women" but "size of the arteries". Those women and men with smaller arteries do less well with angioplasty.

f. There are particularly "female" concerns involved in pharmacokinetics of some drugs in women. These include the influence of the cycling menstrual status on drug pharmacokinetics, the effect of menopausal status, the influence of concomitant supplementary estrogen administration, both oral contraceptive pills (OCPs) and HRT, on drugs and whether the drug clearance and use is affected by the phase of the menstrual cycle.[7,16]

Women metabolize some common substances, such as alcohol, differently from men.

Table 1.3. Interaction of OCPs with some other drugs

- Cause decreased clearance
  - Imipramine
  - Diazepam
  - Chlordiazepoxide
  - Phenytoin
  - Caffeine
  - Cyclosporine
- Increase clearances by inducing drug metabolism
  - Acetaminophen
  - Aspirin
  - Morphine
  - Lorazepam
  - Temazepam
  - Ibrate
- Reduce the effectiveness of OCPs
  - Carbamazepine
  - Phenytoin
  - Antibiotics rifampin, ampicillin

Data from Department of Health and Human Services. Food and Drug Administration. *Guidelines for the Study and Evaluation of Gender Differences in the Clinical Evaluation of Drugs.* FDA, Washington, DC, 1993.

Pregnancy

Pregnant women have larger volumes of distribution and total body water and fat levels. They may need higher doses of drugs such as antibiotics to reach therapeutic levels. Pregnancy induces a decrease in pepsin activity and gastric acid secretion, with a slower gastric emptying time in later trimesters, although intestinal motility is greater. High steroid levels affect hepatic metabolism of drugs.[15]

Pregnant women may need higher doses of drugs such as antibiotics to reach therapeutic levels.

Specific examples

1. Drug differences: Drugs, especially those that are metabolized or used in the liver, in the cytochrome P450 system, which is also affected by estrogen, OCPs, HRT, and other female hormones may act differently in women (Table 1.3).

2. Seizure medications:
   a. Most drugs for seizures are metabolized in the liver. Estrogen-containing OCPs and other hormones are known to affect the metabolism of most of these drugs; the drugs also reduce the effectiveness of OCPs.
   b. Women on antiseizure medication often have reduced fertility, menstrual cycles, and hormone levels, including disturbances in luteinizing hormone (LH), growth hormone, prolactin, and androgen levels.[16] Women with epilepsy were only 37 percent as likely to have ever had a pregnancy, in one study.[17]
   c. Epileptic women are more likely to have poorer bone health and failure of hormonal contraception. The failure rate of OCPs in epileptic women is more than four times that in nonepileptic women.[18]
   d. Most of the older antiseizure drugs including hydantoin are fetal teratogens, while the newer drugs such as gabapentin, oxcabazepine, tiagabine, and topiramate have not been well studied in pregnant women. Steroid hormones, including estrogen and progesterone, affect the seizure threshold.
   e. In double blind randomized controlled trials, women have responded better to gabapentin than men, both as a first-line and as an additional drug for seizures.[16]
   f. Antiepileptic drugs, especially phenytoin, phenobarbital and carbamezine, have been known to affect bone metabolism and induce hypocalcemia and these effects occur more often in women.
3. Antidepressants: Studies have suggested that antidepressant levels vary during the menstrual cycle and a constant level of drug may require varying the dose.[2]
4. Antipsychotic drugs: Antipsychotic drugs are more often prescribed for women. Side effects of sexual dysfunction including anorgasmia, menstrual abnormalities and changes in libido occur in women. Levels of lithium excreted by the kidney may be different in women given the same doses as men and should be monitored carefully.
5. Cardiovascular drugs: Although more women than men use antihypertensive medications, most recommendations have been made from studies performed on men under age 65 years. Calcium channel blockers and nitrates may be better choices for angina in women because women usually have smaller coronary arteries in which artery tone is a more important determinant of flow. High blood pressure levels in women may be more responsive to calcium channel blockers and diuretics.

   Side effect profiles may be different. Women who use beta-blockers may have more side effects, including Raynaud's phenomenon and alterations of diabetic responses. Women who take hydralazine are more likely than men to develop drug-induced lupus.

6. OCPs: OCPs can induce changes in the clearance of other drugs (Table 1.3). They alter hepatic metabolism, inhibiting metabolism of caffeine, antidepressants and benzodiazepines.[15]

Conclusions

Women's health care has been ignored or marginalized. Recent changes have attempted to mainstream women and their concerns into health care research. Women are more likely to be caregivers, elderly, poor, alone, and uninsured, making their health care needs different from those of men. Women's immunology, drug use, and metabolism may differ. However, there are more differences among women, making easy conclusions difficult.

REFERENCES

1. Nelson HL. Cultural values affecting women's place in medical care. In Rosenfeld JA, ed., *Women's Health in Primary Care*. Williams & Wilkins, Baltimore, MD, 1997, pp. 9–18.
2. Mann C. Women's health research blossoms. *Science* 1995;**269**:766–70.
3. Council on Ethical and Judicial Affairs, American Medical Association. Gender disparities in clinical decision making. *JAMA* 1991;**266**:599–62.
4. Vagero D. Health inequities in women and men. *BMJ* 2000;**320**:1286–7.
5. Cohen J. Women: Absent term in AIDS research equation. *Science* 1995;**269**:777–80.
6. National Institute of Health. *Guidelines on the Inclusion of Women and Minorities as Subjects in Clinic Research*. NIH, Bethesda, MD, 1994.
7. Department of Health and Human Services, Food and Drug Administration. *Guidelines for the Study and Evaluation of Gender Differences in the Clinical Evaluation of Drugs*. FDA, Washington, DC, 1993.
8. Rich-Edwards JW, Manson JE, Hennekens CH, Buring JE. The primary prevention of coronary heart disease in women. *N Engl J Med* 1995;**332**:1758–66.
9. Rossouw JE, Finnegan LP, Harlan WR, et al. The evolution of the Women's Health Initiative: Perspectives from the NIH. *J Am Med Women Assoc* 1995;**50**:50–5.
10. Ward DH, Carney PA. Caregiving women and the US welfare state: The case of elder kin care by low-income women. *Holistic Nurse Pract* 1994;**8**:44–58.
11. Unlenberg P, Cooney R, Boyd R. Divorce for women after midlife. *J Gerontol* 1990;**45**:S3–S11.
12. Barer BM. Men and women aging differently. *Int J Aging Hum Dev* 1994;**38**:29–40.
13. Fletcher CV, Acosta EP, Styrykowski JM. Gender differences in human pharmacokinetics and pharmacodynamics. *J Adolesc Health* 1994;**15**:619–29.
14. Butler RN, Collins KS, Meier DE, Muller CF, Pinn VW. Older women's health. *Geriatrics* 1995;**50**:39–47.

15. Rosenfeld JA. Pharmacokinetics: The female factor. *The Female Patient* 1997;**22**:53–60.
16. Morrell MJ. The new antiepileptic drugs and women: Efficacy, reproductive health, pregnancy and fetal outcome. *Epilepsia* 1996;(**37**Suppl6):S34–S44.
17. Schupf N, Ottman R. Likelihood of pregnancy in individuals with idiopathic/cryptogenic epilepsy: Social and biologic influence. *Epilepsia* 1994;**35**:750–6.
18. Morrell MJ. Maximizing the health of women with epilepsy: Science and ethics in new drug development. *Epilepsia* 1997;**38**:S32–S41.

Preventive care

2 Preventive care of adolescents

Rebecca Saenz, MD

Caring for adolescent females is both challenging and rewarding. Short and important interventions and counselling can make a significant impact into the health of the adolescent female and create an atmosphere of trust and a healthier lifestyle for adulthood.

Concerns unique to adolescents

1. Adolescents who seek medical treatment can be a difficult social challenge for the practicing family physician. Having rapport with the adolescent from previous well-child visits is both a positive and a negative factor. While adolescents may feel comfortable confiding in someone whom they have known for years, they may feel uncomfortable confiding in the same physician who has also known their parents for years.

2. This situation also creates legal challenges regarding consent for treatment. Each practitioner should have an established policy regarding consent for treatment of adolescents, explained to all adolescent patients and their parents.[1]

   a. Legal issues: The practitioner treating adolescents should be familiar with state and local statutes concerning age of consent and confidentiality of treatment.

   b. Consent: Age of consent varies from state to state in the USA, and may also vary depending on circumstance.

   c. Treatment of minors for most medical problems requires parental consent.

   d. Emancipated minors are those who are considered by the court to be independent of parental authority. Examples are pregnant adolescents and those in the military.

   e. Mature minors are those who are still legally under parental authority, but are judged to be of sufficient maturity to understand the consequences of a given treatment or procedure, for example a 17-year-old college student who requests treatment for strep throat.

    f. Consent is presumed in emergencies.

3. Confidentiality: Many US states have statutes requiring maintenance of confidentiality if an adolescent seeks treatment for pregnancy, sexually transmitted diseases (STDs), substance abuse, or mental health issues.

Normal growth and development

1. Physical growth and development of adolescent females, or puberty, is divided into Tanner stages, and usually follows a predictable pattern.
   a. Breast bud development (Tanner stage 2) is usually the first sign of the beginning of puberty, occurring between ages 8 and 13 years.
   b. Acceleration in rate of increase in height begins at approximately age 9.5 years, with a peak around age 12 years.
   c. Pubic hair growth (Tanner stage 2) begins at around age 11 years.
   d. Menarche occurs at an average age of 13 years, but there is wide variation from age 10 to 16 years. Menarche is usually concurrent with the attainment of Tanner stage 4 development.
2. Psychosocial and cognitive development is generally divided into three stages: early, middle, and late adolescence. Progression in these spheres is less predictable, and stages may overlap somewhat.
   a. Early adolescence (age 12–14 years) is characterized by the shift toward independence, preoccupation with body image, early peer group involvement, and the beginnings of identity development.
   b. Middle adolescence (age 15–17 years) is characterized by conflicts with authority figures and intensification of the above tasks.
   c. Late adolescence (age 18–21 years) is characterized by completion of the four tasks mentioned in (a), solidification of abstract reasoning, and assumption of adult responsibilities.

Recommendations

Organizations

Recommendations for health maintenance for adolescents have been made by several organizations. Most recommendations are based on descriptive studies of causes of morbidity and mortality among this age group and have not necessarily been validated by prospective studies.

1. The American Medical Association first published the *Guidelines for Adoles-*

cent Preventive Services in 1994. A scientific advisory board developed guidelines for health and biopsychosocial screening with representatives from pediatrics, adolescent medicine, child and adolescent psychiatry, health and developmental psychology, health education, and preventive medicine. Twenty-four recommendations are cited.[1]

2. The Maternal and Child Health Bureau, Health Resources and Services Administration, and Medicaid published *Bright Futures: Guidelines for Health Supervision of Infants, Children, and Adolescents* in 1994.[2]

3. The US Preventive Services Task Force: *Guide to Clinical Preventive Services*, 2nd edition, published in 1996, includes 26 recommendations for adolescents and young adults up to 24 years of age[2] (Appendix 2.1).

Health maintenance issues

1. Since most adolescents do not present routinely for screening visits, the physician should seize opportunities to incorporate screening questions and anticipatory guidance into acute visits whenever possible. One recent study demonstrated that nearly half of a population of adolescents attended a preventive health visit when an invitation was initiated by the family physician's office, and attendance rate was higher for adolescent females than for adolescent males.[3]

2. Interviewing adolescents:
   a. Confidentiality should be assured and maintained except in cases of abuse, which are legally mandated to be reported.
   b. Rapport regarding sensitive issues can be established by using such phrases as, "I ask all my patients . . .".
   c. The importance of active listening cannot be underestimated.

3. "Checkups": All guidelines recommend periodic health maintenance visits to assess growth and development, facilitate healthy behaviors, and screen for both physical and psychosocial problems.[4,5]

4. Screening tests: Recommendations for routine screening tests to be performed include the following:
   a. Weight, height, body mass index, and blood pressure should be checked at each visit.
   b. Laboratory studies that might be indicated include random cholesterol, HIV antibody, Papanicolaou smear (Pap smear), *Chlamydia* screen, and tuberculin skin test.
   c. Selective screening for vision problems, scoliosis, diabetes mellitus, hearing loss, orthopedic problems, allergies, reactive airway disease, and STDs should be performed as indicated.

Table 2.1. Recommended immunizations for adolescents

- Hepatitis B series, if not previously immunized
- Tetanus, if more than 10 years since last booster
- Measles, mumps, rubella (MMR), if second dose not already given
- Pneumoccocal pneumonia, if chronic disease state
- Varicella, if disease or immunization not previously documented
- Annual influenza, if requested
- Poison ivy desensitization, if requested
- Additionally, the CDC now recommends hepatitis A vaccination in adolescents at risk of acquiring this disease

Data from Centers for Disease Control and Prevention (CDC). Guidelines for treatment of sexually transmitted diseases. *MMWR Morb Mortal Wkly Rep* 1998;**47**(RR-1):1–111. Preventive Services Task Force: *Guide to Clinical Preventive Services*, 2nd edn. Williams & Wilkins, Baltimore, MD, 1996.

5. Immunizations recommended for the adolescent age group are included in Table 2.1.

When one is working with adolescents, confidentiality must be assured and maintained except in cases of abuse, which must be reported.

Sexuality

Sexuality is often an uncomfortable topic for family physicians to discuss with their adolescent patients, and one which parental views may influence. Non-judgmental, open-ended questions should be used, and some graphic definition of terms used may be necessary.

The first pelvic examination

1. Explain everything, including that intolerable discomfort is reason to stop.
2. Use a Pederson or smaller speculum, particularly if the patient is not yet sexually active.
3. Lubricate well. With Thin Prep™ Pap smears, lubrication is less problematical. Even with traditional Pap smears, lubricant artifact is less problematical than the psychological consequences of a painful first gynecological examination.
4. If the patient is unable to tolerate speculum, a Pap smear can be done by guiding a cytobrush to the cervical os along a gloved finger.

Table 2.2. Screening tests for sexually transmitted diseases

- DNA probe or culture for gonorrhea and *Chlamydia*
- Wet preparation for *Trichomonas*
- Pap test for HPV
- Serum for RPR and HIV
- Culture for HSV, if indicated

HPV, human papillomavirus; RPR, rapid plasma reagin; HIV, human immunodeficiency virus; HSV, herpes simplex virus.

5. Bimanual can be done using one finger instead of two.
6. Recommendations for Pap smears are the same as for women over the age of 21 years:
    a. At the initiation of sexual activity or at age 18 years, whichever comes first.
    b. Yearly thereafter, unless the patient is at extremely low risk for cervical cancer, at the physician's discretion.

> Recommendations for Pap smears for adolescents include one at the initiation of sexual activity or at age 18 years, whichever comes first, and then yearly thereafter, unless there is extremely low risk of cancer.

Recommendations for STD screening

Yearly, or more often if at high risk (Table 2.2). Recommendations for treatment may be found in Chapter 15.

Contraception and STD prevention

1. Consistent abstinence is the most reliable way to prevent pregnancy and STDs. It has no side effects.
2. Injectable or implantable contraceptives prevent pregnancy, but not STDs. They are convenient, do not require daily compliance, and are not event specific. Side effects may include irregular menses or amenorrhea.
3. OCPs prevent pregnancy, but not STDs. They are convenient and not event specific. They do require daily compliance to be effective. Many pills have other health benefits, such as regulation of menses, elimination of premenstrual syndrome, and positive influences on the hormonal factors that exacerbate acne.
4. Diaphragms prevent pregnancy and reduce likelihood of some, but not all, STDs. They should be used with spermicidal jelly for maximum effectiveness. They must be fitted and prescribed by a physician, and a weight gain or loss of

Table 2.3. Abused substances that need screening at adolescents' visits

- Tobacco
- Ethanol, especially while driving or engaging in recreational activities
- Anabolic steroids
- Inhalants

more than 10 lbs (4.5 kg) requires refitting. They are event specific, and may therefore be viewed as inconvenient.

5. Condoms (both male and female) both prevent pregnancy and reduce the likelihood of acquiring STDs. They can be obtained without a prescription, but are event specific, and therefore may be viewed as inconvenient.

6. Current recommendations are for abstinence. If the adolescent female is already sexually active, or has decided to become so, oral contraceptives may be prescribed, together with counselling about proper use of condoms.

> Current recommendations for contraception in adolescents are for abstinence. If the adolescent female is already sexually active, oral contraceptive pills with counselling about proper use of condoms may be prescribed.

Special issues

Substance abuse

All guidelines recommend screening for substance abuse with open-ended questions, and anticipatory counselling regarding avoidance of all abusable substances. Random urine drug testing, particularly without the adolescent female's knowledge or consent, has no place as a screening tool (Table 2.3).

Eating disorders (see chapter 28)

Body mass index (BMI) should be calculated at each visit, a significant drop being a marker for possible eating disorders. Questions should also be asked regarding body image perception.

1. Dietary counselling: All adolescents should be reminded of the importance of a healthy diet.

2. Screening for overweight: Adolescents whose BMIs are at or above the 85th percentile, but below the 95th percentile, or equal to 30, whichever is smaller, are considered to be at risk for overweight, and should be evaluated by further screening. If any of the second-level screening items are positive, the adoles-

cent should receive appropriate dietary counselling for weight loss.[7] The following factors should be assessed:

   a. Family history of cardiovascular disease, hypercholesterolemia, or unknown family history.

   b. High blood pressure.

   c. High total cholesterol.

   d. Increase of two BMI points since previous year's measurements.

   e. Concern about weight.

3. A multivitamin supplement with folic acid is now recommended for all women of childbearing age, including adolescents.[3]

4. Adequate calcium intake should also be ensured.[3]

Dental health

Daily oral hygiene and regular dental visits should be stressed.

Risk-taking behavior

Since risky behaviors, including daily cigarette use, frequent alcohol use, and sexual intercourse have been cited as risk factors for foregone healthcare in adolescents, these behaviors should be assessed for at every visit.[8]

1. Screening questions: "What do you like to do for fun?" may often yield surprising answers that can be indicative of risk-taking behavior. Specific inquiry should be directed toward driving while intoxicated, number of sexual partners, [5] and toward the current local fads in risky behaviors.

2. Parental influence: Parents should be counselled not to underestimate their influence on their teens' risk-taking behaviors, because parental direction and expectations have been shown to have a powerful effect on reduction of tobacco, alcohol and drug use, sexual activity, and gang membership.[9]

School issues

"How are you doing in school?" can lead to discussions about future plans, lack of which may indicate depression. The discussion can also help to uncover previously undiagnosed learning disabilities, attention deficit and hyperactivity syndrome, or psychological stressors.

Safety

"Do you wear seatbelts and use appropriate safety equipment when participating in sports?" provides an opportunity to remind adolescents of the importance of good protection from traumatic injury.

Conclusion

Adolescents, particularly adolescent females, offer unique challenges to the family physician. Confidentiality should be maintained. Anticipatory guidance for both teens and their parents regarding growth and developmental issues, as well as prevention of risky behaviors, is important.

REFERENCES

1. American Medical Association. *Guidelines for Adolescent Preventive Services (GAPS)*. AMA, Department of Adolescent Health, Chicago, 1994.
2. Green M, ed. *Bright Futures: Guidelines for Health Supervision of Infants, Children, and Adolescents.* National Center for Education in Maternal Child Health, Arlington, VA, 1994.
3. US Preventive Services Task Force. *Guide to Clinical Preventive Services*, 2nd edn. Williams & Wilkins, Baltimore, MD, 1996.
4. Kniiishkowy B, Palti H, Schein M, Yaphe J, Edman R, Baras M. Adolescent preventive health visits: A comparison of two invitation protocols. *J Am Board Fam Prac* 2000;**13**:11–16.
5. Montalto NJ. Implementing the guidelines for adolescent preventive services. *Am Fam Physician 1998;* **57**: 2181–8.
6. Forman SF, Emans SJ. Current goals for adolescent health care. *Hosp Physician* 2000;**35**: 27–42.
7. Himes JH, Dietz WH. Guidelines for overweight in adolescent preventive services: Recommendations from an expert committee. *Am J Clin Nutr* 1994; **59**:307–16.
8. Ford CA, Bearman PS, Moody J. Foregone health care among adolescents. *JAMA* 1999; **282**:2227–34.
9. Nelson BV, Patience TH, MacDonald DC. Adolescent risk behavior and the influence of parents and education. *J Am Board Fam Pract* 1999;**12**:326–43.

Appendix 2.1. Recommendations for adolescents and young adults (aged 11–21 years)

- Leading causes of death
  - Motor vehicle/other unintentional injuries
- Interventions considered and recommended for the periodic health examination:
  - Homicide
  - Suicide
  - Malignant neoplasms
  - Heart diseases

Interventions for the general population
- **Screening**
  - Height and weight
  - Blood pressure
  - Pap test (females)
  - *Chlamydia* screen (females < 20 years)
  - Rubella serology or vaccination history (females > 12 years)
  - Assess for problem drinking

- **Counselling**
- Injury prevention
  - Lap/shoulder belts
  - Bicycle/motorcycle/all-terrain vehicle helmets
  - Smoke detector
  - Safe storage/removal of firearms
- Substance use
  - Avoidance of tobacco use
  - Avoidance of underage drinking and illicit drug use
  - Avoidance of alcohol/drug use while driving, swimming, boating, etc.
- Sexual behavior
  - STD prevention: abstinence; avoid high-risk behavior; condoms/female barrier with spermicide
  - Unintended pregnancy: contraception
  - Diet and exercise
  - Limits to fat and cholesterol; maintenance of caloric balance; emphasis on grains, fruits, vegetables
  - Adequate calcium intake (females)
  - Regular physical activity
  - Regular visits to dental care providers
  - Floss, brush with fluoride toothpaste daily

- **Immunizations**
  - Tetanus-diphtheria (Td) boosters (11–16 years)
  - Hepatitis B

- MMR (measles, mumps, rubella) (11–12 years)
- Varicella (11–12 years)
- Rubella (females > 12 years)

- **Chemoprophylaxis**
  - Multivitamins with folic acid (females planning/capable of pregnancy)

From US Preventive Services Task Force, *Guide to Clinical Preventive Services*, 2nd edn. Williams & Wilkins, Baltimore, MD, 1996.

3 Preventive care of adults (19 to 65 years)

Diane Madlon-Kay, MD

Preventive health care for adult women consists of active intervention and counselling to help to prevent the common causes of death. Screening, counselling, and immunizations can dramatically reduce morbidity and premature mortality in women.

Introduction

Causes of mortality

The five leading causes of death in women in the USA are, to a large extent, preventable, and the risk factors responsible for each cause may be modifiable[1] (Table 3.1). Primary care physicians can specifically intervene in the form of screening, immunizations, and counselling and can dramatically reduce morbidity and premature mortality in women (Appendix 3.1).

Strength of evidence

As with other clinical practices, providers should carefully evaluate individual preventive services before incorporating them into routine practice. In general, preventive interventions should not be used unless they have been demonstrated to be effective in well-designed studies. Expecting every physician to assess the quality of scientific evidence for each preventive service individually is unrealistic. Therefore many authorities, including professional societies, government agencies, ad hoc committees, voluntary associations, academic experts and consensus panels have made recommendations for the prevention of disease. Well-known examples include the CDC, US Preventive Services Task Force (USPSTF) and American Cancer Society (ACS).[2,3] Some organizations' policy statements do not describe the methods used to generate their recommendations. Others, notably the USPSTF, provide a

Table 3.1. The five leading causes of death in women in the USA and associated modifiable risk factors, 1995

Cause of death	Modifiable risk factor
1. Heart diseases	Tobacco use
	Elevated serum cholesterol
	High blood pressure
	Sedentary lifestyle
2. Cancer	Tobacco use
	Improper diet
	Alcohol
	Occupational exposures
3. Cerebrovascular diseases	High blood pressure
	Tobacco use
	Elevated serum cholesterol
4. Chronic obstructive pulmonary disease	Tobacco use
	Occupational exposure
	Environmental exposure
5. Pneumonia and influenza	Tobacco use
	Lack of immunization

detailed description of the methodology used. Therefore, clinicians must be discerning consumers of recommendations made by preventive care authorities. Preventive care recommendations differ. However, major authorities do agree about many preventive services. The clinical preventive services recommended by most US authorities for normal risk adults are shown in Appendix 3.1.[4]

New guidelines

The yearly physical examination, a relatively ineffective ritual, is no longer recommended by most authorities and has been replaced by a variety of screening tests, immunizations and counselling interventions.[5] Services not routinely recommended for asymptomatic normal risk women include the chest X-ray, electrocardiogram, exercise stress test, multiple blood chemistry screens, sputum cytology testing, and multivitamin prophylaxis. The focus of this chapter is on the preventive services recommended by most major authorities that are unique to women.

Screening

Physical examination

The American Medical Association in 1922 first proposed the annual physical examination of healthy persons as effective preventive medicine. However, today, while it is realized that routine visits with the primary care clinician are important, performing the same interventions on all patients, and as frequently as yearly is not a clinically or cost-effective approach to disease prevention. Rather, both the frequency and the content of the periodic health xamination need to be tailored to the unique health risks of the individual patient and should take into consideration the quality of the evidence that specific preventive services are clinically effective.

1. Clinical breast examination (CBE)
   a. Risk: Breast cancer is the most common type of cancer in women and the second leading cause of cancer death in American women.[6] The average lifetime risk of developing breast cancer for a woman in the USA is approximately 1 in 9.[7]
   b. Method: The CBE involves bilateral inspection and palpation of the breasts and the axillary and supraclavicular areas. Examination should be performed in both the upright and supine positions. Palpation must be systematic. One of the best predictors of examination accuracy is the length of time spent by the examiner.
   c. Effectiveness: The sensitivity and specificity of CBE for breast cancer screening varies with the skill and experience of the examiner and with the characteristics of the individual breast being examined. The estimated sensitivity of clinical examination alone is approximately 45 percent. Data from studies using manufactured breast models show that the mean sensitivity among registered nurses was 65 percent, compared with 87 percent for physicians for lumps 1.0 cm in diameter.

   The results of several large studies have convincingly demonstrated the effectiveness of CBE when combined with mammography as screening for breast cancer in women older than age 50 years. The effectiveness of CBE by itself has not been well studied.
   d. Recommendations: Most authorities recommend CBE for women, beginning at a variety of ages and at varying frequencies. Examples include:
      i. USPSTF: All women over age 40 years should receive an annual CBE.[3]
      ii. ACS: Women should have CBEs every three years from age 20 to 39 years. Annual CBEs should be performed on women 40 years of age and older.[8]

The clinical breast examination when combined with mammography in women older than age 50 years is effective in screening for breast cancer.

2. Pelvic organ examination: The pelvic examination is used in the detection of cancers of the female genital tract, namely the ovaries, cervix and endometrium.[6] The pelvic examination is usually performed in conjunction with Pap smear testing for cervical neoplasms. The pelvic examination is considered by many, but not all, major authorities to be a necessary component of the periodic health examination.

   a. Risk and effectiveness:

      i. Ovarian cancer is the fifth leading cause of cancer death in American women. How sensitive and specific a pelvic examination is in detecting ovarian cancer is not well known. However, small, early stage ovarian tumors are often not detected by palpation because of the deep anatomical location of the ovary. Thus ovarian cancers detected by pelvic examination are generally advanced and associated with poor survival. The pelvic examination may also produce false positives when benign adnexal masses are found.

      ii. Approximately 12 800 cases of invasive cervical cancer were diagnosed and 4800 women died of cervical cancer in the USA in 1999. The pelvic examination is much less sensitive than Pap testing for cervical neoplasms.

      iii. Endometrial cancer is not a leading cause of death among North American women, although its incidence is relatively high.[9] Survival rates are relatively good, with 84 percent of all women with endometrial cancer alive after five years. The techniques available for diagnosing endometrial cancer in the asymptomatic woman, unfortunately, are far from ideal. The pelvic examination has never been suggested to be effective in diagnosing endometrial cancer.

   b. Method: The woman should empty her bladder prior to the pelvic examination. A general inspection of the external genitalia should be performed with the woman in the lithotomy position. A speculum should be used to inspect the vagina and cervix. The lubricated index and middle fingers of one hand are placed into the vaginal vault, with the other hand on top of the abdomen for bimanual palpation of the pelvic organs. The hand is partially withdrawn from the vagina and inserted in the rectum to allow for palpation of the rectovaginal septum.

   c. Recommendations: The ACS recommends pelvic examination should be performed every one to three years for women aged 18 to 39 years and annually for women over age 40 years.[2] The USPSTF states it is prudent to examine the uterine adnexa when performing gynecological examinations for other reasons.[3]

The American Cancer Society recommends that women age 18 to 39 years have a pelvic examination every one to three years and then annually after age 40 years.

Specific screening tests

1. Pap smear:
   a. Effectiveness: The effectiveness of early detection of cervical cancer through Pap smear testing and early treatment has been impressive, resulting in a marked decrease in mortality from cervical cancer.[10] The incidence of invasive cervical cancer has decreased 70 percent as a result of screening. However, a large proportion of women, particularly middle-aged, poor, rural and inner city women, have not had regular Pap smears.

      Depending on the technique used, Pap testing has a sensitivity of 50 to 90 percent and a specificity of 90 to 99 percent. A large proportion of false negative Pap smears may be caused by poor technique in performance and inadequate laboratory interpretation. Because of the long lead time from development of precancerous changes to invasive carcinoma (eight to nine years by some estimates) almost all precancerous or early stage malignancies initially missed can still be detected by repeat testing.

   b. Methods: Women should be instructed not to douche on the day of the examination. A Pap smear should not be performed if the patient has significant menstrual flow or obvious inflammation. The Pap smear should be performed before the bimanual examination and before obtaining culture specimens. The speculum should not be lubricated with anything but water. The cervix should be completely visualized. Excess cervical mucus should be gently removed with a swab. A wooden or plastic spatula, preferably Ayres's type, should be used first. The spatula should be firmly yet gently rotated circumferentially around the os at least one turn to obtain a 360° sample. The specimen should be transferred promptly to a slide, or more recently a Thin Prep™ solution. An endocervical brush should then be inserted into the os no deeper than the length of the bristled section. It should be rotated 360° and then the specimen transferred by rolling onto the slide. Specimens should be uniformly applied to the slides without clumping, or a Thin Prep™ preparation used. Fixation should be performed promptly to minimize air drying of the specimen.

   c. Recommendations: All authorities recommend periodic Pap testing.

      i. The USPSTF states that Pap tests should begin with the onset of sexual activity and should be repeated every one to three years at the physician's discretion. They may be discontinued at age 65 years if previous smears have been consistently normal.[3]

      ii. The ACS recommends that all women should begin having annual Pap tests at the onset of sexual activity or at 18 years of age, whichever occurs first. After a woman has had three or more consecutive satisfactory normal annual examinations, the Pap test may be performed less frequently at the discretion of the patient and clinician.[2]

2. Mammography:

   a. Risk: Breast cancer is the most common type of cancer in women and the second leading cause of cancer death in American women, after lung cancer.[11] The strongest risk factor is age, with first deaths occurring at approximately age 30 years. Mortality from breast cancer does not plateau, even in extreme old age.

      Mortality from breast cancer is strongly influenced by the stage at detection. The five-year survival rate is 98 percent for white women found to have localized disease. The five-year survival rate for white women with distant spread is only 23 percent.

   b. Method: The woman should wear pants or a skirt for her mammogram since she will have to undress from the waist up. She should be instructed not to use deodorants, powders, or other topical applications on the breasts or in underarm areas as these may cause artifacts on the mammogram. Because of potential premenstrual breast tenderness, it is preferable to schedule mammography at other times in the woman's menstrual cycle.

   c. Effectiveness: Mammography is the most effective means of early detection for breast cancer, with sensitivity estimates of 70 to 90 percent and specificity estimates of 90 to 95 percent. The results of several large studies have convincingly demonstrated that breast cancer screening by mammography reduces mortality from breast cancer by approximately 30 percent in women older than age 50 years. Most studies have not shown a clear benefit from mammography in women aged 40 to 49 years.

      Despite recommendations that women receive regular screening for breast cancer, too few women use this service. In 1990, two-thirds of US women over age 40 years had not had a screening mammogram in the previous year, and 38 percent had never had a mammogram.[12]

   d. Recommendations: All major authorities recommend mammography but at varying ages. The USPSTF recommends mammography every one to two years for all women, beginning at age 50 years and concluding at approximately age 75 years.[3] The ACS states that women of 40 to 49 years of age should receive screening mammograms every one to two years. Yearly mammography screening is recommended for women of 50 years and older.[8]

3. Breast self-examination (BSE):
   a. Efficacy: Self-examination appears to be a less sensitive form of screening than clinical examination, and its specificity remains uncertain. Among participants in a breast cancer registry, BSE was reported to detect 34 percent of cancers. Although training sessions increase detection rates, they also increase false positive rates.
   b. Recommendations: Major authorities disagree on their recommendations regarding BSE. The USPSTF states that, although the teaching of BSE is not specifically recommended, there is insufficient evidence to recommend any change in current BSE practices. The ACS recommends monthly BSE for all women.

Breast cancer screening by mammography reduces mortality from breast cancer by approximately 30 percent in women older than age 50 years.

Immunizations/prophylaxis

Rubella

Preventing fetal infection and consequent congenital rubella syndrome is the primary objective of rubella immunization. Rubella infection that occurs in early pregnancy may result in abortion, miscarriage, stillbirth, or other congenital abnormalities.[12]

1. Effectiveness: Rubella incidence decreased steadily after rubella vaccine was licenced; fewer than 128 cases occurred in 1995.[4] Fewer than an estimated 6 to 11 percent of young adults remain susceptible to rubella.[12]

2. Method: Women of childbearing age must be assured of immunity against rubella, unless there is laboratory evidence of immunity or a record of vaccination after the first birthday.[13] Susceptible women of childbearing age should not be vaccinated during pregnancy. Instead, they should be vaccinated immediately after delivery. Every woman should receive rubella vaccine in the form of MMR (measles, mumps and rubella).

Hormone replacement therapy

1. Benefits of use:
   a. Osteoporosis: In postmenopausal women, use of supplemental estrogen can reduce the risk of osteoporosis. Osteoporosis contributes to

approximately 1.2 million fractures in the USA annually, two-thirds of which occur in women (see Chapter 33). Women who are older, white, slender, and those who have had a bilateral oophorectomy or early menopause are at increased risk for developing osteoporosis-related fractures.[14]

b. Coronary heart disease (CHD): The use of estrogen to prevent CHD is being investigated in a multicenter prospective trial. CHD causes approximately 30 percent of deaths in women older than age 50 years. A large case-controlled study showed a reduced risk of mortality from all causes for women using postmenopausal HRT.[14]

c. Other symptoms: Estrogen supplementation also improves climacteric symptoms, including decreasing hot flashes, and alleviating genitourinary symptoms such as dryness, urgency, incontinence, and frequency.

2. Risks of use:

a. Endometrial cancer: Use of estrogen supplementation alone for 10 to 20 years in women with an intact uterus leads to an eightfold increased incidence of endometrial cancer. If, however, the woman uses progestin concomitantly, the risk of endometrial cancer decreases to that of women not taking estrogen. Whether use of progestin blunts any potential cardiovascular benefits of estrogen is unclear.[14]

c. Breast cancer: Whether estrogen supplementation increases a woman's risk for breast cancer also remains controversial.[15]

d. Thrombosis: Estrogen increases the risk of venous thromboembolism, but because the dosage used is much lower, the risk is not as great as with OCPs.

3. Method:

a. To prevent irreversible bone loss, estrogen replacement should begin soon after the onset of menopause, except in women with contraindications (Table 3.2) or preferences against its use.

b. An absolute upper age limit for estrogen replacement has not been established.

c. Use of progestin or careful endometrial monitoring is recommended for women with intact uteri.

d. Several different regimens for HRT have been developed. Oral preparations have been studied more extensively for primary prevention than has transdermal or other routes of administration. The most common initial oral dosage in the USA is 0.625 mg of conjugated estrogen taken every day.

In postmenopausal women, use of supplemental estrogen can reduce the risk of osteoporosis.

Table 3.2. Contraindications to estrogen replacement

- Unexplained vaginal bleeding
- Active liver disease
- Chronic impaired liver function
- Recent venous thrombosis
- Carcinoma of the breast, ovary or endometrium

Progestin (medroxyprogesterone acetate, MPA) may be given cyclically or continuously (2.5 to 10 mg daily).

e. The usual dosage for cyclic administration is 5 to 10 mg of progesterone acetate (or equivalent) daily for the first 10 to 14 days of the month. The usual dosage for continuous administration of progesterone acetate is 2.5 mg daily.

f. If progestin is used in a continuous regimen, it causes unpredictable endometrial bleeding in 30 to 50 percent of women. If this occurs, increasing the progestin daily dose can help to achieve amenorrhea. Such bleeding abates after six to eight months of use because of uterine atrophy. Amenorrhea should be achieved in 85 percent of women within 6 to 12 months of progestin use.

g. The most common side effects of estrogen therapy include endometrial bleeding, breast tenderness, nausea, bloating, and headaches. When a progestin is added to estrogen therapy, the most common side effects are bloating, weight gain, nausea, irritability, breast tenderness, and depression. Decreasing the dose of progestin generally can alleviate these symptoms.

The most common initial oral dosage in the USA is 0.625 mg of conjugated estrogen taken every day. Progestin (medroxyprogesterone acetate) may be given cyclically or continuously (2.5 to 10 mg daily).

4. Recommendations: The USPSTF states that, although universal postmenopausal HRT is not recommended, HRT should be considered for asymptomatic women who are at increased risk for osteoporosis, who lack known contraindications, and who have received adequate counselling about potential benefits and risks (Table 3.3).

The most common side effects of estrogen therapy include endometrial bleeding, breast tenderness, nausea, bloating, and headaches. The most worrisome, but rare side effect, includes increased risk of thrombosis.

Aspirin therapy

1. Benefits and efficacy: The Nurses' Health Study found that low dose aspirin

Table 3.3. Individual factors in counselling for hormone replacement therapy

- Coronary heart disease risk factors, such as family history, blood pressure, weight, smoking status and cholesterol
- Osteoporosis risk factors, such as race, body build, physical activity level, bone mineral density
- Breast cancer risk factors, such as personal and family history, late parity (after age 30 years), early menarche (before age 12 years), and late menopause (after age 50 years)
- Patient desire to decrease climacteric symptoms, such as decreased vasomotor and genitourinary tract symptoms
- Tolerance for side effects, such as endometrial bleeding and breast tenderness
- Willingness and ability to participate in follow-up, such as mammography and endometrial sampling

Data from American College of Physicians. Guidelines for counseling postmenopausal women about preventive hormone therapy. *Ann Intern Med* 1992;**117**:1038–41.

significantly decreased the incidence of first myocardial infarction in middle-aged women. Several prospective studies suggest that women, like men, who have risk factors for stroke may benefit from aspirin therapy to reduce the risks. However, a decrease in total cardiovascular mortality for women with aspirin prophylaxis was not proven. There may be an increased risk of hemorrhagic stroke and sudden death with its use. Use of 60 to 65 mg rather than 600 mg of aspirin daily is being studied for risk reduction efficacy and decreased hemorrhagic stroke incidence. The Women's Health Study, a large RCT that is examining the benefit of aspirin prophylaxis, is in progress.

Aspirin use for the primary prevention of colon cancer is also being investigated. Observational studies have shown an association between aspirin use and a reduction in the incidence of colon cancer.

2. Methods of counselling: Women older than age 50 years with risk factors for CHD are the group most likely to derive benefit from primary prevention with aspirin. Risks and benefits of aspirin prophylaxis should first be considered and discussed with each patient. The optimal dosage of aspirin for the primary prevention of heart disease has not been clearly established. The most widely accepted regimens are 325 mg orally daily or every other day.

3. Recommendations: The USPSTF recommendation regarding aspirin prophylaxis refers to men only.[3] The American Heart Association states that care should be exercised before beginning a life-long program of aspirin therapy. The decision to begin taking aspirin should be made only after consultation by each individual with her physician. The individual who begins a regular aspirin regimen should be aware of the side effects of the drug and should report symptoms to her physician. All risk factors for CHD and stroke should

Table 3.4. Women at high risk for sexually transmitted diseases and HIV infection in western Europe and the USA

- Sexually active individuals under age 25 years
- Those who have multiple sexual partners
- Those with a prior history of a sexually transmitted disease
- Those who practice anal intercourse
- Prostitutes
- Users of illicit drugs
- Inmates of detention centers

be determined and a concerted program to reduce those risk factors begun.[16,17]

The Nurses' Health Study found that daily low dose aspirin use significantly decreased the incidence of first myocardial infarction in middle-aged women.

Counselling behavioral changes

Patient behavior changes, although difficult to achieve, may be more valuable for health promotion than many of the screening tests and immunizations that patients receive. In general, patients value the advice of clinicians. Studies show that even brief interventions may have a beneficial effect.

The following counselling recommendations suggest a changing role for both clinicians and patients. The increasing evidence of the importance of personal health behaviors and primary prevention means that patients must assume greater responsibility for their own health. Clinicians may need to develop new skills in helping to empower patients and in counselling them to change certain health-related behaviors.

1. Sexually transmitted diseases (see Chapter 15): Although STDs are less prevalent among women than among men, the medical complications associated with these diseases are more serious in women (Table 3.4). In addition to AIDS and subsequent death, the most serious complications for women are PID, increased risk of cervical cancer, ectopic pregnancy, congenital infections, delivery of premature and low birth weight infants, and fetal death. The poor, medically underserved, and minority groups incur a disproportionate share of STDs and subsequent disabilities.

The most serious complications of sexually transmitted diseases are pelvic inflammatory disease, increased risk of cervical cancer, ectopic pregnancy, congenital infections, delivery of premature and low birth weight infants, and fetal death.

Table 3.5. Counselling for prevention of sexually transmitted diseases and AIDS

- Every patient's risk for STDs should be determined with a thorough sexual and drug history
- Patients should be informed that HIV is transmitted by sexual intercourse, sharing needles, and infected blood. Providers should dispel myths about HIV transmission
- All patients should be advised that any unprotected sexual behavior poses a risk for STDs
- All patients should be counselled that STDs are best prevented by: abstinence, limiting sexual relationships to those between mutually monogamous partners known to be HIV negative, avoiding sex with high risk partners, avoiding anal intercourse, and using latex condoms if having sex with anyone other than a single mutually monogamous partner known to be HIV negative
- All sexually active patients should be counselled about the effective use and limitations of condoms
- All patients should be counselled to avoid injection drug use

From Hearst N. AIDS risk assessment in primary care. *J Am Board Fam Pract* 1994;**7**:44–8.
STD, sexually transmitted disease.

2. Human immunodeficiency virus:
   a. Risks: HIV infection is now the third leading cause of death for women aged 25 to 44 years.[4] For African-American women in this age group, HIV infection ranked as the second leading cause of death, and for Hispanic women in the USA, it is the third leading cause.[12]

      During the past decade, the HIV epidemic in the USA has evolved from one occurring primarily among homosexual men to one that is affecting many different population subgroups disproportionately.[14] Although most cases of AIDS continue to occur in men, the impact of the disease on women is growing (Table 3.4).

      As the rate of heterosexual transmission of the virus increases, more women are being placed at risk of being infected. As many as 80 000 women of reproductive age in the USA could be infected with HIV. Minority women have been disproportionately affected by the AIDS epidemic. Of the AIDS cases reported among women in 1992–3, 76 percent were among nonwhite women. Worldwide, more women than men will soon be affected with AIDS. Although HIV infection is preventable, the changes in behavior that are needed to prevent it have not been easily achieved.
   b. Methods of counselling: See Table 3.5.

HIV infection is now the third leading cause of death for women aged 25 to 44 years.

    c. Recommendations:

        i. The USPSTF recommends that clinicians take a complete sexual and drug use history for all adults.

        ii. Sexually active patients should be advised that abstaining from sex or maintaining a mutually faithful monogamous sexual relationship with a partner known to be uninfected are the most effective strategies to prevent infection with HIV or other STDs.

        iii. Patients should also receive counselling about the indications and proper methods for using condoms and spermicides in sexual intercourse and about the health risks associated with anal intercourse.

        iv. Intravenous drug users should be encouraged to enroll in a drug treatment program and should be warned against sharing drug equipment or using unsterilized needles and syringes.

3. Unintended pregnancy:

    a. Risks: In 1988, US women aged 15 to 44 years reported that 35 percent of their births in the preceding five years were unintended.[18] Most of the unintended births were mistimed; that is they occurred sooner than wanted. However, as many as one-third of unintended pregnancies end in therapeutic abortion.

    b. Modern contraceptives are safe and effective. Primary care clinicians are the main source of authoritative information and advice on responsible family planning practices for patients.

    c. Recommendations: The USPSTF recommends that clinicians obtain a complete sexual history from all adult patients. Sexually active women who do not want to become pregnant should receive detailed counselling on methods to prevent unintended pregnancy.

4. Injury and violence prevention:

    a. Unintentional injuries are the sixth leading cause of death in women in the USA and the leading cause of death for those aged 1 to 34 years.[19,20] Motor vehicle crashes cause half of the unintentional injury deaths. Most motor vehicle trauma is related to alcohol use and/or failure to use safety belts.

    b. Injury to women as a result of violence is one of America's most widespread health problems, yet one of the least reported. Partner abuse has been estimated to occur in up to 25 percent of all familial relationships. More than 1 million women seek medical assistance each year for injuries caused by battering.

Unintentional injuries are the sixth leading cause of death in women in the USA and the leading cause of death for those aged 1 to 34 years.

Table 3.6. Counselling women about spousal violence

- Women should be asked directly whether they have ever been physically abused
- The clinician thus acknowledges the problem and affirms that battering is unacceptable
- Information about available community, social and legal resources, legal rights and a plan for dealing with the abusive partner should be made available to these women

     c. Recommendations: The USPSTF recommends the following counselling.

        i. Patients who use alcohol or other drugs should be warned against engaging in potentially dangerous activities while intoxicated.

        ii. Counselling on other measures to reduce the risk of unintentional household or environmental injuries from falls, drownings, fires, or burns, poisoning, and firearms is also important.

        iii. All patients should be urged to use occupant restraints for themselves and others, and to wear safety helmets when riding motorcycles.

        iv. Routine screening interviews or examinations for evidence of violent injuries are not recommended.

        v. The American Medical Association recommends that all women patients should be screened for domestic violence[20] (Table 3.6).

5. Osteoporosis:

     a. Risk: More than 25 million Americans have osteoporosis, and each year more than 1.3 million fractures occur as a result (see Chapter 33).

     b. Recommendations: The USPSTF states that there is insufficient evidence to recommend for or against routine screening for osteoporosis with bone densitometry in postmenopausal women. All postmenopausal women should be counselled about hormone prophylaxis and advised of the importance of smoking cessation, regular exercise and adequate calcium intake. For those high risk women who would consider estrogen only to prevent osteoporosis, screening may be appropriate to assist treatment decisions.

     c. Methods: The National Osteoporosis Foundation recommends a comprehensive program to prevent osteoporosis in women of all ages that includes adequate calcium and vitamin D intake, weight-bearing exercises, a healthy lifestyle with no smoking and limited alcohol consumption, and medication when appropriate. A bone mineral density test is the only way to detect bone loss before a fracture occurs. A bone mineral density test is indicated when risk factors are present and a decision must be made regarding osteoporosis medications to reduce fracture risk.[4]

Partner abuse has been estimated to occur in up to 25 percent of all familial relationships.

d. Counselling: The most effective management for osteoporosis is the prevention of osteoporosis through counselling about dietary and behavioral practices to maximize the peak bone mass achieved by the third decade and to slow the rate of bone loss after that period.

All patients should be advised to consume adequate amounts of calcium and vitamin D,[21,22] to avoid smoking and excessive alcohol intake, and to exercise. Weight-bearing activities such as walking and stair climbing promote achievement of peak bone mass and delay bone loss. Perimenopausal women should be advised of the probable risks and benefits of HRT.[21] For all older persons, the risk of falls should be assessed and appropriate counselling to implement precautionary measures such as removal of throw rugs and installation of hand rails next to stairs and in the bathroom should be provided.

There should be evaluation of the presence of clinical risk factors to identify individuals who may profit from more precise evaluation of bone mineral content as a procedure for selection and monitoring of specific therapy. The drugs currently approved by the Food and Drug Administration for the prevention of osteoporosis (estrogen replacement therapy and alendronate) and for the treatment of osteoporosis (estrogen replacement therapy, alendronate, and calcitonin) should be discussed with patients.[22] The protective effects of all therapies appear to be lost soon after discontinuation of therapy.

> A comprehensive program to prevent osteoporosis in women of all ages includes adequate calcium and vitamin D intake, weight-bearing exercises, a healthy lifestyle with no smoking and limited alcohol consumption, and medication when appropriate.

Conclusions

Prevention for adult women is primarily counselling, screening, and interventions to prevent cardiovascular diseases, cancer, and infection. Lifestyle changes are a potent force for prevention of disease in women.

REFERENCES

1. Landis S, Murray T, Bolden S, Wingo P. Cancer statistics, 1999. *CA Cancer J Clin* 1999;**49**:8–31.
2. Mettlin C, Dodd GD. The American Cancer Society guidelines for the cancer-related checkup:

An update. *CA Cancer J Clin* 1991;**41**:279–82.

3. US Preventive Services Task Force. *Guide to Clinical Preventive Services*, 2nd edn. Williams & Wilkins, Baltimore, MD, 1996.

4. *Clinician's Handbook of Preventive Services*, 2nd edn. US Public Health Service, Washington, DC, 1998.

5. Oboler SK, LaForce FM. The periodic physical examination in asymptomatic adults. *Ann Intern Med* 1989;**110**:214–26.

6. Harris JR, Lippman ME, Veronesi U, Willett W. Breast cancer. [First of three parts.] *N Engl J Med* 1992;**327**:319–28.

7. Richert-Boe KE, Humphrey LL. Screening for cancers of the cervix and breast. *Arch Intern Med* 1992;**152**:2405–11.

8. Dodd GD. American Cancer Society guidelines on screening for breast cancer: An overview. *CA Cancer J Clin* 1992;**42**:177–80.

9. Mettlin C, Jones G, Averette H, Gusberg SB, Murphy GP. Defining and updating the American Cancer Society guidelines for the cancer-related checkup: Prostate and endometrial cancers. *CA Cancer J Clin* 1993;**43**:42–6.

10. Koss LG. The Papanicolaou test for cervical cancer detection. A triumph and a tragedy. *JAMA* 1989;**261**:737–43.

11. Davis DL. Mammographic screening. *JAMA* 1994;**271**:152–3.

12. Horton JA, ed.: *The Women's Health Data Book*, 2nd edn. Elsevier, Washington, DC, 1995.

13. ACP Task Force on Adult Immunization and Infectious Diseases Society of America. *Guide for Adult Immunization*, 3rd edn. American College of Physicians, Philadelphia, 1994.

14. American College of Obstetrics and Gynecologists. *Hormone Replacement Therapy*. ACOG Educational Bulletin no. 247, 1998.

15. Henrich JB. The postmenopausal estrogen/breast cancer controversy. *JAMA* 1992;**268**:1900–2.

16. AHA Medical/Scientific Statement. Aspirin as a therapeutic agent in cardiovascular disease. *Circulation* 1993;**87**:659–75.

17. AHA/ACC Scientific Statement: Consensus Panel Statement. Guide to preventive cardiology for women. *Circulation* 1999;**99**:2480–4.

18. Forrest JD. The delivery of family planning services in the United States. *Fam Plann Perspect* 1988;**20**:88, 90–5, 98.

19. Rosenberg ML, O'Carroll PW, Powell KE. Let's be clear. Violence is a public health problem. *JAMA* 1992;**267**:3071–72.

20. American Medical Association diagnostic and treatment guidelines on domestic violence. *Arch Fam Med* 1992;**1**:39–47.

21. Levinson W, Altkorn D. Primary prevention of postmenopausal osteoporosis. *JAMA* 1998;**280**:1821–2.

22. Khosla S, Riggs BL. Treatment options for osteoporosis. *Mayo Clin Proc* 1995;**70**:978–82.

Appendix 3.1. US Preventive Services guidelines in preventive care for all women aged 25–64 years

- Leading causes of death
  - Malignant neoplasms
  - Heart diseases
  - Motor vehicle and other unintentional injuries
  - Human immunodeficiency virus infection
  - Suicide and homicide

Interventions for the general population

- **Screening**
  - Blood pressure
  - Height and weight
  - Total blood cholesterol (age 45–65 years)
  - Pap test
  - Fecal occult blood test and/or sigmoidoscopy (⩾ 50 years)
  - Mammogram ± clinical breast examination (age 50–69 years)
  - Assess for problem drinking
  - Rubella serology or vaccination history (women of childbearing age)

- **Counselling**
  - Substance use
    - Tobacco cessation
    - Avoid alcohol/drug use while driving, swimming, boating, etc.
  - Diet and exercise
    - Limit fat and cholesterol; maintain caloric balance; emphasize grains, fruits, vegetables
    - Adequate calcium intake
    - Regular physical activity
  - Injury prevention
    - Lap/shoulder belts
    - Motorcycle/bicycle/all-terrain vehicle helmets
    - Smoke detector
    - Safe storage/removal of firearms
  - Sexual behavior
    - STD prevention: avoid high-risk behavior; condoms/female barrier with spermicide
    - Unintended pregnancy: contraception
  - Dental health
    - Regular visits to dental care providers
    - Floss, brush with fluoride toothpaste daily
  - Immunizations
    - Tetanus-diphtheria (Td) boosters
    - Rubella (women of childbearing age)
  - Chemoprophylaxis
    - Multivitamin with folic acid (women planning or capable of pregnancy)
    - Discuss hormone prophylaxis (peri- and postmenopausal women)

4 Preventive care for older adults

Jeannette South-Paul, MD, Deborah Bostock, MD, and Cheryl Woodson, MD

Primary preventive measures for older women must be accomplished early in life to make an impact later in life. Prevention for the older person includes maintaining quality of life, preserving function, preventing collapse of family support systems, and maintaining independence in the community.

Primary preventive measures are optimally accomplished early in life to make an impact later in life.

Goals of preventive care for the older woman

1. The percentage of US adults older than age 65 years is growing rapidly and expected to almost double between 1995 and 2030 (12.8 to 20 percent).[1]
2. Life expectancy for women is longer than that of men, at all ages older than age 65 years. By age 85, only 45 men will be alive for every 100 women.[2] This significantly changes the social environment in which older women live. Understanding the specific needs and circumstances of an individual woman helps to guide preventive health decisions.
3. The annual physical examination encompasses screening and preventive counselling. Both primary preventive measures (i.e., interventions targeted at preventing specific conditions in asymptomatic persons) and secondary preventive measures (i.e., screening for early detection and treatment of modifiable risk factors or preclinical disease) are described.

General assessment

Well-being/living situation/independence
1. Health status assessment and primary and secondary prevention encompass more than a periodic physical examination. A multidimensional assessment

Table 4.1. Checklist of assessment areas for maintaining healthy geriatric patients

Injury prevention
- Use of safety belts or helmets
- Smoke detectors (in place and working)
- Hot water temperature at $\leqslant$ 48.8 °C (120 °F)
- Smoking near bed or upholstery
- Poor lighting
- Obtrusive furniture
- Slippery floors and loose rugs
- Handrails and grab bars
- One-leg balance (5 seconds)
- "Get Up and Go" test*
  *The patient rises from a sitting position, walks 3 m (~ 10 ft), turns and returns to the chair to sit. The test is positive if these activities take more than 16 seconds.

Sensorium
- Snellen eye chart
- Ophthalmology examination
- Hearing Handicapped Inventory for the Elder – Screening version
- Pure tone audiometry

Nutrition
- Nutritional Health Screen
- Tooth brushing, flossing and dental visits

Immunizations
- Tetanus and diphtheria toxoid
- Influenza vaccine
- Pneumoccal vaccine

Sexuality
- Review of chronic conditions and medications
- Initiation of discussion about sexuality

Continence
- Review of chronic conditions and medications
- Initiation of discussion about incontinence
- Focused physical examination (pelvis, rectum)

Mental status (consider one of the following)
- Mini-Mental State
- Clock Test
- Informant Questionnaire on Cognitive Decline in the Elderly
- Geriatric Depression Scale
- Yale Depression Screen
- Questioning about suicide

Social issues
- Changes in living arrangements, finances or activities
- Caregiver support or burnout
- Advance directives
- Family training in cardiopulmonary resuscitation
- Activities of Daily Living
- Instrumental Activities of Daily Living
- Performance Test of Activities of Daily Living

focusing on mental health, physical health, basic functioning, social functioning, and economic well-being provides a complete picture of the older woman (Table 4.1).

2. Early in the evaluation, establishing the older woman's marital status, her current living arrangements and household partners, and whether she has experienced the loss of a spouse or long-time friend is important. Is she currently working or active in group activities outside the home?

3. The accuracy of the history depends on adequate mental and affective functioning of the patient. The accuracy of historical information gathered

from the older woman, family member or friend, and the consistency of the information between sources, provide clues regarding the older woman's cognitive function and whether she can remain independent.

Caregiving responsibilities

1. Older women often have substantial responsibilities for caring for spouses, siblings, children, and grandchildren. More than 15 million adults currently provide care to relatives.[3] Of all caregivers for disabled elders, 70 percent are women and 30 percent of these are older than age 74 years.[4]
2. Caregiving taxes physical, social, emotional, and financial resources, and can significantly affect the health and functional status of the caregiver. The combination of loss, prolonged distress and the physical demands of caregiving increase the caregiver's risk for physical and emotional health problems.[3]
3. Caregivers who provide support to their spouses and report caregiving strain are 63 percent more likely to die within four years than noncaregivers.[3]
4. Significant levels of depression are seen in caregivers of Alzheimer's patients. Assistance is available through support groups and information accessible through the Internet: www.alz.org and www.alzheimers.com
5. Reducing caregiving demands by providing respite care or other relief for the caregiver may mitigate the strain so that the caregiver and cared-for family member can remain independent longer.

> Caregiving taxes physical, social, emotional, and financial resources, and can significantly affect the health and functional status of the caregiver.

Presence of chronic disease

1. With aging, the older woman becomes more susceptible to chronic illness and disease. For example, the incidence of degenerative joint disease is increased in older women. This causes an increased incidence of knee pain, which is associated with a diminished quality of life.[5]
2. There is a higher incidence of all chronic diseases, especially diabetes mellitus and hypertension, in minority groups.[6]
3. The presence of common chronic health problems is associated with lower levels of cancer screening – presumably because of the time commitment required by the clinician to care for these chronic illnesses, negatively impacting on preventive services.[7]

Access to care

Insurance coverage/underinsurance

1. In the USA, underinsurance is the inability to pay out-of-pocket expenses despite having insurance, and usually implies inability to use preventive services also. Medicare-eligible citizens may be unable to afford medical expenses not covered by Medicare. Many elderly recently joined Medicare Health Maintenance Organizations (HMOs) to obtain added benefits, including prescription benefits, and have been confused and abandoned by the failure and break-up of these Medicare HMOs.

2. The underinsured category also includes unemployed persons age 55 to 64 and those not provided with coverage through their jobs. They are not yet eligible for Medicare and must pay high individual health premiums when they can obtain some form of group coverage. Women are more likely to be underinsured because they are more likely to be divorced and no longer covered by husband's insurance or underemployed in a parttime job that does not provide medical insurance. Lack of health insurance is associated with delayed health care and increased mortality.

3. Underinsurance also may result in adverse health consequences.[8] There is a dose–response relationship between the level of insurance coverage and receipt of preventive services.

4. Women access the health care system more frequently than do men. They receive more health services and prescriptions, undergo more examinations, laboratory tests, and blood pressure checks than men.

5. However, when US physicians were surveyed recently regarding making the diagnosis of coronary artery disease and recommending coronary angiography and/or revascularization procedures, they were significantly less likely to make these recommendations for women and minority groups.[9]

> Lack of health insurance is associated with delayed health care and increased mortality.

Mobility

1. Those women most likely to get screening and preventive services have a usual source of care and no limitations in mobility.[10]

2. This is evident in the higher risk for delayed diagnosis of breast and cervical cancer in disabled women.[11]

Language/acculturation

1. Low level of acculturation results in a lower likelihood of receipt of preventive

services.[12] Cultural explanatory models are important in describing the woman's willingness to receive care. Eliciting this information is easier when the clinician and the older woman have a comfortable relationship. Otherwise, the clinician may be unaware of why therapies prescribed are unsuccessful or why the woman fails to follow advice.

2. Religion is a significant part of the culture of racial and ethnic communities representing a range of socioeconomic status. Physical health, depressive symptoms, and hypertension improved, and tobacco and alcohol use decreased as a woman's religious involvement increased in ethnic communities.[13]

> Those women most likely to get screening and preventive services have a usual source of care and no limitations in mobility.

Emotional/mental status/cognitive functioning

1. Depression: Depression is the most commonly diagnosed mental illness in older adults in the primary care setting, although it often goes unnoticed.[14] Major depression is seen in 1 to 5 percent and significant depressive symptoms in up to 25 percent of community-dwelling older people. Older women receive more antidepressants each year than men, though this difference decreases as they get older.[15]

   a. Older adults with major depression who are seeing primary care physicians have significantly higher medical costs (reflecting more outpatient visits, laboratory tests, X-rays, inpatient days, and specialty medical visits) than controls matched for age, gender, and chronic medical illness.[16]

   b. Older caregivers demonstrate significantly higher levels of depressive symptoms, anxiety, and lower levels of perceived health than do their noncaregiving counterparts.[16]

   c. In addition to depression, stress-related symptoms are common in older adults. Lower stress levels are evident in retirees than in those approaching retirement,[17] or in their working counterparts.

2. Cognitive dysfunction:

   a. Cognitive decline in the very old has been underestimated and must be assessed carefully and regularly (Table 4.2).[18]

   b. A complete mental status examination includes an evaluation of level of consciousness, attention, language capabilities, memory, proverb interpretation, comparisons, calculations, writing, constructional ability.

> Older adults with major depression who are seeing primary care physicians have significantly higher medical costs.

Table 4.2. Laboratory testing for cognitive dysfunction

Basic metabolic testing includes:
- Thyroid function
- Electrolyte levels
- Complete blood count

When suggested by history or examination:
- Erythrocyte sedimentation rate
- Testing for syphilis
- Imaging studies
- Magnetic resonance imaging

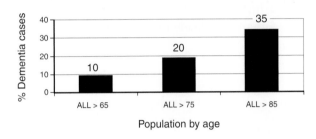

Figure 4.1.   Percentage of elderly with dementia, by age.

    c. Condensed mental status screening tools can substitute for the complete mental status examination and detect cognitive deficits that are often seen in dementia syndromes.

    d. Deficits often occur without a change in level of consciousness, are significantly different from patient's baseline results, and always result in some impairment of function.[19]

    e. The average age of onset of dementia is 69 years (Figure 4.1).

    f. Dementia imposes heavy responsibilities on family and resources and must be distinguished from delirium (reversible cognitive deficits).

    g. Brief mental status tests may evaluate intellectual functioning only or also include a functional assessment. Two commonly used tests are the Pfeiffer Short Portable Mental Status Questionnaire and the Folstein Mini Mental State Examination.[20] None of these tools has complete diagnostic accuracy and they may fail to identify subtle changes in highly functioning elderly. Basic testing is included in Table 4.1.

    h. When there are negative results in both the metabolic work-up and the

Dementia imposes heavy responsibilities on family and resources and must be distinguished from delirium.

mental status examination for patients with functional impairment, formal neuropsychological testing is necessary. The results can also assist in care coordination by suggesting beneficial environmental adaptations.

3. Family support:
   a. The caregiving ability and availability of family and friends must be determined to identify who could help the elder in the event of an illness, accident, or other acute event that would limit self-care ability.
   b. Caregivers also can provide valuable information regarding subtle changes in functioning or cognition.

4. Social network:
   The older woman's involvement in the community reflects her ability to make and sustain relationships and also defines a support system outside the family. The active woman is unlikely to be severely handicapped by mental and emotional conditions.

5. Religious involvement:
   a. After adjusting for physical and mental health conditions, social connections and health practices, older women who attend church at least once weekly had a better chance of survival.[21]
   b. The positive effects of religion have been seen in all age groups. Fewer depressive symptoms occur in women who have a denominational affiliation, whereas women with no or low frequency of church attendance have more current smoking and daily drinking.[13]
   c. Religious participation has short- and long-term influence on functioning in the elderly, especially those who are disabled, including the following:
      i. Attendance at services is a strong predictor of better functioning;
      ii. Health practices, social ties, and indicators of well-being reduce, but do not eliminate, these effects; disability has minimal effects on subsequent attendance.
   d. Older adults who reside in deteriorated neighborhoods experience more physical health problems than older people who dwell in more favorable living environments.[22] Data from a nationwide longitudinal survey of older people suggest that the noxious impact of living in a dilapidated neighborhood on changes in self-rated health over time is offset completely for older adults who are deeply religious.

6. Sexuality:
   a. Like younger adults, older adults are sexual beings. Assumptions of sexual activities or lack thereof based upon age alone are unwarranted. Even in

Older women who attend church at least once weekly had a better chance of survival.

the presence of significant ongoing health problems, appropriate sexual history questioning of all older women is helpful.

b. Issues include lack of availability of partners (widows or spouses with significant health problems), physiological changes associated with age (mucosal dryness in postmenopausal women) and changes in relationships with aging. As with younger patients, discussions of sexual activity include inquiries and education on risky sexual behaviors.

Older adults who reside in deteriorated neighborhoods experience more physical health problems than do older people who dwell in more favorable living environments.

Functional assessment

Activities of daily living/instrumental activities of daily living

1. Periodic health examination provides an opportunity to detect functional problems that can decrease life expectancy. Classifying the older woman by functional ability is more helpful than classifying her by age (Table 4.3).

2. Instrumental activities of daily living (IADLs) are those that require the patient to use integrative thought processes and complex musculoskeletal coordination to perform the necessary daily tasks of life (e.g., working, shopping, cooking, managing money, driving or arranging transportation, using the telephone) (Table 4.4).

3. Basic activities of daily living (ADLs) are those that are necessary to maintain personal care (e.g., bathing, dressing, maintaining continence, transferring or walking, toiletting, eating).

4. Multiple instruments exist for research and social service purposes, but the most commonly used clinical instrument is the Katz Index of Activities of Daily Living.[23]

Ambulation/activity patterns

1. More than 40 percent of women older than age 65 report a sedentary lifestyle that is associated with many chronic illnesses.[24] Maintenance of regular leisure-time activity results in lower lipid levels, coronary artery disease, diabetes mellitus, and hypertension.

Table 4.3. Index of Activities of Daily Living

Name:

Date of evaluation: _____

For each area of functioning listed below, check the description that applies. (The word "assistance" applies to supervision, direction or personal assistance.)

Bathing (sponge bath, tub bath, or shower)

Receives no assistance (gets in and out of bathtub by self if tub is usual means of bathing)	Receives assistance in bathing only one part of the body (such as back or legs)	Receives assistance in bathing more than one part of the body (or is not bathed)

Dressing (gets clothes from closets and drawers, including underclothes and outer garments, and uses fasteners, including braces, if worn)

Gets clothes and gets completely dressed without assistance	Gets clothes and gets dressed without assistance, except for assistance in tying shoes	Receives assistance in getting clothes or in getting dressed, or stays partly or completely undressed

Toiletting (going to "toilet room" for bowel and urine elimination, cleaning self after elimination and arranging clothes)

Goes to "toilet room", cleans self and arranges clothes without assistance (may use an object for support, such as cane, walker or wheelchair, and may manage night bedpan or commode, emptying in morning)	Receives assistance in going to "toilet room", in cleaning self or in arranging clothes after elimination, or in using night bedpan or commode	Does not go to "toilet room" for the elimination process

Transfer

Moves in and out of a bed and chair without assistance (may use object for support, such as cane or walker)	Moves in and out of a bed and chair with assistance	Does not get out of bed

Table 4.3. (*cont.*)

Continence

Controls urination and bowel movement completely by self	Has occasional "accidents"	Supervision helps keep urine or bowel control; catheter is used; or person is incontinent

Feeding

Feeds self without assistance	Feeds self, except for needing assistance in cutting meat or buttering bread	Receives assistance in feeding or is fed partly or completely using tubes or intravenous fluids

Adapted with permission from Katz S. Assessing self-maintenance: Activities of daily living, mobility, and instrumental activities of daily living. *J Am Geriatr Soc* 1983;**31**:721–7.

2. Regular exercise improves neurobehavioral function.[25]
3. Strength training is important for maintenance of strength, physical function, bone integrity and psychosocial health.[26]

> Regular exercise improves neurobehavioral function.

Diet/nutrition

1. Approximately 21 to 45 percent of women between ages 65 and 74 years are overweight.[27] Diet affects the development of most of the chronic diseases that are also impacted by exercise patterns. In addition, stroke, constipation, and diverticular and dental disease are all influenced by diet.
2. This may be the appropriate time in the history to ask about the use of vitamins and nutritional supplements. They serve as a potential source of symptoms and drug interactions.
3. Accurate weights at the clinical visit are important, rather than relying on the stated weight. Unfortunately the national norms do not include data on older people.
4. Significant weight loss (1 to 2 percent of body weight in one week, 5 percent in one month, or 10 percent in six months) may reflect many diseases (Table 4.5), poor dentition, cognitive impairment, respiratory dysfunction, poor hand-to-mouth coordination, a need for assistance in purchasing or preparing foods or other factors affecting the amount of food consumed (such as elder abuse).[19]

Table 4.4. Instrumental Activities of Daily Living (self-rated version)

For each question, circle the points for the answer that best applies to your situation.

1. Can you use the telephone?	
Without help	3
With some help	2
Completely unable to use the telephone	1

2. Can you get to places that are out of walking distance?	
Without help	3
With some help	2
Completely unable to travel unless special arrangements are made	1

3. Can you go shopping for groceries?	
Without help	3
With some help	2
Completely unable to do any shopping	1

4. Can you prepare your own meals?	
Without help	3
With some help	2
Completely unable to prepare any meals	1

5. Can you do your own housework?	
Without help	3
With some help	2
Completely unable to do any housework	1

6. Can you do your own handyman work?	
Without help	3

Table 4.4. (*cont.*)

With some help	2
Completely unable to do any handyman work	1

7. Can you do your own laundry?

Without help	3
With some help	2
Completely unable to do any laundry at all	1

8a. Do you take any medicines or use any medications?

Yes (If "yes", answer question 8b)	1
No (If "no" answer question 8c)	2

8b. Do you take your own medicine?

Without help (in the right doses at the right time)	3
With some help (take medicine if someone prepares it for you and/or reminds you to take it)	2
Completely unable to take own medicine	1

8c. If you had to take medicine, could you do it?

Without help (in the right doses at the right time)	3
With some help (take medicine if someone prepares it for you and/or reminds you to take it)	2
Completely unable to take own medicine	1

9. Can you manage your own money?

Without help	3
With some help	2
Completely unable to handle money	1

Adapted with permission from Lawton MP, Brody EM. Assessment of older people: Self-maintaining and instrumental activities of daily living. *Gerontologist* 1969;**9**:279–85.

Table 4.5. Causes of significant weight loss

Definition: 1 to 2 % of bodyweight in 1 week, 5% in 1 month, or 10% in 6 months.

- Chronic diseases
- Chronic infections
- Diabetes
- Cancer
- Poor dentition
- Cognitive impairment
- Respiratory dysfunction
- Poor hand-to-mouth coordination
- A need for assistance in purchasing or preparing foods
- Other factors affecting the amount of food consumed (such as elder abuse)

From Bignotti DD, Evans JM, Fleming KC. *The Geriatric Patient*, 7th edn.
ABFP Reference Guides. American Board of Family Practice, Lexington, KN, 1999.

Risk assessment (Appendix 4.1)

Risk of elder abuse

1. As many as 2.5 million older adult persons are abused each year and the number of cases is likely to increase as this population grows. Elder abuse exists in many forms: physical, emotional, financial, and sexual; neglect and self-neglect.
2. Most states have mandatory reporting; however, it may infringe on the autonomy of competent geriatric individuals. Supportive assessment and management focuses on both the patient and the caregiver for problem solving.
3. Physicians infrequently report elder abuse. This may be caused by unfamiliarity with reporting laws, fear of offending patients, concern about time limitations, and the belief that they do not have appropriate evaluation skills. In the USA, reporting suspected abuse directly to the appropriate state agency facilitates the coordination of thorough long-term assessment and management.
4. Older women and men have similar abuse rates. Abuse is best correlated with the emotional and financial dependence of the caregivers on the geriatric victims. Relatives, usually spouses, most commonly abuse older patients.
5. No specific screening tools have been found to be clearly effective in identifying elder abuse victims. A few direct questions in the course of routine history taking may provide the physician with insight into those patients at risk (US Preventive Services Task Force (USPSTF) class C).[20] Helpful questions include: "Are you afraid of anyone at home?", "Have you been struck, slapped, or kicked?" or "Do you ever feel alone?".[28]

Elder abuse is best correlated with the emotional and financial dependence of the caregivers on the geriatric victims, and relatives, usually spouses, most commonly abuse older patients.

Risk for substance abuse

1. Substance abuse, including alcohol and tobacco abuse, afflicts the older patient as well as the young. The periodic examination is the logical time to screen for substance abuse and provide appropriate counselling. Emphasizing the relatively short-term rewards of smoking cessation, such as decreasing the risk of stroke, can be persuasive for the older person struggling with tobacco abuse.

2. Referral to a specific program is more helpful for the patient than merely suggesting she discontinue tobacco use. However, more women and more elderly quit smoking "cold-turkey" and on their own than using a program. Recognize the multiple ways other than cigarettes (snuff, pipes, etc.) that an older woman can use tobacco.

3. The four-question CAGE instrument (see Chapter 27) can be very helpful in identifying alcohol abuse or dependence. It is less sensitive for early problem drinking, heavy drinking or drinking in any women or the elderly than it is with men.

More women and more elderly quit smoking "cold turkey" and on their own than using a program.

Risk of injury

1. Safety belts: Older adult persons are less likely to be involved in a motor vehicle accident (caused by decreased driving distances and lower speeds). Older women and their passengers still benefit from the use of lap/shoulder belts at all times even in the presence of air bags (USPSTF class A).[29] For some small, frail women, air bags can pose a potential risk of injury.

2. Falls: Falling is a common, serious problem in older individuals. Falls are the leading cause of nonfatal injuries and unintentional injury deaths in older persons in the USA. Screening for falls may include asking the patient whether she has fallen in the past year or whether she is afraid of falling. Gait assessment and rehabilitation can be offered to such women. These measures have been shown to reduce the risk of falling and subsequent injuries.[28]

Table 4.6. Ten-minute screen for geriatric conditions

Problem	Screening measure	Positive screen
Vision	Ask this question: "Because of your eyesight, do you have trouble driving a car, watching television, reading or doing any of your daily activities?" If the patient answers "yes", test each eye with the Snellen eye chart while the patient wears corrective lenses (if applicable)	"Yes" to question and inability to read at greater than 20/40 on the Snellen eye chart
Hearing	Use an audioscope set at 40 dB. Test the patient's hearing using 1000 and 2000 Hz	Inability to hear 1000 or 2000 Hz in both ears or inability to hear frequencies in either ear
Leg mobility	Time the patient after giving these directions: "Rise from the chair. Then walk 6 m (20 feet) briskly, turn, walk back to the chair and sit down."	Unable to complete task in 15 seconds
Urinary incontinence	Ask this question: "In the past year, have you ever lost your urine and gotten wet?" If the patient answers "yes", ask this question: "Have you lost urine on at least 6 separate days?"	"Yes" to both questions
Nutrition and weight loss	Ask this question: "Have you lost 4.5 kg (10 lb) over the past 6 months without trying to do so?" If the patient answers "yes", weigh the patient	"Yes" to the question or a weight of less than 45.5 kg (100 lb)
Memory	Three-item recall	Unable to remember all 3 items after 1 minute
Depression	Ask this question: "Do you often feel sad or depressed?"	"Yes" to the question
Physical disability	Ask the patient these six questions: "Are you unable to do strenuous activities, like fast walking or bicycling?" "Are you unable to do heavy work around the house, like washing windows, walls or floors?"	"Yes" to any of the questions

Table 4.6. (*cont.*)

Problem	Screening measure	Positive screen
	"Are you unable to go shopping for groceries or clothes?" "Are you unable to get to places that are out of walking distance?" "Are you unable to bathe – sponge bath, tub bath or shower?" "Are you unable to dress, like put on a shirt, button and zip your clothes, or put on your shoes?"	

Adapted with permission from Moore A, Siu AL. Screening for common problems in ambulatory elderly: Clinical confirmation of a screen instrument. *Am J Med* 1996;**100**:438–43. Copyright 1996, with permission from Excerpta Medica Inc.

Periodic medical care

Examination frequency

All elders benefit from a periodic examination that focuses on prevention. However, with accurate record keeping, this evaluation can be accomplished through serial visits as the older woman is monitored for chronic diseases. This approach is consistent with the current USPSTF guidelines (Table 4.6).

Immunizations

1. Older adults are often inadequately immunized. Formal documentation of remote vaccine history is often unavailable. A review of immunization history and documentation can be performed during the periodic examination (Table 4.7).
2. Influenza vaccine: Annual influenza vaccine is recommended for all older adults, particularly those who are chronically ill or at high risk of contracting influenza, such as those patients in institutions (assisted living centers, nursing homes, boarding and daycare homes) (USPSTF class B).[29] The vaccine is effective in reducing hospitalizations, deaths, associated complications and health care costs from influenza.[30]

Table 4.7. Recommended immunizations for older women

- Influenza vaccine annually
- Pneumococcal polysaccharide vaccine once after age 65 years for all immunocompetent adults
- Tetanus-diphtheria vaccine every 10 years or a single booster at age 65 years

3. Pneumococcal polysaccharide vaccine: A single immunization is recommended for all immunocompetent adults age 65 years and older (USPSTF class B).[29]

   Universal revaccination is unnecessary as the protection afforded by the vaccine persists for up to nine years or more. The American College of Physicians does recommend revaccination for patients who have received the vaccine before age 65 years and more than six years have passed since the initial vaccine.[31]

4. Tetanus: Although tetanus is an uncommon disease in developed nations, more than 60 percent of cases occur in patients older than age 60 years. The standard recommendation is a combined tetanus-diphtheria (Td) given every 10 years for all patients (USPSTF class A).[29]

   A single Td booster at age 65 years may be a cost-effective alternative, given current compliance with the 10-year guideline.[32] A complete primary series of three toxoid doses over 6 to 12 months is necessary for those patients who have never been vaccinated.[29]

Screening (Table 4.8)
1. Hypertension:
   a. Impact: Elevated blood pressure occurs in 60 percent of non-Hispanic whites, 71 percent of non-Hispanic African-Americans, and 61 percent of Mexican-Americans older than age 60 years.
   b. Systolic rather than diastolic blood pressure is a better predictor of coronary artery disease, cardiovascular disease, heart failure, stroke, end-stage renal disease, and all-cause mortality than diastolic blood pressure in the elderly. Primary hypertension is the most common form of hypertension in older persons.[33]
   c. Blood pressure measurements at least every two years for adults with diastolic blood pressures less than 85 mmHg and systolic blood pressures below 130 mmHg are recommended.[33]
   d. Annual blood pressure measurements are recommended for persons with diastolic blood pressures 85 to 89 mmHg or systolic blood pressures 130 to

Table 4.8. Recommended screening for older women

Disease	Recommended screening	Comments
Hypertension	BP measurements every 2 years for BP < 130/85 BP measurements annually for BP 130–139/85–89	Measure blood pressure both standing and sitting to assess for orthostatic changes
Breast cancer	Clinical breast examination annually Mammography every 1–2 years	Encourage monthly self breast examination
Cervical cancer	Pap smears every 1–3 years	Consider discontinuing screening if repeated Pap smears are normal
Colon cancer	Annual fecal occult blood test Flexible sigmoidoscopy every 3–5 years	
Depression	Geriatric Depression Scale	5-item version reduces administration time
Cognitive impairment	Mini Mental Status Examination	
Hyperlipidemias	Screening of asymptomatic women not recommended	May consider screening otherwise healthy women with major risk factors for CHD
Thyroid disease	TSH	Especially women with symptoms of cognitive or affective deficits
Incontinence	Direct questioning	
Osteoporosis	Dual energy X-ray absorptiometry for high risk women	
Hearing loss	Periodic direct questioning about potential hearing loss	Handheld audioscopes may be more sensitive
Vision loss	Periodic Snellen acuity testing	

BP, blood pressure; CHD, coronary heart disease; TSH, thyroid-stimulating hormone.

139 mmHg. Persons with higher blood pressures require more frequent measurements.

e. Older individuals are more likely than younger individuals to exhibit an orthostatic fall in blood pressure and hypotension. Therefore, measure

Systolic rather than diastolic blood pressure is a better predictor of coronary artery disease, cardiovascular disease, heart failure, stroke, end-stage renal disease, and all-cause mortality than diastolic blood pressure in the elderly.

blood pressure in both the standing and sitting positions in older individuals.

    f. Treating hypertension in the elderly is important and does decrease their risk of morbidity and mortality. Effects of nonpharmacological first-line therapy (i.e., weight reduction, increased physical activity, sodium restriction, decreased alcohol intake) on cardiovascular morbidity and mortality are less well studied.[29]

2. Breast cancer:

    a. The USPSTF recommends routine screening every one to two years with mammography and annual clinical breast examination (CBE) for women aged 50 to 69 years.[29]

    b. There is insufficient evidence to recommend for or against routine mammography or CBE for women age 70 years or older, although recommendations for healthy women older than age 70 may be made on other grounds (e.g., those with a past history of malignancy). Women who have had one mammogram after age 70 years are much less likely to die of breast cancer. Continuing mammography screening after 69 years results in a small gain in life expectancy and is moderately cost-effective in those with high bone mineral density, but more costly in those with low bone mineral density.[34]

    c. Older women with low bone mineral density have a lower risk of breast cancer (presumably caused by decreased exposure to estrogen) and may benefit less from continued screening.[35]

    d. Data regarding the sensitivity of monthly breast self-examination (BSE) in detecting breast cancer are extremely limited. Sensitivity may be approximately 15 percent. Sensitivity for detecting breast cancer rises to 26 percent if the women are also screened by CBE and mammography.[36]

    e. Factors that have been associated with inadequate screening are advanced age, poor cognitive function, and nursing home residence.[37]

3. Cervical cancer:

    a. For those older women in whom repeated Pap smears have been normal, further screening does not appear to be beneficial. Those women with no prior screening, previously inadequate screening or for those women

Treating hypertension in the elderly is important and does decrease their risk of morbidity and mortality.

The USPSTF recommends routine screening every one to two years with mammography and annual clinical breast examination for women aged 50 to 69 years.

    engaging in high risk sexual behaviors, screening with Pap smears every one to three years is recommended.

b. Women who have undergone hysterectomy for noncervical cancer diagnoses, with complete removal of the cervix do not benefit from Pap smear screening.[29]

c. There is insufficient evidence to provide for or against an upper age limit to Pap smear screening. The USPSTF and the American College of Physicians offer guidelines to cease screening after age 65 years, while the Canadian Task Force recommends ceasing after age 69 if prior screening has been normal (USPTFP class C).[29]

4. Colon cancer:

a. Colon cancer is the second most common form of cancer in the USA and has the second highest mortality. Although its peak incidence is between ages 70 and 80 years, none of the available studies focuses on the geriatric population.

b. Digital rectal examination (DRE) is of little value in screening for colon cancer, since fewer than 10 percent of colorectal cancers can be palpated.

c. Annual fecal occult blood testing (FOBT) in asymptomatic patients has a high rate of false positives. The positive predictive value is only 2 to 11 percent for carcinomas and 20 to 30 percent for adenomas in patients older than age 50 years. The predictive value may be higher in older patients caused by the higher prevalence of colorectal cancers in these age groups. Two recent studies have shown reductions in mortality in patients offered FOBT every one to two years.[38] All positive results need to be further evaluated with appropriate testing (colonoscopy, air contrast barium enema).

d. Screening with sigmoidoscopy, with or without FOBT, is recommended every three to five years by most authorities, although intervals of 10 years may also be adequate (USPSTF class B).[29]

e. Sigmoidoscopy with longer (60 cm) flexible sigmoidoscopes has been shown to have greater sensitivity and is better tolerated by the patient than rigid sigmoidoscopy.

5. Depression/cognitive impairment:

For those older women in whom repeated Pap smears have been normal, further screening does not appear to be beneficial.

Table 4.9. Geriatric Depression Scale (short form)

For each question, choose the best answer for how you felt over the past week.

1. Are you basically satisfied with your life?	Yes/NO
2. Have you dropped many of your activities and interests?	YES/No
3. Do you feel that your life is empty?	YES/No
4. Do you often get bored?	YES/No
5. Are you in good spirits most of the time?	Yes/NO
6. Are you afraid that something bad is going to happen to you?	YES/No
7. Do you feel happy most of the time?	Yes/NO
8. Do you often feel helpless?	YES/No
9. Do you prefer to stay at home, rather than going out and doing new things?	YES/No
10. Do you feel you have more problems with memory than most?	YES/No
11. Do you think it is wonderful to be alive now?	Yes/NO
12. Do you feel pretty worthless the way you are now?	YES/No
13. Do you feel full of energy?	Yes/NO
14. Do you feel that your situation is hopeless?	YES/No
15. Do you think that most people are better off than you are?	YES/No

The scale is scored as follows: 1 point for each response in capital letters. A score of 0 to 5 is normal; a score above 5 suggests depression.
Adapted with permission from Sheikh JI, Yesavage JA. Geriatric Depression Scale (GDS): Recent evidence and development of a shorter version. *Clin Gerontol* 1986;**5**:165–72.

a. Office screening tools: The ideal depression-screening tool for older persons is both accurate and easy to administer. The original 30-item Geriatric Depression Scale (GDS) was developed by M. Brink and J.A. Yesavage in 1982 and condensed to a 15-item version by J.I. Sheikh in 1986 with improved efficiency and no loss of accuracy.[39] Most recently, a 5-item version of the GDS has been developed resulting in a marked reduction in administration time (Table 4.9).[40]

b. Education and cultural background moderate Mini Mental Status Examination (MMSE) results. College-educated women perform better on these examinations and racial and ethnic minorities do more poorly, almost entirely related to lower socioeconomic status and poorer educational attainment.[41]

6. Hyperlipidemias:

a. Current recommendations for screening of asymptomatic women older than age 65 years are conflicting. Although hyperlipidemia is strongly associated with atherosclerotic heart disease, little correlation has been shown between elevated total or low-density lipoprotein (LDL) cholesterol and long-term heart disease risk or mortality in women older than age 65 years.

b. Currently the American College of Physicians and USPSTF do not recommend cholesterol screening in asymptomatic women older than age 65. Individualized screening of otherwise healthy women with major risk factors for CHD (smoking, hypertension, and diabetes) is a class C recommendation.[29] Screening with fasting or nonfasting samples is appropriate. The ratio of total to high density lipoprotein (HDL) cholesterol appears to be the best predictor of coronary risk in older patients.[42]

7. Thyroid disease:

a. Although there is a high prevalence of thyroid disorders in older patients, especially women, no benefits of thyroid screening have been shown in clinical trials.

b. Asymptomatic elevations in thyroid-stimulating hormone (TSH) or low thyroxine (T_4) levels have been found in up to 15 percent of women older than age 60 years.[43] Subclinical thyroid disease is also described, especially in patients with cognitive and affective deficits.

c. With reasonable assay costs, screening for mild thyroid failure at the periodic health examination may be cost effective. The US and Canadian Task Forces agreed that it might be reasonable to test high risk patients, especially women, and those with possible symptoms (class C recommendation).[29]

d. A TSH assay alone is a reasonable test, with subsequent follow-up of abnormal values.

Screening for colon cancer with sigmoidoscopy, with or without fecal occult blood testing, is recommended every three to five years.

Table 4.10. Risk factors and indications for bone density screening

• Age	• Caucasian or Asian race
• Smoking	• Sedentary lifestyle/immobility
• Estrogen deficient states	• Excessive alcohol intake
• Low body weight	• Long-term medications (e.g. glucocorticoids,
• Calcium deficient diet	phenytoin, excessive thyroxine)
• Nulliparity	• Fracture
• Family history of osteoporosis	

Data taken from AACE clinical practice guidelines for the prevention and treatment of postmenopausal osteoporosis. *Endocrine Pract* 1996;**2**:157–71.

    e. Screening every five years has been suggested as an appropriate interval.

8. Incontinence:

    a. Urinary incontinence is a common, disruptive, and potentially disabling condition. Women, more commonly than men, experience urinary incontinence with increasing frequency with age and level of institutionalized care. Significant problems with incontinence may lead to social isolation, with resultant decline in physical well-being and quality of life (see Chapter 21).

    b. Simple, direct questioning in the routine history taking will often reveal symptomatic urinary incontinence. Because urinary incontinence is curable or treatable in many elderly women it is essential that specific questions be included in the periodic examination.

9. Osteoporosis (see also Chapter 33):

    a. Approximately 1.3 million osteoporosis-related fractures occur each year in the USA. Seventy percent of fractures in those 45 years or older are types related to osteoporosis.

    b. Osteoporosis is defined as a bone mineral density 1 to 2.5 standard deviations (SD) below the normal mean.[44] However, it is not necessary to obtain such measurements in order to initiate treatment (see Chapter 33).

    c. Dual energy X-ray absorptiometry (DEXA) is recognized as the safest, most accurate, and most precise modality for measuring bone density in the clinical setting and is the gold standard. If the patient already has evidence of vertebral fracture, the diagnosis of osteoporosis is present and treatment is indicated.

    d. Randomized trials show that estrogen and calcium supplementation are effective in preserving bone density in postmenopausal women.

    e. Benefits of hormonal prophylaxis on bone mass and fracture risk appear greatest when treatment is begun close to menopause (before period of

Table 4.11. Prevention, diagnosis and treatment of osteoporosis

Prevention is achieved by maintaining:
- Balanced, calcium-rich diet from adolescence onward
- Regular, weight-bearing exercise
- Stable estrogen levels
- Avoidance of tobacco, alcohol, certain medications
- Chemoprophylaxis (bisphosphonates – alendronate) if at risk

Diagnosis
- History and assessment of risk factors are the most important elements of diagnosis
- Clinical manifestations
  - Early: upper- or mid-thoracic back pain associated with activity, aggravated by long periods of sitting or standing, easily relieved by rest in the recumbent position
  - Late: common osteoporotic fracture sites: vertebrae, forearm, femoral neck, proximal humerus, dorsal kyphosis (dowager's hump)
  - Bone density screening: DEXA preferred, quantified computed tomography (much more expensive and greater radiation exposure), plain films (if positive, consistent with 50 percent bone loss)

Treatment
- All women should receive estrogen and calcium unless specifically contraindicated. Other therapies available include weight-bearing exercise, balanced nutrition, as well as consideration of the following:
  - Antiresorptive agents – estrogen, bisphosphonates, raloxifene, calcium, calcitonin
  - Bone forming agents – sodium fluoride
  - Miscellaneous – vitamin D metabolite (especially in those with limited sun exposure)

DEXA, dual energy X-ray absorptiometry.

rapid bone loss) and continued for longer periods (more than five years) (Table 4.10).[29]

    f. Prevention, diagnosis and screening methods are listed in Table 4.11.

10. Sensory impairment:

    a. Hearing loss: Hearing impairment occurs with increasing prevalence as patients age. Presbycusis is the most common cause, with approximately 33 percent of patients aged 65 years and older suffering objective hearing loss. Periodic questioning about potential hearing loss is a rapid and inexpensive screen for hearing impairment. Handheld devices (audioscopes) may be more sensitive but there is inconclusive evidence to support routine audiometry testing (USPSTF class B).[29]

    b. Vision loss: Visual impairment is a common problem among older patients, with potentially serious complications in general health and quality of life. Presbyopia, cataracts, age-related macular degeneration (ARMD) and glaucoma are the most common causes of visual impairment. Routine screening with Snellen acuity testing is recommended for older women (USPSTF class B).[29] Screening asymptomatic patients with ophthalmo-scopy by the primary care physician is a class C[29] recommendation. No specific frequency for screening is recommended.

11. Polypharmacy:

a. Polypharmacy is the rule rather than the exception for older patients. Multiple chronic illnesses, self-medication, and the physiopharmocologi-cal changes with aging can lead to adverse reactions and drug interactions that may go unrecognized in the older patient.

b. Incorporating a medication review into the periodic health examination and then again frequently in follow-up visits can help to avoid adverse drug reactions. Inquiring about all medications taken, including over-the-counter medications, vitamins, herbals and alternative/complementary therapies is helpful. Asking the patient to bring in the entire content of her medicine cabinet can be illuminating. Expired drugs, medications for illnesses no longer requiring treatment and prescriptions from multiple providers are frequently noted.

c. Encouraging the patient to use a pharmacy with database capability can help to reduce the likelihood of drug–drug interactions or adverse effects of multiple drug regimens. A good relationship between the physician and pharmacist can also be beneficial in avoiding adverse reactions or drug–drug interactions.

> The ratio of total to high density lipoprotein cholesterol appears to be the best predictor of coronary risk in older patients.

Chemoprophylaxis

Aspirin

Aspirin prophylaxis for stroke and myocardial infarction prevention has been well studied in men. There is as yet, inconclusive evidence to recommend for or against aspirin prophylaxis in older women. Individual patients may bene-fit from such intervention but potential risks (gastrointestinal bleeding or cerebral hemorrhage) must be weighed (USPSTF class C).[29]

Postmenopausal therapies

1. Osteoporosis prevention (see also Chapter 33):

a. HRT, alendronate, and raloxifene are all efficacious, but individual risk profiles determine which is best for a given patient.[45] HRT and weight-bearing exercise are the most important therapies for maintaining adequate bone density.

b. Conjugated equine estrogens in doses of 0.625 and 1.25 mg/day and transdermal estrogen (0.05 mg) are equally effective in reducing bone loss in postmenopausal and oophorectomized women.[46] Progesterone should be used in addition in women with intact uteri, and should be started at 2.5 mg daily. The dose can be increased to 10 mg daily to produce amenorrhea. The drugs can be given cyclically or continuously.

c. Calcium supplementation produces beneficial effects on bone mass throughout postmenopausal life and may reduce fracture rates by as much as 50 percent.[47]

d. Bisphosphonates (alendronate) are effective for preventing bone loss associated with estrogen deficiency, glucocorticoid treatment, and immobilization.[48]

2. Coronary artery disease prevention (see also Chapter 29):

a. There is a benefit for coronary artery disease prevention from HRT, given no contraindications.[45]

b. For women with at least one coronary artery disease risk factor, HRT should extend life expectancy, with some gains exceeding three years.

3. Alzheimer's disease prevention:

The impact of estrogen replacement therapy on cognitive functioning over time is unclear. Current and past users of HRT performed better on initial MMSE in one prospective cohort study, but not in randomized controlled trials.[49]

Conclusion

By attending to the differing risk factors of older women and following a systematic periodic evaluation (not necessarily at one visit), physicians can assist older women in maintaining their health and functional status. Secondary prevention issues can also be addressed and the appropriate preventive or therapeutic interventions highlighted.

REFERENCES

1. Desai MM, Hennessy CH. Surveillance for morbidity and mortality among older adults – United States, 1995–1996. *MMWR Morb Mortal Wkly Rep* 1999;**48**:7–25.

2. Speroff L. Preventive health care for older women. *Int J Fertil Menopausal Study* 1996;**41**:64–8.

3. Schulz R. Caregiving for children and adults with chronic conditions. *Health Psychol* 1998;**17**:107–11.

4. Ineichen B. Measuring the rising tide: How many dementia cases will there be by 2001? *Br J Psychiatry* 1987;**150**:193–200.

5. Andersen RE. Prevalence of significant knee pain among older Americans. *J Am Geriatr Soc* 1999;**47**:1435–8.

6. Casper M, Rith-Najarian S, Groft J, Giles W, Donehoo R. Blood pressure, diabetes and body mass index among Chippewa and Menominee Indians. *Public Health Rep* 1996;**111**:37–9.

7. Fontana SA, Helberg C, Love RR. The delivery of preventive services in primary care practices according to chronic disease status. *Am J Public Health* 1997;**87**:1190–6.

8. Faulkner LA, Schauffler HH. The effect of health insurance coverage on the appropriate use of recommended clinical preventive services. *Am J Prevent Med* 1997;**13**:453–8.

9. Schulman KA, Berlin JA, Harless W et al. The effect of race and sex on physicians' recommendations for cardiac catheterization. *N Engl J Med* 1999;**340**:618–26.

10. Caplan LS, Haynes SG. Breast cancer screening in older women. *Public Health Rev* (Israel) 1996;**24**:193–204.

11. Nosek MA, Howland CA. Breast and cervical cancer screening among women with physical disabilities. *Arch Phys Med Rehab* 1997;**27**:440–3.

12. Harmon MP. Acculturation and cervical cancer: Knowledge, beliefs, and behaviors of Hispanic women. *Women Health* 1996;**24**:37–57.

13. Matthew DA , McCullough ME, Larson DB et al. Religious commitment and health status: A review of the research and implications for family medicine. *Arch Fam Med* 1998;**7**:118–24.

14. Wooley DC. Geriatric psychiatry in primary care: A focus on ambulatory settings. *Getriatr Psychiatry* 1997;**20**:241–60.

15. Mamdani M, Herrmann N, Austin P. Prevalence of antidepressant use among older people: Population based observations. *J Am Geriatr Soc* 1999;**47**:1350–3.

16. Unutzer J, Patrick DL, Simon G et al. Depressive symptoms and the cost of health services in HMO patients age 65 and older: A 4 year prospective study. *JAMA* 1997;**277**:1618–23.

17. Midanik LT, Soghikian K, Ransom LJ, Tekawa IS. The effect of retirement on mental health and health behaviours. The Kaiser Permanente Retirement Study. *J Gerontol B Psychol Sci Soc Sci* 1995;**50**:S59–S61.

18. Brayne C, Spiegelhalter DJ, Dufouil C et al. Estimating the true extent of cognitive decline in the old. *J Am Geriatr Soc* 1999;**47**:1283–8.

19. South-Paul JE, Woodson CE. Optimal care of older women. *Postgrad Med* 1992;**91**:439–58.

20. Gallo JJ, Anderson L. *Handbook of Geriatric Assessment.* Aspen, Rockville, MD, 1988.

21. Koenig HG, Hays JC, Larson DB et al. Does religious attendance prolong survival? A 6 year follow-up study of 3968 older adults. *J Gerontol A Biol Sci Med Sci* 1999;**54**:370–6.

22. Krause N. Neighborhood deterioration, religious coping, and changes in health during late life. *Gerontologist* 1998;**38**:653–64.

23. Katz SFA, Moskowitz RW, Vignos PJ. Studies of illness in the aged. The index of ADL: A standardized measure of biological and psychological function. *JAMA* 1963;**185**:914–19.

24. Caspersen CJ, Christenson GM, Pollard RA. Status of the 1990 physical fitness and exercise objectives: Evidence from NHIS 1985. *Public Health Rep* 1985;**101**:587–92.

25. Okumiya K, Matsubayashi K, Wada T, Kimura S, Doi Y, Ozawa T. Effects of exercise on neurobehavioral function in community dwelling older people more than 75 years of age. *J*

Am Geriatr Soc 1996;**44**:569–72.

26. Taunton JE, Martin AD, Rhodes EC, Wolski LA, Donelly M, Elliot J. Exercise for the older woman, choosing the right prescription. *Br J Sports Med* 1997;**31**:5–10.

27. Kamimoto LA, Easton AN, Maurice E, Husten CG, Macera CA. Surveillance for five health risks among older adults – United States 1993–1997. *MMWR Morb Mortal Wkly Rep* 1999;**48**:89–130.

28. Bignotti DD, Evans JM, Fleming KC. *The Geriatric Patient*, 7th edn. ABFP Reference Guides. American Board of Family Practice, Lexington, KN, 1999.

29. US Preventive Services Task Force. *Guide to Clinical Preventive Services*, 2nd edn. Williams and Wilkins, Baltimore, MD, 1996.

30. Nichol KL, Margolis KL, Wuorenma J, Von Sternberg LV. The efficacy and cost effectiveness of vaccination against influenza among elderly persons living in the community. *N Engl J Med* 1994;**331**:778–84.

31. American College of Physicians. Immunizations. Guide for Adult Immunization. ACP, Philadelphia, 1994.

32. Balestra D, Littenberg B. Should adult tetanus immunization be given as a single vaccination at age 65? *J Gen Intern Med* 1993;**8**:405–12.

33. *The Sixth Report of the Joint National Committee on Prevention, Detection, Evaluation and Treatment of High Blood Pressure.* NIH publication no. 98-4080. National Institutes of Health, Bethesda, MD, 1997.

34. Kerlikowske K, Salzmann P, Phillips KA, Cauley JA, Cummings SR. Continued screening mammography in women aged 70 to 79 years. *JAMA* 1999;**282**:2156–63.

35. Zhang Y, Kiel DP, Kreger B et al. Bone mass and the risk of breast cancer among postmenopausal women. *N Engl J Med* 1997;**336**:611–17.

36. O'Malley MS. Screening for breast cancer with breast self-examination. *JAMA* 1987;**257**:2197–203.

37. Marwill SL, Barry PP. Patient factors associated with breast cancer screening among older women. *J Am Geriatr Soc* 1996;**44**:1210–14.

38. Mandel J, Bond JH, Church TR et al. Reducing mortality from colorectal cancers by screening for fecal occult blood. *New Engl J Med* 1993;**328**:1365–71.

39. Sheikh JI, Yesavage JA, Brooks JO III et al. Proposed factor structure of the Geriatric Depression Scale. *Int Psychogeriatr* 1991;**3**:23–8.

40. Hoyl MT, Alessi CA, Harker JO et al. Development and testing of a five item version of the Geriatric Depression Scale. *J Am Geriatr Soc* 1999;**47**:873–8.

41. Butler SM, Ashford JW, Snowdon DA. Age, education and changes in the Mini Mental Status exam scores of older women: Findings from the Nun Study. *J Am Geriatr Soc* 1996;**44**:675–81.

42. Kinosian B, Glick H, Garland G. Cholesterol and heart disease: Predicating risks by level and ratios. *Ann Intern Med* 1994;**121**:641–7.

43. Rosenthal M, Hunt WC, Garry PJ, Goodwin JS. Thyroid failure in the elderly: Microsomal antibodies as discriminant for therapy. *JAMA* 1987;**258**:209–13.

44. Kanis JA, Melton LJ III, Christiansen C et al. The diagnosis of osteoporosis. *J Bone Miner Res* 1994;**8**:1137–41.

45. Col NF, Pauker SG, Goldberg RJ et al. Individualizing therapy to prevent long-term consequences of estrogen deficiency in post-menopausal women. *Arch Intern Med* 1999;**59**:1458–66.

46. Lindsay R, Hart DM, Clark DM. The minimum effective dose of estrogen for prevention of

postmenopausal bone loss. *Obstet Gynecol* 1984;**63**:759–63.

47. Aloia JF, Vaswani A, Yeh JK et al. Calcium supplementation with and without hormone replacement therapy to prevent postmenopausal bone loss. *Ann Intern Med* 1994;**120**:97–103.

48. Watts NB. Treatment of osteoporosis with biphosphonates. *Endocrinol Metab Clin North Am* 1998;**27**:419–39.

49. Matthews K, Cauley J, Yaffe K, Zmuda JM. Estrogen replacement therapy and cognitive decline in older community women. *J Am Geriatr Soc* 1999;**47**:518–23.

Appendix 4.1. US Preventive Services Clinical Guidelines (ages 65 and over)

Leading causes of death

- Heart disease
- Cerebrovascular disease
- Obstructive lung disease
- Pneumonia/influenza
- Lung cancer
- Colorectal cancer

Screening	Counselling	Immunizations	High risk groups	
			Examinations	Counselling
History	Diet and exercise	Tetanus-	Auscultation for	Injury prevention
Prior	Fat (especially	diphtheria (Td)	carotid bruits	Prevention of falls
symptoms of	saturated fat),	booster	Complete skin	Safety belts
transient	cholesterol,	Influenza vaccine	examination	Smoke detector
ischemic attack	complex	Pneumococcal	Complete oral	Smoking near
Dietary intake	carbohydrates,	vaccine	cavity	bedding or
Physical	fiber, sodium,	Hepatitis B	examination	upholstery
activity	calcium	vaccine	Palpation of	Hot water heater
Tobacco/	Caloric balance		thyroid nodules	temperature
alcohol/drug	Selection of		Glaucoma testing	Discussion of
use	exercise		by eye specialist	estrogen
Functional	program		Tuberculin skin	replacement
status at home	Substance use		test (PPD)	therapy
Physical	Tobacco		Electrocardiogram	Discussion of aspirin
examination	cessation		Pap smear	therapy
Height and	Alcohol and		Fecal occult blood	Skin protection from
weight	other drugs		test	ultraviolet light
Blood pressure	Limiting		Sigmoidoscopy	Depression
Visual acuity	alcohol			symptoms
Hearing and	consumption			Suicide risk factors
hearing aids	Driving/other			Abnormal
Clinical breast	dangerous			bereavement
examination	activities while			Changes in cognitive
	under the			function
	influence			Medications that
				increase risk of
				falls
				Signs of physical
				abuse or neglect

5 Cigarette smoking and cessation

Jo Ann Rosenfeld, MD

Cigarette smoking is one of the most modifiable causes of death and disease. Helping smoking cessation is one of the most important messages and actions physicians can perform for their patients. Earlier in this century, women started smoking at older ages and in smaller numbers than men, but now numbers, percentages, years of smoking history, and complications of smoking in women are approaching those of men. In addition, fewer women may be quitting smoking, making the message more critical.

Epidemiology

1. Twenty-two million adult women in the USA are cigarette smokers and, although more men smoke, the difference in percentages is narrowing. In 1994, 28 percent of men and 23 percent of women considered themselves smokers in the USA.
2. Twenty-one to 23 percent of women smoked in a large prospective UK heart disease study of more than 12 000 individuals.[1]
3. Smoking contributes to 17 percent of all women's deaths and significantly to at least one-third of all cancer deaths in the USA[2] (as compared to 45 percent in men). Tobacco-related deaths in women will double in the next 30 years.[2] The cumulative risk of death from lung cancer by age 75 years in the UK in one large case-controlled study rose from 1 percent to 10 percent in female smokers from 1950 to 2000, as compared with a rise from 6 to 16 percent in male smokers.[3] In Denmark where 18 percent of women smoke heavily, the risk of tobacco-related deaths in women increased steadily, from fewer than 1% of all deaths in 1950 to 25 percent in 1990.[4]
4. Smoking rates are increasing in women, because of both increasing numbers and decreasing quitting rates in women.
5. Young women and men are smoking at increasingly early ages and women

have lower quit rates. This is concerning because 73 percent of teens who smoke become regular smokers.

6. Smoking rates differ by race, educational levels, and social groups. Poor and rural women and those who live in the southeast of the USA are more likely to smoke.

7. Although overall fewer women are quitting smoking, there has been a decline in smoking prevalence in a few specific groups – women aged 20 to 24 years, those women with fewer than 12 years' education, and among African-American women and high school seniors.

8. Cessation has almost halved the number of lung cancers.[3]

More women are smoking, fewer are quitting and up to one-third of all cancer deaths in women are related to smoking.

Effects of smoking

Smoking affects many organ systems deleteriously, including respiratory, cardiovascular and immune systems, causing complications for both women and men. Smoking affects the liver and the cytochrome P450 system in which both endogenous and exogenous estrogen (OCPs, HRT) and many other drugs are metabolized. Thus, smoking in itself has an antiestrogen effect (Table 5.1 and Figure 5.1).

Cardiovascular disease

Smoking is a risk factor for coronary artery disease, myocardial infarctions and cardiovascular-related deaths. In a five-year prospective study in three communities with more than 7000 elderly individuals, among women who smoked, the relative risk of cardiovascular mortality was greater than 1.8. Quitting reduced the rate to that of nonsmokers.[5] A metaanalysis of 19 studies found that even passive smoking increases the relative risk of ischemic heart disease to 1.3.[6]

Smoking is a risk factor for coronary artery disease, myocardial infarctions, and cardiovascular-related deaths.

Respiratory system

Cigarette smoking causes chronic obstructive pulmonary disease and lung cancer. In 1987, lung cancer surpassed breast cancer as the leading cause of cancer death in women. In one prospective mortality study in the 1980s,

Table 5.1. Strength of evidence that smoking affects risk of certain conditions

Complication	Increased risk	Proven by prospective study or RCT	Does stopping smoking reduce risk?	Comments
Lung cancer	Yes – Single cause of excessive death of smokers Fourfold increased risk in women who smoke	Prospective studies of large populations	Yes	
Osteoporotic fractures	Yes – 17 percent at age 60 yr Hip fractures: RR = 1.3 of all smokers; RR = 1.6 if smoke > 25 cigs./day	NHS – prospective	Yes, after 10 years	May be related to weight gain
Stroke	Yes – 2 × the risk of ischemic stroke and 4 × the risk of hemorrhagic stroke	NHS – prospective	Yes	
Breast cancer	Yes – Smokers of > 30 years have 2 × risk of breast cancer Breast cancer occurred at earlier age in smokers	Prospective in women with breast lumps or pain	Unknown	
Incontinence	Yes – 2 × risk	Retrospective case control	Unknown	
Fertility	Yes Half rate of fertilization in IVF program	Prospective noncontrolled small numbers	Unknown	
Coronary artery disease	Yes – 2 × the mortality in smokers	Prospective	Yes	

RCT, randomized controlled study; NHS, Nurses' Health Study; RR, relative risk; IVF, in vitro fertilization.

smoking caused 85 percent of excessive cancer deaths in women who smoked; over three-quarters of all the excessive death was caused by lung cancer.[7]

Stroke

Smoking and passive smoking increase the risk of ischemic stroke and the risk is dose related. The more cigarettes smoked, the higher is the risk of stroke. The Nurses' Health Study (NHS) found that a woman who smokes more than 40 cigarettes a day doubles her risk of stroke. Smoking cessation will decrease

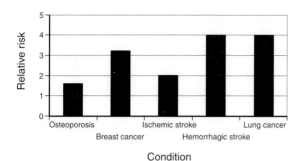

Figure 5.1.   The effect of smoking on other conditions – increase in relative risk of developing other conditions.

this risk; two years after quitting, the increased risk is gone.[8] Smokers also have an increased fourfold risk of hemorrhagic stroke.[9]

Bone

Cigarette smoking increases the risk of developing osteoporosis and the risk of OP fractures in some studies.

1. In the NHS, a 17 percent increase in risk of hip fractures was found for current smokers at age 60 years.
2. Also, there was a dose–response effect between smoking and hip fracture. Current smokers had a higher hip fracture rate than did women who never smoked and the risk increased with the numbers of cigarettes smoked daily (Figure 5.1).
3. Further, quitting smoking led to a decline in the increased risk, but not until 10 or more years following cessation. This may be partially explained by the weight gain accompanying smoking cessation.[10]
4. However, in the Framingham Study, this relationship was not found. In an evaluation of more than 2500 women, smoking was not related to an increase in the risk for hip fracture.[11]

Early menopause and decreased fertility

Through its antiestrogen effects, cigarette smoking may decrease fertility.

1. Within five years of trying to get pregnant, twice as many smokers as non-smokers fail to conceive after quitting smoking.[12]
2. In a small study of women younger than age 40 years in an in vitro fertilization

program, almost twice as many eggs from nonsmokers than from smokers successfully fertilized.[12]

3. On average, women smokers go through menopause one to three years earlier than nonsmokers.[13]

Breast cancer

The prevalence of breast cancer in smokers was approximately three times that of nonsmokers. In a British observational study of more than 3000 women who had a mammogram for a reason – lump or tenderness – at every age from 30 to 80 years, smokers had an increased risk of breast cancer.[14] If the woman smoked for more than 30 years, the breast cancer prevalence was 15 percent (as compared with 10 to 11 percent in all women) and the average age of presentation was eight years earlier than in women with breast cancer who did not smoke.

The prevalence of breast cancer in smokers was approximately three times that of nonsmokers.

Cervical cancer

Women who smoke, and even those exposed to passive smoking, have an increased incidence of cervical cancer and cancer precursors. This may be caused by the tobacco-induced changes in the immune system.

Incontinence

Women who smoke have a twofold greater risk of stress incontinence and detrusor instability, perhaps caused by increased incidence of cough.[15]

Smoking cessation

Quitting improves risks

Quitting smoking reduces many of the increased risks, especially of cardiovascular disease and stroke. The NHS found that former smokers had a 24 percent decrease in risk for cardiovascular disease within two years of quitting, and returned to nonsmoker mortality risk 10 to 14 years after quitting.[16] A prospective 10-year study found that even smoking cessation in the elderly reduces the relative risk of all causes of mortality by one-third.[17]

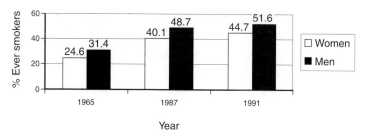

Figure 5.2.   Percentage of ever smokers who have quit smoking, by gender. (Data from Wetter DW, Kenford SL, Smith SS, et al. Gender differences in smoking cessation. *J Consult Clin Psychol* 1999;**67**:555–62.)

> Quitting smoking reduces many of the increased risks, especially of cardiovascular disease and stroke.

Differences in women quitting smoking

1. Rates: Smoking prevalence rates in women are declining slower than in men. However, until the 1990s, few studies had analyzed women's quitting rates and patterns (Figure 5.2).
    a. In the Framingham Study, men and women were equally likely to report quitting successfully for at least one year (42 versus 41 percent), after excluding men who switched to pipes or cigars. However, women who were heavy smokers (more than two packs per day) and older women were less likely to quit than all male smokers.
    b. In many studies, women are less likely to quit smoking successfully, and the causes of gender differences are not well known.[18]
2. Patterns: Men and women have similar rates of attempting to quit smoking (Figure 5.2),[12] but men abstain for longer periods.[18] Women and men have similar short-term patterns of quitting; similar percentages are able to quit for 1 or 30 days. However, in the long term more men than women were able to abstain.[12] Women who smoke heavily are the least likely to quit.
3. Reasons for differences:
    a. Some studies suggest that, in women, nicotine may enhance the feeling of satiety and block perceptions of muscle tension more than for men. Women may be more likely to rely on smoking as a coping aid and to regulate affect.
    b. Women may have a greater physical and emotional dependence on cigarettes as compared with men and measured by when they have their first cigarette, even when they smoke only a few cigarettes daily.[19]
    c. Women have different withdrawal symptoms. Women who have more withdrawal symptoms are more likely to relapse.[19]

d. Women were more likely to be concerned about weight gain after quitting. Eighty percent of smokers increase their weight when they stop smoking.[20] Especially in young women, this may be a major problem. Some women use smoking to control weight.[21]

e. Smokers' diets are different and less healthy and female smokers have different diets as compared with nonsmoking women. Heavy smokers eat less vegetables, carbohydrates, fiber, beta-carotene and fruit, and drink more alcohol and coffee. Women who are current smokers eat less cereals, vegetables, and iron. Over time as smokers quit, they increase their total carbohydrates and decrease alcohol, perhaps accounting for weight gain.[22]

f. In women, social isolation may be a greater factor for smoking or smoking may cause isolation in women. More women who smoke lack social support for quitting, particularly those who live with smokers. In a metaanalysis of 55 studies of social support and health, social support was positively related to smoking cessation and improved health in women.[23]

g. Men were more likely to relapse at work and then requit, whereas women relapsed at home or during negative emotional situations.

Women may be more likely to rely on smoking as a coping aid.

h. Living with smokers: Women were less likely than men to quit and to relapse once they quit if they lived with smokers.[13] Pregnant women who lived with smokers were only one-fifth as likely to quit smoking as other pregnant women who smoked.[24]

Women were less likely than men to quit and to relapse if they lived with smokers.

Smoking cessation advice

Although physicians feel they frequently offer smoking cessation advice, patients' perceptions are often different. In a primary care setting, most patients have been told only once or counselled for only brief periods. Only half of patients consider that smoking is a health problem. Although patients regard their primary care physician's advice highly, only 30 percent of smokers who have seen their physicians in the previous year recall the doctor giving antismoking advice.[25] Table 5.2 shows methods of incorporating smoking cessation into daily office practice.

Methods of quitting smoking

1. Counselling: Even small amounts of counselling in primary care situations

Table 5.2. Ways in which primary care physicians can help smoking cessation

- Create a smoke-free office
- Ask the following questions of patients at every opportunity:
  - Do you smoke?
  - How much?
  - How soon after awakening do you have your first cigarette?
  - Are you interested in stopping smoking?
  - Have you tried before? If so, what happened?
- Use self-administered questionnaire to assess patient's smoking behavior
- Use a sticker on the charts of smokers to remind them to talk about smoking cessation each visit
- Advise each patient, individually, to stop smoking
- Assist patients in stopping:
  - Help establish quit date
  - Offer educational materials
  - Consider prescription of nicotine gum and patches or antidepressants
  - Consider signing stop-smoking activity
  - Refer patient to cessation groups
- Ask patient if she has stopped each visit
- Close follow-up

From US Public Health Services. Smoking cessation in adults. *Am Fam Physician* 1995;**51**:1914–18.

does help individuals to quit. The time for counselling need not be longer than a regular visit. Older people and those more dependent on nicotine are more likely to quit with just physician counselling alone.

2. Behavioral modification: Women do better in programs using behavioral modification and individualized attention than they do in minimal contact programs using educational materials or psychotherapy.[13]

3. Exercise: Exercise can be used as an aid to quitting smoking. Using exercise has been shown to reduce stress and the fear of weight gain. In a RCT that only included women, those who exercised and quit did not gain weight during the exercise weeks, as compared with those who quit but did not exercise. However, when they stopped exercise, in the following 12 weeks, they did gain weight. Almost double the number of individuals in the exercise group were able to quit. However, only 15 percent of the control and 26 percent of the exercise group were abstinent at end of treatment and only 8 percent of the control group and 16 percent of the exercise group were still abstinent one-year post treatment.[26]

4. Gum: Nicotine gum is better than placebo in achieving smoking cessation.

5. Several studies have shown that nicotine gum use with a diet and behavioral

therapy works better than gum alone, especially in women.[27] A 16-week RCT of 247 motivated women who had quit smoking and started again, compared two groups, one who used gum, behavior control and diet, and a second group who used gum and behavioral therapy without a diet. After 16 weeks, 50 percent had stopped in diet group (weight dropped an average of 2.1 kg) as compared with only 35 percent in non-diet group (weight gained average 1.6 kg). After one year, abstinence rates were 28 percent in the diet group and 16 percent in the no-diet group.[28]

6. Transdermal nicotine patch: The transdermal patch enhances smoking cessation, and increases the six-month quit rates. In a RCT in which approximately 60 percent of control and treatment groups were women, 18 percent quit with nicotine patch use as compared with 10 percent of controls. Fourteen percent with patch use were still abstinent at one year as compared with 8.7 percent without.[29]

7. Special programs for women who quit smoking:
   a. External controls to help to quit smoking, such as no smoking areas and increased cost of cigarettes, are essential, but may not help women.
   b. Programs must be designed for women with special needs such as rural homemakers.
   c. Addressing special needs such as weight gain or spousal smoking must be included in programs for women.
   d. Marketing approaches that target women quitting are important. Tobacco control must become a woman's issue. Cigarette advertisements targeting women should be discouraged.

Exercise can be used as an aid to quitting smoking.

Pregnancy and smoking

1. Between 30 and 50 percent of pregnant women and 28 to 62 percent of pregnant adolescents smoke.[30] However, recent studies suggest that pregnant women were less likely to smoke in 1996 than in 1987, but the change reflected reduced smoking rates overall, rather than increased quitting rates.[31]

2. Smoking causes severe deleterious effects on pregnancy (Table 5.3). Women who smoke while being pregnant have a two times greater mortality ratio.[32]

3. Quitting smoking during pregnancy:
   a. Pregnant women who smoke must be counselled and urged to quit smoking as soon as possible.

Table 5.3. Deleterious effects of smoking on pregnancy

Increased risks of:
- Preterm labor
- Abruption
- Spontaneous abortion
- Previa
- Polyhydramnios
- Low Apgar scores
- Low weight in baby – increase of two times the incidence of low birth weight with number of cigarettes smoked during the third trimester[a]
- Prematurity
- Increased perinatal mortality
- Sudden infant death syndrome (SIDS)
- Otitis media in child

[a]From English PB, Eskenazi B, Christianson RE. Black–white differences in serum cotinine levels among pregnant women and subsequent effects on infant birthweight. *Am J Public Health* 1994;**84**:1439–42.

b. The effect of smoking on the risk of damage to the infant may be dose related. Women must be counselled to cut down, if they cannot quit.

c. Pregnant women who smoked were more likely to quit if they received their prenatal care from a private physician.[31]

d. Approximately 40 to 50 percent of pregnant women who smoke quit during pregnancy, and another third cut down. Older women, women planning to breast feed and/or those who were better educated were more likely to quit.[33] However, more than half who did quit, resumed smoking after the pregnancy, many increasing their daily cigarette consumption.[34]

Smoking and exogenous estrogen

OCPs

Women who use estrogen-containing OCPs, are older than 35 years and smoke have an increased risk of thrombosis (deep venous thromboses, strokes) and death. Smoking and being older than age 35 years is a contraindication for use of estrogen-containing OCPs.

Hormone replacement therapy

Smoking should be strongly discouraged in postmenopausal women, but smoking in itself is not a contraindication for use of HRT.

Conclusions

Cigarette smoking is a potent potentially modifiable risk factor for many diseases that cause death in women, including heart and lung disease and cancers. Women have been quitting smoking at lower rates than men and in different patterns, and different methods may be needed to help women give up the habit.

REFERENCES

1. Wood DA, Kinmonth AL, Davies GA et al. Randomised controlled trial evaluating cardiovascular screening and intervention in general practice: Principal results of British family heart study. *BMJ* 1994;**308**:313–20.

2. Shopland DR, Eyre HJ, Pechacek RF. Smoking attributable cancer mortality in 1991: Is lung cancer now the leading cause of death in smokers in the United States? *J Natl Cancer Inst* 1991;**83**:1142–8.

3. Peto R, Darby S, Deo H et al. Smoking, smoking cessation, and lung cancer in the UK since 1950: Combination of national statistics with two case-control studies. *BMJ* 2000;**321**:323–9.

4. Juel K. Increased mortality among Danish women: Population based register study. *BMJ* 2000;**321**:349–50.

5. LaCroix AZ, Lang J, Scherr P et al. Smoking and mortality among older men and women in three communities. *N Engl J Med* 1991;**324**:1619–25.

6. Law MR, Morris JK, Wald NJ. Environmental tobacco smoke exposure and ischaemic heart disease: An evaluation of the evidence. *BMJ* 1997;**315**:973–80.

7. Stellman SD, Garfinkel L. Proportions of cancer deaths attributable to cigarette smoking in women. *Women Health* 1989;**15**:19–28.

8. Colditz GA, Bonita R, Stampfer MJ et al. Cigarette smoking and risk of stroke in middle aged women. *N Engl J Med* 1988;**318**:937–41.

9. Terent A. Increasing incidence of stroke among Swedish women. *Stroke* 1988;**19**:598–603.

10. Cornuz J, Feskanick D, Willet WC, Colditz GA. Smoking, smoking cessation and the risk of hip fracture in women. *Am J Med* 1999;**106**:311–14.

11. Brand FN, Kiely DK, Kannel WB, Myers RH. Family patterns of coronary heart disease mortality: the Framingham Longevity Study. *J Clin Epidemiol* 1992;**45**:169–74.

12. Rosevear SK, Holt DW, Lee TD, Ford WC, Wardle PG, Hull MG. Smoking and decreased fertilisation rates in vitro. *Lancet* 1992;**340**:1195–6.

13. Gritz ER, Nielsen IR, Brooks LA. Smoking cessation and gender: The influence of physiological, psychological and behavior factors. *J Am Med Womens Assoc* 1996;**51**:35–42.

14. Bennicke K, Conrad C, Sabroe S, Sorensen HT. Cigarette smoking and breast cancer. *BMJ* 1995;**310**:1431–3.

15. Bump RC, McClish DK. Cigarette smoking and urinary incontinence in women. *Am J Obstet Gynecol* 1992;**167**:1213–18.

16. Kawachi I, Colditz GA, Stapfer MH et al. Smoking cessation in relation to total mortality rates in women. A prospective cohort study. *Ann Intern Med* 1993;**119**:992–1000.

17. Paganini-Hill A, Hsu G. Smoking and mortality among residents of a California retirement community. *Am J Public Health* 1994;**84**:992–5.

18. Wetter DW, Kenford SL, Smith SS et al. Gender differences in smoking cessation. *J Consult Clin Psychol* 1999;**67**:555–62.

19. Royce JM, Corbett K, Sorensen G, Ockene J. Gender social pressure and smoking cessation: The community intervention trial. *Soc Sci Med* 1997;**44**:359–70.

20. Pirie PL, Murray DM, Luepker RV. Gender differences in cigarette smoking and quitting in a cohort of young adults. *Am J Public Health* 1991;**81**:324–7.

21. Ward KD, Klesges RC, Zbikowski SM, Bliss RE, Garvey AJ. Gender differences in the outcome of an unaided smoking cessation attempt. *Addictive Behav* 1997;**22**:521–33.

22. Morabia A, Curtin F, Berstein MS. Effect of smoking and smoking cessation on dietary habits of a Swiss urban population. *Eur J Clin Nutr* 1999;**53**:239–43.

23. Schwarzer R, Leppin A. Social support and health: A meta-analysis. *Psychol Health* 1989;**3**:1–15.

24. Nafstad P, Botten G, Hagen JA. Partner's smoking: A major determinant for changes in women's smoking behaviour during and after pregnancy. *J Public Health* 1996;**110**:379–85.

25. Coleman T, Lakhani M, Wilson A. Managing smoking cessation. *BMJ* 1999;**318**:138–9.

26. Marcus BH, Albrecht AE, King TK et al. The efficacy of exercise as an aid for smoking cessation in women. *Arch Intern Med* 1999;**159**:1229–34.

27. Pirie PL, McBride CM, Hellerstedt W et al. Smoking cessation in women concerned about weight. *Am J Public Health* 1992;**82**:1238–43.

28. Danielsson T, Rossner S, Westin A. Open randomised trial of intermittent very low energy diet together with nicotine gum for stopping smoking in women who gained weight in previous attempt to quit. *BMJ* 1999;**319**:490–4.

29. Daughton D, Susman J, Sitorius M et al. Transdermal nicotine therapy and primary care. *Arch Fam Med* 1998;**7**:425–30.

30. Albrecht SA, Cornelius MD, Braxter B et al. An assessment of nicotine dependence among pregnant adolescents. *J Subst Abuse Treat* 1999;**16**:337–43.

31. Ebrahim SH. Trends in pregnancy related smoking rates in the United States, 1987–1996. *JAMA* 2000;**283**:361–6.

32. Rantakillio P, Laara E, Koiranen M. A 28 year followup of mortality among women who smoked during pregnancy. *BMJ* 1995;**311**:477–80.

33. Waldron I, Lye D. Employment, unemployment, occupation, and smoking. *Am J Prev Med* 1989;**5**:142–9.

34. Christmas JT, Knisely JS, Dawson KS, Dinsmoor MJ, Weber SE, Schnoll SH. Comparison of questionnaire screening and urine toxicology for detection of pregnancy complicated by substance use. *Obstet Gynecol* 1992;**80**:750–4.

6 Nutrition

Jo Ann Rosenfeld, MD

Good nutrition is essential for healthy living. Eating wisely can be primary prevention for many diseases and it is a part of the treatment for many medical disorders from heart disease to hypertension.

Introduction

1. Nutrition is basic and important. Yet, seldom do discussions about nutrition take place in physicians' offices. The physician should be ready to counsel the patient about her diet. If the physician is uncomfortable, consultation with nutritionists can be obtained.

2. Research: Much of the data on nutrition and nutritional therapy (supplementation or elimination) has been anecdotal. Recording accurate diet records is difficult and observing results from nutritional therapy may take years or decades. The best data are from large surveys such as the Nurses' Health Study (NHS) or the National Health and Nutrition Examination Survey (NHANES), but these relationships are often merely correlations and causation is difficult to determine precisely.

3. Nutrition as therapy: Many medical conditions require the use of specialized diet or diet therapy. Obesity, anorexia, diabetes, hypertension, hyperlipidemia, kidney stones, gout, and other diseases need specialized nutritional counselling. Women who have chronic obstructive pulmonary disease (COPD) or cancer have increased calorie requirements. Vegetarian women may need advice about maintaining a well-rounded diet.

4. Obesity: Obesity is epidemic in the USA. Approximately 35 percent of women and 25 percent of children and adolescents are obese.[1] Health risks and mortality increase as body mass index increase, including a higher risk of hypertension, dyslipidemias, diabetes mellitus, and CHD mortality.

5. Obesity is difficult to treat. Those individuals who finish weight loss programs lose an average of 10 percent of body weight. Two-thirds of these regain the

Table 6.1. Risk factors for nutritional problems for women

- Demographic values
  - Adolescent
  - Elderly
  - Pregnant
- Social
  - Poverty
- Habits
  - Cigarette smoking
  - Substance abuse
  - Frequent dieting
  - Frequent missing meals
  - Living away from home
- Dietary habits
  - Vegan
- Medical problems
  - Mental retardation
  - Chronic obstructive pulmonary disease
  - Pica
  - Chronic medical illness
  - Depression or chronic psychiatric illness
  - Use of medications including phenytoin
  - Mental retardation
  - Cancer
  - Problems with swallowing or chewing – dentition problems
  - Stroke
  - Dementia
- Gynecological factors
  - High parity
  - Menorrhagia

weight within one year, and almost all regain it within five years.[1]

6. Undernutrition or malnutrition is rare, but more prevalent in low income women in their childbearing years who may have diets deficient in protein, vitamins A and C, iron, calcium and folic acid. Approximately 6 percent of African-American women and 5 percent of non-Hispanic whites had iron deficiency.[2]

7. Women at high risk for nutritional problems are listed in Table 6.1. Women with these risk factors may need nutritional counselling or consultation.

Obesity is epidemic in the USA.

Table 6.2. The American Cancer Society 1996 nutrition guidelines for prevention of cancer

- Choose most food from plant sources
- Eat five or more servings of fruits and vegetables daily – fruits or vegetables in every meal and for snacks
- Include breads, cereals, grains, rice, pasta and beans several times a day
- Limit intake of high fat foods
- Choose foods low in fat and limit consumption of meats, especially high fat meats
- Be physically active
- Maintain a healthy weight
- Limit consumption of alcohol
- Artificial sweeteners do not increase the risk of cancer

Data from American Cancer Society 1996 Advisory Committee on diet, nutrition and cancer prevention. Guidelines on diet, nutrition and cancer prevention: Reducing the risk of cancer with healthy food choices and physical activity. *CA Cancer J Clin* 1996;**46**:325–41.

Basic diet

1. A healthy diet for all women and men should be a low fat, moderate salt intake diet.
2. Basic suggestions include maintaining a good weight, eating a variety of foods, eating a low fat, low saturated fat diet, eating five or more servings of vegetables and fruits daily, and moderating use of sugars, salt, and alcoholic beverages.
3. The recommended diet for adult women who are not pregnant, lactating, or trying to gain or lose weight is 1200 to 1500 calories (1 kcal $\approx$ 4 kJ) daily, with less than 30 percent of the calories from fat. Salt intake should be approximately 3 to 4 g daily, with 1000 mg of calcium daily for premenopausal and 1500 mg of calcium daily for adolescents and postmenopausal women.
4. The American Cancer Society has published guidelines for the importance of nutrition in cancer prevention (Table 6.2).[3]

The recommended diet for adult women who are not pregnant, lactating, or trying to gain or lose weight is 1200 to 1500 calories daily, with less than 30 percent of the calories from fat.

Basic diet for special groups

Adolescents

1. Adolescents need more calories and have a higher calcium requirement of 1500 mg daily.

2. Adolescents often eat a less healthy diet because of peer pressure, easy availability of fast food, pressure to be thin, and lifestyles that include few regular mealtimes and sitting down to eat.
3. African-American adolescents are at a higher risk of eating poorly.
4. Anorexia and bulimia (see Chapter 28) are also significant dietary problems for adolescents in whom psychological therapy is essential.

> Because of social factors, peer pressure, pressure to remain thin and chaotic lifestyles, adolescents are a high risk for nutritional and eating disorders.

Pregnancy and lactation (see Chapter 13)

Elderly:

1. Elderly individuals, especially those who live alone, may have mechanical, social, physical or psychological problems maintaining a good diet and adequate nutrition. Inability to get to a market, inadequate resources to buy a balanced diet, difficulty shopping, difficulty cooking, fear of lighting a stove, difficulty opening jars or cans, and isolation, all contribute to poor nutrition in the elderly.
2. Asking questions such as "Who helps you shop?" and "How often do you cook yourself a hot dinner?" may reveal such problems.
3. Overcoming these difficulties may include "Meals-on-Wheels," using flip-top cans, helping organize services for obtaining groceries or preparing foods together. Using a microwave has helped many elderly remain in good health and on their own.

> Elderly individuals, especially those who live alone, may have mechanical, social, physical or psychological problems maintaining a good diet and adequate nutrition.

Diet as therapy (Table 6.3)

Vegetarianism

1. A prospective study of more than 6000 vegetarians and 5000 control women and men followed for more than five years in the UK showed that vegans had lower cholesterol levels and lower total death rates (RR = 0.8) and mortality rates for death by heart disease (RR = 0.72) and cancer (RR = 0.61), after adjusting for smoking, body mass index (BMI) and social class. This reduction in risk was more significant for women.[4]

Table 6.3. Effect of diet on risk of disease and death

Risk factor	Diet				
	Low fat	Low salt	Vegan	Vitamins	Fruits/Vegs.
Total death rates			Lowers		
CV mortality		Lowers	Lowers		
CV disease	Lowers	Lowers		E lowers	
Hypertension		Lowers			
Cholesterol	Lowers		Lowers		
Menstrual disorders			Lowers	B6 or B12 affects	
Lung cancer					Lowers
Colon cancer	High fat increases risk				Lowers
Breast cancer	High fat increases risk				
Endometrial cancer	High fat increases risk				

CV, cardiovascular.

2. Vegans also had a 50 percent reduced risk of needing an emergency appendectomy, and a higher risk of iodine deficiency.[4]
3. Although cross-sectional surveys suggest vegetarian women have more menstrual disturbances, a prospective study found that, when controlled for weight, vegetarian women had fewer menstrual disturbances, if their weight was stable.[5] Vegetarian women may have a lower BMI.

Diabetes

Diet is an important part of diabetes therapy (see Chapter 30).

Hypertension

1. Dietary modifications have a definite and important place in the therapy of hypertension. A low salt, low cholesterol diet can improve blood pressure and decrease cardiovascular morbidity and mortality.
2. Weight loss is important and evidence exists that a loss of 5 to 10 kg, or 10 percent of weight, may allow for sufficient improvement in blood pressure levels to allow for withdrawal of antihypertensive medications. A weight loss of more than 10 kg will reduce the individual's risk of hypertension by 26 percent.[6]

3. Sodium reduction will also help and the reduction in sodium intake does not have be considerable. Moderating sodium intake by not adding salt and moderating use of processed and salty foods can reduce salt intake from 15 g to 5 to 7 g daily. In one placebo-controlled RCT, changing regular salt to low sodium, high potassium, high magnesium mineral salt reduced systolic blood pressure (SBP) by an average of 7.6 mmHg and diastolic blood pressure by (DBP) an average of 3.3 mmHg in 100 men and women aged 55 to 75 years.[6]

Heart disease

1. A low cholesterol, low saturated fat diet reduces the risk of CHD.
2. Vitamin E: The NHS found a small but reduced risk of CHD in women who used vitamin E supplements (see Chapter 29).[7] Four hundred to 800 IU daily is the suggested preventive dose needed to prevent low density lipoprotein (LDL) cholesterol oxidation.[8]
3. Homocysteine: Women who have elevated levels of homocysteine (>15 mmol/L) have an increased risk of heart and thromboembolic disease.[9] Women who supplemented their diet with folic acid, vitamins B6 and B12 had reduced levels of homocysteine and an observational study suggests that such supplementation may help cardiovascular disease prevention (see Chapter 29).[10]
4. Nut intake: Two studies – the Seventh Day Adventist[11] and the Iowa Women's Health Study[12] – suggest that increased intake of nuts is related to a reduction in risk of developing CHD and mortality from ischemic heart disease.

A low cholesterol low saturated fat diet reduces the risk of coronary heart disease.

Cancer

1. Lung cancer: Individuals who have a greater intake of fruits and vegetables have a lower risk of lung cancer.[3] Eating foods rich in beta-carotene may protect against lung cancer, although trials of supplementation have shown that male smokers taking beta-carotene supplements have higher rates for lung cancer.[13]
2. Obesity has been reported to increase the risk of colon cancer.[14] While vegetable consumption is considered to be protective against colon cancer, very recent epidemiologic data showed that while Japanese vegetable consumption stayed the same, an increase in cereals intake paralleled the decline in colon cancer.[15]

3. In the NHS, a twofold higher risk of colon cancer was seen in women who consumed the highest quartile of animal fat.[16]

Increased consumption of fruits and vegetables has been associated with reduction in risk of colon cancer.

Breast disease

1. Fibrocystic breast disease: Anecdotal and observational evidence suggest that diet therapy, in the form of elimination diets may help fibrocystic breast disease. Case-controlled studies of the elimination of caffeine, chocolate, cigarette smoking and alcohol, and the addition of extra vitamins A and E to treat fibrocystic disease have failed to show decreased nodularity or pain.[17,18]
2. Breast cancer: The relationship between high fat intake and body fat and the risk of breast cancer remains disputed.[19] Before menopause, women who are obese may have a reduced risk of breast cancer.[20]

Osteoporosis: For dietary calcium needs, see Chapter 29.

Menstrual disorders

1. Dysmenorrhea: A variety of diet therapies has been suggested. A double blind crossover study of 42 adolescent women who took additional omega-3 poly-unsaturated fats found some relief of dysmenorrhea with treatment.[21] Oral B1 (thiamine) 100 mg daily has also been suggested for treatment of dysmenorrhea.
2. Chronic pelvic pain: Without RCT proof, a high bulk low fat diet has been suggested to improve the symptoms of chronic pelvic pain.
3. Premenstrual syndrome (PMS): Suggested treatments include exercise and changes in diet – caffeine restriction, carbohydrate consumption, and decreased alcohol. A metaanalysis of the use of vitamin B6 (pyridoxine 100 mg daily) that combined 9 studies and 940 patients found that use of pyridoxine improved depressive symptoms (RR = 1.69) and improved PMS symptoms (RR = 2.32).[22] Some small crossover RCTs suggest that a low fat vegetarian diet may reduce premenstrual symptoms.[23]
4. Endometrial cancer: High fat diets and being obese have been associated with an increased risk of endometrial cancer.[24]

Use of vitamin B6 (pyridoxine 100 mg daily) improved depressive and other symptoms in women with premenstrual syndrome.

Conclusion

A healthy diet can be preventive and therapeutic. A low fat moderate salt diet with increased calcium diet should help most women.

REFERENCES

1. Stern JS, Hirsch J, Blair SN. Weighing the Options: Criteria for Evaluating Weight Management programs. *Obesity Res* 1995;**3**:591–605.
2. Nutrition and women. *Int J Gynecol Obstet* 1997;**56**:71–81.
3. The American Cancer Society 1996 Advisory Committee on diet, nutrition and cancer prevention. Guidelines on diet, nutrition and cancer prevention: Reducing the risk of cancer with healthy food choices and physical activity. *CA Cancer J Clin* 1996;**46**:325–41.
4. Appleby PN, Thorogood M, Mann JI, Key TJA. The Oxford vegetarian Study: An overview. *Am J Clin Nutr* 1999;**70S**:525S–531S.
5. Barr SI. Vegetarians and menstrual cycle disturbances: Is there an association? *Am J Clin Nutr* 1999;**70S**:549S–554S.
6. Geleijnse JM, Wetteeman JC, Bak AA Breijen JH, Grobee DE. Reduction in blood pressure with a low sodium, high potassium, high magnesium salt in older subjects with mild to moderate hypertension. *BMJ* 1994;**309**:436–40.
7. Stampfer MJ, Hennekens CH, Manson JE et al. Vitamin E consumption and the risk of coronary disease in women. *N Engl J Med* 1993;**328**:1444–9.
8. Faggiotto A, Poli A, Catapano AL. Antioxidants and coronary artery disease. *Curr Opin Lipidol* 1998;**9**:541–9.
9. Boushey CJ, Beresford SAA, Omenn GS, Motulsky AG. A quantitative assessment of plasma homocysteine as a risk factor for vascular disease: Probable benefits of increasing folic acid intakes. *JAMA* 1995;**274**:1049–57.
10. Rimm EB, Willett WC, Hu FB. Folate and vitamin B6 from diet and supplements in relation to risk of coronary heart disease in women. *JAMA* 1998;**297**:359–64.
11. Fraser GE, Sabate J, Beeson WL, Strahan TM. A possible protective effect of nut consumption on risk of coronary heart disease: The Adventist Health Study. *Arch Intern Med* 1992;**152**:1416–24.
12. Kushi LH, Folsom AR, Prineas RJ et al. Dietary antioxidant vitamins and death from coronary heart disease in postmenopausal women. *N Engl J Med* 1996;**334**:1156–62.
13. The Alpha Tocopherol Beta-carotene Cancer Prevention Study Group. The effect of vitamin E and beta-carotene on the incidence of lung cancer and other cancers in male smokers. *N Engl J Med* 1994;**330**:1029–35.
14. Murphy TK, Calle EE, Rodriguez C, Khan HS, Thun MJ. Body mass index and colon cancer mortality in a large prospective study. *Am J Epidemiol* 2000;**152**:847–54.
15. Kono S, Ahn YO. Vegetables, cereals and colon cancer mortality: Long-term trend in Japan. *Eur J Cancer Prev* 2000;**9**:363–5.
16. Willett WC, Stampfer MJ, Colditz GA et al. Relation of meat, fish and fiber intake to the risk of colon cancer in a prospective study among women. *N Engl J Med* 1990;**323**:1664–72.

17. Lubin F, Ron E, Wax Y et al. A case control study of caffeine and methyl xanthines in benign breast disease. *JAMA* 1985;**253**:2388–92.

18. Marchant DJ. Controversies in benign breast disease. *Surg Oncol Clin North Amer* 1998;**7**:285–98.

19. Willett WC. Goals for nutrition in the year 2000. *CA Cancer J Clin* 1999;**49**:331–52.

20. Tretli S. Height and weight in relation to breast cancer morbidity and mortality: A prospective study of 570,000 women in Norway. *Int J Cancer* 1989;**44**:23–30.

21. Harel Z, Biro FM, Kottehahn RK, Rosenthal S. Supplementation with omega-3 polyunsaturated fatty acids in the management of dysmenorrhea in adolescents. *Am J Obstet Gynecol* 1996;**174**:1335–8.

22. Wyatt KM, Dimmock PW, Jones PW, Shaugh O'Brien PM. Efficacy of vitamin B-6 in the treatment of premenstrual syndrome: Systematic review. *BMJ* 1999;**18:**1375–81.

23. Barnard ND, Scialli AR, Hurlock D, Bertron P. Diet and sex-hormone binding globulin, dysmenorrhea, and premenstrual symptoms. *Obstet Gynecol* 2000;**95**:245–50.

24. Hill HA, Austin H. Nutrition and endometrial cancer. *Cancer Causes Control* 1996;**7**:19–32.

7 Exercise

Rebecca Jaffe, MD

The health benefits of exercise are well established.[1,2] Mortality rates decrease as physical activity increases. Active people often outlive inactive people even when they begin exercise later in life.

Introduction

1. A consensus statement about the amount of exercise necessary to confer health benefits was published in *Physical Activity and Health: A Report of the Surgeon General.*[3] The consensus states that children and adults should perform at least 30 minutes of moderate intensity activity almost daily. The activity can be divided into three or fewer parts.
2. The studies currently published are flawed in their abilities to accurately assess the physical activity of women.[4] Nonetheless, regular sustained exercise is essential and the benefits far outweigh any risks. Many of the larger studies have been done on a predominantly male population; however, those studies including women tend to show comparable results on health.[5]

Children and adults should perform at least 30 minutes of moderate intensity activity almost daily.

The benefitsof exercise

Physiological
1. There are many benefits to regular exercise. The immediate physiological effects include stimulation of catecholamine, lowering in blood glucose levels, and improved sleep, both in quality and quantity.
2. Best reported benefits are the cardiovascular effects of exercise. Many retrospective studies have demonstrated the decrease in the risk and rate of heart

disease for exercising individuals. One of the largest studies to demonstrate the benefit of moderate as well as vigorous exercise is the Iowa Women's Health Study.[6] Even nonstrenuous activity and walking have demonstrated reduction in risk for myocardial infarction (MI).

3. Improved serum lipid levels are seen in individuals who exercise regularly. These include a reduction in serum triglyceride levels, elevations in HDL cholesterol and a decrease in LDL cholesterol. The HDL benefits can begin with exercise less than necessary for physical fitness and improve with increases in activity levels.[7]

4. There are beneficial effects of regular physical activity on the lowering of blood pressure. Moderate exercise improves both the resting systolic and diastolic pressures. The higher the intensity of regular physical activity, the lower the blood pressure readings. Exercise seems to be an effective nonpharmacological treatment for mild to moderate hypertension.

5. There is a direct correlation between weight and mortality in middle-aged women.[8]

6. Studies that have examined the relationship between the risk of certain cancers and physical activity found an increased risk of endometrial cancers and other cancers among the least active women.[9]

   a. However, there is one study of ovarian cancer in which the opposite was found. In this study, the women with more vigorous activity had a higher risk of ovarian cancer.[10]

   b. More active women are at a relative decreased risk of breast cancer.[11] Higher levels of activity may decrease the woman's exposure to estrogen and progesterone.

   c. Similarly, there are numerous studies to support the finding that regular physical activity can decrease a woman's risk of colon cancer and possibly adenomas.[12]

Improved serum lipid levels are seen in individuals who exercise regularly.

Treatment

1. Obesity: Exercise is the only nonpharmacological method of effective weight control and prevention of obesity. This energy expenditure not only increases calorie consumption it also can suppress appetite. This benefit allows for the best success toward weight loss. Engaging in regular exercise helps to ensure continued success at maintaining weight loss rather than the up and down effect of fad dieting.

Exercise treats obesity and suppresses the appetite.

2. Glucose intolerance: Physical activity, even when no observed weight loss is noted, is associated with improvement in glucose tolerance and insulin sensitivity.[13] There appears to be a direct effect as well as the effect of decreased intraabdominal fat.

3. Diabetes: Patients with both type I and type II diabetes mellitus will benefit from regular exercise, with resulting improvement in glycemic control. Prevention of type II diabetes may be possible with exercise; however, more data are needed to quantify and qualify the optimal regime. The actual effect on type I diabetes probably comes from improvement in the cardiovascular risk profile (better blood pressure, higher HDL).[14]

4. Osteoporosis: Improved bone health is seen among women who exercise. There are many factors that influence the incidence of osteoporosis. Genes, diet, hormones and the environment all play an important role. Physical activity is one of the environmental factors that can influence peak bone mass and maintenance of current bone density.[15] Weight-bearing exercise that specifically stimulates bone growth is vital to bone health. The Surgeon General's report on physical activity concludes that weight-bearing exercises such as walking, jogging, tennis, rowing, aerobic and strength training are essential for normal skeletal development during childhood and adolescence and for achieving and maintaining peak bone mass in young adults.

Improved bone health, glucose control and perhaps even prevention of type II diabetes mellitus may occur with exercise.

5. Osteoarthritis: Even women with osteoarthritis benefit from regular physical activity.[16] There is improvement in their symptoms of pain and improvement in balance and coordination, which helps to prevent falls. The development and maintenance of muscular strength, endurance and joint flexibility aid in the overall bone health seen in active women.

6. Alcoholism: Possibly of anecdotal importance is the higher rate of abstinence in alcoholics who continue to exercise regularly at a moderate level of activity.

7. Gall bladder disease: Some studies report a decreased risk of cholecystectomy in regularly exercising women.[17]

Weight-bearing exercises such as walking, jogging, tennis, rowing, aerobic and strength training are essential for normal skeletal development.

Psychological

1. Exercise also provides psychological benefit. Very immediate benefits include improvement in ability to relax, reduced stress and anxiety and enhanced mood.
2. Long-term psychological benefit provides the exercising individual with a general feeling of well-being. These exercisers appear to have a higher self-esteem.[18]
3. Women who suffer from premenstrual syndrome report improvements of their symptoms with regular moderate aerobic exercise.
4. The improved mental health includes sometimes significant improvements in depression and anxiety neurosis symptoms as demonstrated by objective inventory evaluations.
5. Cognitive improvements postpone the age-related declines in central nervous system speed and reaction time. Motor control and performance allows for the acquisition of new skills no matter what the age of initiation of regular activity.

> Exercise provides a long-term feeling of well-being in the participants.

Social benefits

1. Regular physical activity provides for immediate social benefits. The dedication to the consistent exercise is empowering to individuals. This allows for greater independence and self-sufficiency in women who participate. There is also enhanced social and cultural integration; these women interact more with the people around them. This is of both short-term and long-term benefit.
2. For the long term, women who exercise withdraw less from society. The ability to form new friendships and widened social and cultural networks is yet another positive attribute. There is the acquisition of new roles and the ability to maintain current roles. And lastly there is enhanced intergenerational activity seen in communities where regular exercise exists.

Studies of current inactivity

1. In 1988, the CDC stated that 59 percent of American women led a sedentary lifestyle. In a survey five years later, only 24.8 percent of female high school

students exercised for 20 minutes at least three times the two weeks before the survey.

2. Patients reported that they are more likely to engage in healthy behaviors when their physician makes a specific recommendation. In a 1990 survey, fewer than 20 percent of health care providers discussed regular exercise with their patients; a newer survey in 1998 saw that percentage increase to 49 percent of the physicians discussing the importance of exercise with their patients.[19]

3. In the USA 36.4 percent of women have a BMI of $\geqslant 27\,kg/m^2$ and 16.2 percent have BMIs $\geqslant 30$. In addition, 26 percent of American children are overweight and 10 percent severely obese. Exercise could help to address this tragedy.

Revised exercise recommendations

1. In 1994, the CDC and ACSM (American College of Sports Medicine – a membership organization of health researchers and providers) collaborated on a recommendation for exercise. They stated that every adult should do 30 or more minutes of moderate intensity physical activity spread over the course of the day during most days of the week.

2. ACSM revised this general statement in 1998 to be more specific.[20] They addressed cardiorespiratory fitness and weight control, muscular strength and flexibility. For cardiovascular activities, the recommendation states that the activity should be three to five days a week for 20 to 60 minutes at an intensity that achieves 55 to 90 percent of maximum heart rate. Multiple short spurts through the day rather than all at one time can achieve this minimal goal.

3. There are studies to indicate that three 10-minute bouts of physical activity are almost as effective as a continuous 30-minute routine.[21]

4. For muscular strength, the recommendation was that resistance training be done, to include one set of 10 exercises that work the major muscle groups; this should be done two or three days a week.

5. Flexibility training should be stretching to include ballistics, static and proprioceptive neuromuscular facilitation. This should be done two to three days a week, with at least four repetitions per major muscle group.

For cardiovascular fitness, exercise that is performed three to five days a week for 20 to 60 minutes at an intensity that achieves 55 to 90 percent of maximum heart rate should be accomplished.

Table 7.1. Activities that use 3 to 6 METs

- Walking briskly, 5 to 6 km/hour (3–4 miles per hour)
- Cycling for pleasure, more than 16 km/hour (10 miles per hour)
- Swimming, moderately
- Racquet sports
- Golf, carrying clubs
- General calisthenics
- Fishing, standing
- Mowing lawn, general house cleaning
- Stair climbing

MET, metabolic equivalent.

Definition of moderate physical activity

When exercise physiologists speak about moderate physical activity, they speak of exercise that consumes 3 to 6 metabolic equivalents (METs) (Table 7.1). One MET is the amount of oxygen that is consumed by the body at rest. METs are multiples of the resting metabolic rate. In the average person, 1 MET burns 1 kcal per minute (1 kcal ≈ 4 kJ).

Barriers to exercise

Barriers

When individuals are interviewed as to why they do not exercise on a regular basis, four reasons are consistently reported. These include lack of time, embarrassment at taking part in physical activity, an inability to exercise vigorously and a lack of enjoyment in exercising.

Readiness for exercise

Discussing exercise with an individual is similar to discussing any behavior change from quitting smoking to losing weight. Individuals are in one of five stages of change.

1. The first is the *precontemplation phase* where the person is clearly not interested in exercise. These individuals need to be educated about the risks and benefits of regular physical activity.
2. Next is the *contemplation phase* where the individual is considering a program. Here, there needs to be emphasis on the positive impacts of exercise.
3. In the *preparation phase*, the woman is ready to initially commit to exercise.

Table 7.2. Medical history needed before exercising

- Evaluation of cardiac risk
  - Patient age
  - Family history of cardiac problems including sudden death before the age of 50 years
  - Hypertension
  - Poor lipid profiles
  - Smoking
  - Diabetes
  - Obesity
  - Sedentary lifestyle
  - Cardiac symptoms, and other previous significant history
- Orthopedic status including
  - Any previous injuries and/or surgeries
  - Chronic problems involving any specific joints
- A personal history of exercise would include previous successful and unsuccessful programs, as well as information regarding pain or urine leakage with exercise
- Medications including beta-blockers and calcium channel blockers
- Previous weight management attempts
- Weight fluctuations including childbearing history

These women need to be encouraged and reinforcement of the benefit which will enrich their lives needs to be reiterated.

4. When the individual is in the *action phase,* they have already begun a program and they should be commended regularly.
5. Finally, those in the *maintenance phase* are currently already physically active and should be encouraged to continue for the rest of their lives.

Initial assessment before a program

Most adults do not need to see a physician before embarking on an exercise program. The ACSM recommends that women older than age 50 years who plan a vigorous program (more than 6 METs) or who have any chronic disease should consult a physician before commencement of their program.[22]

Most adults do not need to see a physician before embarking on an exercise program.

History

Individuals who choose to embark upon a rigorous exercise program should have a medical screening (Table 7.2).

Receptivity

Patient considerations need to be addressed, such as long- and short-term goals. Exercising preferences and access can be assessed by questions such as "What sounds appealing?", "What is available to you both physically and conveniently?", "What is affordable?", "Do you own any home exercise equipment?", "Is there access to exercise, either equipment or classes in the community?".

Fitness evaluation

1. A fitness evaluation would include checking both blood pressure and pulse.[23] Body composition can be assessed via body fat analysis. This could include hydrostatic weighing, bioelectrical impedance or caliper measurements. BMI or circumference measurements can be used in place of body fat analysis if necessary.

2. Flexibility can be tested by sit and reach, trunk extension and various range-of-motion tests. Tight muscle groups that are identified can be addressed with a stretching program. This gives an opportunity to introduce proper stretching technique, where one can feel the stretch, but no pain is experienced. Emphasis is made on constant hold for 20 to 30 seconds, with *no* ballistics. The best time to do stretching is after exercise when muscle blood flow is best.

3. Cardiovascular endurance should be evaluated with a maximal stress test if the woman is over age 50 years and has any one risk factor. These major risk factors include cigarette smoking, hypertension (blood pressure $> 160/90$), serum cholesterol over 239 mg/dL, diabetes, family history of cardiac disease before age 65 years, and known pulmonary, cardiac or metabolic disease. If an individual is not at risk, then a submaximal stress test may be considered. This does not require a physician and can be done by a trained professional in the health club or office setting. A bicycle, treadmill or step can be employed and blood pressure and pulse are monitored through stages of the test and during recovery. Perceived exertion ratings are also monitored.

4. Muscular strength and endurance are more difficult to assess. There is no one good test that applies. Measuring the strength of each specific muscle would be difficult to do. A one-repetition maximum is done on some major muscle groups. This is the weight that an individual can lift only one time. There are standardized muscle endurance tests which involve abdominal curls, push ups, flexed arm hang, bench and leg press over a specified time span. Age-related norms give one an idea of ability.[23]

Table 7.3. Sample exercise prescription

- *Goal:* Cardiovascular condition, increase energy
- Mode: Aerobic activities including swimming, jogging, cycling, stairstep, rowing, aerobic class, walking, hiking, or dance
- Frequency: 3 to 4 times per week
- Duration: 15 to 60 minutes (does not include warm up and cool down)
- Intensity: 55 to 90 percent of maximal heart rate or rate of perceived exertion of 13 to 17 METs

- *Goal:* increase strength, muscular endurance, change body shape
- Mode: weight training (free weights, Universal, Cybex, bands)
- Frequency: 2 to 3 times per week or every other day
- Duration: 8 to 12 repetitions, 1 to 3 sets (fewer repetitions and higher weights for hypertrophy, more repetitions and less weight for endurance)
- Intensity: to momentary muscular fatigue (do not increase until routine is easy during 2 consecutive workouts)
- Exercise intensity: The standard heart rate goal is 70 to 85 percent of maximum expected heart rate with a ± 15 beat variance. If reducing body fat is the goal, then a lower intensity and longer duration is recommended

MET, metabolic equivalent.

Designing an exercise program

Planning

In assisting a woman in her initiation of an exercise program it is important to match goals, needs and activities. Help to establish ideal recommendations, identify obstacles and facilitate problem solving. The health professional can identify equipment and clothing needs, identify support systems, create a tracking system for progress (calendar). If necessary an initial system of rewards (e.g., massage) for completing stated goals can be worked out. A contract for behavior and/or exercise may be executed at the outset of the program to serve as a summary and reminder of what the agreed upon design contained.

Exercise prescription

The actual exercise prescription traditionally contained five components: the goal, activity mode, training frequency, duration of exercise, and the intensity of exercise.[24] An example is given in Table 7.3.

Perceived exertion rating (RPE)

This is a 20-point scale, which was initially reported by G. Borg (Table 7.4).[25]

Table 7.4. Borg's rating of perceived exertion (RPE)

RPE scale value (METs)	Perception
6	
7	Very, very light
8	
9	Very light
10	
11	Fairly light
12	
13	Somewhat hard
14	
15	Hard
16	
17	Very hard
18	
19	Very, very hard
20	

MET, metabolic equivalent.

From Borg G. Perceived exertion as an indication of somatic stress. *Scand J Rehab Med* 1970;**2**:92–8.

With this scale, an individual can assess his or her exertion. It has been demonstrated that there are direct correlations between the level on the RPE scale and with $O_{2\,max}$ and MET rate. And so with the perceived exertion rate one can estimate the level of functional exercise. A healthy person, exercising at an RPE of 12–15, is exercising at 4 to 6 METs and at a heart rate of approximately 130–160 beats per minute.

Rate of progession in cardiovascular conditioning

When advising a woman on her program, one would increase duration to 30 minutes before increasing intensity. Increase time or distance by no more than 10 percent per week. Encourage variety to avoid boredom and prevent overuse. Three kilometers (two miles) three times a week appears to convey protection.

Weight loss tips

The focus should be on increasing energy expenditure, between 1000 and 3000 kcal/week. To decrease the risk of orthopedic injury, a combination of weight and nonweight bearing exercises should be instituted. Supplementary resistance training may increase lean body mass. A single, long bout of exercise is better than multiple short bouts (better utilization of free fatty acids).

Aerobics

Aerobics burns calories; leg lifts and curls just tone muscles. Regular aerobics combined with a hypocaloric low fat diet is the best method to lose weight maximally.

Project PACE

Project PACE stands for *p*hysician-based *a*ssessment and *c*ounselling for *e*xercise. It provides a comprehensive approach to counselling patients about physical activity. It comes with a physician's manual as well as material to use with a counsel, to include a physical activity questionnaire (assess readiness) along with three interactive counselling protocols. A starter kit can be purchased. An adolescent program is also available (see website http://shs.sdsu.edu/pace/).

Special considerations

Exercise and menses

There is absolutely no reason to alter exercise during the menses. As a matter of fact, some people use exercise as a treatment for cramps and premenstrual syndrome. Tampons and good support bras seem to make this time of month accessible to regular exercise.

Exercise and pregnancy

1. In February 1994, the ACOG (American College of Obstetricians and Gynecologists) published their newest recommendations with regard to pregnancy and exercise.[26] In the absence of obstetric or medical complications, most women can exercise moderately to maintain cardiopulmonary and muscular fitness throughout pregnancy and the postpartum period. *Moderation* is the key. Exercise at a moderate level of physical activity should help the mother and fetus and perhaps make delivery and labor tolerable. Use perceived exertion in all activities and keep the level for most pregnant women at 17 METs or lower.
2. Women who exercised vigorously before pregnancy can probably continue at that level or just below that level during their pregnancy.[27]

3. No exercise should be done in the supine position once the woman is in the second or third trimester. The pregnant exerciser should be taught the warning signs of impending problems as well as how to avoid activities with potential for injury or abdominal trauma.

4. The risk of hyperthermia is mentioned in the ACOG recommendations. Adequate hydration is emphasized. And resumption of a program after delivery should be done slowly.

> Most women can exercise moderately to maintain cardiopulmonary and muscular fitness throughout pregnancy and the postpartum period.

Exercise and youth

1. In youth, especially for those who are not skeletally mature, the emphasis is on fun, submaximal weight training. Even though some of the gains may not be appreciated until after puberty, exercise patterns established in adolescence usually reflect female adult participation.

2. Elementary school age children should participate in at least 30 to 60 minutes of age-appropriate physical activities from a variety of sources daily. Extended periods of inactivity are inappropriate for children. Adolescents can exercise aerobically like adults. Strength training depends on their skeletal maturity.[28]

Exercise and menopause

Menopause is a good opportunity to reintroduce the idea of regular physical activity. There is no documented harm and much written about the benefits. Emphasis on flexibility and stretching goes along with the aerobics.

Exercise and the elderly woman

1. There is no time like the present to start to exercise no matter when that point in time happens to fall. Clearly, there are benefits to continuing or starting an exercise regimen. For example, there is a decrease in body fat that is ''normally'' seen with aging. At any age, women are capable of accomplishing much with physical activity.

2. Exercise will decrease cholesterol, decrease diastolic blood pressure, help bone density and prevent falls. The benefits are seen at all ages.

> Exercise will decrease cholesterol, decrease diastolic blood pressure, help bone density and prevent falls in elderly women.

Exercise and the disabled woman

1. Multiple sclerosis is a common neurological disorder affecting primarily young to middle-aged women. Most of these women can exercise, heat may exacerbate symptoms and so swimming may be a good form of participation.
2. Wheelchair athletic competition is becoming much more popular as is disabled athletic participation in all arenas. Each case is unique and deserves consideration if safe and the participant is willing.[29]

Potential problems with exercise

Injury

Whenever one is more physically active, the risk of increased injury does exist. However, proper techniques, as well as knowing one's limits, including the environment, will help to keep injuries down. Multiple musculoskeletal injuries may occur as a consequence of exercise, including shoulder problems, and stress fractures. Heat injury is also a risk.[30]

Sudden death

With any exertion there is always the risk of sudden death; this risk is extremely small especially if good screening has occurred before the onset of the program.[31]

Coronary risk

In individuals older than age 40 years, coronary artery disease may occur. Remember that even four cigarettes per day will increase a person's risk by 2.4. However, more than 80 percent of myocardial infarctions occur at rest and not during exercise.

Female athlete triad

Athletic amenorrhea and those who suffer with the female athlete triad are at risk.[32] This should not be a deterrent for those who are not exercising at all.

Conclusions

Exercise is beneficial as a lifestyle habit and as a therapy for a variety of conditions including depression, cigarette smoking, cardiovascular fitness, osteoporosis, and arthritis.

REFERENCES

1. Paffenbarger RS, Hyde RT, Wing AL, Hsieh CC. Physical activity, all-cause mortality, and longevity of college alumni. *New Engl J Med* 1986;**314**:605–13.

2. Leon AS, Connett J, Jacobs DR Jr. et al. Leisure time physical activity levels and risk of coronary heart disease and death: The Multiple Risk Factor Intervention Trial. *JAMA* 1987;**258**:2388–95.

3. Physical Activity and Health: *A Report of the Surgeon General.* Rockville, MD. US Department of Health and Human Services, DHHS publication no. CDC (S/N 017-023-00196-5), 1996. (Available from website http://www.cdc.gov/nccd/php/sgr/sgr.htm).

4. Ainsworth B. Challenges in measuring physical activity in women. *Exerc Sports Sci Rev* 2000;**28**(2):93–6.

5. Manson JE, Lee IM. Exercise for women: How much pain for optimal gain? *New Engl J Med* 1996;**334**:1325–7.

6. Kushi LH, Fee RM, Folsom AR et al. Physical activity and mortality in postmenopausal women. *JAMA* 1997;**277**:1287–92.

7. Greendale GA, Bodin-Dunn L, Ingles S, Haile R, Barrett-Connor E. Leisure, home and occupational physical activity and cardiovascular risk factors in postmenopausal women. *Arch Intern Med* 1996;**156**:418–24.

8. Manson JE, Willet WC, Stampfer MJ et al. Body weight and mortality among women. *New Engl J Med* 1995;**33**:677–85.

9. Olson SH, Vena JE, Dorn JP et al. Exercise, occupational activity, and risk of endometrial cancer. *Ann Epidemiol* 1997;**7**:36–53.

10. Mink PJ, Folsom AR, Sellers TA, Kushi LH. Physical activity, waist-to-hip ratio, and other risk factors for ovarian cancer: a follow-up study of older women. *Epidemiology* 1996;**7**:38–45.

11. Thune I, Brenn T, Lund E, Gaard M. Physical activity and the risk of breast cancer. *New Engl J Med* 1997;**336**:1269–75.

12. White E, Jacobs EF, Dailing JR. Physical activity in relation to colon cancer in middle-aged men and women. *J Epidemiol* 1996;**144**:42–50.

13. Van Dam S, Gillespy M, Notelowitz M, Martin D. Effect of exercise on glucose metabolism in postmenopausal women. *Am J Obstet Gynecol* 1988;**159**:82–6.

14. Haapanen N, Milunpalo S, Vuori I et al. Association of leisure time physical activity with the risk of coronary heart disease, hypertension and diabetes in middle-aged men and women. *Int J Epidemiol* 1997;**26**:739–47.

15. Puntilla E, Kroger H, Lakka T et al. Physical activity in adolescence and bone density in peri- and postmenopausal women: A population-based study. *Bone* 1997;**21**:363–7.

16. van Barr ME, Assendelft WJJ, Dekker J et al. Effectiveness of exercise therapy in patients with osteoarthritis of the hip or knee: A systematic review of randomized clinical trial. *Arthritis Rheum* 1999;**42**:1361–9.

17. Leitzmann MF, Rimm EB, Willett WC et al. Recreational physical activity and the risk of cholecystectomy in women. *New Engl J Med* 1999;**341**:777–84.

18. Ross CE, Hayes D. Exercise and psychologic well-being in the community. *Am J Epidemiol* 1988;**127**:762–71.

19. *Melpomene Summer Institute Newsletter*, Minneapolis, MN, 1999.

20. American College of Sports Medicine. Guidelines for exercise. *J Exerc Sci Sports Exerc* 1988;**30**:124–34.

21. DeBusk RF, Stenestrand U, Sheehan M, Haskell WL. Training effects of long vs short bouts of exercise in healthy subjects. *Am J Cardiol* 1990;**65**:1010–13.

22. Pate RR, Pratt M, Blair SN. Physical activity and public health: A recommendation for the Centers for Disease Control and Prevention and the American College of Sports Medicine. *JAMA* 1995;**273**:402–7.

23. American College of Sports Medicine: *ACSM's Resource Manual for Guidelines for Exercise Testing and Prescription.* Lea & Febinger, Philadelphia, 1998.

24. Stuhr, R. Exercise prescription for women. In Agostini R, ed., *Medical and Orthopedic Issues of Active and Athletic Women.* Hanley & Belfus, Philadelphia, 1994, pp. 56–67.

25. Borg G. Perceived exertion as an indication of somatic stress. *Scand J Rehab Med* 1970;**2**:92–8.

26. American College of Obstetricians and Gynecologists. *ACOG Home Exercise Programs. Exercise During Pregnancy and the Postpartum Period.* Technical Bulletin no. 189, 1994.

27. Warren MR. Exercise in women: Effects on reproduction system and pregnancy. *Clin Sports Med* 1991;**10**:131–9.

28. *Physical Activity for Young People, Research Digest.* President's Council on Physical Fitness and Sports. Series 3 no. 3, 1998.

29. *Physical Activity and Fitness for Persons with Disabilities. Research Digest,* President's Council on Physical Fitness and Sports, series 3 no. 5, 1999 (website http://www.indiana.edu/-preschal).

30. Wiggins DL, Wiggins ME. The female athlete. *Clin Sports Med* 1997;**16**:593–612.

31. Vuori I, Makarainen M, Jaasheiainer H. Sudden death and physical activity. *Cardiology* 1981;**68**(Suppl):1–8.

32. Nattiv A, Agostini R, Drinkwater B, Yeager K. The female athlete triad. *Clin Sports Med* 1994;**13**:405–18.

Psychosocial health

Psychosocial health of well women through the life cycle

Cathy Morrow, MD

Primary care providers are uniquely able to assess the psychosocial health of women. While most individuals who seek care are "patients" – those who require or request care for specific problems – women are more frequently seen when they are well. Whether for Pap smears, prenatal care, or general physical examinations, family practitioners will more likely encounter healthy women throughout their lives. Psychosocial health is the substrate from which a woman adapts to the complex world that is her life. As such, whether seen in illness or in health, the primary care provider always has an abiding interest in the psychosocial state in which the individual presents herself.

Definitions

Psychosocial health is not easily defined. For purposes of this chapter, a few broad definitions will be useful.

1. "Psychosocial" refers generally to the psychological status of an individual within the context of their social environment.
2. "Well woman" refers both to the absence of disease and the experience of health. This implies a broad definition of health to include cognitive, emotional, physical, psychological, spiritual, and environmental factors.
3. Assessment of, and screening for, psychosocial health has an intangible quality that is deeply intertwined with the provider–patient relationship. The life and clinical experience of the provider has a profound impact on decisions about the value, methodology, and approach toward assessment of psychosocial health. Some providers feel this is not an essential role for the clinician and others see the relationship as a potentially powerful tool toward understanding the individual, enhancing the relationship with the patient and potentially favorably influencing her future health.

4. Less well explored is the potential for affecting the provider's own satisfaction with the daily work of supplying medical care to diverse peoples. Undoubtedly, all agree that it can be delightfully refreshing to provide medical care for a "well" person. Less clear are what the parameters of that care might include.

5. Each provider brings to the examination room a set of knowledge, beliefs, and experiences rooted in his or her own upbringing, family system, and education and training experiences. Depending on the era of the provider's training, his/her own knowledge base about the normal psychological development of women (and men) will vary widely.

6. Many physicians, nurse practitioners and physician assistants have had little to no educational background in normal women's psychological development. Their approach to and understanding of psychosocial issues might then be limited to their own family's system and their clinical experience. Other providers might have had extensive training in traditional psychology that, historically, has viewed women's psychological development as deviating from that of men.

7. In the past two decades, feminist thinkers have advanced alternative theories about women's psychological development that have influenced the thinking and approach of mental health and primary care providers. For some practitioners exposure to the "biopsychosocial model" came during their clinical training and is rooted in family systems theory and thinking. The practitioner's knowledge base, wherever rooted, significantly affects his/her ability to attend to psychosocial issues in a woman's life. All practitioners should be fully aware of the strengths and limitations of their own experience in this regard.

> The doctor–patient relationship is a potentially powerful tool toward understanding the individual, enhancing the relationship with the patient and potentially favorably influencing her future health.

Theories of early psychological development

1. Theoretical constructs of psychological development have been rooted for much of this century in theories based on observations and studies of men. Theories designed to describe normal psychological development of men thus resulted in the description of women's development as aberrant or arrested.[1]

2. While extensively debated over the decades, the works of Sigmund Freud and Erik Erickson remain, to this day, the underlying sets of assumptions about

the earliest psychological development of infants and young children. These principles emphasize separation, autonomy, and independence of the infant from the (mother) caregiver, with evolution toward emphasis on generativity, the development of rules and universal principles. Pediatric and family medicine texts continue to offer these understandings as norms for early childhood development.[2]

3. Accepting that these constructs may be relevant for male infants and children, they leave behind female infants and children as problems that need explaining. As such, these theories often concluded that females were wanting, less evolved, and less capable of achieving the highest levels of development.[1]

4. In the 1970s, women psychologists and psychotherapists began to critique and expand upon ideas of early female psychological development. Rather than an approach that tended to see what it was not, relative to male development, these theorists began to describe how the experience of attachment, separation, growth, and individuation might be different for women. These ideas assumed femaleness to be uniquely itself, rather than as "other". Further, the truth that caregivers to infants and children were overwhelmingly female was bound to be relevant. Might not, these theorists argued, the experience of attachment and separation differ for male and female infants, particularly in light of the powerful gender identification that highlights caregivers and the cultures from which they come? These questions ultimately led to a theory of development that has relationship at its core.

5. This relational approach to developmental theory holds that being-in-relation is the core experience for female infants and children. In other words, attachment is the norm, particularly in light of the mother from whom separation is not required. Given the sameness to, or identification with, the mother caregiver, the process is more likely of relationship to than separation from.

6. By this formulation, ideas of empathy, relationship, connectedness, and mutuality come to the forefront of the development process and remain there throughout a woman's life,[3] in contrast to ideas of separation, autonomy and independence. Thus, "relationship is seen as the basic goal of development: i.e. the deepening capacity for relationship and relational competence. . . . [O]ther aspects of self (e.g. creativity, autonomy, assertion) develop within this primary context . . . There is no inherent need to disconnect or to sacrifice relationship for self development."[4]

7. In adolescence, therefore, relational theory would describe a transformation

---

Theories designed to describe normal psychological development of men thus resulted in the description of women's development as aberrant or arrested.

Table 8.1. Requirements of a relational theory of women's development

- It must incorporate a historical and social context
- It must be applicable to women without limiting their development to their biology
- It must consider the centrality of work as well as family to women's lives
- It must be broad enough to consider women who make a variety of choices: single, without children, with children, working, in-career, noncareer, lesbian, heterosexual

in the pattern of the parent–child bond rather than a break in the bond. "Adolescent identity formation is realized in individuated relationships in which differences are freely expressed within a basic context of connectedness."[5] Female adolescents traverse the complex terrain of individuation within the context of relatedness. They must forge new identities while remaining rooted in the mutuality of their families. The emphasis on friendships during this time does not necessarily imply a separation from the family of origin, but rather a new context in which to be individuated and broaden the range of their relationships.[6] These are formidable challenges and important times for psychosocial assessment and care.

> The experience of attachment, separation, growth and individuation might be different for women. Attachment is the norm.

Women's psychological development

1. Relational theory sees women in a context broader than that assigned by their reproductive abilities or gender-driven caregiving roles. If development is understood as unfolding from infancy onward via one's affiliations, there will be a much broader context from within which to understand women as they are self-defined rather than as role or gender defined. Being "self-defined" means recognizing that women are both self-defined and in relationship to others, whatever the context of that "other" might be.
2. Relational theory, therefore, would suggest that autonomy means being in relation and caring, but it does not matter which is dependent or oppressive.[2] Lucy Candib asks us to consider what is requisite to create a working model of adult development for clinical practice (Table 8.1).[2]
3. It must take racism into consideration in looking at women's experience of color. Moreover, such a model must consider development within the context of relationships rather than separate from them, and it must view critically the idea that development consists in striving toward the goal of male-defined autonomy.[2]

4. This discussion of relational theory attempts, with broad brush strokes, to describe a methodology for thinking about psychosocial issues in women's lives. It is, for purposes of this chapter, a brief and superficial overview. The interested reader is strongly encouraged to understand more deeply by reading any of the references cited, but particularly relevant to the practicing clinician is the excellent discussion found in Medicine and the Family by Lucy Candib.

> Relational theory suggests that autonomy means being in relation and caring, but it does not matter which is dependent or oppressive.

Principles of psychosocial care for women

1. The busy provider, hustling through a day packed with sick patients and interspersed with physicals on well children and adults, has her doubts about all this. For many, taking care of ill people and performing well care with the requisite attention to preventive counselling and screening, and doing this well, is more than a day's work. Nonetheless, it is also true that when family practitioners enter the examination room and ask "How are you?," they begin the process of providing good psychosocial care.

2. The principles of good psychosocial care are both simple and complex. A caring, attentive ear that remains alert to the woman's own understanding of her life in relation to self, to others and to the systems and institutions that comprise her life is a beginning. Fuelled by genuine interest and curiosity, good psychosocial care has, at its heart, a deep and abiding respect for women, their enormous strengths and vulnerabilities. It is dependent upon relationship: that that exists and is developing each moment of an encounter. For most providers, this is knowledge acquired over time, both in the general sense and in the specific.

3. The broader culture has not inculcated providers with a sense of deep respect for women. Many come to the practice of medicine with biases and stereotypes about the roles and capabilities of women. Even if physicians are raised in families with positive messages about women, the surrounding culture has muddled that message to some extent.

4. The psychosocial care of women respects relationships as fundamental and is

> The broader culture has not inculcated providers with a sense of deep respect for women.

capable of viewing the world through relational lenses. It avoids judgment and labelling and is willing to accept a world view different from one's own. It demands some fearlessness about feeling and asks us to rethink the more traditional medical rules about boundaries. It will, at times, call for emotional investment on the provider's part and remains open to that possibility. Nonetheless, thoughtful psychosocial care fully respects appropriate boundaries.

5. Good psychosocial care is sensitive to the dilemmas faced by women in the culture and does not trivialize them. Respect for the burdens placed by assumptions and prescribed roles that have oppressed women is critical.

6. Good psychosocial care does not fail to acknowledge these hard realities and appreciate the power of them, and it does not shirk from addressing them. It respects the enormous diversity of women's lives and does not make assumptions of normalcy. It remains sensitive to the dilemmas faced by women within the medical culture and seeks to improve upon them.

7. If the relational model is used to consider health care, the major risk factors threatening psychosocial health become more apparent. Those events and influences that lead to major disconnection will be the most likely to disturb the well-being of an individual woman. The potential dislocations that occur as a result of social change, coupled with the significant mobility of the culture, provide enormous opportunity and potential for major disconnection.

8. Disconnections such as death (particularly of a child), job loss, divorce, partnership dissolutions, domestic violence, trauma, or illness may threaten a woman's sense of herself and her world. Women remain particularly at risk for economic dislocation, whether by earning less then men for equivalent work, or through divorce, partnership dissolution, or spousal death. Her psychological and biological health are all at substantial risk during such times. Her sense of control over her environment and life is potentially seriously threatened. Her ability to process, grieve, and ultimately grow through such events is predicated upon her own internal and external support systems that may facilitate, or may threaten, her survival.

9. A helpful model for considering the coping styles of women facing major disconnections is that of resiliency, the ability to rebound from adversity. Steven and Sybil Wolin have described seven features of the resilient individual from their work with survivors of troubled families (Table 8.2).[7] These features will cluster in varied fashion depending on the personality and circumstances of the loss or disconnection faced, and a given woman may utilize one or several of these qualities in coping. For the provider, assessment of the ability and diversity of such strategies may highlight risks and illumi-

Table 8.2. Seven features of the resilient individual

- Insight
- Independence
- Relationships
- Creativity
- Humor
- Morality
- Initiative

Taken from Wolin S, Wolin S. *The Resilient Self: How Survivors of Troubled Families rise above Adversity.* Villard Press, New York, 1993.

> The potential dislocations that occur as a result of social change, coupled with the significant mobility of the culture, provide enormous opportunity and potential for major disconnection. Women remain particularly at risk for economic dislocation, whether by earning less than men for equivalent work, or through divorce, partnership dissolution, or spousal death.

nate strengths, while suggesting other potential strategies for improved coping.

10. Knowledge of the individual, her experience with previous coping strategies that were successful or not, and awareness of the presence or absence of support may all serve to help the provider care for, and work with, an ill woman. A past experience of acceptance by the provider is very powerful. Knowledge that she will be accepted for her coping strategy rather than lectured to about what she "should" do is powerful.

11. Well-meaning friends and cultural mores often dictate powerfully to women how they should cope or grieve. Mores about acceptable grief, whether temporal or topical, often tyrannize women. A climate of acceptance, a sense that she is right to do it her way, in her own time, is very powerful. Avoiding a tendency to immediately medicate signs and symptoms of psychological distress may also be valuable and appropriate. Many women will benefit from a steadying hand from their provider rather than a prescription.

12. Yet the provider should exercise caution about minimizing and downplaying distress. Supporting women through periods of reactive depression, overwhelming grief, and intense feeling without judging or pathologizing can be among the most important and powerful clinical interventions physicians will ever perform.

> Avoiding a tendency to immediately medicate signs and symptoms of psychological distress may also be valuable and appropriate. Yet, the provider should exercise caution about minimizing and downplaying distress.

13. Of course, there are circumstances when prescriptions, active interventions, and referrals are absolutely necessary. The clinical judgment of the provider must always be alert for the signs and symptoms of major depression, suicidality, and life-threatening behaviors. In fact, an environment of trust and relationship improves the likelihood that dangerous disconnections will be more readily identified by the provider and interventions more readily accepted.

14. Many women have had their feelings and concerns minimized in the medical setting. Some arrive to these environments primed to be ignored or to have their feelings discounted. Lesbian women and women of color have often been the victims of insensitive care. Women are much more likely than men to have had their behavior and symptoms labelled. Providers who are inclined toward curiosity rather than judgment, understanding instead of diagnosis, and mutuality rather than doctor–patient, may find they are more successful at providing good psychosocial care.

> Women are much more likely than men to have had their behavior and symptoms labelled.

Psychosocial health through the life cycle: adolescents

1. Providing humane, thoughtful psychosocial care to the young woman during this period of enormous transition and growth is exciting and often very challenging for the provider. The stakes inevitably are high and there is significant content in screening, assessment, and risk factors that the provider is attempting to cover. The adolescent often does not really want to talk, and there are still all the medical aspects of the visit with which to contend.

2. The 1990s have brought an explosion of work, both scholarly and popular, about the risks and transitions for adolescent girls in the Western culture. Galvanizing public attention to the issue, the American Association of University Women study of 1990 looked at 3000 young girls and boys aged 9 to 15 years. The results clearly identified the costs and risks of coming of age in America within a patriarchal cultural and educational system. The study found that the passage to adolescence was particularly treacherous for girls, marked by decreased confidence, decreasing abilities in mathematics and science, and an increasingly critical attitude toward their own body.

3. Female adolescents experienced increased feelings of depression, hopelessness, and vulnerability, with a rate of suicide attempt four to seven times higher than that of boys.[8]

Table 8.3. Psychosocial relational adolescent screening

A. Tell me about your important relationships. Who matters in your life right now? Mom? Dad? Friends? Siblings? Pets?

B. How do you feel about your body now? Do you like it? Why or why not? Sports, exercise, diet, etc.

C. How do you feel about school? Work, if any? Other? e.g., Church, volunteering?

D. What are your recreations? Hobbies? Drugs? Alcohol?

E. Have there been any big losses in your life since I saw you last? Conflicts? Problems or obstacles that you felt like you couldn't solve?

F. How about successes? Accomplishments?

G. Tell me about your dreams? Goals? Aspirations?

4. Relationally speaking, the girls begin to lose their voice. The pressures and messages about being female in a Western culture sufficiently quieted the strong and confident younger girls as they learned to be nice, get along, and accommodate others. "At the crossroads of adolescence, the girls in the study describe a relational impasse that is familiar to many women: a paradoxical or dizzying sense of having to give up relationship for the sake of "relationships."[6]

5. Thoughtful psychosocial care can be provided by attending to this fact. By caring about and creating relationships with the adolescent girls, physicians come to know them and identify those risks that arise from this dissociation from self. The clinician can seek to identify relationships that may be sources either of strength and support or discord and vulnerability.

6. Table 8.3 presents one series of inquiries that may be used as screening questions regarding relationship. A question might lead to a series of others that illuminate a conflict or highlight a strength. Keeping an ear attuned to a sense of disconnection, whether from parents, friends, school, or others can provide the tip-off to other questions to pursue in more depth. Listening to the adolescent's version of her relationship with others helps one keep away from the land mines of assumptions, whether about sexuality, values, or "normalcy".

7. Adolescent girls value relationship. They describe most anxiety about abandonment and they may be most at risk when they abandon themselves,[1] dissociate from their own confident younger girl voices in order to accommodate to the pressures and expectations of the culture around them.

Passage to adolescence was particularly treacherous for girls, marked by decreased confidence, decreasing abilities in mathematics and science, and an increasingly critical attitude toward their own body.

8. Studies that have attempted to isolate correlates of psychosocial health through these turbulent years have identified active participation in all-girl sports teams as a positive factor.[9] Sports involvement helps not only with body image issues as girls come to view their bodies as competent and strong, but ongoing support of other girls in relationship to themselves can help in weathering the doubt and self-negation so ubiquitous during this time.

9. A study of resilient adolescent teens who became mothers identified relationships, insight, and initiative as the positive correlates of coping well with this major transition.[10]

10. An additional strategy can be called responsibility/rebellion. This may be a quality particularly valuable for adolescents. Young women were determined to prove that they would not fail or do poorly as all the surrounding systems predicted.

> Sports involvement helps with body image issues as girls come to view their bodies as competent and strong, and by providing ongoing support of other girls.

11. Given the value placed on relationship, the primary care provider should appreciate the relationship with an adolescent over time and not despair of the limited "progress" that seems to be made in any given individual visit. Many a provider has been surprised and pleased to learn how strongly the young girl identifies them as "my doctor".

12. Creating the environment of trust necessary for a productive care relationship with an adolescent if the provider also cares for the extended family is challenging. Issues of confidentiality need to be addressed directly and adhered to faithfully for the provider to sustain credibility with the adolescent. Identification as "my doctor" will be facilitated by seeing the adolescent alone.

> The primary care provider should appreciate the relationship with an adolescent over time and not despair of the limited "progress" that seems to be made in any given individual visit.

Adult women

1. As women emerge from adolescence into adulthood, issues of relationship persist, but the complexities of attaining a livelihood, sustaining oneself, and possible partnering come more directly to the fore.

2. Many young adult women will be continuing to traverse tasks of adolescence, while many others will have long since been pushed prematurely into assum-

Table 8.4. Developmental tasks facing adult women

- Solidifying a self identity independent of one's family of origin yet remaining in relation to them
- Creating independence as a single person or in a relationship
- Participating in many and varied adult relationships at home and work. Possible partnering/marriage
- Supporting self and potentially others
- Considering becoming, or choosing not to become, a parent
- If raising children, establishing and maintaining a secure environment in which to raise them
- Continued extended family involvement, establishing newly configured adult relationships with parents
- Finding balance between work, family, and social responsibilities
- Balancing own personal, emotional, psychological, spiritual and health needs

ing sets of responsibilities normally thought of as adult. The developmental tasks faced in adulthood are numerous (Table 8.4). These broadly apply to most women in a Western culture but will be affected powerfully by ethnicity, culture, and circumstance.

3. Few women, if any, follow a smooth developmental trajectory. Economic forces will shape this trajectory tremendously; poverty is consistently identified as a major source of psychosocial stress.

4. Sexual orientation may have significant influence on the accessibility of social supports upon which one might depend. Changing social mores may affect how openly a woman remains single, is lesbian, or adopts children of color, and lives her life. Job and legal changes may allow closeted women to live more openly than previously, or the reverse may occur.

5. Threats of violence, harassment, and intimidation are daily facts of life for millions of women. Constructing a model for "normalcy" in women's lives is not reasonable. There are simply as many variations as there are women. Table 8.5 presents some suggestions for psychosocial screening questions that may facilitate a deeper discussion of these issues.

6. Research that explores psychosocial correlates of health has highlighted attributes that may be relevant for the provider. One large study examined psychosocial factors and their relationship to CHD in 750 women between the ages of 45 and 64 years. Women who developed angina and CHD were two to three times more likely to score higher on scales measuring type A behavior (emotional lability, ambitiousness, and "noneasygoing"), suppressed hostility and anger, tension and anxiety.[11] A follow-up study examining this same group 20 years later revealed similar findings but added low educational level,

Table 8.5. Psychosocial relational adult screening

- Who do you care for at this time? Children? Partner? Siblings? Parents? Extended family?
- How do you care for yourself? Who helps care for you? Where do you go for help when you need it?
- Tell me about work (in or out of home). Does it nourish/stress you? Is the balance right?
- Are there other environments besides home/work that matter to you? Church? School? Volunteer work?
- Tell me about your successes and accomplishments.
- How about losses? Conflicts that were difficult to resolve or remain a source of a lot of distress?
- Do you feel as though your life is under your control?

lack of vacations, and perceived financial status among employed women as risk factors.[12] Measurable associations exist between divorce, lower socio-economic class, lower educational attainment, and limited social supports, on the one hand, and cardiovascular disease, cardiac arrhythmias, sleep disturbance, depression, and anxiety, on the other.[13,14]

7. Conversely, overall health has been shown to have strong correlations with role satisfaction (particularly work related),[15] higher socioeconomic class, caring for a family, strong social supports, high self-esteem, and larger social networks.[16,17,18]

8. Clear differences exist in mortality between lowest and highest income women and educational attainment level. Many argue that the higher rates of morbidity and mortality found in low income groups are explained solely by differences in health-related behaviors such as alcohol and tobacco consumption. While no doubt a factor, other studies refute these as the major etiology and find that education level, social stresses, and social roles at work and home are independent risk factors.[19,20]

9. Women are the caregivers in the culture; this role can be a source of great satisfaction, identity and fulfillment, but can also be the source of enormous stress and frustration.

   a. How caregiving affects women will be highly dependent on a host of associated factors: support systems, relief from the role, degree of caregiving, presence of more than one generation requiring caregiving, and the nature of the caregiving relationships, to name a few.

   b. The fulltime working woman (some 65 percent of women) who is responsible not only for young children but also aging parents or relatives is at high risk of being overwhelmed by these responsibilities.

   c. Relationships with those being cared for may be warm and loving or may be fraught with anger, unresolved issues, and confusion.

d. The provider should be aware of the caregiving responsibilities of their patients and how these will affect psychosocial and overall health. Providers can serve not only as a source of this needed caregiving but also assist women in realistic assessment of the demands upon them, and assist with finding alternatives where needed.

Constructing a model for "normalcy" in women's lives is not reasonable.

Older women

1. Although poverty is an enormous issue in the psychosocial life of any woman, with elderly women this issue becomes more important. Women older than 65 years constitute the fastest growing segment of the population and comprise the significant majority of that total population.

2. By the year 2012, people aged 65 years and older will comprise 14 percent of the total population in the USA, twice the number in 1956.[21] Moreover, women comprise an even higher percentage of the elderly poor (72 percent), and twice as many African-American women as white women live in poverty. Elderly women are half as likely as men to have pensions and four times more likely to become indigent and require Medicaid for nursing home or other care.[22]

3. As women age, life cycle tasks evolve significantly. There is enormous diversity of life experience, health status, economic conditions and overall social supports that each individual woman experiences. Many providers will first come to know women during this time; the frequency of visits tends to increase with the development of health problems. Eighty percent of elderly women older than age 65 years have at least one chronic health condition.

4. Attention to psychosocial health may reap significant benefits. The aging woman may have more time for reflection, more knowledge about herself and life, and be less driven by sociocultural norms of success and achievement. It has the potential to be a time of enormous satisfaction. A lifetime of caregiving for others may be turned, finally, toward the self. Women may need permission to do so, and may benefit from support and encouragement to see the value in evolving roles.

5. It can be deeply unsettling to no longer be needed in familiar roles. What is perceived as a time of freedom and independence to some can be a source of depression and loss for others.

6. Major financial changes, whether caused by retirement, death of a supporting partner, or divorce can dramatically alter the course of an older woman's life.

Eighty percent of elderly women older than age 65 years have at least one chronic health condition.

Statistically, a woman in America who reaches age 65 years can expect to live another 19 years, a lengthy period of time to finance and survive, if at or near poverty.[22]

7.   Several psychosocial challenges are likely to present themselves as women age. Loss of partners, loved ones, spouses, and siblings may place a woman at risk of isolation, living alone, and marked diminution of social supports.

8.   Women who have enjoyed lifelong independence may find themselves facing gradual dependence secondary to physical decline. The profoundly mobile society may mean that children, grandchildren, and other potential sources of support may be substantial distances away. Retirement from work may be associated with pleasure and joy in newfound freedom or may result in a loss of sense of identity, value and importance.

9.   In Western culture, aging women are not usually revered and beloved for their wisdom and past work, though surely these family systems exist as places of support for some. The individuals' ethnicity will influence, to some extent, how older women are valued within a family and community. The culture and providers tend to focus on loss in the elderly.

10. As chronic medical conditions mount, numbers of prescriptions increase, and visits to the office become regular, both the provider and the individual can lose sight of the health that does remain. Gains of this time in a woman's life should be celebrated. A new grandchild, volunteer work that is meaningful, travel, pleasure in time spent with loved ones all contribute to the health of an aging individual. These should be acknowledged and celebrated in the course of the care as surely as the blood pressure should be monitored.

11. Isolation is one of the greatest psychosocial risk factors, and can lead to, or be a symptom of, depression. Recognition by the provider that an aging individual is becoming isolated can be an important step in preventive care.

12. End-of-life issues are challenging for all providers, and perhaps even more so with patients with whom family practitioners have developed strong, psychosocially rich relationships. Yet the fruits of long relationship can be realized powerfully in such times. All wish for a peaceful death. If the provider genuinely knows the patients, then she or he genuinely knows their wishes.

13. Inevitably, except for sudden unexpected deaths, the process of physical decline, diagnosis, work-up, and treatment often moves women away from the primary care world and into specialty centers and intensive care settings for a time. Primary providers can lose touch with their patients, yet this is a time when their continued presence can be quite valuable. Occasionally, the provider will be the only individual who has had direct, clear conversation

about the woman's wishes toward the end of life. Often, though, patients return to the responsibility of their primary care physicians to die.

14. Confusion and conflict within families, particularly gatherings of those from distances may demand the distinct voice of the provider who has had these conversations. It is a component of good psychosocial care to assist the extended family in these times, and it honors the provider's relationship with the individual. Countless patients have experienced a sense of abandonment by providers as the time for medical intervention passes and the time arrives for allowing the inevitable to occur. "A peaceful death can only be possible if it is understood that the power of death in the end triumphs over human science and artifice, and that only a stepping aside to allow it to happen can be faithful to the force of nature and the respect owed to patients."[23] Family practitioners must remain present in order to see these relationships through, to facilitate that stepping aside if need be, and to continue the process of providing good psychosocial care to those left behind.

Isolation is one of the greatest psychosocial risk factors, and can lead to, or be a symptom of, depression.

Conclusions

Providing excellent psychosocial care to women throughout the life cycle is one of the most complex and rewarding tasks a primary provider will undertake. The attention, time, and focus given by the provider to the broad spectrum of emotional, developmental, economic, cultural, and social issues that will impact on one's health will be time well spent. Women, by virtue of their unique caregiving, childrearing, and employment responsibilities have special concerns that require care and attention by the provider. Respect and appreciation for the value of psychosocial care will lead not only to better care of patients but also to better satisfaction for providers.

This chapter has focused on the psychosocial health care of women and suggested shifts in the paradigm of the approach in order to meet the needs of women that may be unique to them. However, many feel that the precepts and principles of relational thinking are relevant to both genders and support an overall approach that is more sensitive to the needs and realities of all. Viewing one's patients, regardless of gender, through a relational lens offers the possibility of humanism as a guiding ideal for medicine. Perhaps, as family practitioners care for the caregivers in the culture, this ideal might be better realized throughout medicine.

REFERENCES

1. Gilligan C. In *A Different Voice: Psychological Theory and Women's Development*. Harvard University Press, Cambridge, MA, 1982, pp. 8–12.

2. Candib L. *Medicine and the Family*. Basic Books, New York, 1995, pp. 4–13.

3. Jordan JV et al. Women's Growth in Connection: Writings from the Stone Center. Guilford Press, New York, 1991.

4. Surrey JL. Relationship and Empowerment. In Jordan JV et al., ed., *Women's Growth in Connection, Writings from the Stone Center*, Guilford Press, New York, pp. 153–67, 1991.

5. Grotevant HD, Cooper CR. Individuation in family relationships: A perspective on individual differences in the development of identity and role-taking skill in adolescence. *Hum Dev* 1988:**29**:93–4.

6. Brown LM, Gilligan C. *Meeting at the Crossroads: Women's Psychological and Girls' Development*. Harvard University Press, Cambridge, MA, 1992.

7. Wolin S, Wolin S. *The Resilient Self: How Survivors of Troubled Families rise above Adversity*. Villard Press, New York, 1993.

8. American Association of University Women. *Shortchanging Girls, Shortchanging America*. AAUW, Washington, DC, 1991.

9. Pipher M. *Reviving Ophelia*. Ballantine Books, New York, 1995, pp. 266–7.

10. Carey G, Ratliff D, Lyle RR. Resilient adolescent mothers: Ethnographic interviews. *Fam Syst Health*, 1998;**6**:347–64.

11. Haynes SG, Feinleib M, Kannel WB. The relationship of psychosocial factors to coronary heart disease in the Framingham Study. *Am J Epidemiol* 1980;**3**:37–58.

12. Eaker ED, Pinsky J, Castelli WP. Myocardial infarction and coronary death among women: Psychosocial predictors from a 20 year follow-up of women in the Framingham Study. *Am J Epidemiol* 1992;**135**:854–64.

13. Horsten M, Erickson M, Perski A, Wamala SP. Psychosocial factors and heart rate variability in healthy women. *Psychosom Med* 1999;**61**:49–57.

14. Owens JF, Matthews KA. Sleep disturbances in healthy middle aged women. *Maturitas* 1998;**30**:41–50.

15. Rosenfeld JA. Maternal work outside the home and its effect on women and their family. *J Am Med Women Assoc* 1992;**47**:47–53.

16. Thomas SP. Psychosocial correlates of women's health in middle adulthood. *Issues Mental Health Nurs* 1995;**16**:285–314.

17. Denton M, Walters V. Gender differences in structural and behavioral determinants of health: An analysis of the social production of health. *Soc Sci Med* 1999;**48**:1221–35.

18. McQuaide S. Women at midlife. *Social Work* 1998;**43**:21–31.

19. Lantz PM, House JS, Lepkowski JM, Williams DR, Mero RP, Chen J. Socioeconomic factors, health behaviors, and mortality: Results from a nationally representative prospective study of US adults. *JAMA* 1998;**279**:1703–8.

20. Gottlieb NH, Green LW. Life events, social network, life-style, and health: An analysis of the 1979 National Survey of Personal Health Practices and Consequences. *Health Educ Q* 1984;**11**:91–105.

21. Butler RN, Oberlink M, Schechter M. *The Elderly in Society: An International Perspective*. Brocklehurst's Textbook of Geriatric Medicine and Gerontology, 5th edn. Churchill Livingstone, New York, p. 1445, 1998.

22. Goldstein MZ. Gender issues in geriatric psychiatry. In Sadock BJ, Sadock VA, eds., *Kaplan and Sadock's Comprehensive Text of Psychiatry*, 7th edn. Lippincott, Williams & Wilkins, New York, 1999, p. 3174.

23. Callahan D. The value of achieving a peaceful death. In Cassel CK, Cohen HJ, Larson E et al. *Geriatric Medicine*, 3rd edn. Springer-Verlag, New York, 1997, pp. 1035–42 (see p. 1038).

LIVERPOOL
JOHN MOORES UNIVERSITY
AVRIL ROBARTS LRC
TEL. 0151 231 4022

Sexuality

9 Sexuality and sexual dysfunction through the life cycle

Patricia Lenahan, MA, and Amy Ellwood, MSW

Sexuality is a significant aspect of all individuals' lives. Physicians and health care professionals, who provide longitudinal care to individuals and families, have both an opportunity and a responsibility to provide appropriate counselling, anticipatory guidance and education for their patients regarding sexual concerns occurring throughout the life cycle.

Introduction

Sexual issues are frequently ignored in practice, for a variety of reasons. Physicians must be aware that sexual behavior, in addition to procreation, serves many other functions related to physiological and psychological development. Sexuality provides individuals with a way to express their feelings, demonstrate caring, and communicate and develop intimacy with another person. As such, sexual expression becomes a source of pleasure and fulfillment. For couples, it is a powerful form of communication.

Medical concerns

Physicians have the responsibility to address the sexual concerns of their patients. Many women regard their physicians as experts in the area of human sexuality. There are many medical and developmental concerns that will impact on sexual behavior, and questions may concern psychosexual development, contraception, STD counselling and the impact of various illnesses, such as depression, substance abuse, physical disability, and diabetes, on sexuality. These provide a springboard for physician inquiry into the sexual health of their patients. Many illnesses impact on sexual behavior and if not discussed, will be ignored.

Physician reluctance

While most practitioners have had some training in taking sexual histories during medical school, many physicians are reluctant to pursue this issue with their patients. Embarrassment, fear, and uncertainty about useful recommendations contribute to this reluctance. Developing an awareness of one's own attitudes, feelings, and beliefs about sexual functioning is vital.

> Many physicians are reluctant to discuss sexuality with their patients because of embarrassment, fear, and uncertainty about useful recommendations.

Cultural obstacles

When obtaining sexual histories and eliciting concerns of a sexual nature, considering the age, culture, and religious background of the individual patient is essential. Discussion of sexual matters may be viewed as inappropriate and elicit embarrassment or anger. For other women, the opportunity to address their sexual issues may come as a welcome relief.

Sexuality and adolescence

Adolescence is a time of great physiological, emotional, and psychological change. It is a time of exploration, emancipation, and a search for self-identity and intimacy.

Initiation of sexual intimacy

For many adolescents, sexual intimacy is one aspect of accomplishing this transition.

1. Statistics from the CDC estimate that, in the USA, more than three-quarters of boys and two-thirds of girls have had sexual intercourse by their senior year in high school.[1] Adolescents who began having sex before age 13 years were more likely to have had multiple partners.[2]

2. The onset of sexual intimacy varies among adolescents. Peer pressure, feelings of love, curiosity, and wanting to be grown up are among the reasons frequently cited by teenagers for initiating sexual experimentation.[3] Family factors such as divorce or single parent homes and abuse also contribute to the early onset of sexual activity.[4] Environmental and behavioral factors such as drug and alcohol use, delinquency, and decline in school grades have also been linked to premature sexual experimentation among adolescents.[5]

3. Physicians may overlook the issue of emerging and possibly confusing sexuality in gay and lesbian adolescents. Approximately 10 percent of all adolescents may experience interpersonal struggles related to sexual identity issues.[6]

Sexuality, STDs and unplanned pregnancy

1. Since relatively few adolescents admit to planning sexual encounters, they are less likely to utilize any type of contraceptive.[7] Lack of comfort with their bodies, self-image and embarrassment may also interfere with an adolescent's willingness to consider contraceptives, thus increasing the potential for STDs or pregnancies.[8]
2. Adolescents may be reluctant to discuss sexual issues with their physicians. Although most teenagers respond positively to physician inquiries about sexual issues, many do not identify confidentiality as a major concern.[9]
3. Adolescents, especially those who begin their sexual activity at a younger age, are more likely to have multiple partners over time, exhibiting a type of serial monogamy, which also places them at higher risk for STDs or pregnancy.

Physician interaction

Exploring the adolescent's understanding of sexuality (including sexual dreams, fantasies, homosexual thoughts, masturbation), hormonal changes, reproduction, contraception (including how to say ''no''), and prevention of STDs is important. Physicians can also offer reassurance to adolescents concerned about body image changes and fears related to body development such as breast size. They can explore with the adolescent her understanding of sex versus love and any guilty feelings about sex and/or masturbation. Assessing for any other risk-taking behaviors, such as drug or alcohol use, that often accompany premature sexual activity is important also. It is a time to debunk the sexual myths such as the need for simultaneous orgasms with her partner and clitoral versus vaginal orgasms. Physicians have numerous opportunities to provide information and education regarding safer sexual practices, family planning, and sexual fulfillment during pregnancy.

Pregnancy

Pregnancy creates numerous physical and psychological changes in the woman and in the couple's relationship. They must now consider another life in addition to their own. For the woman, body image changes, physical

LIVERPOOL JOHN MOORES UNIVERSITY
LEARNING SERVICES

Table 9.1. Changes that may accommodate sexual relations during pregnancy

- Use of pillow(s) under the woman's head and back or reclining – shortness of breath may occur when the woman is lying prone on her back
- Alternative positions – side-to-side, woman on top
- Sex without penetration

discomfort, and fears for the safety of the fetus may affect her interest in sexual activity during pregnancy.

Changes in desire and function

1. Sexual desire decreases during the first trimester, increases during the second trimester, and decreases again in the final trimester. Some studies have linked advanced pregnancy to decreased sexual desire and satisfaction.
2. For couples wanting to continue sexual intimacy throughout pregnancy, the physician may recommend positional changes that are more comfortable for the woman and can accommodate the growing fetus (Table 9.1).
3. Unless the woman is at high risk for, or develops, premature labor, there is no medical reason except discomfort to stop having sexual relations during pregnancy.

Unless the woman is at high risk for or develops premature labor, there is no medical reason to stop having sexual relations during pregnancy except discomfort.

Post partum

1. Following delivery, most research shows that women gradually return to their former levels of sexual desire and interest, although physiological factors such as vaginal bleeding or dyspareunia may contribute to decreased sexual interest during the postpartum period. Fatigue, psychological concerns and stress may also have a negative impact upon the resumption of sexual activity in the new mother.[10]
2. Other factors such as role overload may affect sexual desire.
3. The man's fear about hurting his partner may impact on the couple's resumption of sexual activity. Family physicians can be very helpful to couples during this life phase transition. Doctors can offer guidance regarding ways to cope with the numerous adjustments a couple may experience when becoming parents and how they can balance fulfillment of sexual intimacy needs with the demands of a new baby.

Medical problems and sexuality

Cancer

1. The word cancer elicits a variety of feelings in patients and their families. The diagnosis of cancer has a profound effect upon the woman, her partner, and her family. Loss, fear, anxiety, and depression are common responses to the diagnosis. Loss may be related to expectations of fertility or experienced as becoming less whole, less feminine, and more vulnerable to the exigencies of life. Fears associated with the treatment, pain, loss of control, desirability, and death are frequent responses. Those cancers that affect sexual organs can be traumatic for the patient and her partner. Since cancer provokes crises in the lives of many women, exploring the nature and quality of significant relationships in the woman's life is important.

2. Partners of cancer patients also experience reactions to the illness that may include fear of hurting the patient, irrational fears of contamination or contracting the disease, or a decreased sense of desirability. Communication between partners is crucial at this point. The family physician can facilitate communication between the partners. He or she can provide information on the treatment and outcome and explore their understanding of what cancer means to them.

3. Pain, or the anticipation of experiencing pain, may have a negative effect on the woman's interest in sexual intimacy. Premature resumption of sexual intimacy, before the woman is ready physically, psychologically, and emotionally, may occur in order to relieve anxiety about her partner's perceived sexual needs and a need to affirm her desirability as a woman.

> Pain, or the anticipation of experiencing pain, may have a negative effect on the woman's interest in sexual intimacy.

Gynecological cancers

1. While the sexual consequences of gynecological cancers vary according to the treatment used, dyspareunia is more common among women who have had radiation rather than surgical interventions.[11]

2. Vaginal dilators may be recommended for women experiencing dyspareunia following radiation treatment or surgical interventions. Use of the dilator two or three times a week may reduce anxiety related to pain and enable the woman to resume sexual activity more comfortably and experience penetration without pain.[12]

Dyspareunia is more common among women with gynecological cancer and disease who have had radiation rather than surgical interventions.

Breast cancer

1. A diagnosis of breast cancer has numerous psychological, emotional, relational, and sexual ramifications for the woman and her family. Cultural views of the breast as a symbol of femininity and attractiveness and, conversely, as a source of life and nutrition, play a role in how a woman and her partner respond to the diagnosis.

2. Assessing the woman's self-concept, her body image, and her sense of femininity when discussing treatment options are important. Women also fear the response of their partners to potentially disfiguring surgeries. Earlier studies have addressed the importance of involving the partner in the treatment of breast cancer patients.[13] The adjustment process can be improved by encouraging the partner to view the surgical site early, discussing issues of revulsion or avoidance (of the breast and the partner), and addressing concerns about sexual activity causing pain.

3. Sexual dysfunction occurs frequently among breast cancer patients.[14] However, the source of this dysfunction has not been linked solely to the diagnosis and treatment of breast cancer. The sequelae of treatments, premature menopause, depression, the impact of medications and chemotherapies, and preexisting sexual problems may all contribute to dysfunction in the breast cancer patient.

4. Studies indicate that a relationship exists between menstrual status and sexual functioning in the woman who has breast cancer. Chemotherapy-induced menopause that causes vaginal dryness and other hormonal changes exacerbates sexual problems.[15] Women who have had chemotherapy and younger women who have premature menopause are more likely to have problems with sexual functions.

5. Women who have undergone reconstructive surgery following mastectomy often complain of loss of sensation and pain in the breast.[16] Direct stimulation of the breast is no longer as pleasurable and may affect the quality of the sexual interactions between the woman and her partner. Women who have had reconstructive surgery are more likely to experience significant sexual problems than those who have undergone lumpectomies.

Women also fear the response of their partners to potentially disfiguring surgeries.

Women who have had reconstructive surgery are more likely to experience significant sexual problems than those who have undergone lumpectomies.

Disability

1. While a significant number of studies have addressed the sexual concerns and functioning of individuals who have suffered spinal cord injuries, little research has been conducted to assess the sexual health needs of persons born with physical and intellectual disabilities.[17] Societal attitudes toward sexual expression among people with intellectual disabilities have not been favorable. Families, fearing exploitation and abuse, may shield their impaired children from obtaining any sexual knowledge or keep them from participating in appropriate sex education programs.

2. Clearly, an assessment of the intellectual capabilities of the individual is needed to determine the person's ability to consent to sexual overtures. Similar problems may arise among individuals with congenital physical disabilities. In both cases, the family physician must address the concerns of the parents, provide education, anticipatory guidance to the child or young adult, and encourage responsible sexual behavior.

3. Appropriate confidentiality is important also. Treading the difficult line between giving the nonindependent woman her appropriate confidential information and consultation and helping her work within her family system may be challenging. Understanding guardianship and family relations will help.

Chronic illness

Many individuals begin to experience the onset of chronic illness during the fifth and sixth decades of life. Diseases such as cardiac and circulatory problems, diabetes, arthritis, osteoporosis, chronic obstructive pulmonary disease, hypertension, neurological disorders, and depression, among others, have a profound impact on sexual functioning (Table 9.2).

1. Heart disease:

   a. The effects of cardiac illness on men have been well researched. Few studies, however, have addressed the specific issues of women following a cardiac event and their unique counselling needs. Women may receive less counselling, including referral to cardiac rehabilitation, than men do. Often, this is a time in which individuals receive information about returning to work, exercise, and other activities, including sex.

   b. Resumption of sexual activity following a cardiac event may elicit fear and anxiety in a person. Women may choose to avoid returning to their

Table 9.2. Effect of medical diseases on sexuality in women

Disease	Effect
Cancer	
Gyn. cancers	Fertility concerns, fear of partner rejection, pain, dyspareunia
Breast cancer	Altered self-image and fears of loss of sexuality
	Sexual dysfunction
	Loss of sensation and pain in the breast
Chemotherapy-induced menopause	Vaginal dryness
Heart disease	Fear of restarting sexual intercourse, chest pain
Hypertension	Medications often cause dysfunction
Diabetes	Orgasmic difficulty
Renal failure	Anhedonia, decreased vaginal lubrication, and anorgasmia, hypoactive sexual desire disorders
Spinal cord injuries	Loss of self-esteem, perceptions of body image, social role, penetration difficult
Decreased mobility	Decreased ability to participate
Multiple sclerosis	Decreased libido, delayed and decreased lubrication, decreased orgasmic capacity
Arthritis	Reduced mobility, detrimental effect on sexual function
Scleroderma	Vaginal dryness, dyspareunia, and decreased orgasmic function

Gyn., gynecological.

previous level of sexual activity fearing a reinfarct or death. Symptoms such as chest discomfort, shortness of breath, and excessive sweating have been identified as deterrents to the resumption of sexual activity in women.[18]

c. Women can resume when climbing two flights of stairs no longer causes anxiety or chest pain. Education regarding the impact of the sexual response cycle on cardiac function is essential.

d. For example, explaining the number of metabolic equivalents (METs) used during sex compared with common daily activities can help to reduce anxiety (see Chapter 7). Patients must understand the need to avoid heavy eating and drinking prior to sex in order to reduce the potential stress on the heart. Patients should be advised to discontinue sexual activity if they become short of breath, experience chest pain, or become too anxious, and to notify their physician of their symptoms immediately. Reassurance and education can help to reduce anxiety among women with cardiac disease.

2. Hypertension: Medications utilized to control hypertension may affect the sexual response cycle negatively (Table 9.3).

Table 9.3. Some medications that may affect sexual functioning in women

Medication	Effect
Amphetamines	Decreased or no orgasm
Antipsychotics	
Phenothiazines, butyrophenones	Decreased desire, hypoactive sex drive
Antihypertensive medication	
ACEIs	Decreased arousal
Beta-blockers	Decreased arousal, desire
CNS-active drugs, clonidine, methyl dopa, reserpine	Decreased arousal, anorgasmia
Thiazides, spironolactone	Decreased arousal, desire
Antihistamines	
H2-blockers	Decreased sex desire, decreased arousal
Danazol	Decreased or increased sexual desire
Narcotics	Decreased sex desire, decreased arousal, decreased orgasm
Sedatives	Decreased sex desire, decreased arousal, decreased orgasm
Benzodiazepines	Anorgasmia, decreased desire
Antidepressants	Decreased sex desire, decreased arousal, decreased orgasm, delayed orgasm
MAO inhibitors	
Tricyclics	
?SSRIs	
Alcohol	Decreased arousal, decreased orgasm

ACEI, angiotensin-converting enzyme inhibitors; CNS, central nervous system; MAO, monoamine oxidase; SSRIs, selective serotonin reuptake inhibitors.

For additional information refer to Crenshaw TL, Goldberg JP, eds. *Sexual Pharmacology: Drugs that Affect Sexual Function.* WW Norton, New York, 1996.

3. Diabetes:
   a. While impaired or decreased sexual functioning is a complication of diabetes in men, the sexual impact of diabetes on women is not as well defined. Fewer than 30 studies that focus on the sexual concerns of diabetic women have been conducted. One of the first studies by Kolodny indicated that women with diabetes suffer significant orgasmic difficulty.[19] Few studies conducted since then have replicated this information. Results of

Women can resume sexual relations when climbing two flights of stairs no longer causes anxiety or chest pain.

subsequent research present contradictory and inconclusive data about the effects of diabetes on female sexual function.[19]

b. However, neuropathies do not contribute to sexual dysfunction in female diabetics.[20]

c. Numerous psychosocial problems have been linked to diabetes. These psychosocial and psychological issues may interfere with, or exacerbate difficulties in, sexual functioning.

d. Renal failure has been linked to several types of sexual dysfunction in women. Anhedonia, decreased vaginal lubrication, and anorgasmia have been associated with women patients on dialysis.[21] Additionally, women with chronic renal failure often have a hypoactive sexual desire disorder.[22] The source of this dysfunction may be multifactorial illness, medications, and psychological issues.

5. Spinal cord injuries:

   a. Spinal cord injuries result in multiple losses for the patient and her partner. Self-esteem, perceptions of body image, social role and feelings of dependence are all affected. The degree of the impairment dictates the degree of effect on sexual function. Muscle spasticity may make penetration difficult.[23] Therefore, an assessment of the patient's sensory capacity and mobility are important in offering anticipatory guidance. Recommendations may include encouraging the patient to improve self-esteem and self-image and to make advance preparations for sexual intimacy by attending to bowel and bladder care before initiating sex in order to avoid any accidents, which may have significant psychological consequences.[24]

   b. The timing of the sexual activity may also be important to avoid fatigue or spastic responses.[25] Sensate focus exercises may be helpful to the patient with spinal cord injuries, and her partner, in establishing communication and in determining sensory capabilities.

6. Decreased mobility problems:

   a. Diseases that result in decreased mobility, such as multiple sclerosis, arthritis, or autoimmune disorders, often contribute to sexual inactivity. Joint stiffness, decreased flexibility, pain, muscle spasms, and other symptoms affect an individual's ability to engage in sexual activity.

   b. Multiple sclerosis has been associated with decreased libido, delayed and decreased lubrication, decreased orgasmic capacity, and anorgasmia in a significant number of women.[26] Fatigue, spasticity, contractures, loss of manual dexterity, and incontinence may contribute to sexual problems.[27] The use of assistive devices, muscle relaxants, and vibrators may help to alleviate the distress and disability caused by contractures, muscle weakness, and spasms.

Table 9.4. PLISSIT model

P – Permission giving
LI – Limited information
SS – Specific instructions
IT – Intensive treatment

Developed by Annon JS, *The Behavioral Treatment of Sexual Problems: A Brief Therapy.*
Harper and Row, New York, 1976.

   c. Bowel and bladder training programs may be recommended when incontinence is a problem.

   d. For some patients, the use of corticosteroids has produced improvement in sexual functioning.[28]

7. Arthritis:

   a. Arthritis, a common disease in older individuals, can cause reduced mobility, joint stiffness and pain both having a detrimental effect on sexual function.

   b. Timing of sexual activity to coincide with optimal physical mobility and pain relief, along with specific suggestions such as positional changes (e.g., side by side), symptom relief (medications), and advanced preparation (warm baths or use of hot tubs) can aid the arthritic woman to maintain her sexual identity.

8. Scleroderma: Scleroderma is another disorder that can have negative effects on sexual functioning. Studies of women with scleroderma and Sjögren's syndrome have been shown to have high rates of sexual dysfunction. Common problems include vaginal dryness, dyspareunia, and decreased orgasmic potential. Other changes such as joint pain, contractures, and muscle weakness may interfere with a woman's ability to masturbate.

9. Treatment and facilitation:

   a. Physicians can best assist their patients to maintain healthy sexual functioning by taking a sexual history and exploring the patient's sexual concerns, fears, and expectations. Utilizing a PLISSIT model (Table 9.4), physicians can elicit patient's concerns and understanding and give appropriate information.[29]

   b. Physicians may suggest positional changes (side to side), environmental changes (placement of pillows, use of waterbeds, etc.), and alternative activities to intercourse such as hugging, caressing, cuddling, and masturbation. A thorough sexual history and an understanding of the patient are needed before making any recommendations. Both the patient and her partner must be willing to consider suggestions regarding alternative positions or practices.

c. Good communication between the partners is essential. Individuals or their partners who have significant concerns or reservations about changing their sexual practices may be encouraged to discuss their feelings and to explore any cultural, religious, or personal factors that may be affecting their decisions.

d. Referrals to certified sex therapists, and to chronic disease support groups and organizations may be helpful.

> Sensate focus exercises may be helpful to the patient with spinal cord injuries, and her partner.

Medications and sexuality

Effects

Medications can cause many effects that interfere with an individual's usual sexual functioning.

Specific medications

Because the list of medications that may cause sexual dysfunction is extensive and because the effects are often idiosyncratic, discussing potential sexual side effects with patients on medication is important. When medication with possible sexual side effects is necessary, specific adaptations to enhance the possibility of sexual arousal can be suggested, including reducing the number and dosage of drugs and changes in the timing of the medication. Additionally, physicians can advise their patients to have intercourse at a time when the drug's effect is least disruptive (Table 9.3).

Selective serotonin reuptake inhibitors

1. Selective serotonin reuptake inhibitors (SSRIs) are the medications of choice for many depressed individuals. These drugs have been linked to decreased libido and anorgasmia in women and may affect every phase of the sexual response cycle.

2. With patient with depression, whether the disease or the medications are causing the changes in desire is difficult to separate. A small study of 14 women found that desire and arousal problems in women improved with use of SSRIs.[30] Obtaining sexual histories from patients before initiating treatment

with SSRIs will help the practitioner to identify sexual dysfunctions associated with the medications and those that were preexisting. Administration of the Rush Sexual Function Inventory, designed specifically to assess sexual problems in depression, may be helpful.

Since depression itself frequently results in anhedonia, decreased sexual desire, decreased frequency of sexual activity, and a lowered sense of sexual satisfaction, it is essential to assess the patient's premorbid level of functioning and interest in sex before associating the dysfunction with the medication.

3. Treatment:
   a. Recent literature reviews have addressed the possibility of using sildenafil to treat sexual dysfunction associated with SSRIs.[31] Other studies have examined bupropion and herbal remedies such as yohimbine and gingko biloba as possible ways of treating sexual side effects of antidepressants.[32]
   b. Drug holidays may be considered when the patient is using an SSRI with a shorter half-life. However, caution should be used before making this recommendation since drug holidays may have the potential for causing discontinuation syndromes. Drug holiday proposals also require good communication between the partners and decreases spontaneity.

Alcohol

1. The use of alcohol has been associated with risk-taking behaviors in women.[33] The disinhibition effect of alcohol may result in a subjective sense of increased arousal and desire, but does not affect performance in a positive way.
2. Various studies also report that alcoholic women have high rates of sexual dysfunction. There is some connection between alcoholism and sexual abuse histories, which may complicate the understanding of the etiology of the dysfunction.
3. Hypoactive sexual desire, orgasmic dysfunction, and dyspareunia have been reported in large samples of women in alcoholic treatment programs.[34]

Midlife

Women in later midlife, age 40 to 60 years, can use guidance regarding the impact of chronic illness and medications on sexual functioning. Women at this stage of life are frequently experiencing changes in family structure and the psychological and psychosocial adjustments this demands. Women may express fears regarding their partner's fidelity and anxiety about their perceptions of themselves as less feminine and less desirable. Physicians can provide their patients with information regarding the physiological changes that occur with aging, including menopause, and explore the patient's sexual beliefs about the appropriateness of sex at her age.

Physiological changes

1. Many physiological changes associated with aging affect the sexual response cycle of the older woman. Estrogen-deficient vaginitis and reduced lubrication are common complaints associated with aging. The thinning and drying of the vaginal walls may result in dyspareunia and bleeding. The use of artificial lubricants can reduce the symptoms and pain.[35]

2. As women age, the excitement phase occurs much more slowly. Women in their reproductive years generally achieve lubrication in about 10 to 15 seconds during the excitement phase. For the postmenopausal woman, it may take up to five minutes or more for lubrication to occur. More direct genital stimulation is needed during the arousal or excitement phase for the woman and her partner as well.

3. The plateau phase may also become longer. For many women aged 50 to 70 years, the duration of the orgasmic phase becomes shorter and orgasms may be experienced as painful. Contractions may be spasmodic, rather than rhythmic and pleasurable. With a decreased number of uterine contractions per orgasm, some women may be unaware that orgasm has occurred. Vasocongestion, nipple erection, and breast tumescence are all decreased.[20] Despite all these changes, women retain the potential to return to the excitement phase at any point during resolution and to experience multiple orgasms.[36]

> The thinning and drying of the vaginal walls may result in dyspareunia and bleeding.

Sexual history

Obtaining a sexual history from elderly women may be embarrassing for many clinicians. While the elderly woman is less likely to complain about sexual problems than younger patients, overcoming this sense of embarrassment and asking their older patients about sexual function is important. Also, educating the older patient about the physiological changes helps.

Interest

1. Most studies of older people demonstrate that interest in sexual intimacy continues into advanced old age. Prevalence varies by area, country, and population asked; from 30 percent of community-dwelling US women older than age 65 years to 95 percent of community-dwelling older Danish women

have regular intercourse. According to a lengthy study conducted by the Consumers' Union,[37] most women over age 65 years engaged in sexual activity at least once a week. On the whole, older women report less sexual activity than men do, correlating with the availability of a socially sanctioned partner.[38]

2. The most important correlation between continued sexual activity in older women is availability of a healthy partner. Women marry older men, who may develop chronic illnesses or die before them. Women who are widowed, divorced, or unmarried are less likely to continue their sexual activity. Various studies have noted a sharp decrease in sexual interest and activity among women in their late 60s. For many women, this may be a source of considerable frustration. Societal expectations, cohort effect, and misconceptions about the physiological effects of aging on sexuality contribute to this distress. The apparent aspects of aging, wrinkles and gray hair, may result in feelings of decreased sexual attractiveness.[20]

3. For women without sexual partners, masturbation may be an option.

4. However, sensitive inquiry about sexual beliefs, practices, and concerns will be needed before any recommendations can be made. Providing education and debunking the sexual misconceptions will enable her to make informed decisions.

5. For the "younger" geriatric patient, William Masters and Virginia Johnson have suggested, in general publications, various factors that may contribute to a lack of sexual responsiveness: monotony, preoccupation with career and finances, physical and mental fatigue, overindulgence in food and drink, and fear of failure of sexual performance. Other factors that have been identified as contributing to a decline in sexual activity among the elderly include: overall life stressors, socioeconomic issues, patterns of disinterest in sexual activity as a young adult, and institutionalization resulting in a lack of privacy for those individuals who reside in assisted living or extended care facilities.

Various factors in middle age may contribute to a lack of sexual responsiveness: including monotony, preoccupation with career and finances, physical and mental fatigue, overindulgence in food and drink, and fear of failure of sexual performance.

Facilitation

The woman and her partner may ask for or require help in facilitating continued sexual intercourse.

1. Positional changes, side-to-side or least ill partner on top, may help. Using several pillows for the prone partner can also facilitate sexual relationships.

2. Arthritis and stiffness can make sex difficult. Asking the partners to come into the office in comfortable clothes and/or sweatsuits and trying different positions to help them find comfortable ones may help. Using nonsteroidal antiinflammatory drugs (NSAIDs) or acetaminophen (Tylenol) or nitroglycerin before sex may help.

3. Suggesting refraining from alcohol and heavy meals and attempting sex when not fatigued may help older couples continue to have satisfaction with sexual relations.

4. Reviewing drugs used by both partners may show the possibility of eliminating or reducing a drug that may affect sexual functioning.

5. Lubrication by exogenous creams may help.

Elderly

Dementia

Dementia and Alzheimer's disease present special difficulties for the older woman and her partner. Common sexual consequences of Alzheimer's disease include anhedonia, impotence, incontinence and anorgasmia. During the early and middle stages of the disease, however, sexual intimacy remains a viable option for couples.

1. Yet some individuals will withdraw from their partners prematurely as a result of guilty feelings about continuing the sexual relationship in light of the cognitive impairment, as a result of role changes, distaste for sexual or physical intimacy because of poor hygiene, or as a means of coping with the increasing demands of caregiving.[39]

2. Desexualization of the demented spouse often helps the caregiver to meet the very personal and intimate caregiving demands.[40]

3. Also, for some individuals, touch is no longer perceived as pleasurable or soothing. As the disease progresses, physical touch and intimacy may result in increased agitation or anxiety.

4. A score of less than 15 on the Mini Mental Status Examination generally indicates that an individual is unlikely to understand the nature of sexual activity and, therefore, is unable to give consent.[40]

5. While overt and inappropriate sexual behavior of Alzheimer's patients is much rarer than believed, caregivers may be at risk for sexual abuse or rape by their demented spouses. Family physicians need to explore this issue gently with the caregiver. Such circumstances may result in the filing of elder abuse charges.

Sexual relationships in long-term facilities

1. Older women residing in assisted living and extended care facilities may lose their privacy and may experience a loss of sexual freedom as a result.

2. Sexual intimacy between married or unmarried and consenting individuals may present difficulties for facility staff who are concerned about safety and legal issues. Family members may also object to the expression of intimacy between their aging relatives and other residents of the facility. Again, the family physician can serve an important role in addressing the concerns of both the family and the older patient.[41]

3. Practitioners can advocate for their patients in allowing privacy and conjugal visits or permitting medically stable individuals to have home visits. Family physicians also serve a vital role in educating nursing home staff about the sexual needs of their patients.[42]

Common sexual dysfunctions

In assessing sexual problems, considering all aspects of the patient's life is important. Often by considering the phase in which the sexual dysfunction occurs, the woman and physician may find ways of improving satisfaction with sexual life (Table 9.5).

Decreased sexual desire

1. According to the DSM-IV (*Diagnostic and Statistical Manual of Mental Disorders*, fourth edition), hypoactive sexual desire disorders (HSDs) are characterized by persistent or recurrent absence of sexual fantasies and desires that are not associated with other axis I or medical conditions.

2. This is a commonly diagnosed disorder with a prevalence rate ranging from 1 to more than 30 percent in women. Because the etiology of HSD is multifactorial, a thorough physical, psychological, and sexual history is essential.

3. A variety of treatments have been recommended for individuals with HSD. These treatments range from more insight-oriented approaches to cognitive-behavioral ones. Despite the therapeutic orientation of the counsellor, most treatment regimens for HSD involve the use of sensate focus techniques. These exercises are designed to increase sexual communication between the partners and to identify impediments to sexual arousal and enjoyment. As such, the initiation of sensate focus exercises may prompt a crisis for the patient who must now confront her sexual fears or concerns.

Table 9.5. Common medical causes of sexual dysfunction

	Decreased sexual desire	Problems with arousal	Problems with orgasm
Medical conditions	Serious or chronic illness CNS disease	Vascular disease Menopause Diabetes Alcoholism	Diabetes Vascular disease Chronic illness
Medications	Antipsychotic drugs Phenothiazines Butypherones Cimetadine and ?other anthistamines Narcotics Tricyclic antidepressants ?SSRIs Antihistamines Anticholinergic Beta-blockers	Beta-blockers Thiazide diurectics ACEIs CNS-active antihypertensives Antihistamines Benzodiazepines	Narcotics Sedatives Alcohol Tricyclic antidepressants ?SSRIs Alcohol Benzodiazepines
Life stresses	Sexual trauma Rape, abuse Depression Anger and difficulties in relationships Negative body image Chronic stress Fatigue	Stress Fatigue Anxiety Inadequate stimulation	Inadequate stimulation Fear of loss of control Lack of knowledge

For abbreviations, see Table 9.3.

Sexual arousal disorders

1. Sexual arousal involves both physiological and psychological factors.
2. Physiologically, vaginal lubrication occurs during the excitement phase of the sexual response cycle while psychological factors include a more subjective perception of sexual pleasure.[43]
3. Prevalence of this disorder varies according to the type of research conducted. It is generally acknowledged that women with a diagnosis of cancer have higher rates of arousal disorders. According to some studies, women with a history of sexual abuse or trauma experience significant sexual arousal and aversion disorders.
4. Treatment approaches for sexual arousal disorders frequently include sensate focus techniques and masturbation training. Other therapists recommend

assertion training for women who have been noninitiators of sexual intimacy. This technique encourages the woman to identify times when she is interested in sexual activity and to be comfortable in rejecting advances at times when she is tired or stressed.

Orgasmic disorders

1. A variety of factors – inability to relax, inconvenient timing of sexual activity, lack of communication, limited sexual knowledge, body image distortions, absence of sufficient foreplay, and lack of sexual interest – have been associated with orgasmic problems in women.[44]

2. At the same time, many women have been socialized by their cultures, or their age cohorts, to view sex as a spousal "duty," not as an act to be enjoyed or considered pleasurable.[45] Sexual "scripts" such as the "good girl" image, may contribute to orgasmic difficulties as well. This contrasts with current social and cultural values that emphasize a woman's responsibility to achieve her own sexual satisfaction.

3. Primary care physicians can assist their patients through education (sexual response cycle, sexual anatomy), and referral to appropriate therapists.

4. Treatment of orgasmic disorders generally involves an assessment of body image and introduction to masturbation. Self-help books such as *Becoming Orgasmic*[46] and *For Yourself*[47] are useful adjuncts to treatment.

> A variety of factors – inability to relax, inconvenient timing of sexual activity, lack of communication, limited sexual knowledge, body image distortions, absence of sufficient foreplay, and sexual disinterest – have been associated with orgasmic problems in women.

Vaginismus

1. The prevalence of vaginismus, the involuntary contraction of the vaginal muscles preventing penetration, has been found to be underreported by many sex therapists, due, in part, to the lack of consistency in statistical reporting. Some studies indicate that women in other countries present with complaints of vaginismus far more frequently than women in the USA.[48]

2. The etiology of vaginismus is considered to be variable depending upon the type of disorder. Theories about the cause of vaginismus abound and range from the physiological to the psychoanalytical and psychosomatic. Thus primary vaginismus has been associated with long-term negative feelings and fears about sex, near phobic fears about becoming pregnant or acquiring a venereal disease, and general sexual misinformation.

3. Women with secondary vaginismus are those who are more likely to have experienced sexual trauma such as childhood molestations, have a history of painful sex, and have marital or relational distress.

4. In assessing the possible cause of the vaginismus, the practitioner should explore the woman's attitudes, beliefs, and early experiences with sexual expression. Understanding parental beliefs about sexuality also may be significant. Since women who experience vaginismus can be sexually responsive to a certain degree and may experience orgasm, it is necessary to obtain a complete sexual history to determine the presence/absence of arousal, sexual interest, and the presence or absence of sexual fantasies.

5. This will help the physician to differentiate the type of vaginismus and to determine whether the source of the disorder is situational and partner specific.

6. Treatment of vaginismus is fairly consistently applied despite the varied theoretical orientations of the therapists. Education (sexual anatomy), sensate focus techniques focused on genital self-exploration, relaxation exercises, gradual introduction of dilators, and involvement of the partner through support and communication exercises are the essential aspects of treatment recommended by many therapists. Again, hypnosis may also be considered.

Conclusions

Sexuality is a natural part of human existence, yet there is considerable variability in the ways in which individuals express themselves sexually. This variability may be mediated by age, culture, religion, marital status, or experiential factors.

Normative changes – physiological, psychological, and emotional – occur in the sexual life cycle of the individual. The onset of illness or chronic disease may have a significant impact on how and when a person engages in sexual activity.

REFERENCES

1. Centers for Disease Control and Prevention. *Pregnancy, Sexually Transmitted Diseases, and Related Risk Behaviors Among US Adolescents.* Adolescent Health State of the Nation Monograph Series, no. 2, CDC Publication no. 099-4630. CDC, Atlanta, 1994.

2. Durbin M, DiClemente RJ, Siegel D et al. Factors associated with multiple sex partners among junior high school students. *J Adolesc Health* 1993;**14**:202–7.

3. Alexander E, Hickner B. First coitus for adolescents: Understanding why and when. *J Am Board Fam Pract* 1997;**10**:96–103.

4. Goodson P, Evans A, Edmundson E. Female adolescents and onset of sexual intercourse: A theory-based review of research from 1984 to 1994. *J Adolesc Health* 1997;**21**:147–56.

5. Orr DP, Beiter M, Ingersoll G. Premature sexual activity as an indicator of psychosocial risk. *Pediatrics* 1991;**87**:141–7.

6. Braverman PK, Strassburger VC. Adolescent sexual activity. *Clin Pediatr* 1993;**56**:658–68.

7. Gilcrest V. Preventive health care for the adolescent. *Am Fam Physician* 1991;**43**:869–79.

8. Millstein SG, Moscicki A. Sexually transmitted disease in female adolescents: Effects of psychosocial factors and high risk behaviors. *J Adolesc Health* 1995;**17**:83–90.

9. Strasburger VC, Brown RT. Adolescent sexuality and health-related problems. In *Adolescent Medicine: A Practical Guide.* Little, Brown and Co., Boston, MA, 1991, pp. 232–48.

10. Reamy KJ, White SE. Sexuality in the puerperium: A review. *Arch Sexual Behav* 1987;**16**:165–86.

11. Shover LR. *Sexuality and Cancer: For the Woman with Cancer, and her Partner.* American Cancer Society, New York, 1990.

12. Auchincloss SS. After treatment: Psychosocial issues in gynecologic cancer survivorship. *Cancer* 1995;**76**(10 Suppl):2117–24.

13. Frank D, Dornbush RL, Webster SK, Kolodny RC. Mastectomy and sexual behavior: A pilot study. *Sexuality Disabil* 1978;**1**:16–26.

14. Myerowitz BE, Desmond KA, Rowland JH, Wyatt GE, Ganz PA. Sexuality following breast cancer. *J Sexual Marital Ther* 1999;**25**(3):237–50.

15. Ganz PA, Rowland JH, Desmond KA, Meyerowitz BE, Wyatt GE. Life after breast cancer: Understanding women's health-related quality of life and sexual functioning. *J Clin Oncol* 1998;**16**:501–14.

16. Wilmott MC, Ross JA. Women's perception: Breast cancer treatment and sexuality. *Cancer Prac* 1997;**5**: 353–9.

17. McCabe MP. Sexual knowledge, experience and feelings among people with disability. *Sexuality Disabil* 1999;**17**:157–70.

18. Hamilton GA, Seidman RN. A comparison of the recovery period for women and men after an acute myocardial infarction. *Heart Lung* 1993;**22**:308–15.

19. Kolodny RC. Sexual dysfunction in diabetic females. *Diabetes* 1971;**20**:557–9.

20. Meston CM. Aging and sexuality. *West J Med* 1997;**167**:285–90.

21. Kaiser FE. Sexuality in the elderly. *Geriatr Urol* 1996;**1**:99–109.

22. Toorians AW, Janssen E, Laan E et al. Chronic renal failure and sexual functioning: Clinical status versus objectively assessed sexual response. *Nephrol Dialysis Transplant* 1997;**12**:2654–63.

23. Berard EJ. The sexuality of spinal cord injured women: Physiology and pathophysiology. A review. *Paraplegia* 1989;**27**:99–112.

24. Garden FH. Incidence of sexual dysfunction in neurologic disability. *Sexuality Disabil* 1991;**9**:39–47.

25. Lemon MA. Sexual counseling and spinal cord injury. *Sexuality Disabil* 1993;**11**:73–97.

26. Lundberg PO, Hulter B. Female sexual dysfunction in multiple sclerosis: A review. *Sexuality Disabil* 1996;**14**:65–72.

27. Bezkor MF, Canedo A. Physiological and psychological factors influencing sexual dysfunction in multiple sclerosis: Part I. *Sexuality Disabil* 1987;**8**:143–6.

28. Mattson D, Petrie M, Srivastava DK, McDermott M. Multiple sclerosis: Sexual dysfunction and its response to medications. *Arch Neurol* 1995;**52**:862–8.

29. Annon JS. *The Behavioral Treatment of Sexual Problems: Brief Therapy*. Harper and Row, New York, 1976.

30. Piazza PA, Markowitz JC, Kocsis JH et al. Sexual functioning in chronically depressed patients treated with SSRI antidepressants: A pilot study. *Am J Psychol* 1997;**154**:1757–9.

31. Shen WW, Urosevich Z, Clayton DO. Sildenafil in the treatment of female sexual dysfunction induced by selective serotonin reuptake inhibitors. *J Reprod Med* 1999;**44**:535–42.

32. Gitlin MJ. Effects of depression and antidepressants on sexual functioning. *Bull Menninger Clin* 1995;**59**:232–48.

33. Ericksen KP, Trocki KF. Sex, alcohol and sexually transmitted diseases: A national survey. *Fam Plann Perspect* 1994;**26**:257–63.

34. Beckman LJ, Ackerman KT. *Women, Alcohol, and Sexuality: Recent Developments in Alcoholism*, vol. 12. *Women and Alcoholism*. Plenum Press, New York, 1995.

35. Brooks TD. Sexuality in the aging woman. *The Female Patient* 1993;**18**:27–34.

36. Kaplan HS. Sex, intimacy, and the aging process. *J Am Acad Psychoanal* 1990;**18**:185–205.

37. Brecher EM, ed. *Love, Sex, and Aging: A Consumers' Union Report*. Little Brown and Co., Boston, MA, 1984.

38. Mooradian AD, Greiff V. Sexuality in older women. *Arch Intern Med* 1990;**150**:1033–8.

39. Davies HD, Zeiss A, Tinklenberg JR. 'Til death do us part: Intimacy and sexuality in the marriages of Alzheimer's patients. *J Psychosoc Nurs* 1992;**30**:5–10.

40. Hanks N. The effects of Alzheimer's disease on the sexual attitudes and behaviors of married caregivers and their spouses. *Sexuality Disabil* 1992;**10**:137–51.

41. Mulligan T, Modigh A. Sexuality in dependent living situations. *Clin Geriatr Med* 1991;**7**:153–60.

42. Richardson JP, Lazur A. Sexuality in the nursing home patient. *Am Fam Physician* 1995;**51**:121–4.

43. O'Donohue W, Dopke CA, Swingen DN. Psychotherapy for female sexual dysfunction: A Review. *Clin Psychol Rev* 1997;**17**:537–66.

44. Tiefer L. A feminist critique of the sexual dysfunction nomenclature. *Women Ther* 1988;**7**:5–21.

45. Morokoff P. Sex bias and POD. *Am Psychol* 1989;**44**:73–5.

46. Heiman JR, Lopiccolo J. *Becoming Orgasmic*. Prentice Hall, New York, 1998.

47. Barbach L. *For Yourself: The Fulfillment of Female Sexuality*. Anchor Press/Doubleday, Garden City, NY, 1975.

48. O'Donohue W, Geer JH, eds. *Handbook of Sexual Dysfunction: Assessment and Treatment*. Allyn and Bacon, Boston, MA, 1993.

10 Contraception

Kathryn Andolsek, MD

Contraception is an inherent part of good health care and good preventive care for women. Fertility is not a disease, and therefore, contraception is not a purely medical concern but an area for collaborative care in which the woman asks for information and help in planning her pregnancies.

Introduction

1. The "modern" birth control era began in the USA in 1912 with Margaret Sanger's programs.[1] Table 10.1 provides a historical timeline of contraception in the USA.[2]

2. The proportion of reproductive age women using contraception and the percentage of women using contraception at "first intercourse" continue to increase. The percentage of sexually active women not using contraception has declined among most major ethnic groups including African-Americans, Hispanics, and whites.

3. Despite these successes, nearly half of the over six million pregnancies in the USA each year are "unintended". Half of the unintended pregnancies occur in the three million women who do not use contraception. The remaining half of unintended pregnancies occurs in the 39 million women who use contraception but experience a method failure.[2]

4. Women who do not use contraception and have an unintended pregnancy are equally as likely to have a therapeutic abortion as to continue the pregnancy and have a live birth. Effective contraception for more women would help to reduce the number of abortions.[3]

5. Family size continues to decline; this increases the number of years that contraception is necessary for each woman. The average American family had 7.0 children in 1800, 3.5 children in 1900 and 2.0 children in 1972. The average woman will need to practice contraception for more than 20 years, if she

Table 10.1. Timeline for US contraception

Year	Event
1914	Margaret Sanger arrested for distributing birth control information
1916	First birth control clinic, Brooklyn, NY, closed after 10 days
1925	First manufacture in USA of diaphragms
1928	Timing of ovulation established
1937	American Medical Association endorses birth control
1937	North Carolina was first state to include birth control in a public health program
1960	First birth control pill approved by FDA
1960	Intrauterine device approved by FDA
1965	Supreme Court (*Griswold* vs. *Connecticut*) declares state laws prohibiting contraceptive use by married couples unconstitutional
1972	Medicaid funding for family planning services authorized
1973	Supreme Court legalizes abortion (*Roe* vs. *Wade*)
1990	Norplant approved by FDA
1992	Depo Provera approved by FDA
1993	Female condom approved by FDA
1997	Emergency use of OCPs approved by FDA

Modified from Milestones in family planning: United States 1900–1997. *MMWR Morb Mortal Wkly Rep* 1999;**48**:1073–80.

wishes only two children. Most women will use several different contraceptive methods to meet this need.

6. Clinicians should be prepared to make every visit a "contraceptive" visit. They should assess the woman's need for contraception, satisfaction with her current method(s) and desire for change(s). Counselling about effective contraceptive methods receives a grade of "B" from the US Preventive Services Task Force, indicating there is at least fair clinical evidence supporting this practice.[4]

7. Couples need to consider many factors when selecting a contraceptive method (Table 10.2). There is no one "perfect" contraceptive method and the decision is reached by compromising among various factors. Most couples desire a highly efficacious, reliable, safe, inexpensive method. Ethnicity and socioeconomic status also influence contraceptive failure and success.

8. Contraceptive methods have a "theoretical" failure rate as well as an "actual observable" failure rate experienced by "real life" users. Table 10.3 lists the

Nearly half of the pregnancies in the USA each year are "unintended".

Table 10.2. Factors important in the selection of a contraceptive method

- Efficacy
- Safety
- Cost
- Accessibility
- Acceptability to partners
- Degree of involvement from both members of the couple
- Ease of use
- Reversibility
- Tolerability of side effects
- Presence of noncontraceptive benefits
- Mechanism of action

Table 10.3. Percentage of US women experiencing contraceptive failure during first 12 months of use, corrected for abortion underreporting

Method	% Failure
Total	13.1
Implant	2.0
Injectable	3.5
Oral contraceptive	8.5
Diaphragm/cervical cap	13.2
Male condom	14.9
Periodic abstinence	21.8
Withdrawal	26.0
Spermicides	28.2

Data from Fu H, Darroch JE, Haas T, Ranjit N. Contraceptive failure rates: New estimates. In *1995 National Survey of Family Growth Family Planning Perspectives* 1999;**31**(2):56–63.

percentage of US women experiencing contraceptive failure, by method, during the first 12 months of use, corrected for underreporting of abortion.[5]

9. Contraceptives are safe and, fortunately, almost all contraceptives result in less morbidity and mortality than does pregnancy for women younger than age 45 years.

   a. OCPs may be riskier than a pregnancy for women older than age 45 years who smoke cigarettes. There are "safer" contraceptive methods for them.

   b. Women with chronic conditions such as diabetes mellitus, heart disease, hypertension, and collagen vascular diseases may have higher morbidity and mortality from some contraceptive methods than do women without these conditions. However, they may also have a greater risk from pregnancy and pregnancy-related complications, so the "risk" from the method of contraception needs to be weighed against the risk of pregnancy.

10. Access to the desired contraceptive method is an important ingredient in its success. Some methods are available "over the counter"; others require a clinician visit. Both partners must find the method "acceptable" and commit to the necessary level of involvement required for its success. For example, condoms require participation of the man; injectable progesterone does not.

> Almost all contraceptives result in less morbidity and mortality than does pregnancy for women younger than age 45 years.

11. The ease of use is important for many women. For some, a one-time decision, such as subdermal progesterone is easier than a method that requires a "decision" and a "behavior" with each act of intercourse, such as a diaphragm. Some women will find a "permanent" method desirable; others prefer methods with more immediate reversibility.

12. Virtually all methods have side effects. The perceived benefits must outweigh the adverse effects. Some of these effects are medically significant, such as uterine perforation associated with intrauterine device (IUD) insertion. Others are "nuisance", such as weight gain from injectable progesterone. "Nuisance" symptoms should not be disregarded as "less significant" because they may be highly significant to the women and impact on the adherence necessary for the success of the regimen.

13. Some side effects are, in fact, desirable benefits. Many barrier methods combine protection from sexually transmitted infections and diseases with their contraceptive effect. The incidence of some cancers may be reduced with use of some methods. Dysmenorrhea, iron deficiency anemia, and acne can be decreased in users of oral contraceptives.

14. Some individuals are concerned with the method's mechanism of action, especially methods that may work by affecting "postfertilization" mechanisms. This is very important to individuals with ethical or religious views that would preclude them interfering with the process once fertilization of the egg by the sperm had occurred.

15. There is no one "ideal" contraceptive method. Table 10.4 lists the contraceptive choices for women in 1995.[6] Nine percent of users combine more than one method. Some do this to "improve" the success of contraception. Others

> Both partners must find the method "acceptable" and commit to the necessary level of involvement required for its success.

Table 10.4. 1995 contraceptive choices for US women

Method	% Who use method
Tubal sterilization	27.7
Oral contraceptive	26.9
Male condom	20.4
Vasectomy	10.5
Withdrawal	3.0
Injectable	3.0
Periodic abstinence	1.9
Diaphragm	1.9
Other	1.8
Implant	1.3
IUD	0.8
Female condom	< 1.0
Total	100

IUD, intrauterine device.
Data from Piccinino LJ, Mosher WD. Trends in contraceptive use in the United States: 1982–1995. *Fam Plann Perspect* 1998;**30**:4–10.

"Nuisance" symptoms should not be disregarded as "less significant" because they may be highly significant to the women and impact on the adherence to contraceptive method.

want to get some enhanced efficacy and to gain an additional benefit. The most common combination of contraceptives is the condom and the OCP.

16. Knowledge of contraceptive status is critical even for the "noncontraception" office visit. For example, prescribing retinoic acid (Accutane®) for a sexually active woman with acne vulgaris should only occur if she is known to consistently use a reliable method of contraception.

17. Finally, even if the patient is not interested in contraception, discussing the nature and frequency of sexual activity with patients provides an opportunity to assess the risk of common STDs.

    a. If the woman is "at risk", counselling can include safe sex practices such as abstinence. Barrier methods, such as the male and female condoms may be recommended as a strategy to decrease risk while providing some contraceptive benefit.

    b. Screening for cervical dysplasia can be performed.

    c. Screening for sexually transmitted infections such as gonorrhea, chlamydia, syphilis, hepatitis B and HIV may be recommended.

    d. If, on the other hand, the woman is interested in becoming pregnant, she

There is no ideal contraceptive method.

    may benefit from preconception assessment and counselling, such as folic
    acid supplementation.
  e. Primary prevention with hepatitis B vaccination can be offered.
  f. Office visits can provide an opportunity to discuss the availability of emerg-
    ency contraception or "EC" (see below) because even the woman who uses
    contraception may experience method "failure". Women may choose to
    keep a prescription for EC "on hand" in much the same way as women
    with infrequent asthma may opt for a rescue inhaler or parents with
    toddlers keep ipecac.

Knowledge of a woman's contraceptive status is critical even for the "noncontraception" office visit.

Emergency contraception

In the USA, EC has been used infrequently.[7] Usually, it has been limited to
emergency rooms for victims of rape, to college student health centers, or to
Planned Pregnancy offices.[7] EC can be combined with virtually all other
methods to provide a back-up if there is known "method failure" such as a
broken condom. In addition, EC provides some protection for the "nonuser"
who has an episode of unprotected intercourse.

Office visits can provide an opportunity to discuss the availability of emergency contraceptives because even
the woman who uses contraception may experience method "failure".

Method

EC hinders or delays ovulation and may affect implantation.[8] It does not
interrupt or disrupt an already established pregnancy.

Effectiveness

On average, eight of 100 women will become pregnant from a single act of
unprotected intercourse. EC results in 1 to 3 pregnancies per 100 women,
depending upon the method chosen and its timing.[9] Half of all unintended
pregnancies could be avoided if EC were widely available.[10] Currently, available methods of EC include oral hormones similar to those available in many
OCPs and the Copper T® intrauterine device.[11]

Table 10.5. Medications used as emergency contraception

Medication	Dose	Description
Diethylstilbestrol	25 to 50 mg × 5 days	Older method with high rate of nausea/vomiting; better methods currently available
Ovral[R]	2 tablets; repeat in 12 hours	Original "Yuzpe" method
Lo Ovral[R]	4 tablets; repeat in 12 hours	Consider prophylactic antiemetic
Nordette[R]	4 tablets; repeat in 12 hours	Consider prophylactic antiemetic
Alesse[R]	5 tablets; repeat in 12 hours	Consider prophylactic antiemetic
Levlen[R]	4 tablets; repeat in 12 hours	Consider prophylactic antiemetic
Triphasil[R]	4 tablets; repeat in 12 hours	Consider prophylactic antiemetic
TriLevlen[R]	4 tablets; repeat in 12 hours	Consider prophylactic antiemetic
Preven[R]	2 tablets; repeat in 12 hours	Marketed specifically as emergency contraception with a pregnancy test included
Plan B[R]	1 tablet; repeat in 12 hours	Levonorgestrel only
Ovrette[R]	20 tablets; repeat in 12 hours	

Emergency contraception hinders or delays ovulation and may affect implantation.

Doses and medication

1. In the past, diethylstilbestrol in a dose of 25 to 50 mg daily for five days was used. While efficacious, it was associated with an unacceptably high incidence of nausea and vomiting.

2. Danazol has also been used, in a single dose of 800 mg, but has significant side effects of nausea, vomiting, breast tenderness and allergic reactions.

3. Some clinicians informally prescribed combinations of available birth control pills "off label". In 1997, the US Food and Drug Administration (FDA) recognized that seven currently available OCPs could be safely and effectively used as EC.[12] These include the medications listed in Table 10.5. The major value of these regimens is that the woman may already have these products "on

hand''. The drawback is that they require taking a relatively large number of tablets.

4. Recently, two products marketed specifically for EC have been developed. Although they can be started within 72 hours of unprotected intercourse, they are more successful if used immediately. There have been virtually no contra-indications. Emergency oral contraception is of such short duration and utilizes such a low hormonal dose that it is not thought to pose a risk for women at risk of stroke, deep vein thrombosis, or cardiovascular disease, even those who are not usually considered candidates for combination oral contra-ceptives. For almost all of these women, their risk from an unintended pregnancy would be far greater than their risk from the medication.

5. Levonorgestrel or the Copper T® IUD is recommended for women who absolutely must avoid estrogen completely. Some change in the next menstrual cycle (amount, duration, timing) occurs in about 10 percent of women.

6. Preven®, available since 1998, consists of four tablets each composed of 0.25 mg of levonorgestrel and 0.05 mg of ethinylestradiol.[13]

   a. Two tablets are taken initially; the second two are taken in 12 hours.

   b. Side effects include nausea, vomiting, headache, dizziness, fatigue, and breast tenderness.

   c. Prophylactic antiemetics are recommended: meclizine 25 to 50 mg one hour before and repeated at 24 hours or diphenhydramine 25 to 50 mg one hour before and repeated in four to six hours. However, they are not effective if used after nausea develops.

   d. If the woman vomits within a few hours of taking her dose, whether the does needs to repeated is uncertain. Some experts feel the nausea is an estrogen-mediated central nervous system effect and if she has enough of an effect to be nauseated she is also achieving sufficient contraceptive benefit. Other experts recommend repeating the dose, following use of an antiemetic.

   e. Preven®, as it is currently marketed, also contains a urine pregnancy test. However, there have been no adverse effects on pregnancy demonstrated, even for women later found to be pregnant at the time Preven® was used. The pregnancy test is therefore felt to be an unnecessary step by some. If the woman does perform the pregnancy test, and the results are ''negative'', she needs to be specifically counselled that this does not indicate that she does not need the medication and that she needs to go ahead and use the tablets as prescribed.

7. Plan B® became available in 1999.

   a. It consists of two tablets of levonorgestrel, 0.75 mg. One tablet is taken initially and the second tablet is taken in 12 hours. It can be used within 72 hours but is more successful the closer in time to the episode of unprotected intercourse it is initiated.

b. Plan B® has fewer side effects and is somewhat more efficacious than Preven®. The incidence of nausea is 23 percent compared with 51 percent; the incidence of vomiting is 6 percent compared with 19 percent. Neither a pelvic examination nor a pregnancy test is necessary before use.

c. The Copper T® IUD requires a visit to a clinician and is, therefore, not as "convenient" as oral methods. Its "window" of efficacy is longer and it can be inserted within five days of unprotected intercourse. It has the advantage of providing continuing contraception for the woman who desires it.

d. Mifepristone has also been used as an EC, although it is not currently available in the USA. It may be the most efficacious among the oral emergency contraceptive options. It prevents 85 percent of the pregnancies expected to occur without treatment. The only side effect is delayed onset of the next menses. Dosages of 600 mg, 50 mg and 10 mg are similarly efficacious. The smallest dose results in the lowest incidence of side effects.[14,15]

8. Providers may consider counselling women about EC and encouraging them to have a method "on hand". Women who do not use regular contraception, women who have a history of a past unintended pregnancy, and those who use contraceptive methods with a high rate of method failure may find this particularly beneficial.

9. Women who use EC should be given additional opportunities to consider whether a more permanent or better method of contraception is warranted.

> Although emergency contraception can be started within 72 hours of unprotected intercourse, it is more successful if used immediately.

Abstinence

Abstinence is the only 100 percent effective contraceptive, if used 100 percent of the time. In reality, it may be difficult to practice. Patients may benefit from practical suggestions about how to implement abstinence in situations in which they feel pressured. This includes the word "choice" and "role plays". Once adolescents have had a sexual experience, they may be more open to reconsidering "abstinence" and should be offered this as a potential choice.[16]

Fertility awareness

1. Fertility awareness methods identify the relatively few "fertile days" of each menstrual cycle.[17] The couple then avoids genital sexual contact during those days. The number of days can range from 7 to 15 days each cycle. Many couples prefer these methods because no hormones, chemicals or appliances interfere with their lovemaking.

2. "Calendar" rhythm, the method that predicts the fertile days by "extrapolating" from the length of the previous menstrual cycles, is unreliable.

3. The sympathothermal methods of natural family planning take advantage of predictable physiological changes that coincide with ovulation or the immediate period just prior to ovulation. "Thermal" refers to the characteristic temperature elevation associated with progesterone.

4. Just prior to ovulation a woman's temperature declines approximately 0.1 to 0.2 degrees C from her usual baseline and then rises 0.5 to 0.6 degrees C and remains elevated for 12 to 15 days until the onset of menstruation. These changes are best assessed by taking the "basal body temperature", or the temperature each morning at the same time daily before arising, eating, drinking, or smoking.

5. Other conditions may affect temperature including febrile illness and alcohol consumption. Women can also use nonprescription kits that measure the presence of urine leutenizing hormone. However, these kits are expensive.

6. "Sympatho" includes the predictable physiological changes associated with ovulation such as Mittelschmerz pain (mid cycle ovulatory pain), moliminal symptoms (breast tenderness) and changes in cervical consistency. For many couples, the most consistent "symptom" is the predictable changes in cervical mucus that correlates with various portions of the menstrual cycle. Classes taught by experienced health educators or couple-to-couple instruction help couples to reliably recognize and interpret mucus changes and establish the days that require "abstinence". The couple who wishes to identify the time of peak fertility can also use these methods.

7. Lactational amenorrhea is another of these methods described in greater detail under "Special populations" (see p. 176).

"Calendar" rhythm, the method that predicts the fertile days by "extrapolating" from the length of the previous menstrual cycles, is unreliable.

Coitus interruptus/withdrawal

1. Coitus interruptus (CI)/withdrawal is the withdrawal of the man's penis from the vagina prior to ejaculation. Failures most commonly occur with lack of clear communication and because sperm are present in the preejaculatory seminal fluids released before withdrawal. Although the failure rate is high, it is better than "no method".
2. Couples may benefit from knowledge regarding EC.

Although the failure rate of withdrawal is high, it is better than "no method".

Spermicides/sponges

1. Methods: Spermicides are chemicals that are "toxic" to sperm.[18] They either kill or inactivate sperm, without harming either partner. Most contain nonoxynol-9 or octoxynol-9 as the active ingredient.
2. They can be used by themselves or in combination with condoms, diaphragms, or cervical caps.
3. STD prevention: They may reduce the risk of acquiring some sexually transmitted infections, but, unfortunately not HIV. In fact, some experts suggest that the risk of HIV transmission may increase because of the associated local irritation of tissue. A recent report from South Africa found that women who used vaginal gel with condoms became infected with HIV at approximately a 50 percent higher rate than women who used the placebo gel.[19]
4. Spermicides are available as gels, creams, jellies, foam, film, and suppositories. Creams may contain a higher concentration of the active ingredient. No clinical trials have compared the efficacy of one product to another and choice is usually dependent on partners' preferences. Suppositories and tablets dissolve in less than 30 minutes and are generally effective for less than one hour. Either partner may develop a hypersensitivity to these products.
5. Sponge: The sponge provides a physical barrier that contains spermicide and provides protection for 24 continuous hours. Sponges should be moistened with water prior to insertion. They are more effective in nulliparous than in parous women. The Today® sponge has not yet been marketed in the USA. In the meantime, a similar product, Protectaid®, can be ordered from Canada. See http://www.birthcontrol.com/orderpage.html

Table 10.6. Compounds that impair latex integrity

• Butoconazole	• Ticonazole
• Miconazole	• Conjugated estrogens (cream)
• Baby oil	• Estradiol (cream)
• Butter	• Cold creams
• Cocoa butter	• Mineral oil
• Hand lotion	• Massage oil
• Petroleum jelly	• Vegetable oil
• Shortening	• Suntan oil
• Rubbing alcohol	

Table 10.7. Lubricants compatible with condoms: safe lubricants

• Egg white	• Glycerine
• Nonoxynol-9	• Saliva
• Water	• Aloe-9
• KY^R jelly	• Astroglide^R
• Gynol II^R	• Prepair^R
• Ramses personal lubricant^R	• Probe^R

Condoms

1. STD prevention: Some types of condom provide some protection against sexually transmitted infections, in addition to contraception. All condom materials do not provide the same protection. Animal-based condoms do not protect against HIV. Latex products offer less protection against human papillomavirus and herpes simplex virus.
2. Cervical cancer effect: Condoms decrease the risk of cervical cancer by as much as 50 percent, probably because of their impact on sexually transmitted infections.
3. Efficacy: The addition of spermicidal products increases their efficacy. Products that impair latex integrity should be avoided. See Table 10.6.
4. Lubricants that are compatible with condoms are listed in Table 10.7.
5. Female condoms became available in the early 1990s. The most common has two flexible rings on each end of a polyurethane sheath. The one ring inserts into the vagina similarly to a diaphragm. The other end remains on the vulva. Female condoms should be removed immediately following intercourse and before standing.
6. In laboratory studies, HIV transmission has been prevented but there are no

clinical studies available. One study in Africa has suggested that use of female condoms, in addition to male condoms, by women with husbands with AIDS may further reduce the transmission rate.[20]

7. Latex sensitivity is not an issue, because they are not made of latex. Oil-based products can be used.

8. The availability of EC should be discussed because condoms can break (1/100), slip (5/100), leak (3.5 to 10/100) and be used inconsistently. Some couples report less sexual sensitivity.

9. Latex-sensitive individuals cannot use latex condoms.

Diaphragm

1. Method: Diaphragms were invented in the USA in the 1860s and first used in a family planning clinic in the Netherlands in the 1880s. Most diaphragms are composed of soft latex. They are available in sizes from 50 to 100 mm in 2.5 mm and 5.0 mm increments. Diaphragms must be properly fitted and several varieties including a coil spring, flat spring, arching spring, or hinged spring are available.

2. Use: They are placed anteriorly just under the symphysis pubis and the posterior fornix, acting as a physical barrier to sperm. Spermicidal cream or gel is applied to the rim. The diaphragm is inserted up to two hours before intercourse. If intercourse is repeated, additional spermicide is inserted without removal of the diaphragm; it should be left in place for a minimum of six to eight hours following intercourse. They are less effective with increased episodes of intercourse.

3. As with condoms, products that affect latex integrity should be avoided (Table 10.6). Soap and water can be used in cleansing. The women should be instructed and correct insertion, placement, and removal demonstrated. Diaphragms should not be used during menses because toxic shock syndrome can occur if they are left in place for more than 24 hours.

4. The risk of urinary tract infections is increased twofold in women who use diaphragms. If they occur, a smaller diaphragm or one with a different rim can substituted.

5. Diaphragms are more effective than the sponge or the cap for parous women.

6. They should be refitted yearly and following pregnancy, miscarriage, abortion, pelvic surgery, or weight change of more than 4.5 kg (10 lbs).

Diaphragms are more effective than the sponge or the cap for parous women.

Cervical cap

The cervical cap is essentially a smaller diaphragm that fits snugly over the cervix providing continuous contraceptive protection for 48 hours. Although not necessary, the addition of spermicides improve efficacy. Because they are made from latex, they are damaged by oil-based lubricants. Although the Prentif Cavity Rim Cervical Cap is available in the USA, many clinicians are unfamiliar with it.

Oral contraceptive pills

1. OCPs are hormonal methods of birth control. There are two general varieties: the combination OCPs that consist of an estrogen (usually 20 to 50 μg ethinylestradiol) and progesterone (levonogestrel, norethindrone, desogestrel, norgestimate) or the progestin-only pills that contain only progesterone. By comparison, the estrogen dose in pills available 25 years ago was 50 to 80 μg and higher.
2. Combination OCPs are further classified as "monophasic" (fixed dose of estrogen and fixed dose of progestin); "biphasic" (fixed dose of estrogen with one of two different progesterone doses) or triphasic (fixed concentration of estrogen and three increasing concentrations of progesterone). One oral contraceptive varies the dose of estrogen throughout the cycle with a single fixed dose of progesterone. There are no documented clinically significant differences among these combination pills.
3. Progestin-only pills or "mini pills" contain one of two different kinds of progesterone. They are used by fewer than 1 percent of OCP users. They are less effective than combination OCPs and very sensitive to the timing of the doses. Ideally, they should be taken at the same time of day each day. A back-up contraceptive should be instituted if the dose is delayed by more than three hours. Menses may be irregular or absent.
4. Newer OCPs have been developed that offer additional options in dosing. "Very low dose estrogen" pills contain less than 20 μg. Although very low dose estrogen pills minimize the risk of thrombosis compared with older estrogen doses greater than 50 μg, they have not been proven to be safer than OCPs with an intermediate estrogen dose of 30 to 50 μg. They are associated with more breakthrough bleeding, which may be problematic for patients.
5. New OCPs using new progestins, such as norgestimate and desogestrel, are referred to as third-generation progestins. They have fewer of the androgenic

Table 10.8. Conditions that appear to be decreased in incidence or severity by oral contraceptives

• Ectopic pregnancy	• Premenstrual syndrome	• Menstrual flow
• Endometrial cancer	• Dysmenorrhea	• Toxic shock syndrome
• Ovarian cancer	• Hirsutism	• Risk of hospitalization
• Ovarian cysts	• Uterine fibroids	• Rheumatoid arthritis
• Benign breast disease	• Endometriosis	• Osteoporosis
• Acne		

> There are no documented clinically significant differences among combination pills.

side effects such as acne and hair loss. Thus these newer progestins have fewer side effects. They do not affect weight or blood pressure. They cause negligible changes in blood glucose, plasma insulin or lipids. A few years ago they were thought to possibly increase the risk of thromboembolism; however, the evidence is inconclusive.

6. OCPs offer many noncontraceptive benefits.[21] The newer progestin-containing OCPs increase high density lipoprotein cholesterol. Perimenopausal users of OCPs with 50 µg of estrogen increase bone density and reduce their risk of hip fracture by 44 percent. Triphasic pills combining norgestimate are as efficacious as topical tretinoin, benzoyl perdioxide, and topical or systemic antibiotics for treating women with moderate acne vulgaris. Table 10.8 lists other conditions ameliorated or lessened by the use of oral contraceptives.

7. OCPs protect against reproductive cancers of the endometrium and ovary.
   a. The risk of ovarian cancer is decreased by 40 percent among OCP users and this benefit persists for up to 20 years following discontinuation of the pill. Women who use OCPs for ten or more years reduce the risk of ovarian cancer by 80 percent. *BRCA*-positive women experience similar reductions in risk.
   b. The risk of endometrial cancer is decreased by 40 percent in women who use OCPs for at least two years and a decrease of 60 percent if OCPs are used for at least four years.

8. The link between OCP use and breast cancer is less conclusive. A 1996 collaborative analysis of over 53 000 women with breast cancer enrolled in 53 studies from 25 countries concluded that "ever users" of OCPs had a 1.07 relative risk of breast cancer unrelated to dose or duration of use. OCP users had a lower risk of metastatic disease (RR = 0.88 compared with nonusers).[22]

> Progestin-only OCPs are less effective than combination OCPs and very sensitive to the timing of the doses.

Table 10.9. Category 1: Conditions for which there are no restrictions to oral contraceptive use

• > 21 days postpartum	• Current or recent history of PID	• Cervical ectropion
• Postpartum with 2nd or 3rd trimester abortion	• Current or recent history of STD	• Carrier status, viral hepatitis
• History of gestational diabetes	• Vaginitis without purulent cervicitis	• Uterine fibroids
• Varicose veins	• Increased risk of STD	• Past history of ectopic pregnancy
• Mild headaches	• HIV positive or at high risk for HIV infection or AIDS	• Obesity
• Irregular vaginal bleeding patterns without anemia	• Benign breast disease	• Thyroid conditions
• Past history of PID	• Family history of breast cancer or endometrial or ovarian cancer	

STD, sexually transmitted disease; PID, pelvic inflammatory disease.

New OCPs using new progestins, such as norgestimate and desogestrel, are referred to as third-generation progestins and have fewer side effects.

---

9. For most women, pregnancy and/or abortion have higher risk factors than oral contraceptives. In attempting to assist the individual woman and her clinician in decision-making, the World Health Organization has replaced a single list of "contraindications" with four categories of increasing "precautions" for using oral contraceptives.[23]

   a. Category 1 consists of conditions for which no restrictions to pill use are necessary. Category 2 contains medical conditions for which the advantages of OCPs outweigh the known risks. Category 3 includes conditions for which the clinician is asked to exercise caution but not necessarily to refrain from prescribing. Only category 4 conditions are felt to be so significantly linked to OCP use that clinicians and patients should refrain from use (Tables 10.9 to 10.12).

   b. Thromboembolism, found in category 4, is not related to the dose of hormone but instead to the duration of use. There is a decreased risk over time.

   c. Some medical conditions may worsen with the use of oral contraceptives. If this occurs, an oral contraceptive with a lower estrogen dose or progestin-only oral contraceptive can be substituted.

Table 10.10. Category 2: Advantages of oral contraceptive pill use should outweigh risk

• Severe headaches after initiation of OCP	• BP 140/100 to 159/109	• Conditions predisposing to medication noncompliance
• Diabetes mellitus	• Undiagnosed breast mass	• Family history of lipid disorders
• Major surgery without prolonged immobilization	• Cervical cancer	• Family history of premature myocardial infarction
• Sickle cell disease or sickle cell hemoglobin C disease	• Age > 50 years	

BP, blood pressure; OCP, oral contraceptive pill.

Table 10.11. Category 3: Conditions for which caution should be exercised in the use of oral contraceptives

• < 21 days postpartum	• > 35 years + smoke < 20 cigarettes/day	• Gall bladder disease
• Lactation 6 weeks to 6 months	• History of breast cancer with no recurrence in the past 5 years	
• Undiagnosed vaginal or uterine bleeding	• Interacting drugs	

Table 10.12. Category 4: Conditions for which oral contraceptive use should be avoided

• Venous thromboembolism	• Breast cancer	• Headaches + focal neurological symptoms
• Cerebrovascular or coronary artery disease	• Pregnancy	• Major surgery with prolonged immobilization
• Structural heart disease	• < 6 weeks postpartum in lactating mother	• > 35 years + smoke > 20 cigarettes/day
• Diabetes with complications	• Liver disease	• BP > 160/100 or with concomitant vascular disease

BP, blood pressure.

   d. Women with well-controlled diabetes mellitus, hypertension, and hyper-triglyceridemia (triglyceride < 750 mg/dL) should be followed closely but most will do well on OCPs.

   e. OCPs are generally contraindicated in women over 35 years of age who smoke cigarettes. Newer OCPs with low doses of estrogen or progestin-only pills are associated with less risk of heart disease for these women.

   f. Women who have migraines may have problems with OCPs. If a woman's migraines are controlled, she may try a lower dose estrogen or progestin-only OCP. If headaches worsen, OCPs should be discontinued and another method used.

10. Side effects:

   a. Most women will experience breakthrough bleeding (BTB) within the first three months of OCP use.

      i. If pregnancy has been excluded, BTB is not necessarily a reason to change pills.

      ii. Breakthrough bleeding is more likely with progestin-only oral contraceptives.

      iii. It may be managed with NSAIDs, a change to combined OCPs, a second- or third-generation OCP, or 10 to 13 days of oral estrogen.

   b. If the patient develops hair thinning or acne, a low androgenic progestin such as desogestrel or norgestimate can be considered.

   c. Most women using OCPs will have a blood pressure rise of less than 5 mmHg, which generally resolves within three months of discontinuing the pill.

   d. Mood changes and fatigue are usually related to the progestin. A change to a different progestin or a decrease in dose may ameliorate symptoms.

   e. Some women prefer amenorrhea to continued end-of-cycle bleeding. This will usually be accomplished by continuing directly onto the active pills from the next pack once a pack is completed and neither "stopping the pills for seven pill free days" nor using the "placebo" pills.

   f. Women with uncomfortable premenstrual symptoms that occur during the pill free or placebo days may benefit from continuing directly with another active pill from the next pill pack.

11. Missing pills: If a woman misses one pill she should take two pills the next day and continue with the rest of the pack as usual. If she misses two pills in the

Breakthrough bleeding is more likely with progestin-only oral contraceptives.

first two weeks of the cycle she should take two pills each day for two days and then complete the pack as usual using a back-up method of contraception. If she misses two pills in the third week or misses additional pills, the pack should be discarded and a new pack used. She should use a back-up method of contraception for at least seven days.

12. Teratogenic effects: Teratogenic effects have probably been overstated in the past. If a woman inadvertently becomes pregnant while using OCPs, the pills should be discontinued but therapeutic abortion is not necessary.

Mood changes and fatigue are usually related to the progestin.

13. Vacations and subsequent fertility:
    a. Pill-free periods are unnecessary. When she wishes to conceive, she need only discontinue the pill.
    b. Over 50 percent of women will become pregnant in three months and 80 percent in one year.
    c. Folic acid supplementation is desirable preconception because OCPs may deplete folic acid stores.
    d. The woman does not need to wait three months after discontinuing the pill before conception.
14. Medications: OCPs may affect, or be affected by, the concurrent use of other medications especially seizure medication and some antibiotics.
15. Pathophysiology: Although the primary mechanism of OCPs is to inhibit ovulation, secondary mechanisms also occur, especially with the low dose pills, progestin-only pills, and inconsistent use of OCPs. These include "post-fertilization" effects. W. L. Larimore and J. B. Stanford suggest that the evidence is compelling enough that patients should be fully informed about the mechanisms of action so that individuals with reservations involving postfertilization mechanisms have the opportunity to make a truly informed decision.[24]

Women do not need to wait three months after discontinuing the pill before conception.

Injectable progestin

Impact

Approximately 1 percent of US women elect to have injectable depot medroxyprogesterone acetate (DMPA).

Method

Intramuscular DMPA (150 mg) provides effective contraception for 12 weeks. The drug should be deposited in the gluteal or deltoid muscle using a 21- or 23-gauge needle within five days of the onset of menses and a negative pregnancy test. The site should not be massaged following injection. There is an increased risk of pregnancy if the injection is delayed to 14 weeks and if given beyond 12 weeks a back-up contraceptive should be used for two to four weeks.

Postuse fertility

Fertility usually returns in four to nine months but may take as long as 18 months. Duration of use is not related to the length of time before fertility returns.

> Fertility usually returns in four to nine months after cessation of injected progestins, but may take as long as 18 months.

Injectable progestin

This is particularly effective if temporary excellent contraception is required as during the use of isotretinoin or other medicines, or while waiting for confirmation of vasectomy success.

Side effects

1. Menstrual disturbances are common. Bleeding can be treated with NSAIDs, combined combination oral contraceptives, or 10 to 13 days of oral estrogen.
2. Amenorrhea is common. Over half of women develop amenorrhea within the first year and three-quarters after the second year.
3. Weight gain is a problem for many women. The average weight gain is 2 kg (5 lbs) during the first year of use and 5+ kg (11+ lbs) during the second year.
4. Overweight and obese women have lower efficacy rates.
5. Other side effects include bloating, decreased libido, dizziness, mood changes, acne, palpitations, depression, breast tenderness, and headache. Total cholesterol and LDL may increase; HDL decreases.
6. Bone mineral density may be reduced in women younger than age 20 years. Duration of use also plays a role and women who use this method for more than five years are at particular risk.
7. There is a high rate of discontinuation from this method, perhaps

because it is associated with irregular bleeding, weight gain, and increased headaches.

Bone mineral density may be reduced in women younger than age 20 years.

Alternatives

The availability of alternative contraceptive strategies should be discussed at each visit. Adolescents, in particular, may simply not return for a subsequent injection and yet fail to substitute an effective contraceptive.

There is a high rate of discontinuation from this method.

Subdermal implantable progestin contraceptive

Method

The Norplant® system contains six flexible elastic capsules that release 50 to 80 µg levonorgesterel the first year and 30 and 35 µg per year for each of the following four years. They are inserted in the soft tissue just above the elbow and provide continuous contraception for five years.

Future developments

A newer method studied in Europe and Asia that uses only one or two rods may be approved within the next few years (Implanon® or Uniplant®).

Efficacy

The efficacy is very high. Only 0.05 percent of women experience an unintended pregnancy within the first year of use. It should be removed and replaced, if continued contraception is desirable, after this five-year period.

Postuse fertility

Its effect is quickly reversible. A woman's fertility returns within 24 to 72 hours of removal.

Cancer effects

The overall progestin dose is one-quarter to one-tenth of that found in typical combined oral contraceptives. Women who use the Norplant® system have a lower risk of endometrial and ovarian cancer, PID, ectopic pregnancy, anemia, and pain from endometriosis. Norplant users have experienced no documented effects on their risk of breast or cervical cancer and no change in average blood cholesterol, glucose, blood coagulation parameters, or liver function tests.

Side effects

Side effects include an average of 2 kg (5 lbs) weight gain and irregular menses. Persistent irregular bleeding may be managed by NSAIDs, OCP use, or one week of 1.25 mg of conjugated estrogen orally (or its equivalent).

Warnings

1. It is less effective for women over 70 kg (154 lbs), women concomitantly using carbamazepine, phenytoin, phenobarbitol, or rifampin, and during the fifth year.
2. Contraindications include active liver disease or tumors, active thrombophlebitis, known or suspected breast cancer, undiagnosed abnormal gynecological bleeding, pregnancy, or hypersensitivity to the drug.
3. A major drawback to this method is its higher initial cost. The Norplant Foundation (tel. + 1 800 760 9030) may provide financial help for disadvantaged women. Most women request removal before the end of five years and there have been some liability concerns involving its insertion and removal.

> Norplant users have experienced no documented effects on their risk of breast or cervical cancer and no change in average blood cholesterol, glucose, blood coagulation parameters or liver function tests.

Intrauterine devices

Efficacy

IUDs are the most cost-effective efficacious methods of contraception if used for at least two years.[25] IUDs are the most widely used reversible contraceptive worldwide. However, in the USA, fewer than 1 percent of women use IUDs, even though user satisfaction is greater than with any other contraceptive method.

Method

The two IUDs currently available in the USA are both T shaped and have monofilament tails. They can be inserted at any time of the menstrual cycle.

The copper variety may be used as an "emergency contraceptive method" if inserted within five days of unprotected intercourse.

Pathophysiology

Copper IUDs prevent fertilization by creating sterile inflammation within the endometrium. This inflammation is spermicidal. Progesterone-releasing IUDs thicken cervical mucus, impeding the movement of sperm. They inhibit sperm survival and also affect implantation.

Side effects

1. The most significant side effect is PID, occurring in 0.3 percent of IUD users. IUD users acquire PID, either during the insertion process and/or from sexual activity. To decrease this risk, IUDs are not indicated if either the woman or her partner have multiple sexual partners and are therefore more likely to develop sexually related PID.[26,27]

2. PID associated with IUD insertion rarely occurs beyond the first three weeks of IUD use. The incidence of PID decreases from 10/1000 within the first 20 days to 1/1000 after 21 days. The routine use of 200 mg of doxycycline or 500 mg of azithromycin administered orally one hour before insertion has not been consistently demonstrated to decrease the rate of infection.

3. Antibiotic prophylaxis for subacute bacterial endocarditis is appropriate for women with valvular heart disease as prophylaxis. Prophylactic antibiotics are unnecessary for women with mitral valve prolapse.[28]

4. Complications include uterine perforation and expulsion. Uterine perforation during insertion is rare. The expulsion rate is 2 to 10 percent within the first year. There is a higher risk of expulsion in nulliparous women and in women with severe dysmenorrhea or excessive blood flow. If a woman experiences expulsion, she has a 30 percent risk of having a second IUD expelled.

5. Copper IUDs reduce the risk of ectopic pregnancy. The rate of ectopic pregnancy is 90 percent lower than in women who use no form of birth control. The rate of ectopic pregnancies is slightly increased in women who use the progesterone-releasing IUD and the use of this IUD is contraindicated in women with a history of ectopic pregnancy. If a woman becomes pregnant while using the IUD, there is a 6 percent risk of an ectopic pregnancy if she uses a copper device and a 23 percent risk if she uses a progesterone-releasing IUD.

Intrauterine devices are the most cost-effective efficacious methods of contraception if used for at least two years.

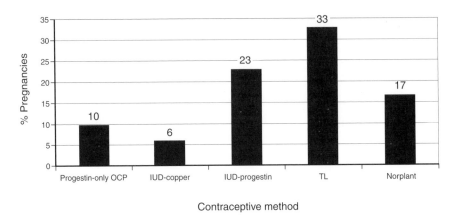

Figure 10.1.   Percentage of pregnancies likely to be ectopic, if the woman becomes pregnant while using a contraceptive method. OCP, oral contraceptive pill; IUD, intrauterine device; TL, tubal ligation.

6.   A woman who conceives while wearing an IUD should be assumed to have an ectopic pregnancy until proven otherwise. This is true of many of the other contraceptive methods as well. Women who become pregnant while using other contraceptive methods are also more likely to have an ectopic pregnancy. A woman who conceives using the subdermal implants has a 17 percent chance the pregnancy is ectopic. A women using progestin-only OCPs who conceives has a 10 percent chance of an ectopic pregnancy and a women with tubal sterilization who conceives has a 33 percent chance (Figure 10.1).

7.   An IUD user who has an intrauterine pregnancy has a 50 percent risk of a spontaneous abortion. This risk can be reduced by the early removal of the IUD, if necessary under ultrasound guidance.

Copper intrauterine devices reduce the risk of ectopic pregnancy.

Contraindications

Nulliparity is not a contraindication to IUD use, although any potential IUD user should be counselled about the potential risk of PID and subsequent sterility.

Contraindications to IUD use are listed in Table 10.13.

Nulliparity is not a contraindication to use of intrauterine devices.

Types of IUDs

1.   The Copper T 380A® is effective for 10 years. Its failure rate is 0.6 percent in the first year of use. It can be used as EC, if inserted within five days of

Table 10.13. Contraindications to use of intrauterine devices (IUDs)

- Pregnancy
- Active or history of pelvic inflammatory disease
- Genital actinomycosis
- High risk of sexually transmitted disease (multiple sexual partners or a partner with multiple sexual partners)
- Uterine or cervical malignancy
- Undiagnosed abnormal uterine bleeding
- Postpartum endometriosis or infected abortion within the preceding three months
- Some immunosuppressed women should also avoid IUDs, such as women with AIDS, because of an increased risk of pelvic inflammatory disease
- The copper IUD is also contraindicated in women with Wilson's disease or copper allergy

intercourse. If used postpartum, it should be inserted within 10 minutes of delivery of the placenta or at six to eight weeks.

2. The progesterone-releasing IUD decreases menstrual flow and dysmenorrhea by 50 percent. There is a greater risk of ectopic pregnancy than with the copper IUD. It requires annual reinsertion and its first-year failure rate is 1.5 to 2 percent.

3. The levonorgestrel-releasing IUD is not currently available in the USA, but is expected soon. It is the most effective of the currently available IUDs. Its first-year failure rate is 0.3 percent. It decreases the risk of PID and can be used to treat both menorrhagia and amenorrhea. It can be used as the progesterone in women who take estrogen for HRT.

Follow-up

1. Patients who do not practice safe sex are probably not good candidates for IUDs.

2. If PID develops, the IUD should be removed.

3. If the patient cannot feel the IUD string and it cannot be visualized, an ultrasound can be used to evaluate whether the IUD is still present and within the uterine cavity.

4. There is no consensus regarding the management of *Actinomyces* reported on a Pap smear of a woman with an IUD. If she is asymptomatic, many clinicians would leave the IUD in place unless there is evidence of upper tract disease. Others would prescribe a two-week course of penicillin.[29] Many experts would also remove the IUD as soon as possible.

Sterilization

Female sterilization

1. Female sterilization has the advantage of being a single decision. It is a safe procedure. Anesthesia, sepsis and hemorrhage primarily cause the mortality rate of 1 to 2 per 100 000. Fortunately, the risk of complications is less than 1 percent.

2. As many as 6 to 22 percent of women report subsequent "regret" over this decision, although only 1 percent choose to reverse the procedure.[30,31] It should be considered a permanent nonreversible option. Although it is possible to reverse the procedure, it is technically difficult and expensive and medical insurance does not typically reimburse this expense. The success rate for subsequent pregnancy is 43 to 86 percent and assisted reproductive technologies are frequently required.

3. The likelihood of regret is increased in women who have been provided with inadequate counselling, women younger than age 30 years, in women who have had postpartum procedures, and among women who have experienced a change in their marital status or relationships. Women seeking this method should be counselled about the availability of other methods, such as OCPs and IUDs that are effective if used consistently, and more easily reversible.

> Sterilization should be considered a permanent nonreversible option.

4. The failure rate is greater than was once appreciated.[32] Consistent use of OCPs or IUDs is more efficacious than tubal ligations. An average of 18.5/1000 women will become pregnant within the 10 year period following sterilization. One-third of the pregnancies that occur are ectopic. The highest risk of pregnancy is among young women sterilized with bipolar coagulation (54.3/1000) or by clip occlusion (52.1/1000).

5. Postpartum tubal ligations are less effective than ligations performed at other "interval" periods. The clinician should have a low index of suspicion in ordering a pregnancy test in the evaluation of an individual with relevant symptoms or signs. A pregnant patient with a previous tubal ligation should be assumed to have an ectopic pregnancy unless proven otherwise.

> A pregnant patient with a previous tubal ligation should be assumed to have an ectopic pregnancy unless proven otherwise.

Male sterilization

1. Male sterilization is the most cost-effective contraceptive method, with a

failure rate of 0.1 to 4 percent. Compared with tubal ligation it is less expensive, results in fewer complications and surgical risks, necessitates a briefer recovery time with less time away from work and poses no long-term health risk.

2. One-half to two-thirds of men will develop sperm antibodies, but their significance is not known.

3. Reversibility is difficult and it should be assumed to be a permanent method. Success of reversal is related to the length of time from the original procedure. The overall success rate is 16 to 79 percent.

> Male sterilization is the most cost-effective contraceptive method with a failure rate of 0.1 to 4 percent.

Special populations

Adolescents[33]

1. Abstinence: Increased abstinence accounted for one-quarter of the drop in the US teen pregnancy rate observed between 1988 and 1995. This decline was caused by lower pregnancy rates among sexually experienced women aged 15 to 19 years, and not because of a rise in abortions. Abstinence, if chosen by the adolescent, should be supported and accompanied by specific peer negotiating strategies. Abstinence programs may help adolescents to postpone first intercourse. It may also be a valid method for teens who have been sexually active to defer further activity.

2. EC: Counselling regarding the availability of EC may provide a back-up method should abstinence not always succeed.

3. Hormonal therapy:
   a. OCPs are excellent choices because teens may benefit from noncontraceptive effects such as more regular periods, less dysmenorrhea, and improved acne.
   b. IUDs are generally avoided.
   c. Injectable DMPA may adversely affect bone density and the associated weight gain may be less well tolerated among adolescents.

4. Condoms should be encouraged to enhance contraception and to provide some protection from STDs. EC should be offered.

5. Abuse: Ten percent of young women report that their first intercourse was either "not voluntary" or "rape". Because coerced sex in this age group is prevalent, clinicians should be vigilant for signs and symptoms of potential abuse.

> Oral contraceptive pills are excellent choices for teens because they may benefit from noncontraceptive effects such as more regular periods, less dysmenorrhea, and improved acne.

Postpartum women

1. Two-thirds of couples resume sexual relations within the first postpartum month; ninety percent within the second month. Because ovulation may occur within three to four weeks and before the first menses, contraception should be initiated either immediately postpartum or within the first few weeks.
2. Although there are theoretical concerns regarding postpartum hypercoaguability, there are no definitive clinical data that justify withholding combined OCPs until two weeks postpartum.
3. IUDs are less likely to be expelled if inserted within 10 minutes following the delivery of the placenta. IUDs should be inserted at six to eight weeks postpartum, if not inserted immediately.

Breast-feeding women[34,35]

1. Lactation provides an excellent and reliable contraceptive method, with a failure rate of 0.5 to 1.5 percent for women who exclusively breast feed at least every four hours and have no menstrual bleeding. Pumping is not an effective substitute for suckling.
2. Another contraceptive method should be initiated if supplemental feedings are given, if there is any decreased frequency of feeds or when the baby reaches six months of age.
3. Spermicides, condoms, and barrier methods are acceptable choices, although diaphragms should be fitted or refitted at approximately six weeks postpartum.
4. Fertility awareness methods may require closer scrutiny of physiological parameters. The basal body temperature may not be reliable in the setting of the normal sleep disruption of the newborn period.
5. Progestin methods (Norplant, progesterone IUD, Depo Provera, and progestin-only pills) are recommended after six weeks postpartum, based upon theoretical concerns and animal studies.
6. The World Health Organization recommends that combined OCPs should be avoided in lactating women within the first six weeks postpartum and used with caution between six weeks and six months. Although the estrogen that is transmitted in breast milk has not been shown to be detrimental to the infant, it does decrease milk supply. The concern is that some mothers may not be

able to compensate by greater milk production. There are essentially no conclusive data in human mothers as to the clinically significant impact of either progestin compounds or combination oral contraceptives.

7. Postpartum sterilization, if chosen, should be performed after the infant's first successful feed, to minimize its impact on lactation, and the mother allowed to nurse again in the recovery room. Alternatively, it can be performed at six weeks postpartum.

Perimenopausal women

1. Many nonsmoking perimenopausal women can continue to use OCPs safely until menopause. The hormone content of OCPs may mask menopausal signs and symptoms. Many women elect to continue OCPs until age 50 to 52 years.

2. To determine whether a woman is menopausal, she can end a pill cycle and use a barrier method of contraception. The serum follicle-stimulating hormone (FSH) should be measured on the seventh pill-free day. If FSH is greater than 30 mIU/mL, she is probably menopausal. A confirmatory FSH can be obtained in six weeks. If this value is also greater than 30 mIU/mL, she can be changed to HRT should she desire, or continue without contraception.

3. The use of OCPs in women over 40 years of age has reduced the risk of hip fracture by 44 percent and strengthened bone density.

Women with disabilities[36]

Women with disabilities may need special attention to their reproductive and contraceptive needs. OCPs are generally safe and effective. Barrier methods may be difficult depending upon the degree of dexterity and motor function. Injectable or subdermal progesteronal agents are efficacious and practical. Surgical interventions may be desirable for women who do not wish to bear children.

Conclusions

Contraception is not a disease but a concern that a couple brings for advice to the physician. Working collaboratively with the woman and her partner, the physician can help them to choose the best method for them, which may not be the most effective one statistically. Close interaction is necessary for good contraception and prevention of unplanned pregnancies.

REFERENCES

1. Connell EB. Contraception in the prepill era. *Contraception* 1999;**59**:7S–10S.
2. Fact sheet with data from The Alan Guttmacher Institute, the National Center for Health Statistics and the Office of Population Affairs of the US Department of Health and Human Services (http://www.ago-usa.org/pubs/fb_contr_use.html).
3. Henshaw SK. Unintended pregnancy in the United States. *Fam Plann Perspect* 1998;**30**:24–9.
4. US Preventive Health Services Task Force. Counseling to prevent unintended pregnancy. In *Guide to Clinical Preventive Services*, 2nd edn. Williams & Wilkins, Baltimore, MD, 1996, pp. 739–54.
5. Fu H, Darroch JE, Haas T, Ranjit N. Contraceptive failure rates: New estimates from the 1995 National Survey of Family Growth. *Fam Plann Perspect* 1999;**31**:56–63.
6. Piccinino LJ, Mosher WD. Trends in contraceptive use in the United States: 1982–1995. *Fam Plann Perspect* 1998;**30**:4–10.
7. Van Look AFA, Stewart F. Emergency contraception. In Hatcher RA, Trussell J, Stewart F et al., eds. *Contraceptive Technology*, 17th edn. Ardent Media, Inc., New York, 1998, pp. 118–36.
8. Glasier A. Emergency postcoital contraception. *New Engl J Med* 1997;**337**:1058–64.
9. Piaggo P, Von Hertzen H, Grimes DA, Van Look PFA. Timing of EC with levonorgestrel or the Yuzpe regimen method. *Lancet* 1999;**353**:721.
10. Cates W Jr., Raymond EG. EC-parsimony and prevention in the medicine cabinet. *Am J Public Health* 1997;**87**:932–7.
11. WHO Task Force on Postovulatory Methods of Fertility Regulation. Randomised controlled trial of levonorgestrel versus the Yuzpe regimen for EC. *Lancet* 1998;**352**:428–33.
12. Trussell J, Rodriguez G, Ellertson C. New estimates of the effectiveness of the Yupze regimen of EC. *Contraception* 1998;**57**:363–9.
13. An emergency contraceptive kit. [Medical Letter.] *Drugs Therapeut* 1998;**40**:102–3.
14. Task Force on Postovulatory Methods of Fertility Regulation. Comparison of three single doses of mifepristone as EC: A randomized trial. *Lancet* 1999;**353**:697–702.
15. WHO Task Force on Postovulatory Methods of Fertility Regulation. Comparison of three single doses of mifepristone as EC: A randomised trial. *Lancet* 1999;**353**:697–702.
16. Kowal D. Abstinence and the range of sexual expression. In Hatcher RA, Trussell J, Stewart F, eds., *Contraceptive Technology*, 17th edn. Ardent Media, Inc., New York, 1998, pp. 137–51.
17. Hilgers TW, Standord JB. Creighton Model NaProEducation Technology for Avoiding Pregnancy: Use effectivness. *J Reprod Med* 1998;**43**:495–502.
18. Raymond E. Contraceptive effectiveness of two spermicides: A randomized trial. *Obstet Gynecol* 1999;**93**:896–903.
19. van Damme L. Advances in topical microbicides. Unpublished paper presented at the XIII International AIDS Conference, 9–14 July 2000, Durban, South Africa.
20. Musaba E, Morrison CS, Sunkutu MR, Wong EL. Long-term use of the female condom among couples at high risk of human immunodeficiency virus infection in Zambia. *Sex Transm Dis* 1998;**25**:260–4.
21. Cerel-Suhl SL, Yeager BE. Update on OCPs. *Am Fam Physician* 1999;**60**:2073–84.
22. Collaborative Group on Hormonal Factors in Breast Cancer. Breast cancer and hormonal contraceptives: Collaborative reanalysis of individual data on 53,297 women with breast cancer and 100,239 women without breast cancer from 54 epidemiological studies. *Lancet* 1996;**347**:1713–27.

23. World Health Organization. *Improving Access to Quality Care in Family Planning: Medical eligibility criteria for contraceptive use.* WHO: Geneva, 1996, pp. 13–26.

24. Larimore WL, Stanford JB. Postfertilization effects of OCPs and their relationships to informed consent. *Arch Fam Med* 2000;**9**:126–33.

25. Kaunitz AM. Intrauterine devices: Safe, effective, and underutilized. *Women's Health Primary Care* 1999;**2**:39–47.

26. Lee NC, Rubin GL, Borucki R. The intrauterine device and pelvic inflammatory disease revisited: New results from the Women's Health Study. *Obstet Gynecol* 1988;**72**:1–6.

27. Skjeldestad FE, Halvorsen LE, Kahn H et al. IUD users in Norway are a low risk for genital *C. trachomatis* infection. *Contraception* 1996;**54**:209–12.

28. Walsh T, Grimes D, Frezieres R et al. Randomised controlled trial of prophylactic antibiotics before insertion of intrauterine devices. IUD Study Group. *Lancet* 1998;**351**:1005–8.

29. Fiorino AS. Intrauterine contraceptive device-associated actinomycotic abscess and *Actinomyces* detection on cervical smear. *Obstet Gynecol* 1996;**87**:142–9.

30. Wilcox LS, Chu SV, Peterson HB. Characteristics of women who considered or obtained tubal reanastomosis from a prospective study of tubal sterilization. *Obstet Gynecol* 1990;**75**:661–5.

31. Rosenfeld JA, Zahorik PM, Saint W, Murphy G. Women's satisfaction with birthcontrol. *J Fam Pract* 1993;**36**:169–73.

32. Peterson HB, Xia Z, Hughes JM, Wilcox LS, Tylor LR, Trussell J. The risk of pregnancy after tubal sterilization. US Collaborative Review of Sterilization Working Group. *N Engl J Med* 1997;**336**:672–7.

33. Darroch JE, Singh S. *Why is Teenage Pregnancy Declining? The Roles of Abstinence, Sexual Activity and Contraceptive Use.* Occasional Report, no. 1. Alan Guttmacker Institute, New York, 1999.

34. Montgomery A. *Contraception in Nursing Mothers: Clinical Update 236.* American Academy of Family Physicians Home Study Self Assessment Program, Kansas City, Missouri, 1999.

35. Hight-Laukaran V, Labbok MH, Peterson AE, Fletcher V, von Hertzen H, Van Look PFA. Multicenter study of the lactational amenorrhea method (LAM): ii. Acceptability, utility and policy implications. *Contraception* 1997;**55**:337–46.

36. Stifel EN, Anderson J. Reproductive and contraceptive considerations for women with physical disabilities. In Rosenfeld JA, ed., *Women's Health in Primary Care.* Williams & Wilkins, Baltimore, MD, 1997, pp. 289–313.

11 Infertility and adoption

Jo Ann Rosenfeld, MD

INFERTILITY

Infertility is the inability of a sexually active couple who desire pregnancy to achieve it after one year.

Impact

1. Approximately 10 to 15 percent of couples have difficulty becoming pregnant. Approximately 9 million American women have impaired fertility, either primary (never having a child) or secondary (trouble having as many children as desired).[1]
2. Family and general physicians can work collaboratively with couples to help them achieve pregnancy. Consultation and referral for reproductive technologies and methods may be needed eventually.

Approximately 10 to 15 percent of couples have trouble achieving pregnancy at sometime in their lives.

Etiology

1. Infertility is a couple's problem. Approximately 40 percent of cases may be caused by ovulation problems. In approximately 10 to 30 percent, there are multiple factors, and male factors make up the remainder (Table 11.1).
2. Chronic disease of either partner may cause infertility.
3. Women's causes of infertility include ovarian and tubal/mechanical factors.
   a. Ovarian failure caused by malnutrition, anorexia, or diabetes can cause infertility.

Table 11.1. Causes of infertility

- Ovulation difficulties
  - Anovulatory cycles – hormonal contraception
  - Hypothalamic/pituitary axis dysfunction
  - Medications
  - Hormonal dysfunction – thyroid, prolactin
- Fallopian tube dysfunction
  - PID, STDs, IUD, after peritoneal infection
- Cervical dysfunction
  - Inimical mucus
- Sexual dysfunction
  - Vaginismus, dyspareunia
  - Erectile dysfunction
- Decreased sperm or sperm motility
  - Medications
  - Varicoele
  - Ductal dysfunction
  - Endocrinopathy
  - Infections – STDs

PID, pelvic inflammatory disease; STD, sexually transmitted disease; IUD, intrauterine device.

b. Ovarian failure can be temporary or permanent (see Chapter 14), and can be caused by an endocrinopathy or polycystic ovary syndrome (PCOS), or be idiopathic.

c. Tubal factors include scarring from endometriosis, PID, or infections, especially gonorrhea or chlamydia.

d. Cervical and uterine factors can include an abnormal uterus (bifid, bicornuate, etc.) or inimical cervical mucus.

e. Use of certain medications, smoking, alcohol, and obesity all reduce women's fertility. A recent retrospective study of more than 400 Danish couples found that drinking as little as one to five alcoholic drinks weekly significantly decreased the likelihood of pregnancy (RR = 0.6) and more than five drinks weekly to less than one-third as likely (RR = 0.3).[2]

4. Men's factors include erectile dysfunction, a low or absent sperm count, abnormal sperm, sperm with altered motility, epidydimal scarring from infections, or medication use.

Use of certain medications, smoking, alcohol, and obesity all reduce women's fertility.

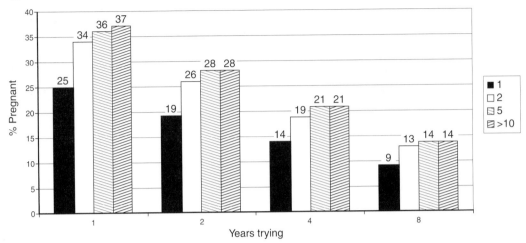

Figure 11.1.   Likehood of getting pregnant by years of trying and sperm count at postcoital test (0 to > 10 motile sperm/mL).

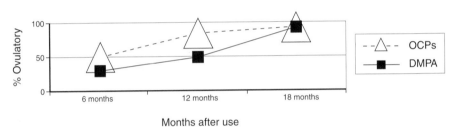

Figure 11.2.   Ovulation after hormonal contraception. OCP, oral contraceptive pill; DMPA, depot medroxyprogesterone acetate.

Evaluation and collaborative treatment

1. The duration of infertility (Figure 11.1) and age of the woman are the most important factors influencing the prognosis for fertility.[3]
2. The history and medication and alcohol use are important factors.
3. After hormonal contraception, ovulation can take months. After discontinuation of OCPs, post-OCP amenorrhea and/or anovulation can last 6 to 12 months. After depot MPA (DMPA), anovulation can last 12 to 24 months (Figure 11.2).
4. A complete physical examination of both the woman and man are essential.
   a. In the woman, medical and medication history, sexual history, gynecological and obstetrical history including pregnancies, abortions, surgeries, episodes of PID or pain, and menstrual history are essential. The physical examination should pay special attention to gynecological examination,

The duration of infertility and age of the woman are the most important factors influencing the prognosis for fertility.

including vaginal, uterine, and bimanual examination. Examination of hair and skin for changes consistent with an endocrinopathy or polycystic ovary syndrome is important.

b. In the man, medical and medication history, sexual history and history of infections or surgery are essential. Physical examination should pay special attention to genitalia. Phimosis and balanitis can cause infected semen that would impede fertilization. Small soft testes may be indicative of impaired spermatogenesis.[3] Varicocoeles may be found in one-quarter of men seeking treatment for infertility.[4]

c. Both partners should be cultured for *Chlamydia*, either by DNA probes or first morning urine specimen cultures.

5. Counselling:

a. Counselling the couple about the normal menstrual and ovulation cycle, about the effect of medications and alcohol on fertility, and about expectations about becoming pregnant are the first steps.

b. General counselling including the following is important:

i. Woman's use of folic acid prophylactically to reduce incidence of spina bifida.

ii. Reducing or quitting smoking and decreasing alcohol consumption should be advised. Smoking also reduces fertility.[5] Few couples seeking fertility counselling know of the need to change certain aspects of their lifestyle, such as quitting smoking and alcohol consumption.[6]

iii. Reduce or change medications (Table 11.2).

iv. The woman should lose weight, if overweight.

v. Stopping the use of vaginal lubricants or gel may cause sperm immobility and impede fertility.[7]

6. Evaluation and treatment (Figure 11.3):

a. The woman should start a three- to six-month basal body temperature log to detect ovulation. Although this seems to be simple, an accurate record takes thoroughness and consistency to achieve. A biphasic curve with 0.4 to 0.5 degree C elevation is consistent with ovulation on the day of degree elevation. Over-the-counter luteinizing hormone (LH) surge predictors to identify ovulation are also available but currently range from $35 to $50 per use.

b. The man should have a semen analysis. Examined within 60 minutes of ejaculation, normal semen contains 2 mL or more of 20 million motile sperm per milliliter or more. The motility of the sperm should show that

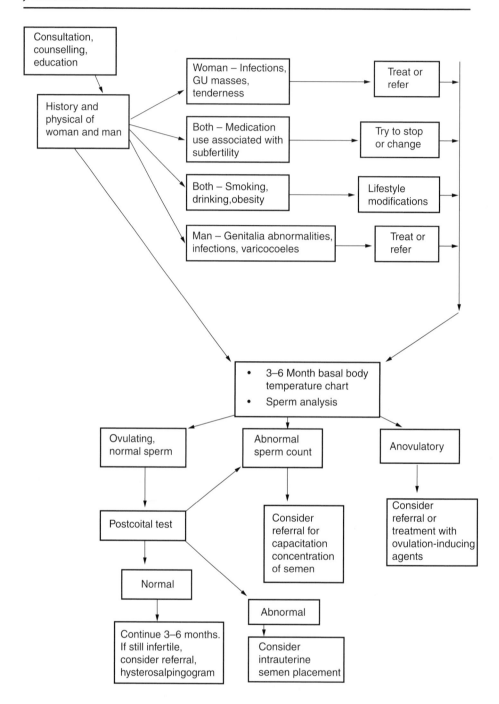

Figure 11.3.   Algorithm for collaborative treatment of infertility by general/family practitioner. GU, genitourinary.

Table 11.2. Substances that decrease fertility

- Medications
  - Nifedipine
  - Sulfasalazine
  - Nitrofuradantoin
  - Tetracycline
  - Cochicine
  - Cancer chemotherapeutic agents
  - Anabolic steroids
- Alcohol
- Smoking

Cigarette smoking reduces fertility.

more than half progress in a forward direction, with more than 25 percent progressing rapidly. Thirty percent or more sperm should have normal forms.[8]

c. If these tests are normal, a postcoital test is suggested. Eight hours after coitus, a cervical specimen is analyzed for sperm motility and normal morphology. However, one RCT found that the use of postcoital tests increased the number of tests but did not improve the overall pregnancy rate.[9]

d. If the woman is not ovulating, the family physician or a consultant can induce ovulation with clomiphene, Pergonal®, gonadotropin agonists or pulsatile gonadotropin-releasing hormone (GnRH) administration. Only physicians with experience using these drugs should start ovulation induction.

i. Clomiphene, a selective estrogen receptor modulator (SERM), is contraindicated in women with liver failure, ovarian cysts, PCOS, and undiagnosed abnormal bleeding or pregnancy. It is associated with multiple births. Treatment is started at 50 mg/day for five days after the start of natural or induced bleeding. Ovulation should occur 5 to 10 days after the final dose, and should be monitored with basal body temperature charts or LH predictors. If ovulation does not occur, the dose can be raised 50 mg in the next cycle. Addition of corticosteroids or estrogen may improve effectiveness.[10]

ii. The next step may be the use of menotropins, including human menopausal gonadotropin (hMG) (Pergonal or Humegon). These can cause high serum estradiol concentrations and ovarian hypertrophy with multiple follicles. These follicles can rupture and cause hemoperitoneum, ascites, and hypovolemia in 8 to 25 percent of women using these drugs.[10] Use of these drugs may require specialist referral.

    iii. Gonadotropin-releasing hormones can be used in pulsatile fashion to induce ovulation.

e. If the semen analysis is abnormal, the man's semen can be capacitated by a variety of methods, concentrating the number of sperm and motile sperm.

f. Alternatively, the sperm can be placed directly into the uterus with a catheter, if the semen analysis is normal and the postcoital test abnormal.

> A woman who is older than age 40 years or who has been trying to become pregnant for more than one year may need a more rapid referral to an infertility specialist.

Indications for more immediate referral for infertility consultant

1. If the woman's age is older than 40 years, or perhaps even 35, an immediate referral may be indicated, especially if the couple have already been trying for more than one year.
2. If a couple has not conceived within three years of stopping contraception, the likelihood of pregnancy in the next year is less than 25 percent,[3] and referral is indicated.
3. Ovarian failure, failure to achieve ovulation within three to six cycles or pregnancy within one year would suggest the need for referral, if the couple is not comfortable using ovulation-inducing drugs.

Specialist function and technology

Anovulation treatment

1. Treated with appropriate ovulation-inducing medications, many women can achieve pregnancy. Medications used for ovulation include clomiphene, gonadotropin agonists or gonadotropin-releasing hormones given in pulses.
2. Women with hyperprolactinemia and amenorrhea-galactorrhea syndrome may be treated with bromocriptine to induce ovulation.
3. Women with PCOS may be treated with metformin, which often induces ovulation. Investigationally, metformin has been studied to examine if it improves the endocrine symptoms of PCOS. Metformin treats insulin sensitivity and causes weight loss. Metformin was given to 43 women with PCOS who were hyperinsulinemic and euglycemic. It was found to cause decreased

weight and BMI and 91 percent resumed menses. The women also had decreased median fasting serum insulin.[11]

4. Women who ovulate and have partners with normal sperm evaluations, especially women with a history of infections may profit from a hysterosalpingogram. This study may identify serious tubal factors for which assisted reproductive technologies will be indicated, or in itself may improve tubal function and help pregnancy.

Assisted reproductive technologies

1. Since the first in vitro fertilization (IVF) baby was born in the UK in 1978, the technologies developed to contribute to fertilization and pregnancy have rapidly increased in effectiveness and complexity. In IVF the egg and sperm are united in a test tube and then the preembryo is transferred to the uterus. GIFT is gamete intrafallopian transfer, where the egg and sperm are placed in the fallopian tube. ZIFT is zygote intrafallopian transfer where the fertilized eggs are placed in the uterus or tubes.

2. The success rates have been increasing, and in some programs reach 25 percent. Actually, the success rates of IVF exceed that of normal conception in a fertile couple in a particular cycle.[3]

3. The success rate for IVF decreases with the woman's age.

4. Ovum donation combined with male partner's sperm and IVF or GIFT can be used for women with premature ovarian failure, ovarian dysfunction caused by cancer, chemotherapy, radiation, maternal chromosomal or genetic abnormalities, or in women who have responded poorly to ovulatory inducers.[8] Older women's eggs are more likely to have mosaicisms, polyploidy and aneuploidy than younger women, and age greater than 40 years may be an indication for ovum donation.

5. Sperm donation can come from the male partner or a male donor. The sperm is then placed in the uterus, or combined with IVF or GIFT. This may be used for male infertility, male ejaculatory dysfunction, after radiation, chemotherapy or surgery for cancer, chromosomal abnormalities or for women without a male partner.[8]

> In vitro fertilization is where the egg and sperm are united in a test tube and then the preembryo is transferred to the uterus.

Psychological effects of infertility

1. Most couples cope well with the rigorous and intricate therapies of infertility.

2. Most couples assume that they will be able to become pregnant when they desire. The inability may lead to frustration, sadness, depression and distancing between the couple. Women who have postponed childbearing to have a career may be used to being in control. When they are unsuccessful at becoming pregnant when they want, they may feel frustrated and angry.

3. The effect of the infertility depends on the age of the couple, the personality and coping styles, preexisting psychopathology, medical causes, and motivations for pregnancy.[8]

4. Infertility can lead to a sense of failure and guilt, that something is wrong with "them" because their body does not function correctly. Body image may be altered.

5. There may be sexual difficulties, avoidance of intercourse, and inability to perform; especially with seemingly "mechanical" tests like postcoital and semen specimens. In one study, up to 5 percent of infertile couples had a history of sexual problems.[12] Anorgasmia, impotence and decreased libido may occur. The spontaneity of sex may disappear.

6. Avoidance of friends and family who have children may occur, further isolating the couple.

7. Psychological counselling before, during and after IVF or other assisted technologies may be indicated. The stress of infertility and its treatment may exacerbate other psychiatric conditions such as mood or anxiety disorders. The ovulation-inducing agents may also exacerbate psychiatric problems or reduce the effectiveness of psychotropic medications.[13]

ADOPTION

Impact

1. Adoption has become a more visible choice. In the USA, approximately 35 000 children are adopted yearly, more than 10 000 from foreign countries.[14]

2. Five percent of children born to unmarried mothers during the 1990s were placed in adoption.[15]

3. Although adoption has become discussed in the media, it is essentially a private choice, both for the birthmother and the adopting family.

The decision to give a child up for adoption is complex, difficult and emotional and may require a physician's counsel.

Caring for the birthmother

1. Although the birthmother no longer may be typically an unmarried adolescent who travels to a distant town to deliver the unwanted child, the decision to place a child for adoption is difficult, disturbing, and emotional. The physician may counsel pregnant or delivered women. The counselling may take time and involvement and additional social service or psychological counsellors.

2. The decision is seldom simple and may change several times in the course of the pregnancy and postnatal time. Financial, social, medical, and personal reasons may all be involved.

3. A complete social, family, medical and personal history is essential, including use of drugs or alcohol. The woman may fear to be explicit.

4. A woman considering placing her child for adoption may be at higher risk for STDs and social problems. She may need additional medical and social supports, even after the placement of her child.

5. Care during delivery should be the same as for all mothers. However, delivery may not be joyful; in fact, the mother may show a sense of grief and bereavement. The mother may not want to see her child or stay on a labor and delivery floor. These wishes should be honored.

6. The adoption may be private or through an agency. Mothers may have significant input into the adoptive parents, even having an "open" adoption. In this, the birthmother may live or visit the adoptive parents before and after adoption.

7. All legal work should be completed in advance.

8. Postpartum, the mother may need social, medical and psychological support.[15]

Care of adoptive mother

1. The adoptive mother may come to the decision to adopt through many avenues, including primary choice or failure of fertility programs. She may be burdened with feelings of failure and grief at the inability to have a child of her own or may choose adoption as a start or addition to her family.

2. The adoptive mother goes through several stages of emotional lability. She and her husband must decide to adopt, deal with the stress, lack of control and insecurity of the adoption process, and deal with the medical, social, and psychological issues of incorporating an adoptive child into the family.

Adoption may be a first or last step, and the woman may have powerful forces for and against adoption and urgency to have a child.[16]

3. The physician may counsel the woman about adoption options, counsel about particular diseases or children with handicaps, treat the child once adopted, help the family to integrate the child into the family, and help to give advice about dealing with the stresses of adoption.

4. Decision: The decision to adopt entails many steps.

    a. Factors such as infertility, failure to produce genetic children, need for children with same genetic make-up, desire to help needy or handicapped children, grief and anger about failure of her own body, single parenting and blended or homosexual parenting, may be part of the decision. Discussing with the mother and her partner the way they came to the decision to adopt will allow the physician to form a therapeutic partnership during this process.

    b. The woman and/or couple must decide if and how they can deal with a special needs or handicapped child, or a child from another ethnic background.

    c. Preadoption counselling may be as important as preconception counselling. The physician should inquire into the mother's daycare and leave options, her insurance status, and back-up. Have the adoptive parents discussed their plans with their family? Adopting older children may need special arrangements for daycare or schooling.

5. Preadoption physical examination.

    a. The physician is often asked to perform the preadoption physical examination. There are some conditions that may make a woman or man hesitant to adopt (Table 11.3).

    b. Any condition that causes an individual to need caregiving themselves, any progressive or terminal disease will probably cause hesitation about ability to adopt a child.

    c. However, it is not the duty of the physician to judge, but to counsel and document. The judge, country, state or adoption agency will have its own requirements. Some countries will not allow a mother older than age 40 years or one who is obese to adopt. In another case, a judge may decide that grandparents or aunts over age 50 years, with some chronic conditions, may be better adoptive parents than strangers.

6. The wait: There is an intensely painful time between the decision to adopt and

The physician may counsel the woman about adoption options, counsel about particular diseases or children with handicaps, treat the child once adopted, help the family to integrate the child into the family, and help to give advice about dealing with the stresses of adoption.

Table 11.3. Medical conditions that may cause hesitation for adoption

Demographic	Age older than 50 years
Medical condition	Any permanent organ failure – liver, renal, heart
	Any progressive or terminal disease – COPD, cancer, AIDS, multiple sclerosis or progressive neurological disease, heart disease, severe type I diabetes
	Any severe disability – blindness, deafness, wheelchair bound, psychiatric illness
Social	History of drug or alcohol abuse
	Family member with progressive disability that may need caregiving
	History of child abuse

COPD, chronic obstructive pulmonary disease.
Data taken from Rosenfeld JA. Caring for the adoptive mother. In Rosenfeld JA, ed., *Women's Health in Primary Care*. Williams & Wilkins, Baltimore, MD, 1977, pp. 363–8.

the arrival of the child. Anticipation, worry, anxiety, legal, and social problems are all factors in this time. Because the woman may be suffering this wait and does not want to tell or burden friends and family, the physician may be need to be available for ventilation and support.

> The physician counsels and observes; she or he does not judge whether the woman is a good candidate to become an adoptive parent.

Fitting the child into the family

1. There will be three types of problem – child illness, social and psychological adaption of the family and child, and handling of discussion of adoption.
2. Foreign or same-country adoptions may have many medical problems, and many unknown problems. These may include infectious diseases, including hepatitis, parasites, AIDS and tuberculosis, malnutrition and lack of immunizations, sexual and physical abuse.
3. The physician can help the family understand cultural differences and obtain help in doing this, including suggesting contacting support and ethnic groups.
4. Sooner or later the family will have to discuss adoption with the child. There are many books, magazines, and support groups that can help. Basically, answering the child's questions honestly is the best method of discussing adoption.

Conclusions

The family physician can often make a positive impact on a couple's quest for fertility, using simple office-based diagnosis and treatment. The physician can help couples through fertility treatment both medically and psychologically, and also through the problems and concerns of adoption.

REFERENCES

1. Jones H. The infertile couple. *N Engl J Med* 1993;**329**:1710–15.
2. Jensen TK, Hjollund NHI, Henricksen TB et al. Does moderate alcohol consumption affect fertility? Follow up study among couples planning first pregnancy. *BMJ* 1998;**317**:505–10.
3. Hargreave TB, Mills A. Investigating and managing infertility in general practice. *BMJ* 1998;**316**:1438–41.
4. Hargrave T, Ghosh C. Varicocele: Does treatment promote male fertility. *Urologe A* 1998;**37**:258–64.
5. Howe G, Westhoff C, Vessey M, Yeates D. Effects of age, cigarette smoking, and other factors on fertility: Findings in a large prospective study. *BMJ* 1985;**290**:1697–700.
6. Olatunbosun OA, Edouard L, Pierson RA. How important is health promotion in the lifestyle of infertile couples? *Clin Exp Obstet Gynecol* 1997;**24**:183–6.
7. Kutteh WH, Chao CH, Ritter JO, Byrd W. Vaginal lubricants for the infertile couple: Effect on sperm activity. *Int J Fertil Menopausal Study* 1996;**41**:400–4.
8. Rosenthal, M. Infertility. In Rosenfeld JA, ed., *Women's Health in Primary Care.* Williams & Wilkins, Baltimore, MD, 1997, pp. 351–69.
9. Oei SG, Helmerhorst FM, Bloemenkamp KWM et al. Effectiveness of the postcoital test: Randomized controlled trial. *BMJ* 1998;**17**:502–5.
10. Carson DS, Bucci KK. Infertility in women: An update. *J Am Pharmaceut Assoc* 1998;**38**:480–8.
11. Glueck CJ, Wang P, Fonataine R, Tracy T, Sieve-Smith L. Metformin induced resumption of normal menses in 39 of 42 (91%) previously amenorrheic women with the polycystic ovary syndrome. *Metabolism* 1999;**48**:511–19.
12. Read J. Sexual problems associated with infertility, pregnancy and ageing. *BMJ* 1999;**318**:587–9.
13. Burt VK, Hendrick VC. *Concise Guide to Women's Mental Health.* American Psychiatric Press, Washington, DC, 1997, pp. 98–9.
14. Quarles CS, Brodie JH. Primary care of international adoptees. *Am Fam Physician* 1998;**57**:2025–32;2039–40.
15. Melina CM, Melina L. The physician's responsibility in adoption, Part I: Caring for the birthmother. *J Am Board Fam Pract* 1988;**1**:50–4.
16. Rosenfeld JA. Caring for the adoptive mother. In Rosenfeld JA, ed., *Women's Health in Primary Care.* Williams & Wilkins, Baltimore, MD, pp. 363–8.

Special issues with lesbian patients

Laura Tavernier, MD, MEd, and Pamela Connor, PhD

Lesbians comprise approximately 5 percent of the female population and have unique and often neglected health care needs.[1] This chapter focuses on the special health care issues associated with the lesbian population. It reviews existing data, as well as proposing strategies for increasing physician recognition and decreasing alienation of the lesbian patient population.[2]

Introduction

1. The distinctive nature of lesbian health care needs does not stem from identifiable biological differences or inherent predisposition to disease processes, but from cultural, social, psychological, and economic factors that have served to marginalize this population from mainstream women's health care.

2. Data regarding lesbian health concerns are scarce. Reasons for the paucity of research are complex.

3. Another difficulty is the invisible nature of the lesbian population. Many lesbians fear stigmatization and discrimination associated with such identification, a finding consistent with all available research in the area. This fear manifests itself when researchers recruit for studies that demand an unbiased representative lesbian population for comparison with their heterosexual counterparts. Given the illusive nature of the lesbian group, recruitment is difficult, thus rendering many of the research studies extremely biased.

4. The absence of comprehensive epidemiological studies regarding lesbian health care needs has led to misunderstanding, mistreatment, and dissemination of misinformation regarding appropriate health care maintenance.

The lesbian population is often invisible, fearing discrimination and stigmatization.

Psychosocial issues

Barriers to health care

1. Invisibility and insensitivity: Lesbians have repeatedly identified, as barriers to appropriate health care, lack of recognition, insensitivity, heterosexist atmospheres, misunderstanding of needs, misinformation, negative attitudes, economic disenfranchisement, and blatant discrimination in health care provision and insurance coverage.[3,4] A 1995 survey found that 55 out of 110 gynecologists (50 percent) stated that they believed that they had never knowingly examined a homosexual woman.[5] In a 1982 survey of all physicians in the San Diego County Medical Society, 23 percent reported themselves as homophobic.[6]

2. Heterosexist bias: Many of the traditional modes of patient–physician communication, such as patient questionnaires and nurse or physician interviews have been heterosexist, which inhibits open communication. Fear of negative consequences has further limited disclosure that would allow more appropriate treatment for lesbians.[7]

3. Health insurance may be a problem because many policies do not allow the inclusion of domestic partners.

Domestic violence

1. Very few studies address lesbian domestic abuse. Most of this literature has used heterosexual data when constructing homosexual partner abuse theories.

2. Theories of human aggression would predict a lower incidence of violence in lesbian relationships. Such theories are based on correlations between power differentials, dominant societal roles, decreased nurturing roles of males, biological predispositions for male aggression, and increased probability of violence.

3. Conversely, biopsychosocial theories would support the hypothesis that rates of domestic violence within lesbian relationships would be similar to that of their heterosexual counterparts. Support of this hypothesis is founded on research, which established that threatened women are equally as capable of aggression as threatened males.[8]

4. Sexual abuse, or victimization within lesbian relationships, is rare, with reported rates of less than 1 percent.[9] Lesbians report being sexually assaulted by males at approximately the same rate as heterosexual women, i.e., approximately 20 percent.[10]

5. The overall prevalence of abuse in lesbian relationships is substantial, with

Table 12.1. Factors that contribute to increased risk for depression and suicide

- Rejection by family, friends, and society
- Verbal and physical abuse by peers
- Homelessness
- Substance abuse

psychological abuse more frequently reported than physical abuse in reviews of available data.[11] The prevalence of psychological abuse in lesbian and heterosexual couple sample populations appears to be similar.[12]

Although sexual abuse within lesbian relationships may be rare, the prevalence of psychological abuse in lesbian and heterosexual couple sample populations appears to be similar.

Depression

1. Data regarding depression in the lesbian population indicate high self-reporting of clinical depression (49 percent) and prior suicide attempts (27 percent).[13] The US Department of Health and Human Services reported that homosexual youths were two to three times more likely to attempt suicide than their heterosexual peers, and accounted for approximately 30 percent of completed suicides.[14]

2. Factors identified as contributing to the increased risk for depression and suicide are listed in Table 12.1.[15] Given the rate of lesbian self-reported depression, the importance of patient–physician trust and disclosure leading to appropriate diagnosis and treatment may have the most significant impact in this area.

3. One study of a general population of lesbians and gay men found that two-thirds reported depression and attributed it to feelings about their sexuality. Eighty-five percent reported verbal insults directed against them because somebody knew or presumed them to be lesbian or gay, and 43 percent stated that they had experienced discrimination or harassment at work. Twenty percent reported that an addiction to alcohol or other drugs was directly related to harassment.[16]

Substance abuse

High rates of reported substance use and abuse among lesbians have been attributed to social rejection, stigmatization, and socialization patterns. Many of these studies relied on sample populations drawn from lesbian bars. This sampling bias is a confounding study variable that weakens study validity and generalization of findings to the general lesbian population.[17] The lesbian population itself has identified substance abuse as a significant health concern. The complexities of substance use and abuse patterns, as well as barriers to treatment, have been documented in recent studies.[18] Barriers to diagnosis and effective treatment are the same as the barriers to health care.[19]

Adolescents

Caught in an already difficult time of finding one's own identity, adolescents with homosexual identities have more difficulties. Confusion about their own desires, homophobia, and frankly inhospitable atmospheres in schools can create depression and anxiety. Studies have shown that gay and bisexual males are at least four times as likely to report a serious suicide attempt, but whether lesbian adolescents have a similar increase in suicide attempts is not known.[20] Other maladaptive behaviors such as running away from home, substance abuse, prostitution and school-related problems may occur. Families and the children themselves may have little information or access to information causing more stress.

Elderly

Elderly lesbians may be in a stable relationship that is mutually supporting, or may be isolated by lack of insurance, status as a widow or surviving spouse, or continued social isolation. Lesbian elderly women have similar concerns of loneliness, failing health, and poverty as nonlesbian elderly women, with the additional concerns of discrimination of age, gender, and sexual orientation. Most elderly lesbians, however, are well adjusted and aging positively.[21]

Health care screening

Cervical cancer screening

1. Misconceptions about the indications for cervical cancer screening of lesbians continue to abound in the medical community.
2. Many lesbians are lead to believe Pap smear screening is unnecessary.[22] From 5 to 9.6 percent of lesbians report never having a Pap smear.[23]
3. Lesbians may be at lower risk for cervical dysplasia and cancer because exclusively homosexual women have an extraordinarily low incidence of STDs, including human papillomavirus (HPV).[24] However, most self-identified lesbians have engaged in heterosexual intercourse before the age of 18

Table 12.2. Factors for cervical dysplasia

- More than four sexual partners
- Age of less than 18 years for the first sexual experience
- Smoking tobacco
- Sexually transmitted diseases
- Oral contraceptive use
- Immunosuppression

years.[25] Additionally, HPV infection has been reported within exclusively lesbian relationships.[26]

4. Risk factors for cervical dysplasia are the same for all women and are listed in Table 12.2. Because cervical dysplasia occurs as frequently in lesbians as in heterosexual women when stratified by risk factors, cervical cancer screening should be performed regularly on all women, with tailoring of the frequency only as indicated with documented normal examinations and accurate assessment of risk factors.

> Lesbians may be at lower risk for cervical dysplasia and cancer because exclusively homosexual women have an extraordinarily low incidence of sexually transmitted diseases, including human papillomavirus.

Breast cancer

1. Self-examination: Monthly breast self-examination has been consistently reported to be lower for the lesbian population than for their heterosexual counterparts, according to the 1987 National Health Interview Survey.[3]
2. Mammography: A comparison of mammography screenings for heterosexual and lesbian women identified a significantly higher rate of mammography screening for lesbians aged 40 to 50 years and older than age 50 years.[27] This finding in and of itself suggests either that lesbians seek health care for breast cancer screening more than the heterosexual population, or that physicians refer more lesbians for screening. The small number of lesbians in these comparison groups makes generalization impossible.
3. Although it has been suggested that lesbians are at a higher risk for breast cancer based on relatively higher BMI and the effects of longer periods of unopposed estrogen on breast tissue, no supporting epidemiological studies exist.

Bone density screening

Data comparing rates of bone density screening between lesbians and heterosexual women are unavailable. Comparison of calcaneal ultrasound measurements (speed of sound (SOS), broadband ultrasound attenuation (BUA), and stiffness index (SI)) between cross-matched heterosexual women and lesbians, revealed no significant difference in bone density. Positive associations across both groups (p < 0.01) were established between BUA and BMI, as well as alcohol consumption.[28]

STDs/HIV

1. Women with a history of exclusively lesbian sexual activity are at lower risk for STDs. Because most women who are self-identified as lesbians have engaged in heterosexual intercourse, the risk of STD infection and transmission is important.
2. There are techniques that result in safer sex. During oral–genital sex, a barrier such as plastic food wrap, condoms, or latex gloves may be used and reduce the likelihood of transmission of sexual disease.
3. One-third of women in the lesbian sample populations are positive for sexually transmitted infection at some point in their lives.[28] STDs and HIV may be transmitted between women by digital to genital, oral to genital, or genital to genital contact, sharing of sex toys, and through artificial insemination.[29]

> Women with a history of exclusively lesbian sexual activity are at lower risk for sexually transmitted diseases.

Family planning and parenting

1. Lesbians who wish to become pregnant have options of heterosexual intercourse or artificial insemination. Many are raising children as single parents or in committed relationships.
2. Obstacles to becoming pregnant are similar for lesbians and single women. These obstacles include social stigmatization, singular financial and emotional support, and insurance practices that preclude reimbursement for fertility services.
3. In addition to the stigmata of single parenthood, lesbians have been regarded as unfit parents by virtue of sexual orientation. Numerous studies examining the psychosocial development of children raised within lesbian households reveal no differences in sexual orientation, gender identity, personality traits, or intelligence as compared with children raised in heterosexual households.[30]

Table 12.3. Questions to be included in revised patient history

- Ask about relationships
  - Are you involved in a significant relationship?
  - Tell me about your living situation. Who shares the household with you?
  - Tell me about the people who are important to you. From whom do you get the most support?
  - Are your relationships satisfying? Are there any concerns you would like to discuss?
- Ask about behaviors
  - Are you sexually active? With men, women, or both?
  - Have your sexual partners in the past been men, women, or both?
  - Have you had a new partner(s) or a change in your sexual activity since your last visit?
  - Do you have any need to discuss birth control?
  - How are you dealing with the issues of "safer sex" and STD risk?

STD, sexually transmitted disease.

Strategies for optimizing lesbian health care

1. The National Institutes for Health have made recent commitments to prospective studies on lesbian health issues; current best knowledge is largely biased and insufficient to answer difficult medical questions. What are well known are methods for optimizing access to, and appropriate utilization of, health care services by lesbians.

2. R. Bell suggests that each practitioner "Be honest with yourself; if you are uncomfortable with gay people, refer the patient to someone else."[31]

3. Make the medical office inviting and comfortable for women of all sexual orientations. Revise your history to be nonheterosexist by including the questions listed in Table 12.3. Preface the history-taking with a statement on the importance of a complete, accurate, history. Accompany this with the reassurance of absolute patient–physician confidentiality.

4. Once acceptance, open communication, and trust are established between the patient and physician, a more detailed history may be undertaken (Table 12.3).

5. In the absence of large bodies of data to support differences in diagnosis and treatment of any minority population, an accurate history, which is dependent on a trusting physician–patient relationship, is essential to legitimate health care practice. Appropriate assessment and management based on an accurate history may be the most effective tool in overcoming barriers to quality health care for lesbians who will otherwise remain marginalized.

Conclusions

There are two major considerations when dealing with lesbian patients – the special concerns of this group and the need to reduce the barriers to health care that lesbians face. There is a need also to increase physician recognition and interaction, and to decrease the woman's alienation from the health care system that often leads to other problems. Special concerns may include depression, substance abuse, adolescent sexual identity problems, and social isolation.

REFERENCES

1. Laumann EO, Gagnon JH, Micheal RT et al. *The Social Organization of Sexuality*. University of Chicago Press, Chicago, 1994.
2. Silvestre, AJ. Gay male, lesbian and bisexual health-related research funded by the National Institutes of Health between 1974 and 1992. *J Homosex* 1999;**37**:81–94.
3. Bradford J, Ryan C. *The National Lesbian Health Care Survey*. National Lesbian and Gay Health Foundation, Washington, DC, 1988.
4. O'Hanlan KA. Lesbian health and homophobia: Perspectives for the treating obstetrician/gynecologist. *Curr Prob Obstet Gynecol Fertil* 1995;**18**:99–133.
5. Good RS. The gynecologist and the lesbian. *Clin Obstet Gynecol* 1976;**19**:473.
6. Matthews HC, Booth MW, Turner JD, Kessler L. Physicians attitudes toward homosexuality: Survey of a California county medical society. *West J Med* 1986;**144**:106–9.
7. Roberts SJ, Sorensen L. Health related behaviors and cancer screening of lesbians: Results from the Boston Lesbian Health Project. *Women Health* 1999;**28**(4):1–12.
8. Fishbein DH. The psychobiology of female aggression. *Criminal Justice Behav* 1992;**19**:99–126.
9. Bradford J, Ryan C, Rothblum ED. National lesbian health care survey: Implications for mental health care. *J Consult Clin Psychol*;**62**:228–42.
10. Koss MP. Detecting the scope of rape: A review of prevalence research methods. *J Interpers Viol* 1993;**8**:198–222.
11. Renzetti CM. Building its second closet: Third party responses to victims of lesbian partner abuse. *Fam Relat* 1989;**38**:157–63.
12. Eastburn J, Sigrist S. Lesbian battering: An exploratory study. Unpublished thesis, GA State University, Sacramento, 1988.
13. Lehmann, JB, Lehmann CU, Kelly, PJ. Development and health care needs of lesbians. *J Women's Health* 1998;**7**:379–87.
14. Remafedi G, French S, Story M, Resnick M, Blum R. The relationship between suicide risk and sexual orientation: Results of a population-based study. *Am J Public Health* 1998;**88**:57–60.
15. US Department of Health and Human Services. *Report of the Secretary's Task Force on Youth Suicide: Alcohol, Drug Abuse and Mental Health Administration*. DHHS publication no. 89-1621, Rockville, MD, 1989.

16. Saunders D, Oxley J, Harvey D. Gay and lesbian doctors. *BMJ* 2000;**320**:2.

17. Skinner WF. The prevalence and demographic predictors of illicit and licit drug use among lesbians and gay men. *Am J Public Health* 1994;**84**:1307–10.

18. Hall JM. An exploration of lesbians' images of recovery from alcohol problems. *Health Care Women Intern* 1992;**13**:181–98.

19. Fifield IH. *On My Way to Nowhere. Alienated, Isolated, Drunk: An Analysis of Gay Alcohol Abuse and An Evaluation of Alcoholism Rehabilitation Services for the Los Angeles Gay Community.* Gay Community Services Center, Los Angeles, 1975.

20. Savin-Williams R. Verbal and physical abuse as stressors in health and risk behaviors among bisexual and homosexual adolescents: Association with school problems, running away, substance abuse, prostitution, and suicide. *J Consult Clin Psychol* 1994;**62**:261–9.

21. Kehoe M. Lesbians over 65: A triply invisible minority. *J Homosex* 1986;**12**:139–52.

22. Ferris D, Batish S, Wright TC et al. A neglected lesbian health concern: Cervical neoplasia. *J Fam Pract* 1996;**43**:581–4.

23. Bradford J, Ryan C, Rothblum ED. National lesbian healthcare survey: Implications for mental health care. *J Consult Clin Psychol* 1994;**62**:228–42.

24. Rankow EJ, Tessaro I. Cervical cancer risk and Papanicolaou screening in a sample of lesbian and bisexual women. *J Fam Pract* 1998;**47**:139–43.

25. O'Hanlon KA, Crum CP. Human papillomavirus-associated cervical intraepithelial neoplasia following lesbian sex. *Obstet Gynecol* 1996;**88**:702–3.

26. Marrazo J. STDs and cervical neoplasia among lesbians: Research review and update. Presentation at the 19th Annual National Lesbian and Gay Health Association Conference. Seattle, WA, July 1996.

27. Lauver DR, Karon SL, Egan J et al. Understanding lesbians' mammography utilization. *Women's Health Issues* 1999;**9**:264–74.

28. Johnson SR, Guenther SM, Laube DW, Kettel WC. Factors influencing lesbian gynecologic care: A preliminary study. *Am J Obstet Gynecol* 1981;**140**:20–9.

29. Carroll, NM. Optimal gynecologic and obstetric care for lesbians. *Obstet Gynecol* 1999;**93**:611–13.

30. Gold MA, Perrin EC, Futterman D et al. Children of gay or lesbian parents. *Pediatr Rev* 1994;**15**:354–8.

31. Bell R. ABC of sexual health. *BMJ* 1999;**318**:452–5.

13 Medical care and pregnancy: common preconception and antepartum issues

Ellen Sakornbut, MD

A general approach to women of reproductive age should include consideration of the possibility of pregnancy. The preconception approach to medical care includes optimization of chronic health problems and risks that may impact negatively on pregnancy. Medical care of women in pregnancy requires understanding of changes in maternal physiology and special risks to the fetus or mother.

The preconception approach to medical care

Preconception counselling

1. Most women do not need special diagnostic testing or therapeutic interventions before the initiation of pregnancy.
2. In general, women without chronic illness may undertake pregnancy with general preventive counselling for a healthy diet, avoidance of substance abuse, regular exercise, and common occupational precautions. This should be a part of preventive care in all young women.

> Most women without chronic disease should be able to undertake pregnancy healthily with advice about a healthy diet, avoiding abuse of substances, taking regular exercise, and common occupational precautions.

Dietary precautions

1. Low levels of serum and red blood cell folic acid have been demonstrated to increase the risk of neural tube defects. In randomized clinical trials, 0.8 mg of folic acid per day decreased the occurrence of neural tube defects and 4 mg of folic acid per day decreased the recurrence of neural tube defects.[1] Lower effective doses were found in nonrandomized trials; current recommendations from the Institute of Medicine and the US Public Health Service recommend 0.4 mg/day in women of childbearing potential.[2] Despite fortification of

cereal grain products with 140 µg of folic acid per 100 g of grain in January 1998, there are concerns that the average daily increase of 0.1 mg of folic acid will be insufficient to achieve the recommended level.

2. A study of low-income women found that significant numbers of women still had diets deficient in folic acid, and most had no knowledge of the foods that they should be eating to achieve a healthy level in their diet.[3]

3. Thus supplementation with a multivitamin or folic acid seems warranted at this time in all women of childbearing potential, and higher levels of supplementation (4 mg/day) in high risk women.[4] These include women with a history of a previous delivery of a child with a neural tube defect, women with a strong family history of neural tube defects, and women on antiepileptic drugs (AEDs).

> Folic acid and a vitamin supplement in all women of childbearing potential is suggested, with higher levels of supplementation (4 mg/day) in high risk women.

Occupational concerns

1. Women with occupational exposures often seek specific information regarding the safety of pregnancy. This complex issue may be viewed from a number of perspectives, including the very personal concerns of the patient for her baby's well-being and her family's economic viability.

2. Although much attention has been focused on maternal occupational exposures, a number of substances appear to cause subfecundity (reduced fertility) or other adverse pregnancy outcomes as a result of paternal exposures.

3. Policies in US industries that exclude women from certain types of job may, therefore, be viewed as discriminatory. From a more general perspective, these exclusionary practices may be shortsighted if they preclude a goal of occupational safety for all workers. Legislative issues have been approached differently in a number of European countries compared with the USA, with special maternity leave status granted to 1 percent and 0.1 percent of women in Denmark and Finland, respectively, whose occupation is judged to be sufficiently hazardous to exclude participation during pregnancy.[5] Table 13.1 provides a brief overview of occupational exposures that are known to be associated with adverse pregnancy outcome.

4. A number of possible exposures have been studied in pregnancy in an effort to decrease associated risk by protective practices. In health care positions, measurements of radiation with exposure to nuclear medicine patients receiving technetium-99m or iodine-131 has led to recommendations on limits for technologists and nursing staff.[6]

Table 13.1. Occupational exposures and pregnancy

Agent	Maternal/paternal exposure	Adverse reproductive outcomes
Herbicides – phenoxy	Paternal	Increased spontaneous abortion OR 2.5–5.0[a]
Pesticides – pyridils, aliphatic hydrocarbons, inorganics, glufosinate	Paternal, maternal	Increased congenital malformations[b], CNS, musculoskeletal, oral clefts
Lead	Maternal	LBW, NTDs[c]
Inorganic mercury vapor	Maternal	Increased congenital malformations[d]
Organic solvents – toluene, chlorphenols, aromatic amines	Maternal	Subfecundity[e], increased congenital malformations[f], fetal growth impairment[g]
Formaldehyde	Maternal	Subfecundity, spontaneous abortions[h]
Radiation	Maternal/paternal	See the text
Anesthetic gases – nitrous oxide, desflurane, sevoflurane	Maternal	Increased spontaneous abortions[i], increase SGA infants[j]
Antineoplastic agents	Maternal	Increased spontaneous abortions[k]
Ethylene oxide	Maternal	Increased spontaneous abortions, preterm birth[l]

CNS, central nervous system; LBW, low birth weight; NTD, neural tube defects; SGA, small-for-gestational age; OR, odds ratio.

[a]Arbuckle TE, Savitz DA, Mery LS, Curtis KM. Exposure to phenoxy herbicides and the risk of spontaneous abortion. *Epidemiology* 1999;**10**:752–60.

[b]Paternal exposure to pesticides and congenital malformations. *Scand J Work Environ Health* 1998;**24**:473–80.

[c]Irgens A, Kruger K, Skorve AH, Irgens LM. Reproductive outcome in offspring of parents occupationally exposed to lead in Norway. *Am J Ind Med* 1998;**34**:431–7.

[d]Elghany NA, Stopford W, Bunn WB, Fleming LE. Occupational exposure to inorganic mercury vapor and reproductive outcomes. *Occup Med (Lond)* 1997;**47**:333–6.

[e]Plenge-Bonig A, Karmaus W. Exposure to toluene in the printing industry is associated with subfecundity in women but not in men. *Occup Environ Med* 1999;**56**:443–8.

[f]Khattak S, K-Moghtader G, McMartin K, Barrera M, Kennedy D, Koren G. Pregnancy outcome following gestational exposure to organic solvents: A prospective controlled study. *JAMA* 1999;**281**:1106–9.

[g]Seidler A, Raum E, Arabin B, Hellenbrand W, Walter U, Schwartz FW. Maternal occupational exposure to chemical substances and the risk for infants small-for-gestational age. *Am J Ind Med* 1999;**36**:213–22.

[h]Taskinen HK, Kyyronen P, Sallmen M et al. Reduced fertility among female wood workers exposed to formaldehyde. *Am J Ind Med* 1999;**36**:206–12.

[i]Smith DA. Hazards of nitrous oxide exposure in healthcare personnel. *Am Assoc Nurse Anesth J* 1998;**66**:390–3.

[j]Bodin L, Axelsson G, Ahlborg G Jr. The association of shift work and nitrous oxide exposure in pregnancy with birth weight and gestational age. *Epidemiology* 1999;**10**:429–36.

[k]Valanis B, Vollmer WM, Steele P. Occupational exposure to antineoplastic agents: Self-reported miscarriages and stillbirths among nurses and pharmacists. *J Occup Environ Med* 1999;**41**:632–8.

[l]Rowland AS, Baird DD, Shore DL, Darden B, Wilcox AJ. Ethylene oxide exposure may increase the risk of spontaneous abortion, preterm birth, and postterm birth. *Epidemiology* 1996;**7**:363–8.

5. Changes in the practice of an occupation may affect risk. A study of hair-dressers examined the high rate of adverse pregnancy outcomes in two time periods, 1986–88 and 1991–93 in hairdressers as compared to sales clerks. However, this study also demonstrated a decline in the higher incidence of spontaneous abortions and low birth weight infants in hairdressers between the two periods.[7] This may be the result of changes in products used by the hairdressers.

6. Exposure to anesthetic gases appears to have diminished among operating room personnel, but exposures may still remain at an unacceptable level for recovery room and surgical intensive care unit personnel caring for recovering postanesthetic patients unless scavenging devices are in operation in these work zones.[8]

7. Radiation:
    a. The issue of occupational exposure to radiation includes workers from several industries.
    b. Lower limits of exposure apply to pregnant women working in fluoroscopy suites than to nonpregnant individuals.
    c. In the USA, these limits apply with voluntary declaration of pregnancy. Appropriate use of protective clothing can limit radiation exposure to recommended levels.[9]
    d. The theoretical risk of cosmic radiation at high altitudes has been included in considering risks encountered by pregnant flight attendants and frequent business travellers. However, little is actually known at this time regarding adverse outcomes.[10] Adverse pregnancy outcomes and childhood malignancy have been studied in workers at nuclear plants. While an increase in stillbirths has been found in offspring with paternal preconception exposure to external ionizing radiation,[11] linkage to childhood cancers seems more clearly demonstrated in mothers with radiation work exposures than it does with paternal preconception exposure.[12]
    e. Additionally, it is important that patients be reassured when studies have failed to demonstrate an association between adverse pregnancy outcomes and occupational exposures. Multiple studies of women working in industry with exposure to electromagnetic fields and video terminals have failed to demonstrate any impact on reproductive health[13] or increase in childhood cancer.[14]

8. Stress:
    a. Occupational stress, especially physical stress, has been widely suspected by physicians and patients of causing adverse pregnancy outcomes, but most women are able to work safely throughout their pregnancies without difficulties. Physical stresses that have been associated with increased rates

of prematurity and low birth weight include prolonged standing, long hours, protracted ambulation, and heavy lifting.[15,16]

b. Studies that examine these issues vary considerably in design and may include confounding factors, thus creating methodological concerns.

c. One study found greater risk of preterm birth, low birth weight, and small-for-gestational age birth in textile workers, food service workers, electrical equipment operators, and janitors when compared with women employed as clerks, teachers, and librarians.[17] Another study found higher rates of preterm deliveries and low birth weight in nurses than in bank workers.[18] A self-report survey of female physicians found higher rates of stillbirth and premature delivery than in the general population.[19]

d. However, a large cohort study of more than 7000 women found only a modest increase in risk of preterm delivery (OR = 1.31) for women whose occupation entailed more than eight hours standing per day. In addition, this study found no increase in low birth weight or preterm delivery with heavy work or exercise after controlling for confounding variables, suggesting that other socioeconomic factors might account for differences in pregnancy outcome.[20]

> Physical stresses that include prolonged standing, long hours, protracted ambulation, and heavy lifting have been associated with increased rates of prematurity and low birth weight.

Chronic medical problems

1. Preconception care of women with chronic illness falls into two categories: the assessment by physician and patient of special risk and the tailoring of care to enhance the safety and optimal outcome of pregnancy. Women should be given the opportunity to understand the extent of risk they may encounter, both to themselves and their babies, during pregnancies complicated by certain chronic conditions, especially chronic cardiovascular, renal, autoimmune, and hemoglobin disorders. See Table 13.2 for a list of disorders with a high risk of maternal complications.

2. Most women will benefit from an understanding that their medical condition should not significantly lessen the chance of successful pregnancy outcome. A number of conditions, including rheumatoid arthritis and multiple sclerosis, demonstrate a tendency to improve during pregnancy. Other conditions, such as inflammatory bowel disease, migraine headaches, and asthma are variable in their clinical course during pregnancy. Women with severe preexisting life-threatening disorders may be managed with good success during pregnancy, including women who have been treated for malignancy and renal transplantation.

Table 13.2. Conditions that pose significant risk to the mother during pregnancy

Condition	Complication
Valvular heart disease, mitral or aortic	Congestive heart failure, pulmonary edema
Marfan's syndrome with dilated aortic root	Aortic dissection
Renal insufficiency related to preexisting diabetes, SLE, HTN, or glomerular disease	Superimposed preeclampsia, CVA
Severe hypertension	Superimposed preeclampsia, abruptio placenta, CVA
Peripartum cardiomyopathy	Congestive heart failure

SLE, systemic lupus erythematosus; HTN, hypertension; CVA, cardiovascular accident.

3. Perinatal consultation may be helpful as a preconception event in a number of high risk medical conditions and in women with an unexplained history of poor reproductive outcomes. A growing list of metabolic problems and hematological disorders are associated with preeclampsia, growth retardation, abruption, and other complications in late pregnancy. These include hyperhomocysteinemia, Factor V Leiden deficiency, Protein C and Protein S deficiency, and the antiphospholipid antibody syndrome. This includes patients with and without preexisting diagnoses of systemic lupus with anticardiolipin antibody or lupus anticoagulant.

4. Treatment of several common disorders should be modified before conception. Asthma generally does not require preconception attention, but patients will frequently have questions about their medications. Heart disease in women of childbearing age encompasses a wide range of conditions, congenital and acquired, with variable risks and prognoses in pregnancy. Women with other neurological disorders, such as paraplegia and mysathenia gravis, may require changes in management, for the most part, during the intrapartum period. Specific preconception issues regarding common chronic disorders are addressed along with antepartum medical care in the latter part of this chapter.

Common conditions that benefit from preconception evaluation and manipulation of treatment include hypertension, seizure disorders, and diabetes.

Assessment of poor pregnancy outcome

1. Consultation with a maternal–fetal specialist should be considered in women with a history of recurrent spontaneous abortion and mid-trimester abortion/

delivery. Recurrent abortion and very preterm birth may be related to uterine structural defects such as müllerian tube defects, uterine leiomyomata, or cervical incompetence. A specific history of preterm premature rupture of membranes may be caused by infection, a modifiable factor, whereas a history of premature labor may be attributable to a number of factors.

2. Patients with recurrent first trimester loss should be offered genetic evaluation. Genetic consultation is applicable for a growing list of preconception concerns, including couples with a previous child with a congenital defect, families with inherited metabolic defects, and couples wherein one partner manifests a genetically transmitted illness.

Common medical issues in the antepartum period

Medication use in pregnancy

1. Throughout the world, medical practitioners became alerted to the potential dangers of medication use in pregnancy with the occurrence of congenital limb defects associated with thalidomide use. Following these events, physicians became much more cautious in using any medication in pregnancy. Several large-scale studies were conducted in the USA by the Collaborative Perinatal Project and the CDC that collected information on drug exposures and outcomes for a large number of medications in many thousands of women. More recently, a number of drug registries have been established to study AEDs, asthma medications, and antidepressants in pregnancy. Ongoing medication surveillance and information services provide both public educational service and data collection, such as the Motherisk program in Toronto.

2. Studies of medication use during pregnancy demonstrate that between 20 and 50 percent of women receive medication other than vitamins and minerals in pregnancy.[21] The most frequently used medications include antibiotics and antinausea medications.

3. The appropriate use of medication in pregnancy hinges on several important clinical principles.

   a. First, practitioners must determine that treatment of an illness or symptoms of an illness is beneficial to the mother and beneficial to the fetus, or, that the risk to the fetus is justified by the potential benefits of treating the mother.

   b. Secondly, accurate information must be available to assess the risk of congenital malformation or other negative impact upon the fetus or pregnancy.

Table 13.3. FDA use-in-pregnancy ratings

Category	Interpretation
A	Controlled studies in pregnant women show no risk to the fetus in any trimester of pregnancy
B	No evidence of risk has been demonstrated in human controlled studies despite adverse findings in animals *or* animal studies show no risk, and human studies are not available
C	Risk cannot be ruled out. Adequate human studies are not available, and animal studies have found risk or are not available. Although there is a risk of harm to the fetus, potential benefits may outweigh risks of use of the medication
D	Positive evidence of risk is demonstrated in human studies. Potential benefits of use may still outweigh risks of use when a safer medication cannot be used or is ineffective for a serious illness
X	Contraindicated in pregnancy because of demonstrated risks that clearly outweigh possible benefits to the patient

Data from Byrd J. Contents of prenatal care. In Ratcliffe SD, Byrd JG, Sakornbut EL, eds., *Handbook of Pregnancy and Perinatal Care in Family Practice.* Hanley and Belfus, Philadelphia, 1996, pp. 21–2.

4. Experts vary in recommendations about medication with some conservative viewpoints expressed caused by concern, not only about teratogenesis, but also about the risk of long-term subtle effects on neurodevelopment.[22] Caution must be balanced, however, with the risk of untreated disease or the intolerability of untreated symptoms. Some medications do not appear to cause malformations, but may be associated with other poor outcome, such as restricted fetal growth, presumably caused by their effects on the utero-placental circulation. Some medications are risky only at certain periods of time within the pregnancy, such as the effect of nonsteroidal antiinflammatory medications on fetal renal function or the risk of kernicterus caused by bilirubin displacement from albumin-binding sites by sulfonamides. Specific knowledge of the mechanism and timing of risk may enhance the clinician's effective utilization of medications in pregnancy.

5. Two systems of classification currently exist for medication use during pregnancy.

   a. Table 13.3 depicts the Food and Drug Administration's (FDA) classification system. This system has been criticized for providing insufficient information about the risks of medications in pregnancy. The requirements to achieve a category A rating are stringent, difficult to achieve, and extremely

Table 13.4. Swedish system of classification for medication in pregnancy

Category A	Drugs that have been used by a large number of pregnant women and have not been shown to produce an increase in malformations or any other harmful effect on the fetus
Category B	Drugs that have been used in a limited number of pregnant women without any definitive disturbance in reproductive outcome
Category C	Drugs that have caused or are suspected of causing disturbance in the reproductive process with potential risk to the fetus without being directly teratogenic
Category D	Known teratogens and other drugs causing permanent damage to the fetus

From Berglund F, Flodh H, Lundborg P, Prame B, Sannerstedt R. Drug use during pregnancy and breast-feeding. A classification system for drug information. *Acta Obstet Gynecol Scand Suppl* 1984;**126**:1–55.

costly to pharmaceutical industries;[23] many medications undergoing FDA approval are not submitted for consideration of category A status because of financial issues. A number of medications that are currently classified as "B" are poorly studied in human pregnancy (e.g., leukotriene receptor antagonists) and should be used only with careful consideration. Other medications currently classified as category C are frequently used in pregnancy for indications and have good safety records.

b. The Swedish catalogue of registered pharmaceutical specialties (FASS) uses a different system to categorize medication, included in Table 13.4.

c. The TERIS protocol for cataloguing teratological information utilizes all available sources of information and assigns ratings of teratogenic risk of "none", "minimal", "small", "moderate", "high", and "undetermined". A 1990 overview of this resource demonstrated that approximately half of the commonly prescribed medications had insufficient information to assess teratogenic risk. Of the drugs that could be rated, over 90 percent were rated as minimal risk or less.[24]

d. Important initiatives underway include drug registries regarding medication for common chronic illness, such as epilepsy and asthma. It is to be hoped that these projects will provide better information for clinicians about the treatment of medical illness in pregnancy.

Between 20 and 50 percent of women receive medication other than vitamins and minerals during pregnancy.

JOHN M~~~~~ ~~~~~~~~~~ (
AVRIL ROBARTS LRC
TEL. 0151 231 4022

Medical care in pregnancy

Physiological changes

1. Physiological changes of pregnancy are listed in Table 13.5, along with poss-
    ible implications for medical care in pregnancy. Most changes are somewhat
    dependent on gestational age. While the most sensitive period with respect to
    congenital malformations occurs during the first trimester in organogenesis,
    the increase in plasma volume, cardiac output, and glomerular filtration does
    not begin to manifest significantly until the second trimester, with peak effect
    noted by 30 weeks' gestation.

2. In general, the fetus poorly tolerates maternal hypotension, hypoxemia, hy-
    povolemia, and acidosis. Thus, while a nonpregnant patient may tolerate
    greater physiological stress, for example mild hypoxemia during an acute
    asthmatic attack, the pregnant woman should be treated vigorously for the
    acute attack with medication and more liberal use of supplemental oxygen.
    More importantly, preventive measures should be undertaken, whenever
    possible, to avoid acute exacerbations of chronic disease, such as diabetes and
    asthma.

Diagnostic measures

1. Diagnostic measures that would normally be employed to evaluate the acute
    complaint can almost always be used in pregnancy. Ultrasound modalities
    (abdominal, renal, breast, and vascular) are considered safe, although there
    may be some decrease in accuracy of venous studies caused by the enlarged
    uterus and inferior vena cava compression. If a renal ultrasound is insufficient
    for evaluation of suspected nephrolithiasis, a single-shot intravenous pyelo-
    gram may be utilized to assist in management.

2. Diagnostic peritoneal lavage and/or computed tomography (CT) scan of the
    abdomen may be indicated in the evaluation of trauma; this modality should
    not be neglected if clinically indicated, since the single greatest cause of
    mortality for pregnant women is motor vehicle accidents.

3. Pneumonia is another illness that may cause both maternal and perinatal
    mortality and morbidity; physicians should not hesitate to utilize chest X-rays
    with shielding as indicated by patient symptomatology.[25]

4. Flexible sigmoidscopy has been studied in all trimesters, with efficacious

> Diagnostic measures that would normally be employed to evaluate the acute complaint can almost always be
> used in pregnancy.

Table 13.5. Physiologic changes of pregnancy and implications for medical care

System	Change	Medical issues
Cardiovascular	Heart rate increases, blood volume increases, increased cardiac output, decreased systemic vascular resistance, and MABP	Detection of shock may be delayed until large volume loss has occurred. Distribution of medication may be altered
Nervous system	?Fluid retention, mechanical effects	Multiple compression neuropathies more common in pregnancy – carpal tunnel, Bell's palsy, meralgia paresthetica
	Decreased seizure threshold, altered medication distribution and metabolism	Increase in frequency of seizures in many patients with epilepsy
Pulmonary	Decrease in FRC, increase in minute ventilation and respiratory rate	Altered interpretation of ABGs, e.g., with asthma, mild compensated respiratory alkalosis normal
Gastrointestinal	Smooth muscle relaxation secondary to progesterone	Constipation
	Multiple changes in bile lithogenicity	Incidence of gallstones increased with parity
	Increased intraabdominal and intragastric pressure, smooth muscle relaxation of lower esophageal sphincter caused by progesterone	Esophageal reflux/"heartburn" symptoms
	Decreased gastric emptying	Increased tendency for aspiration
Hematological	Increased coagulation factors except XI and XIII, which may be decreased, decreased antithrombin III	"Hypercoagulable state"
	Increased WBC, ESR	Interpretation of CBC
Renal	Increased renal plasma flow	Decrease in creatinine, uric acid, increased creatinine clearance
Endocrine	Increased TBG and bound T4 caused by high estrogen state	
	Impaired glucose tolerance, acceleration of starvation ketosis	Maintenance of euglycemia in diabetes requiring close management

MABP, mean arterial blood pressure; FRC, functional residual capacity; ABG, arterial blood gas; WBC, white blood cell; ESR, erythrocyte sedimentation rate; CBC, complete blood count; TBG, thyroxin-binding globulin.

diagnosis of gastrointestinal bleeding and without negative outcomes.[26]

5.   Nuclear medicine studies should be avoided.

6.   Multiple surgical series at this time support the safety and utility of laparascopic surgery during pregnancy.[27] Although timing of surgical procedures in pregnancy is best during the second trimester to decrease the risk of abortion and premature labor, surgical treatment of trauma, appendicitis, and biliary tract disease may not be able to be delayed.

> The best time to perform surgical procedures in pregnancy is during the second trimester to decrease the risk of abortion and premature labor.

Medical care of common acute conditions

1.   Self-limited acute illnesses can often be treated with nonpharmacological measures and/or common symptomatic medications. Table 13.6 lists some symptoms and medications that may be used for a variety of common problems. Table 13.7 includes medications for infection.

2.   Systemic corticosteroids should be used, as indicated, for treatment of severe asthma attacks.

3.   Many antiarrhythmic medications have been used in pregnancy with good outcome.

4.   Genitourinary infections: Pregnant women commonly present with genitourinary infection. Although a number of medications may be designated as category C, topical use of these medications has not been associated with significant absorption, and the risk of use seems minimal. Examples include antifungal preparations for *Candida* vulvovaginitis and limited use of topical corticosteroids. Treatment of symptomatic vaginal trichomoniasis with metronidazole continues to be a concern to some clinicians because of theoretical concerns of teratogenicity, despite metaanalysis and large population-based studies demonstrating no increased risk of defects,[28,29] and long-term population-based studies showing no increase in childhood cancers.[30]

5.   Viral infections: Acute viral infections are often viewed as benign, self-limited conditions outside of pregnancy. During pregnancy, viral illness (such as rubella) may represent a threat to the fetus or a potentially serious threat to the mother's health. The 1918 Spanish influenza pandemic manifested disproportionate mortality in pregnant women.

6.   Herpes: Genital herpes is a common recurrent problem in young women. It is associated with potential neonatal morbidity and mortality, and an increased rate of cesarean delivery. Although prophylaxis with acyclovir to prevent late

Table 13.6. Symptomatic treatment in pregnancy

Symptom	Medication	FDA category	Comment
Pain, fever	Acetominophen	B	No associated defects, fetal hepatotoxicity with maternal overdose
Pain	Codeine, hydrocodone	C	Slight increase defects? Category D with prolonged use
Cough	Dextromethorphan	C	No fetal defects
Pruritus	Diphenhydramine	B	
Nausea, vomiting	Dimenhydrinate	B	
	Promethazine	C	
	Ondansetron	B	
Diarrhea	Loperamide	B	
	Diphenoxylate	C	No associated defects
Heartburn/ dyspepsia	H2 blockers	B	
	Antacids		
	Sucralfate	B	
Constipation	Fiber or Mg laxative		
Eczema/contact dermatitis	Hydrocortisone cream	C	Systemic absorbtion minimal with proper use
Nasal congestion	Pseudoephedrine	C	No associated defects
	Ipatropium bromide nasal spray	B	
Allergic rhinitis	Cromolyn	B	
	Nasal steroids	C	Minimal systemic absorption
	Loratidine	B	
	Fexofenadine	C	

trimester genital herpes infection has not clearly been demonstrated to decrease cesarean deliveries, its use does decrease the number of infections at term.[31] Antiviral prophylaxis decreases the cost of delivery when compared to standard therapy (cesarean for women presenting with active herpes in labor).[32,33]

Table 13.7. Medications for treatment of infection in pregnancy

Medication	FDA category	Comment
Antibacterial		
Penicillins	B	
Cephalosporins	B	
Erythromycin	B	Hepatotoxicity with estolate
Tetracycline	D	Dental staining 2nd, 3rd trimester, hepatotoxicity
Aminoglycosides	C	Fetal ototoxicity
Sulfonamides	B	
Azithromycin	B	
Clarithromycin	C	Defects with animal studies, human studies inconclusive
Metronidazole	B	
Quinolones	C	Cartilage damage in immature animals and humans, ?other defects
Trimethoprim	C	Possible 1st trimester risk (folic acid antagonist)
Nitrofurantoin	B	No fetal defects
Spectinomycin	B	RxGC in penicillin allergy
Antivirals		
Amantadine	C	Possible teratogen
Zidovudine	C	
Oseltamivir	C	
Zanimivir (inhalant)	B	
Rimantadine	C	Embryotoxic in animal studies
Acyclovir	C	No associated defects/adverse effects
Antifungals		
Amphotericin	B	No known defects
Fluconazole	C	Teratogen with continuous dose 400 mg/day, probably very low risk with short course at low dose
Antituberculous		
Ethambutol	B	No associated defects
Isoniazid	C	No clear associated defects, prophylaxis for newborn with vit. K
Rifampin	C	No fetal defects, prophylaxis for newborn with vit. K
Streptomycin	D	Fetal ototoxicity

RxGC, treatment for gonorrhea; vit., vitamin.

7. Hepatitis:
   a. Hepatitis A infection does not pose a threat to the newborn via perinatal transmission.
   b. Hepatitis B infection may be transmitted perinatally, as well as hepatitis C, D, and E. Immunization against hepatitis B and administration of hepatitis B immunoglobulin immediately at birth is protective against perinatal transmission of hepatitis B and D.[34]
   c. Infectivity is related to the concomitant presence of HBsAg and HBeAg (hepatitis Bs and Be antigens). There is approximately 80 to 90 percent transmission if both are present, and 15 percent or less transmission if the mother is HBeAg negative.[35]
   d. Hepatitis C infection is rarely transmitted perinatally. Transmission usually occurs in mothers with concomitant HIV infection or with very high levels of hepatitis C virus RNA. Routine screening is not recommended, since no treatment is available to prevent infection, but women at high risk may warrant evaluation, and pediatric follow-up is warranted if hepatitis C is detected,[36] because of the risk of chronic liver disease in the infant.

Medical care of chronic illness in pregnancy

Diabetes

1. Preconception:
   a. Patients with preexisting diabetes should be euglycemic during the critical period of organogenesis. Congenital abnormalities are increased if first trimester control is poor. For most patients, the chance of a good pregnancy outcome for a diabetic is improved if pregnancy is planned.
   b. Preconception care of type I diabetic women results in earlier prenatal care, lower glycosylated hemoglobin levels, fewer antepartum hospitalizations and fewer hospital days, and decreased intensity and length of stay for newborns. A multicenter prospective study of women who received preconception care versus women who received only antepartum care showed cost savings of more than $(US)30 000 per patient.[37] A study in the UK found that women attending a preconception clinic were more likely to be in a stable relationship and to be nonsmokers. Preconception care improved outcomes and a 50 percent decrease in neonatal intensive care unit admission rate.[38] Therapeutic alliances with diabetic women of childbearing age must start before conception.
   c. For adolescent diabetics, developmental changes and parental control

issues may clash; unprepared pregnancy is a risk for these young women. Physicians must educate both parents and patients about the risks of pregnancy. In this situation, one therapeutic goal may be the establishment of a negotiated agreement between adolescent and parents where graduated autonomy and responsibility for self-care are emphasized.

   d. Type II diabetic patients may not be identified in the medical care system before or during early pregnancy. Patients with gestational diabetes should have normalized glucose status at the six-week postpartum check-up. The identification of unrecognized type II diabetes is enhanced by careful follow-up of all women with a history of gestational diabetes. Screening for diabetes should be considered prior to conception in women with increased risk factors of obesity, unexplained fetal death, strong family history, and a history of macrosomic babies, especially in ethnic groups with a high prevalence of diabetes.

2. Antepartum care:

   a. Screening of patients with increased risk for diabetes: Patients with a preexisting history of any glucose intolerance, morbid obesity, strong family history, or other high risk factor should receive glucose challenge testing (50 g of glucola with one hour blood glucose level) as soon as possible in early pregnancy to screen for undiagnosed type II diabetes.

   b. Most patients with type II diabetes will require insulin during pregnancy; oral agents are not indicated.

   c. Patients who have a prior history of gestational diabetes but are documented with normal glucose testing in early pregnancy may benefit from a prudent diet during pregnancy to avoid excessive weight gain and concentrated fats or simple sugars. These patients should be screened again at 28 weeks as in routine prenatal care.

   d. Normal changes in glucose metabolism in pregnancy: Glucose, amino acids, and ketones pass through the placenta to the fetus. Maternal free insulin and glucagon do not traverse the placenta; fetal insulin secretion and glucagon secretion respond to levels of substrate presented to the fetus. Ketones may be associated with adverse effects upon neurophysiological development of the fetus. The "starvation" state is accelerated with pregnancy, and fasting hypoglycemia occurs after 12 hours in the fasting state, with fasting ketosis occurring as well. The "fed" state in pregnancy is characterized by hyperinsulinemia, hyperglycemia, and diminished sensitivity to insulin by multiple tissues (relative insulin

For most diabetic women, the chance of a good pregnancy outcome is improved if pregnancy is planned.

resistance). This tendency is greatest in the third trimester. Multiple hormones in pregnancy, human placental lactogen, prolactin, estrogen, and progesterone, all contribute to alterations in glucose metabolism and insulin resistance.[39]

Ketones may be associated with adverse effects upon neurophysiological development of the fetus.

3. Diabetes in pregnancy:
    a. All pregnant diabetics, regardless of diabetic type, benefit from home glucose monitoring. Well-controlled gestational diabetics may not need testing more than twice a day, but patients using insulin should self-test four times a day (fasting, before food, and before sleep) and as needed. All patients should keep a log of diet, fingerstick blood sugar, and activity. Treatment goals include avoidance of hypoglycemic spells, fasting blood sugars less than 100 mg/dL, and two-hour postprandial blood sugars of less than 120 mg/dL.
    b. Diabetic women may benefit from mild to moderate exercise as an adjunct to blood sugar control during pregnancy.
    c. Serum alphafetoprotein levels are lower in diabetic women than in those without diabetes, and a lower threshold is set for detection of neural tube defects, usually 2.0 multiples of the mean. Diabetic women should receive careful sonographic assessment of fetal anatomy at between 16 and 20 weeks of pregnancy along with early establishment of gestational age. Although earlier work suggested increased risk of cardiac malformations in pregnancies with initial glycosylated hemoglobin over 8.5 g/dL, recent studies have not supported this conclusion. Some authors recommend fetal echocardiography in all women with preexisting diabetes.[40,41]
    d. Most type I diabetics should be followed during pregnancy with a system that is designed to provide maximal support for diabetic maintenance. Hypoglycemia is more common during the first trimester. Insulin needs increase as pregnancy progresses. If maternal insulin secretion fails to keep pace with glucose levels in pregnancy, resulting fetal hyperglycemia stimulates fetal insulin production and a growth-hormone-like effect on fetal growth. The contribution of strict control to avoidance of fetal macrosomia remains controversial, but some authors suggest that growth acceleration occurring in the late second trimester appears to be triggered by unsatisfactory glucose control in the first half of pregnancy.[42,43]

Diabetic women may benefit from mild to moderate exercise as an adjunct to blood sugar control during pregnancy.

Table 13.8. Factors that relate to prognosis of diabetic women in pregnancy

- Presence or absence of microvascular disease
- Women with microvascular disease (White Class D, E, and FR) are more likely to develop acute hypertensive complications than those without microvascular disease
- Degree of metabolic control
  - Poor first trimester metabolic control increases congenital malformation
  - Poor third trimester metabolic control is more likely to develop polyhydramnios, deliver prematurely, and deliver a large-for-gestational age baby

Data from Reece EA, Francis G, Homko CJ. Pregnancy outcomes among women with and without diabetic microvascular diseases (White's Class B to FR) versus non-diabetic controls. *Am J Perinatal* 1998;**15**:549–55.

e. Tight control should be achieved with one of several possible regimens.

f. Prognostic factors: Women with preexisting diabetes are more likely to experience maternal and neonatal complications than are women without diabetes (Table 13.8). Women with microvascular disease (White Class D, E, and FR) are more likely to develop acute hypertensive complications than those without microvascular disease.

> Women with preexisting diabetes are more likely to experience maternal and neonatal complications than are women without diabetes.

Hypertension

1. Preconception care:

   a. Many women with chronic hypertension experience normal pregnancy outcome.

   b. Mild chronic hypertension (diastolic blood pressure < 100 mmHg) is not significantly associated with increased risks for preeclampsia or severe exacerbations of blood pressure during pregnancy.

   c. Moderate hypertension (diastolic blood pressure 100 to 105 mmHg) is associated with a slightly increased rate of complications. Approximately one-third of patients with diastolic blood pressure consistently > 105 mmHg or those who require high dose or multiple antihypertensives for control experience complications of superimposed preeclampsia. The risk of abruption is also increased.

   d. A prepregnancy creatinine value of > 3.0 mg/dL or blood urea nitrogen (BUN) value of > 30 mg/dL indicates a much greater risk of maternal or fetal complications.

e. These issues may be discussed in preconception counselling, and remediable factors (such as smoking or suspected secondary hypertension) addressed.

f. Hypertensive patients should be switched to a calcium channel blocker, alpha-methyldopa, or hydralazine from angiotensin-converting enzyme inhibitors if they intend to become pregnant. Patients who are on a beta-blocker or thiazide for hypertension need not be switched prior to conception, if they are on acebutolol, pindolol, and oxprenolol. Diuretics are problematic because of associated metabolic abnormalities and volume depletion. They should generally only be used for selected cardiac problems to avoid an effect upon uterine blood flow. The chronic antihypertensive medication with the longest safety record in pregnancy is alpha-methyldopa. Its limitations include sedation at higher doses. Calcium channel blockers have been studied with respect to their effect on uterine blood flow and appear to be relatively safe in the sustained release form. Nicardipine and nifedipine are preferable to verapamil because of possible effects upon the fetal atrioventricular conduction. However, caution must be exercised in the use of calcium channel blockers in the intrapartum setting to avoid severe hypotension, especially in combination with magnesium sulfate.

Hypertensive patients usually undergo normal and healthy pregnancies and should be switched to a calcium channel blocker, alpha-methyldopa, or hydralazine from angiotensin-converting enzyme inhibitors.

2. Antepartum care:

a. Many hypertensive patients merit a trial off medication to see whether blood pressures will normalize by the end of the first trimester. If the patient is able to maintain the normotensive state, this has positive prognostic value and simplifies concerns regarding short- and long-term effects of medication.

b. Hypertensive medication has not been shown to prevent the onset of superimposed preeclampsia, intrauterine growth restriction, or placental abruption. It has been shown to decrease the risk of cerebrovascular accident in pregnancy. Guidelines derived from the Cochrane Perinatal Database recommend institution of hypertensive medication for preexisting hypertension at gestational ages less than 28 weeks with a blood pressure of 140/90 and after 28 weeks for blood pressures of 150/95.[44]

Hypertensive medication has not been shown to prevent the onset of superimposed preeclampsia, intrauterine growth restriction, or placental abruption.

Table 13.9. Common seizure medications and pregnancy

Medication	Fetal effects	Comments
Diphenylhydantoin	Fetal hydantoin syndrome with craniofacial/other abnormalities, coagulopathy in 50 percent of newborns, neurodevelopmental change	Vit. D and calcium supplementation, vit. K last 2 months of pregnancy, monitor newborn, may need dosage increase
Carbemazepine	Craniofacial abnormalities, neurodevelopmental issues, ? less than DPH	Dosage adjustments
Phenobarbital	Lower teratogenic risk	Vit. D, vit. K, sedation in the newborn with breast feeding
Valproic acid	NTDs, cardiac defects, increased with > 1000 mg/d	AFP/genetic amnio/consultative ultrasound
Newer AEDs – lamictal, gabapentin, etc.	Limited published information	Use monotherapy if possible
Trimethadione	> 75 percent anomalies	Stops preconception
Ethosuximide	6 percent anomalies or fewer	Drug of choice for petit mal

DPH, diphenylhydantoin; NTDs, neural tube defects; AFP, alphafetoprotein; vit., vitamin; AED, antiepileptic drug.

Seizure disorders

1. Preconception care:
    a. Patients with seizure disorders will need counselling about the increased risk of birth defects and epilepsy in the offspring of epileptic patients.
    b. In addition, none of the currently used seizure medications is currently without risk. Although some patients who have not had a seizure in years may be considered for a preconception trial off medication, many patients will need AEDs during pregnancy to prevent uncontrolled seizures and their attendant risks. Patients who are being treated for absence or petit mal seizures may "outgrow" their need for medication during adolescence and should be considered for medication discontinuance. Those still needing medication should be switched to ethosuximide because of the high incidence of birth defects from trimethadione.
    c. Of the older AEDs for generalized seizures, the best safety record for

pregnancy belongs to phenobarbital, but many patients will not experience good control of seizures with this medication. Phenytoin has been associated with a syndrome of minor malformations as well as alterations in neurodevelopmental function; carbemazepine has a similar record, although perhaps to a lesser extent, expecially when compared side-by-side with phenytoin. Valproic acid carries a significant risk of malformations, including cardiac and neural tube defects; risk of teratogenesis is dose dependent, with risks increasing at doses over 1000 mg/day. Very little information is available on newer AEDs such as lamotrigine, gabapentin, and lamictal. Table 13.9 contains common seizure medications and known risks and precautions associated with their use.

    d. Patients with a remote history of seizure disorder and no seizures in many years should be considered for a trial off medication before conception. Medication should be adjusted or changed to the safest medication that produces good control of seizures, and monotherapy should be adopted if at all possible. Folid acid should be prescribed for patients on most AEDs at a dose of 4 mg/day.

2.   Antepartum care:

    a. Patients treated with phenobarbital, phenytoin, and primidone therapy need supplemental vitamin D, 1000 mIU/day. A careful ultrasound anatomical survey should be performed at between 16 and 20 weeks' gestation, to evaluate for cardiac, neural tube, renal, gastrointestinal, and limb abnormalities. All patients treated with valproic acid should be evaluated with serum alphafetoprotein (AFP) and considered for a consultative ultrasound scan or for amniocentesis for AFP because of the risk of neural tube defect.

    b. Vitamin K prophylaxis is provided in the later stages of pregnancy to prevent hemorrhagic disease of the newborn.

Asthma

1.   Preconception care:

    a. Severe asthma can be managed during pregnancy with most commonly used medication.

    b. However, at the current time, there is very little information available about human teratogenesis from leukotriene receptor antagonists such as montelukast and zafirlukast and from zileuton. Although the leukotriene receptor antagonists are listed as class B in pregnancy, a more conservative approach at this time would maximize the use of beta-agonists, inhaled steroids, cromolyn, theophylline, and/or systemic steroids as needed. Patients who are not currently stabilized on leukotriene receptor antagonists or 5-lipoxygenase inhibitors and are intending pregnancy should not be started on them. Patients who have achieved good success on these agents and experienced control problems otherwise should be evaluated individually for possible risks and benefits and provided with information to assist in joint decision-making.

2. Antepartum care:
    a. All patients with asthma should receive influenza vaccination if they will be pregnant during the 'flu season. The CDC recommend this to be given outside the first trimester, although influenza vaccination has not been demonstrated to be a teratogen.
    b. Patients with mild asthma should be considered for inhaled corticosteroids, even if they are not currently on such medication, because of several factors:
        i. Approximately 30 to 40 percent of women will sustain increased severity of asthma or need increased medication for control.[45]
        ii. Inhaled steroids have been shown to produce a fourfold decrease of acute attacks in pregnancy.[46]
        iii. Patients may be instructed in home peak flow monitoring and given protocols for self-management and when to contact the physician or come to the emergency room.

> Severe asthma can be managed during pregnancy with most commonly used medications.

Heart disease

1. Preconception care:
    a. Patients with heart conditions who are considering pregnancy range from individuals with no functional impairment, such as women with mitral valve prolapse (MVP), to women with significant structural, functional, and/or electrophysiological disorders of the cardiovascular system.
    b. Patients with MVP on beta-blockers should be considered for adjustment of medication in the antepartum period. Some beta-blockers have been associated with fetal growth restriction. MVP does not appear to have any significant affect on pregnancy outcome, and the degree of prolapse may improve during pregnancy.[47]
    c. Women with repaired congenital heart defects may experience completely normal function or may continue to experience electrophysiological disorders caused by alterations in the conducting system following a complex

repair. With the exception of asymptomatic women who had a successful repair of a ventricular septal defect, atrial septal defect, or patent ductus ligation in childhood, women with a history of complex congenital heart disease should be evaluated by a cardiologist familiar with their condition as a preconception measure. If significant patient risk is present, caused by pulmonary hypertension, continued shunting, or poor cardiac function, the consultant may be able to assist the patient in making a more informed decision regarding pregnancy. This consultant may also be helpful in suggesting whether a significant genetic risk is present for congenital heart disease in the offspring, determining the need for fetal echocardiography. Many of these women will require ongoing cardiology consultation for management during pregnancy.

d. Women with rheumatic valvular heart disease should be evaluated for functional status and receive preconception counselling regarding the risk of pregnancy. Approximately 40 percent of women with valvular heart disease become symptomatic for the first time during pregnancy. Rheumatic fever prophylaxis should be provided (daily penicillin or monthly benzathine penicillin). Patients in whom valvular procedure or replacement is contemplated should generally undergo such procedures before conception, because the increased demands upon the cardiovascular system may cause deterioration during pregnancy. Valvular replacements and other surgeries requiring intraoperative cardiopulmonary bypass are accompanied by high fetal loss rates.[48]

e. Patients with a previous diagnosis of cardiomyopathy, peripartum or otherwise, should be cautioned about cardiac decompensation during pregnancy and the risk of recurrent peripartum cardiomyopathy.[49]

2. Antepartum and intrapartum issues:

a. Subacute bacterial endocarditis prophylaxis should be provided for the intrapartum setting according to standard protocols of the American Heart Association. For most patients, intrapartum prophylaxis will consist of ampicillin and gentamycin. See Table 13.10 for cardiac conditions requiring SBE prophylaxis.

b. Management of individual cardiac conditions during pregnancy are not covered in this chapter. Patients with more than mild disease should be managed with cardiology consultation. Overall management includes close monitoring for maternal congestive heart failure and assessment of fetal well-being, with growth assessment by ultrasound. Clinicians who may attend patients in acute situations should be sensitive to findings such as maternal tachycardia, a state not well tolerated by patients with mitral stenosis and other valvular conditions.

Table 13.10. Cardiac conditions requiring SBE prophylaxis

Prosthetic valves	Valvular disease – MR, MS, AI, AS
Ventricular septal defect (not ASD)	Patent ductus arteriosus
Idiopathic hypertrophic subaortic stenosis	MVP with regurgitation
Marfan's syndrome	Coarctation of the aorta

ASD, atrial septal defect; MR, mitral regurgitation; MS, mitral stenosis; AI, aortic insufficiency; AS, aortic stenosis; MVP, mitral valve prolapse.

Approximately 40 percent of women with valvular heart disease become symptomatic for the first time during pregnancy.

Inflammatory bowel disease

1. Preconception care:
   a. Patients with inflammatory bowel disease may improve or develop more problems during pregnancy, but pregnancy does not appear to affect the long-term course of the disease.
   b. Patients with very active flares or complications just prior to pregnancy tend to have more difficulty during pregnancy.
   c. Methotrexate should be avoided in women trying to conceive because of abortifacient effects and teratogenicity.
2. Antepartum care: Many medications have been used with safety and efficacy during pregnancy. These include sulfasalazaline, 5-aminosalicylic acid drugs, and corticosteroids. Cyclosporin and azathioprine do not appear to be teratogenic, but are associated with growth retardation and prematurity.[50]

Conclusion

Clinicians who provide medical care for women of child-bearing age should be prepared within their clinical roles to provide preconception care and care of medical illness during pregnancy. Incorporating preconception care into primary care of young women enhances the preventive aspects of care and may improve pregnancy outcomes. Approaches to acute clinical problems often need only minor adjustment during pregnancy to assure maternal and fetal safety. Patients with serious chronic medical illness will often benefit from specialist consultation and/or management of their condition. All primary care physicians, emergency department personnel, and other women's health care providers should be familiar with overall principles of medical care during pregnancy to respond well in urgent situations and to facilitate a coordinated approach to pregnant women with complex medical issues.

REFERENCES

1. Lewis DP, Van Dyke DC, Stumbo PJ, Berg MJ. Drug and environmental factors associated with adverse pregnancy outcomes. Part II. Improvement with folic acid. *Ann Pharmacother* 1998;**32**:947–61.

2. Centers for Disease Control and Prevention. Knowledge and use of folic acid by women of childbearing age – United States, 1995 and 1998. *MMWR Morb Mortal Wkly Rep* 1999;**48**:325–7.

3. Kloeben AS. Folate knowledge, intake from fortified grain products, and periconceptional supplementation patterns of a sample of low-income pregnant women according to the Health Belief Model. *J Am Diet Assoc* 1999;**99**:33–8.

4. Locksmith GJ, Duff P. Preventing neural tube defects: The importance of periconceptional folic acid supplements. *Obstet Gynecol* 1998;**91**:1027–34.

5. Tashinken HK, Olsen J, Bach B. Experiences in developing legislation protecting reproductive health. *J Occup Environ Med* 1995;**37**:974–9.

6. Mountford PJ, Steele HR. Fetal dose estimates and the IRCP abdominal dose limit for occupational exposure of pregnant staff to technetium-99 and iodine-131 patients. *Eur J Nucl Med* 1995;**22**:1173–9.

7. Kersemaekers WM, Roeleveld N, Zielhuis GA. Reproductive disorders among hairdressers. *Epidemiology* 1997;**8**:396–401.

8. Byhahn C, Lischke V, Westphal K. [Occupational exposure in the hospital to laughing gas and the new inhalation anesthetics desflurane and sevoflurane]. In German *Dtsch Med Wochenschr* 1999;**124**:137–41.

9. Brateman L. Radiation safety considerations for diagnostic radiology personnel. *Radiographics* 1999;**19**:1037–55.

10. Geeze DS. Pregnancy and in-flight cosmic radiation. *Aviat Space Environ Med* 1998;**69**:1061–4.

11. Parker L, Pearce MS, Dickinson HO, Aitkin M, Craft AW. Stillbirths among offspring of male radiation workers at the Sellafield nuclear reprocessing plant. *Lancet* 1999;**354**:1407–14.

12. Draper GJ, Little MP, Sorahan T et al. Cancer in offspring of radiation workers: A record linkage study. *BMJ* 1997;**315**:1181–8.

13. Robert E. Intrauterine effects of electromagnetic fields – (low frequency, mid-frequency RF, and microwave): Review of epidemiologic studies. *Teratology* 1999;**59**:292–8.

14. Sorahan T, Hamilton L, Gardiner K, Hodgson JT, Harrington JM. Maternal occupational exposure to electromagnetic fields before, during, and after pregnancy in relation to risks of childhood cancers: Findings from the Oxford Survey of Childhood Cancers, 1953–1981 deaths. *Am J Ind Med* 1999;**35**:348–57.

15. Armstrong BG, Nolin AD, McDonald AD. Work in pregnancy and birth weight for gestational age. *Br J Ind Med* 1989;**46**:196–9.

16. Clapp JF III. Pregnancy outcome: Physical activities inside versus outside the workplace. *Semin Perinatol* 1996;**20**:70–6.

17. Savitz DA, Olshan AF, Gallagher K. Maternal occupation and pregnancy outcome. *Epidemiology* 1996;**7**:269–74.

18. Ortayli N, Osugurlu M, Gokcay G. Female health workers: An obstetric risk group. *Int J Gynaecol Obstet* 1996;**54**:263–70.

19. Pinhas-Hamiel O, Rotstein Z, Achiron A et al. Pregnancy during residency – an Israeli survey of women physicians. *Health Care Women Int* 1999;**20**:63–70.

20. Klebanoff MA, Shiono PH, Carey JC. The effect of physical activity during pregnancy on preterm delivery and birth weight. *Am J Obstet Gynecol* 1990;**163**:1450–6.

21. DeVigan C, DeWalle, Cordier S et al. Therapeutic drug use during pregnancy: A comparison in four European countries. OECM Working Group. Occupational Exposures and Congenital Anomalies. *J Clin Epidemiol* 1999;**52**:977–82.

22. Peters PW. Risk assessment of drug use in pregnancy: Prevention of birth defects. *Ann 1st Super Sanita* 1993;**29**:131–7.

23. Sannerstedt R, Lundborg P, Daniellsson BR et al. Drugs during pregnancy: An issue of risk classification and information to the prescribers. *Drug Saf* 1996;**14**:69–77.

24. Friuedman JM, Little BB, Brent RL, Cordero JF, Hanson JW, Shepard TH. Potential human teratogenecity of frequently prescribed drugs. *Obstet Gynecol* 1990;**75**:594–9.

25. Murphy KJ, Kazerooni EA, Braun MA, Weinberg EP, Killam DA, Hendrick WJ. Radiographic appearance of intrathoracic complications of pregnancy. *Can Assoc Radiol J* 1996;**47**:453–9.

26. Cappell MS, Sidhom O. Multicenter, multiyear study of safety and efficacy of flexible sigmoidoscopy during pregnancy in 24 females with follow-up of fetal outcome. *Dig Dis Sci* 1995;**40**:472–9.

27. Gurbuz AT, Peetz ME. The acute abdomen in the pregnant patient. Is there a role for laparoscopy? *Surg Endosc* 1997;**11**:98–102.

28. Czeizel AE, Rockenbauer M. A population based case-control teratologic study of oral metronidazole treatment during pregnancy. *Br J Obstet Gynaecol* 1998;**105**:322–7.

29. Caron-Paton T, Carvahal A, Martin de Diego I et al. Is metronidazole teratogenic? A meta-analysis. *Br J Clin Pharmacol* 1997;**44**:179–82.

30. Thapa PB, Whitlock JA, Brockman Worrell KG et al. Prenatal exposure to metronidazole and risk of childhood cancer: A retrospective cohort study of children younger than 5 years. *Cancer* 1998;**83**:1461–8.

31. Brocklehurst P, Kinghorn G, Carney O et al. A randomised placebo controlled trial of suppressive acyclovir in late pregnancy in women with recurrent genital herpes infection. *Br J Obstet Gynecol* 1998;**105**:275–80.

32. Randolph AG, Hartshoorn RM, Washington AE. Acyclovir prophylaxis in late pregnancy to prevent neonatal herpes: A cost-effective analysis. *Obstet Gynecol* 1996;**88**:603–10.

33. Scott LL, Alexander J. Cost-effectiveness of acyclovir suppression to prevent recurrent genital herpes in term pregnancy. *Am J Perinatol* 1998;**15**:57–62.

34. American College of Obstetricians and Gynecologists. *Viral Hepatitis in Pregnancy.* Technical Bulletin no. 248, 1998.

35. Michielson PP, Van Damme P. Viral hepatitis and pregnancy. *Acta Gastroenterol Belg* 1999;**62**:21–9.

36. Zanetti AR, Tanzi E, Newell ML. Mother-to-infant transmission of hepatitis C virus. *J Hepatol* 1999;**31**(Suppl 1):96–100.

37. Hermann WH, Janz NK, Becker NP, Charron-Prochownik D. Diabetes and pregnancy. Pre-conception care, pregnancy outcomes, resource utilization, and costs. *J Reprod Med* 1999;**44**:33–8.

38. Dunne FP, Brydon P, Smith T, Essex M, Nicholson H, Dunn J. Preconception diabetes care in insulin-dependent diabetes mellitus. *Q J Med* 1999;**92**:175–6.

39. Coustan DR, Gelig P. Diabetes mellitus. In Burrow GN, Ferris TF, eds., *Medical Complications During Pregnancy*. W. B. Saunders Co., Philadelphia, 1988, pp. 34–9.

40. Gladman G, McCrindle BW, Boytin C, Smalthorn JF. Fetal echocardiographic screening of diabetic pregnancies for congenital heart disease. *Am J Perinatol* 1997;**14**:59–62.

41. Shields LE, Gan EA, Murphy HF, Sahn DJ, Moore TR. The prognostic value of hemoglobin A1c in predicting fetal heart disease in diabetic pregnancies. *Obstet Gynecol* 1993;**81**:954–7.

42. Raychaudburi K, Maresh MJ. Glycemic control throughout pregnancy and fetal growth in insulin-dependent diabetes. *Obstet Gynecol* 2000;**95**:190–4.

43. Rey E, Attie C, Bonin A. The effects of first-trimester diabetes control on the incidence of macrosomia. *Am J Obstet Gynecol* 1999;**181**:202–6.

44. Rey E, LeLorier J, Burgess E, Lange IR, Leduc L. Report of the Canadian Hypertension Society Consensus Conference: Pharmacologic treatment of hypertensive disorders in pregnancy. *Can Med Assoc J* 1997;**157**:1245–54.

45. Stenius-Aarniala BS, Piirila P, Teramo K. Asthma and pregnancy: A prospective study of 198 pregnancies. *Thorax* 1998;**43**:12–18.

46. Stenius-Aarniala BS, Hedman J, Teramo KA. Acute asthma in pregnancy. *Thorax* 1996;**51**:411–4.

47. Rayburn WF, LeMire MS, Bird JL, Buda AJ. Mitral valve prolapse. Echocardiographic changes during pregnancy. *J Reprod Med* 1987;**32**:185–7.

48. Khandelwal M, Rasanen J, Ludormirski A, Addonizio P, Reece EA. Evaluation of fetal and uterine hemodynamics during maternal cardiopulmonary bypass. *Obstet Gynecol* 1996;**88**:6667–71.

49. Pearson GD, Veille JC, Rahimtoola S et al. Peripartum cardiomyopathy: National Heart, Lung, and Blood Institute and Office of Rare Disease (National Institute of Health) workshop recommendations and review. *JAMA* 2000;**283**:1183–8.

50. Connell W, Miller A. Treating inflammatory bowel disease during pregnancy: Risks and safety of drug therapy. *Drug Saf* 1999;**21**:311–23.

Genitourinary medicine

14 Menstrual disorders

Kathy Reilly, MD

Normal menstrual function is the result of a complex interaction between the hypothalamus, pituitary gland, ovaries, and endometrium. In addition, a normal outflow tract, including the cervix, vagina and external genitalia is required. Evaluation of the causes of amenorrhea and abnormal bleeding requires that each of these systems be considered and evaluated if indicated. Treatment of these problems depends on the cause, the woman's age, and her desire for fertility.The most common cause of both amenorrhea and abnormal bleeding is anovulation, particularly in adolescents and in perimenopausal women.

Amenorrhea

Definition

Amenorrhea (the absence of menstrual periods for six months) should be evaluated when:

1. An adolescent who has no evidence of growth or development of secondary sex characteristics has no period by age 14 years.
2. An adolescent who has normal development of secondary sex characteristics has no period by age 16 years.
3. An adolescent or her parents have significant concerns regardless of the above criteria.
4. A woman who has been menstruating has absence of periods for at least three cycles or six months.

Importance

1. Amenorrhea occurs in about 5 percent of women of reproductive age.[1] In a Swedish population-based study, the prevalence of amenorrhea for three months was 1.8 percent and for 12 months was 1.2 percent.[2]
2. Amenorrhea is seen in 50 percent of competitive runners, 25 percent of

Table 14.1. Etiology of amenorrhea

- Physiological causes
  - Pregnancy
  - Postpartum amenorrhea
  - Lactation
  - Use of hormonal contraception
  - Posthormonal contraception
- Hypothalamic causes
  - Chronic anovulation
  - Exercise-induced
  - Psychogenic or stress related
  - Anorexia nervosa
  - Bulimia
  - Malnutrition
  - Systemic disease
  - Chronic disease
- Hormonal
  - Hyperprolactinemia
  - Excessive androgens, usually polycystic ovary syndrome
  - Thyroid disease
- Medications
- Galactorrhea

      recreational runners or joggers, and 44 percent of dancers.[3]

3. Amenorrhea and anovulation can cause significant health risks. These include osteoporosis and rapid bone loss. Low and irregular hormone levels can cause infertility, vaginal dryness, and dyspareunia. Hypothalamic amenorrhea may also cause hyperestrogenemia and/or endometrial hyperplasia and cancer.[4]

Etiology (Table 14.1)

1. Physiological causes: There are several physiological causes of primary and secondary amenorrhea.
   a. Pregnancy causes amenorrhea and is the leading cause of primary amenorrhea.
   b. Postpartum amenorrhea can last six to 12 months, but is usually less than three months.
   c. Lactation: Amenorrhea in lactating women usually lasts six to nine months depending on supplementation and infant feeding practices (Table 14.2), and often lasts 6–18 months after cessation of lactation.[5] A woman who breast feeds her child for six months has an average of three months of amenorrhea after breast feeding ceases, whereas a woman who breast

Table 14.2. Factors that prolong lactational amenorrhea

- Longer duration of breast feeding per 24 hours
- Fully breast feeding
- Early first breast feeding
- No supplementation of infant
- Healthy (not-sick) infant
- More previous births
- Low maternal body mass index

Data from WHO Task Force on Method for the Natural Regulation of Fertility. The World Health Organization multinational study of breast feeding and lactational amenorrhea. II. Factors associated with the length of amenorrhea. *Fertil Steril* 1998;**70**:461–70.

feeds her child for 12 months has an average of eight months of postbreast feeding amenorrhea.[6] There are factors that can increase the duration of anovulation and amenorrhea with lactation (Table 14.2).[7]

    d. Use of hormonal contraception – depot MPA (DMPA), Norplant or OCPs – can normally cause amenorrhea.

    e. Posthormonal contraception amenorrhea: After cessation of OCPs, amenorrhea can last six to 12 months; after DMPA, amenorrhea can last 24 months.

2. Hypothalamic causes: In a population-based study of women with adult-onset amenorrhea, excluding anatomical and physiological causes, 32 percent had amenorrhea from hypothalamic causes, including chronic anovulation, exercise-induced, psychogenic, anorexia nervosa, bulimia, malnutrition, systemic disease, or chronic disease. Seventeen percent had chronic anovulation caused by hyperprolactinemia and 35 percent had chronic anovulation caused by excessive androgens, usually PCOS.[8]

3. Medications: Medications, especially psychotropic medications, phenothiazines, haloperidol, tricyclic antidepressants and selective serotonin-reuptake inhibitors can cause amenorrhea.

4. Thyroid disease: Hypothyroidism usually causes oligomenorrhea but can cause amenorrhea. Hypothyroidism can causes hyperprolactinemia as well, because increased thyroxin-releasing hormone (TRH) levels will also suppress prolactin-inhibiting hormone (PIH), luteinizing hormone (LH), follicle-stimulating hormone (FSH), and estradiol production.

5. Galactorrhea: Galactorrhea (secretion from the breast not related to pregnancy) is present in many women with amenorrhea. If galactorrhea is present either historically or on physical examination, a coned-down view of the sella turcica must be included in the evaluation, to evaluate for the presence of a pituitary adenoma.

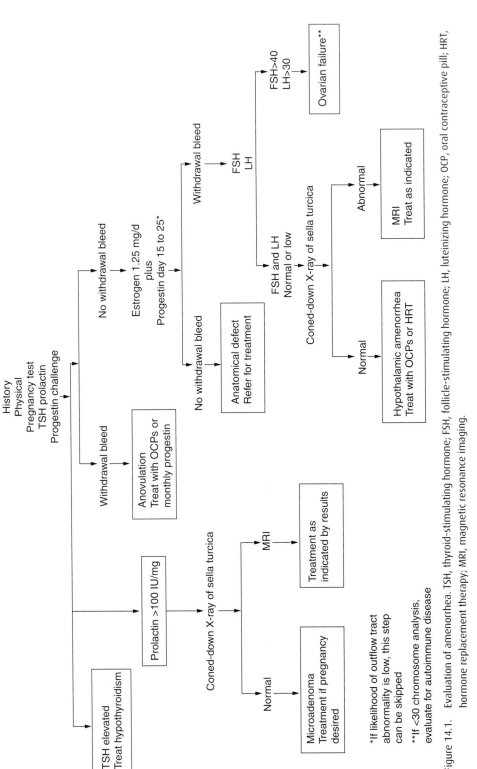

Figure 14.1. Evaluation of amenorrhea. TSH, thyroid-stimulating hormone; FSH, follicle-stimulating hormone; LH, luteinizing hormone; OCP, oral contraceptive pill; HRT, hormone replacement therapy; MRI, magnetic resonance imaging.

Pregnancy is the most common cause of primary and secondary amenorrhea.

Evaluation

1. History: The history obtained in women with amenorrhea should include family history of genetic abnormalities and abnormalities of menstrual function, galactorrhea, recent changes in weight (particularly severe weight loss), psychological dysfunction or stress, and medications and drugs being used. Symptoms of menopause such as hot flashes, vaginal dryness, or night sweats should be elicited.

2. Physical examination: The physical examination should evaluate for evidence of nutritional deficiency, abnormal growth and development and the presence of a normal reproductive tract. Evidence for disease of the central nervous system should be considered.

3. Pregnancy must be excluded in all women with amenorrhea, since this is the most common cause of amenorrhea in women of reproductive age. A urine pregnancy test and physical examination should suffice for pregnancy determination.

4. Laboratory tests: Initial laboratory evaluation includes an immediate in-office urine pregnancy test. If this is negative, a complete blood count (CBC), erythrocyte sedimentation rate (ERS), TSH, prolactin and FSH should be obtained. Further testing depends on results (Figure 14.1).

    a. A high FSH indicates ovarian failure.

    b. If the woman has amenorrhea–galactorrhea, even with a normal prolactin level, a CT scan is indicated because approximately 34 percent of women have been found to have brain tumors.[9]

    c. If these tests are normal and the woman is virilized (hair changes, beard, etc.), PCOS is a likely diagnosis. A testosterone level and an ultrasound scan will detect PCOS. If the testosterone level is very high and the ultrasound normal, an evaluation for an andosterone-secreting tumor in brain, adrenal, ovary or elsewhere must be performed.

    d. If these tests are normal and the woman shows no signs of virilization, a progestin challenge (five days of MPA at 5 to 10 mg) should be accomplished. The woman should have withdrawal bleeding within 10 days of stopping MPA; this would show mild hypothalamic–pituitary axis dysfunction as the cause of the amenorrhea.

5. Evaluation of woman with primary amenorrhea:

a. If the woman has primary amenorrhea and is not pregnant and physical examination shows normal external genitalia, a pelvic ultrasound scan (abdominal and perhaps vaginal) and karyotype are needed.

b. If she has an intact uterus, but no breast development, a high FSH level is consistent with gonadal dysgenesis or Turner's syndrome.

c. A low FSH suggests hypothalamic failure, such as with exercise, anorexia, starvation or bulimia, or gonadotropin deficiency, such as Kallman's syndrome.

d. All women under the age of 30 years diagnosed with ovarian failure should have a karyotype determination, to determine whether they have a mosaic Y chromosome. If mosaicism exists, the woman must have her gonadal areas removed to prevent development of malignancy in areas of testicular tissue.

e. Hypothalamic amenorrhea is a diagnosis of exclusion. It is associated with weight loss, malnutrition, anorexia nervosa, bulimia, exercise, or psychological stress.

All women under the age of 30 years diagnosed with ovarian failure should have a karyotype determination.

Treatment

1. Progestin challenge or withdrawal bleed

    a. The progesterone challenge evaluates whether the uterus has been primed by estrogen. If there is a withdrawal bleed two to seven days after completing the progesterone, the cause of amenorrhea is anovulation.

    b. If the woman does not have a withdrawal bleed, and TSH and prolactin are normal, the next step is to prime the uterus with estrogen (Premarin 1.25 mg/day for 21 days) and with a progestational agent (Provera 10 mg/day for the last week).

    c. If there is no withdrawal bleed, the outflow tract is abnormal. In women who have had previous menstrual periods, adhesions of the endometrial cavity (Asherman's syndrome) may be present, particularly if there is a history of postpartum curettage or severe endometritis.

    d. If Asherman's syndrome is unlikely by history, another month of estrogen and progesterone may be prudent before referring for treatment.

    e. If bleeding occurs following estrogen priming, the next step is to determine whether the problem lies within the ovary (absence of follicles that can respond to gonadotropins, e.g. menopause) or the pituitary (absence of gonadotropins). Measurement of FSH and LH is appropriate at this stage. It is important to wait at least two weeks after administering exogenous hormones before drawing these tests.

   f. If both FSH and LH hormone levels are elevated (FSH >30 IU/L and LH >40 IU/L), the cause of the woman's amenorrhea is ovarian failure or menopause.

   g. Women with normal or low gonadotropins may have either a pituitary or hypothalamic cause for amenorrhea. If the prolactin level is <100 ng/mL and the coned-down view of the sella turcica is normal, no further evaluation is necessary and the woman is said to have hypothalamic amenorrhea.

2. Subsequent treatment: All amenorrheic women need treatment for fertility (if desired), to avoid endometrial hyperplasia, and to prevent osteoporosis.

   a. Fertility: Women with amenorrhea can be placed on ovulation-inducing drugs. However, estrogen or estradiol alone does not induce ovulation and menses. In a placebo-controlled crossover RCT of women with ovarian failure (no menses for six months and high FSH levels), estradiol 2 mg orally each day decreased the woman's LH and FSH levels but did not induce ovulation. An ovulation-inducing agent, such as clomiphene, may be needed.

   b. Endometrial hyperplasia: Women should have withdrawal bleeding or menses either monthly or every three months to avoid the high risk of endometrial hyperplasia and cancer. Use of estrogen at HRT doses combined with progesterone, either orally (5 to 10 mg MPA for 10 days every month or three months) or as a vaginal gel, or use of combination OCPs to promote shedding of the endometrial lining and withdrawal bleeding is essential.[10]

   c. Minimal therapy for anovulation is monthly administration of a progestational agent. MPA can be given at a dose of 10 mg/day for the first 10 days of the month. Alternatives include parenteral progesterone in oil (200 mg), and natural progesterone (Crinone vaginal cream 4%) every other day for six doses.

   d. Levonorgestrel in an intrauterine device has been used extensively in Europe and may be an alternative for women who do not tolerate oral or parenteral progesterone. Women who require contraception can use low dose oral contraceptives or Depo Provera to provide protection of the endometrium as well as prevention of pregnancy.

If both hormone levels are elevated (follicle stimulating hormone >30 IU/L and LH >40 IU/L), the cause of the woman's amenorrhea is ovarian failure or menopause.

e. Osteoporosis: Amenorrheic women are at increased risk of osteoporosis, partially caused by estrogen deficiency. Treatment for osteoporosis must be estrogen in doses higher than normal HRT doses.

f. Therapy for women with a tumor-secreting hyperprolactinoma or idiopathic hyperprolactinemia depends on the size of the adenoma and the woman's desire for pregnancy. Treatment with bromocriptine can produce fertility in 80 percent of women. Women who do not desire pregnancy and whose pituitary tumor is small (less than 10 mm) are usually not given any treatment; rather, they are evaluated periodically to monitor tumor growth. Macroadenomas are usually treated with bromocriptine. Surgery is an option that should be discussed with the woman, since most macro-adenomas require indefinite treatment with bromocriptine.

g. Amenorrhea associated with acute weight loss can usually be reversed with modest weight gain to at least 85 to 90 percent of ideal body weight. Women who are suspected of having anorexia nervosa or bulimia should be referred for appropriate treatment. Exercise-associated amenorrhea is related to body fat and the effect of stress and energy expenditure. Abnormal menstrual function is common when the woman's body fat is less than 22 percent. In women with amenorrhea, a decrease in the level of exercise can lead to a return of menses, without any change in body weight or fat percentage. Exercise-associated menstrual dysfunction is associated with a longer recovery period after musculoskeletal injuries.

h. Hypothalamic amenorrhea: In hypogonadism characterized by neuroendocrine aberrations including altered prolactin, growth hormone (GH), and LH levels, three drugs have been investigated but are not FDA approved for treatment.

   i. Naloxone has been found to increase the LH pulse frequency and amplitude in healthy but not amenorrheic women.

   ii. Naltrexone: In a clinical trial, naltrexone (50 mg orally daily for six months) increased the women's plasma gonadal steroids and menstrual bleeding occurred within 90 days in 24 of 30 women.[11]

   iii. Metoclopramide: Other studies have examined metoclopramide (as a dopamine antagonist) and found that its use increased gonadotropin secretions but not ovulation. A clinical trial of metoclopramide with clomiphene citrate in a few women found that 40 percent ovulated and 60 percent menstruated.

All amenorrheic women need treatment for fertility (if desired), to avoid endometrial hyperplasia, and to prevent osteoporosis.

Table 14.3. Features of polycystic ovary disease

• Oligomenorrhea	• Acne
• Amenorrhea	• Diabetes
• Anovulation	• Abnormal levels of gonadotropins
• Infertility	• Hyperlipidemia
• Hirsutism	• Insulin resistance (60 to 70 percent)
• Obesity	• Elevated total testosterone and androstenidione levels

Prognosis

Seventy-two percent of women with secondary amenorrhea associated with stress or weight loss had spontaneous return of menses after six years.

Polycystic ovary disease

Definition

PCOS is a form of ovarian failure. Many women have cysts on their ovaries seen on ultrasound scan. Not all of them have PCOS. Stein–Levinthal syndrome is a form of PCOS.

Presentation

Although the diagnosis is disputed, PCOS is very common and affects 5 to 10 percent of the US female population. PCOS usually presents with chronic anovulatory bleeding with androgen excess, though definition is not specific.

Symptoms

1. Symptoms include oligomenorrhea, amenorrhea, anovulation, infertility, abnormal levels of gonadotropins, hirsutism, obesity, acne, diabetes, and hyperlipidemia (Table 14.3). These women are usually oligoovulatory rather than amenorrheic.

2. The woman with PCOS often also has insulin resistance with hyperinsulinemia. Experts suspect that the hyperinsulinemia causes abnormal ovarian secretions and this then causes gonadotropin deficiency and oligomenorrhea.[12]

3. Infertility occurs in 74 percent, menstrual irregularity occurs in 51 percent and signs of androgen excess occur in 69 percent of women with PCOS.[12]

Diagnosis

There is no consensus on diagnosis of PCOS. A typical history, ovarian cysts on ultrasound scan and signs of excessive levels of androgens may suggest the diagnosis. High levels of androgens would also support the diagnosis.

Treatment

1. Ovulation can be induced and 80 percent of women have become pregnant with treatment within nine ovulatory cycles.
2. If pregnancy is not desired, the women should be treated for the chronic estrogen exposure unopposed by progesterone that can lead to endometrial hyperplasia, with cyclic, continuous or intermittent progesterone or OCPs.
3. Women with PCOS develop early and male patterns of cardiovascular risk, and should be aggressively counselled to reduce risk factors such as hypertension, smoking, and hypercholesterolemia.[13]
4. Investigationally, metformin has been studied to examine whether it improves the endocrine symptoms of PCOS. Metformin treats insulin sensitivity and occasionally weight loss. Metformin was given to 43 women with PCOS who were hyperinsulinemic and euglycemic. It was found to cause decreased weight and BMI and 91 percent resumed menses. The women also had decreased median fasting serum insulin.[12] Other studies have shown similar effects.
5. Signs of virilization such as hirsutism can be treated with spironolactone 50 to 100 mg up to two times daily.
6. OCPs should be given to decrease estrogen levels and promote withdrawal bleeding to prevent endometrial hyperplasia. Alternatively, MPA (10 mg daily) can be given from day 14 to day 28 of the month.

Abnormal vaginal bleeding

Definitions

1. Although there is significant between-woman variation in the length of each menstrual cycle and the duration of flow, for most women these are stable in the presence of normal ovulation and the absence of anatomical disturbances such as polyps or submucous fibroids. Thus a complaint of increased flow, increased duration of menses, or an acute change in the timing of menses should be evaluated.
2. The usual duration of flow is four to six days, although women may have flow as little as two days or as many as eight days (Table 14.4).

Table 14.4. Definitions of abnormal bleeding patterns

Amenorrhea	More than 6 months without menses
Primary amenorrhea	No menses by age 16
Secondary amenorrhea	No menses for 6 months after initiation of menses
Oligomenorrhea	More than 35 days between menstrual periods
Polymenorrhea	Fewer than 21 days between menstrual periods
Menorrhagia	Regular normal intervals with excessive flow and duration
Metrorrhagia	Irregular intervals with excessive flow and duration

3. Normal volume of blood loss is 30 mL, with more than 80 mL being consider-ed abnormal. Precise measurement of the volume of blood loss is not feasible clinically, and pad counts do not provide accurate measurements of blood loss. Blood loss sufficient to cause anemia should be considered abnormal and should be evaluated.

4. Oligomenorrhea is intermenstrual intervals greater than 35 days and poly-menorrhea is intermenstrual intervals less than 21 days.

5. Menorrhagia is regular normal intervals with excessive flow and duration and metrorrhagia is irregular intervals with excessive flow and duration (Table 14.4).

Epidemiology

The incidence of menstrual disorders is 20.0 per 1000 woman-years in a family practice center.[14]

Etiology (Figure 14.2)

1. The most common causes in a general medical office practice are contracep-tive related in 28 percent, dysfunctional bleeding including perimenopausal bleeding in 40 percent, and cervical pathology in 10 percent.

2. The differential diagnosis depends on the woman's age.

  a. Adolescence:

    1. In adolescence, anovulation caused by the immaturity of the hy-pothalamic–pituitary–ovarian axis is the most common cause. Establish-ment of regular ovulatory bleeding can take up to five years after menarche.[15]

    2. Complications of pregnancy are also a fairly common cause of abnor-mal bleeding in adolescence.

    3. Coagulation disorder, such as von Willebrand's disease or prothrom-bin deficiency may be undetected until the onset of menstrual periods.

    4. Other less likely causes include malignancy, endometriosis, trauma,

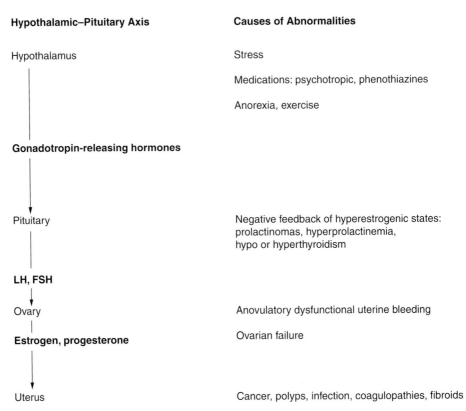

Hypothalamic–Pituitary Axis	Causes of Abnormalities
Hypothalamus	Stress
	Medications: psychotropic, phenothiazines
	Anorexia, exercise
Gonadotropin-releasing hormones	
Pituitary	Negative feedback of hyperestrogenic states: prolactinomas, hyperprolactinemia, hypo or hyperthyroidism
LH, FSH	
Ovary	Anovulatory dysfunctional uterine bleeding
Estrogen, progesterone	Ovarian failure
Uterus	Cancer, polyps, infection, coagulopathies, fibroids

Figure 14.2.   Causes of abnormal menstrual cycles and bleeding. LH, luteinizing hormone; FSH, follicle-stimulating hormone.

infection, anatomical lesions (polyps, fibroids), foreign bodies, systemic illness (including diabetes mellitus) and medications (see Table 14.5).

b. Reproductive age:

1. In women of reproductive age (19 years to mid 40s), the basic differential is the same, although congenital bleeding disorders are not likely to be newly diagnosed in this age group.

2. Pregnancy and its complications must always be considered as a cause of irregular bleeding.

3. Systemic diseases and anatomical lesions are more common as women become older, as is the risk of malignancy of the cervix and endometrium.

4. In women in the perimenopausal years (mid 40s to early 50s) anovulation is a common cause of abnormal bleeding.

c. Perimenopause:

1. In the perimenopausal period, the follicles that remain on the ovary are relatively refractory to stimulation by FSH. The ovaries produce abun-

Table 14.5. Causes of abnormal menstrual periods by age

- Adolescence
  - Anovulation
  - Pregnancy and complications
  - Coagulation disorders
  - Malignancy
  - Endometriosis
  - Trauma
  - Infection
  - Anatomical lesions (polyps, fibroids)
  - Foreign bodies
  - Systemic illness (including diabetes mellitus)
  - Medications
- Reproductive age
  - All of the above, especially
    - Systemic diseases
    - Anatomical lesions
    - Malignancy of the cervix and endometrium
- Perimenopausal years
  - Anovulation
  - Increased risk of endometrial cancer
  - Any of the disorders listed for younger women

dant amounts of estrogen, leading to growth of the endometrium, but since ovulation does not occur, there is absence of progesterone effect and no coordinated shedding of the endometrial lining.

2. Women in this period are also at increased risk of endometrial cancer, and also may have any of the disorders listed for younger women.

Evaluation

1. History:
   a. All women with abnormal vaginal bleeding should be asked about their menstrual history – age at onset, usual bleeding pattern (length of cycle, duration of flow, relative heaviness of flow), presence and severity of dysmenorrhea (if any) – pregnancy history, contraceptive history, and age at menopause (if currently menopausal).
   b. The history of the abnormal bleeding should include the onset, frequency, duration and severity of the abnormal bleeding, presence of any pain and any pattern that is associated with the abnormality.
   c. The woman should list all medications and street drugs taken in the recent past.

    d. The history of previous gynecological disease or pelvic infections should be obtained, as well as symptoms of pregnancy.

    e. Sexual history, including number of recent partners and their risk of STDs should be obtained.

    f. The woman should be asked about fever, chills, lower abdominal pain, and abnormal vaginal discharge.

2. Physical examination:

    a. Although the symptom of abnormal bleeding focuses attention on the genital tract, it is important to evaluate the entire woman in order to assure accurate diagnosis.

    b. Hypotension, orthostatic hypotension, tachycardia and pale conjunctivae suggest the presence of significant anemia. Thyromegaly, or a thyroid nodule, indicate the need to evaluate thyroid function tests.

    c. The skin should be examined for evidence of jaundice (evidence for advanced liver disease), and petechiae, extensive ecchymoses, or hematomas (possible symptoms of coagulopathy).

    d. The vaginal vault should be inspected for evidence of trauma, atrophic vaginitis or foreign bodies. The cervix may show evidence of polyps, erosion, or a lesion suspicious for cancer. A Pap smear should be done whenever there is a complaint of abnormal vaginal bleeding. Bimanual examination may disclose an enlarged, symmetrical uterus (suggests pregnancy complications or adenomyosis), an enlarged, irregular uterus (suggests fibroids) or pain on palpation of the uterus, adnexae or on motion of the cervix (suggests pelvic infection).

3. Laboratory:

    a. A CBC and a pregnancy test should be obtained in all women who have abnormal vaginal bleeding.

    b. If there is any evidence for infection, wet prep, potassium hydroxide and cultures for gonorrhea and chlamydia infections should be done.

    c. If the history and/or examination suggest the possibility of liver disease, liver function tests should be obtained.

    d. A serum TSH should be obtained.

    e. If a coagulopathy is suspected, prothrombin time (PTT) and platelet count should be ordered. These tests should be ordered only if there is serious consideration that there is an abnormality in the appropriate system.

4. Additional diagnostic procedures:

    a. Transvaginal ultrasound has been shown to have excellent sensitivity (0.94 to 0.96) and specificity (0.89) for abnormalities of the endometrium and the uterine cavity (polyps and submucous fibroids).[16,17] This should be obtained if pregnancy is suspected, or definitely on all women of perimenopausal age.

b. Intrauterine polyps and submucous fibroids can also be diagnosed with the use of transvaginal ultrasound. Thus, a transvaginal ultrasound scan should be the first step in evaluating postmenopausal women. Women with an endometrial thickness > 4 mm will require endometrial biopsy and those with structural abnormalities will need hysteroscopy for further evaluation.

c. Hysteroscopy allows direct visualization of the endometrial cavity and is very useful in diagnosing lesions such as endometrial polyps or submucous polyps. Office hysteroscopy is increasingly common.

d. Endometrial biopsy allows histological evaluation of the endometrium. It is done in the office setting, usually without need for any analgesia except NSAIDs for uterine cramping.

e. Dilatation and curettage (D&C) was the procedure of choice in women with abnormal vaginal bleeding for several decades. However, a D&C is not an effective tool to diagnose endometrial polyps or submucous polyps, as compared with transvaginal ultrasound and hysteroscopy.[18] A D&C has been shown to reach less than half of the endometrial lining in 60 percent of 50 hysterectomy specimens and in 16 percent fewer than a quarter.

> Transvaginal sonography has excellent sensitivity and specificity in diagnosing normalcy or abnormal uterine findings in women with abnormal vaginal bleeding.

Diagnosis by age

1. In adolescence, if coagulopathy, pregnancy, and infection are not present, the adolescent woman can be assumed to have anovulatory or dysfunctional bleeding and no further testing is needed.

2. Whether women older than 18 years and younger than age 35 years need any further testing, and, if so, which testing is most appropriate is disputed. Women at increased risk for endometrial cancer (those with a long history of anovulation or severe obesity) (see Chapter 18) should have a transvaginal sonograph (TVS) or an endometrial biopsy to allow histological evaluation of endometrial tissue.

3. In women between 35 years and menopause, an endometrial biopsy has been universally suggested to preclude endometrial cancer. TVS with biopsy may be sufficient to eliminate endometrial cancer as a cause.

4. Postmenopausal women are at high risk for endometrial cancer (see Chapter 18). B. Gull et al. demonstrated that these women do not need endometrial biopsy if their endometrial thickness on transvaginal ultrasound is < 4 mm.[19]

Treatment

1. Treatment of abnormal vaginal bleeding, of course, depends on the etiology. If a cause is identified, treatment is targeted to the cause. Thus thyroid dysfunction or coagulopathy should be treated if present.
2. If a medication is suspected as the cause, the medication should be stopped. Complications of pregnancy are managed appropriately. Cervical and endometrial polyps can be surgically removed, as can submucous fibroids that are symptomatic.
3. If endometriosis is the presumed cause of bleeding, it is managed medically with progestins, danazol, oral contraceptives or gonadotropin-releasing hormone (GnRH) agonists or surgically.
4. Infections are treated with appropriate antibiotics.
5. Endometrial or cervical malignancy is treated surgically.
6. Women in whom a specific abnormality is not found are said to have dysfunctional uterine bleeding (DUB) or anovulatory bleeding, which are diagnoses of exclusion. The goal of treatment in these women is to control acute bleeding, prevent recurrence, preserve fertility, and correct associated disorders, such as anemia.
7. Hormonal therapy: In adolescents and women with acute heavy bleeding, estrogen is most commonly recommended to control severe or emergent bleeding (Table 14.6). Intravenous estrogen at 25 mg every four hours for 12 hours is said to be the treatment of choice, but is difficult to obtain. Conjugated equine estrogen (Premarin) at 1.25 mg every four hours is a good alternative. Bleeding is usually controlled within 24 hours with this high dose estrogen therapy. After the endometrium has been stabilized with high dose estrogen, lower dose estrogen at 1.25 mg per day of conjugated estrogen can be administered for 7 to 10 days, in conjunction with a progestational agent such as MPA at 10 mg/day. The woman should be warned to expect a heavy but time-limited period after stopping the hormones.
8. A treatment for moderate bleeding is to prescribe monophasic oral contraceptives to be taken three to four times per day for a week. The woman may start a new pack of pills after this week, or a heavy, cramping flow after cessation of treatment will follow this week.
9. After control of acute bleeding is obtained, the next goal of therapy is to prevent recurrence of heavy or irregular bleeding. In most adolescents and many adult women, the treatment of choice is monophasic OCPs, taken once daily. If contraception is not required, the adolescent should continue taking OCPs for three months. The woman can then be observed for spontaneous resumption of menses. If amenorrhea is present after three months, the woman can be started on OCPs again, or can take MPA 10 mg daily for 10 to 13

Table 14.6. Hormonal treatment of dysfunctional uterine bleeding

Emergent

1. Intravenous estrogen at 25 mg every 4 hours for 12 hours is said to be the treatment of choice

OR

2. Intravenous conjugated equine estrogen (Premarin) at 1.25 mg every 4 hours is a good alternative

THEN

Estrogen at 1.25 mg per day of conjugated estrogen can be administered for 7 to 10 days, PLUS a progestational agent such as MPA 10 mg/day

Moderate bleeding

1. Monophasic oral contraceptives to be taken 3 to 4 times per day for a week, then start a new pack of pills one pill a day after this week

OR

2. MPA 10 mg daily for 10 days

Mild or recurrent bleeding

1. Monophasic oral contraceptive pills for 3 to 6 months at least

OR

2. MPA 10 mg daily for 10 days each month

OR

3. Depo Provera intramuscularly 150 mg every 3 months

OR

4. Progestin IUD insertion

OR

5. NSAIDs 10 to 15 days per month

MPA, medroxyprogesterone acetate; IUD, intrauterine device; NSAID, nonsteroidal anti-inflammatory drug.

days per month, to permit shedding of the endometrium.

10. If OCPs are contraindicated, or if the woman does not want to take them, therapy with a progestin can be used. Oral MPA (Provera) can be taken for 12 days per month at 10 mg/day, to prevent abnormal accumulation of endometrial tissue. Depo Provera 150 mg i.m. every three months will also prevent further heavy abnormal bleeding and any risk of endometrial cancer. A progestin-containing IUD can also be used to promote atrophy of the endometrial lining.[20]

11. If the woman is perimenopausal, cyclic conjugated equine estrogen, 0.625 to 1.25 mg daily for 25 days with 5 to 10 mg MPA added from days 15 to 25 is an

The treatment of choice for dysfunctional uterine bleeding is monophasic oral contraceptives.

appropriate treatment. OCPs are an alternative treatment for perimenopausal women who do not smoke and have no evidence of vascular disease.

12. NSAIDs have been shown to decrease menstrual blood loss in women with dysfunctional bleeding. They are taken at the onset of bleeding and for the first three to four days of each period.

13. Surgical therapy for dysfunctional bleeding is reserved for women when all other methods fail and the woman has no desire for future pregnancy.

    Endometrial ablation is performed with the use of laser, photovaporization, or electrocautery using hysteroscopic visualization. Endometrial ablation is an outpatient procedure, which results in up to 90 percent of women becoming amenorrheic or having acceptable reduction of vaginal bleeding.

14. Hysterectomy is indicated when there is associated pelvic pathology such as dysplasia, pelvic relaxation, or large fibroids and the woman has no desire for any future pregnancy. The hospital stay is longer for women who have had a hysterectomy than those who have undergone endometrial ablation and the costs are significantly higher.

15. A D&C is frequently used to stop bleeding in women with menorrhagia and hypovolemia. It is effective for this purpose, but does not prevent recurrent abnormal bleeding, unless it is followed by additional hormone treatment.

> Nonsteroidal antiinflammatory drugs have been shown to decrease menstrual blood loss in women with dysfunctional bleeding.

Conclusions

Amenorrhea, oligomenorrhea, and menorrhagia are different clinical syndromes on a spectrum of menstrual irregularity often caused by physiological or pituitary and endocrine disorders. The primary cause of amenorrhea is pregnancy, and pregnancy complications often cause irregular vaginal bleeding. Most often anovulatory or dysfunctional uterine bleeding is the cause of menstrual disorders. With a minimum of diagnostic tests, the physician can impact on and improve menstrual cycles and bleeding.

REFERENCES

1. Ronnerdag J, Odlind, V. Health effects of long-term use of the intrauterine levonorgestrel-releasing system. A follow-up study over 12 years of continuous use. *Acta Obstet Gynecol Scand* 1999;**78**:716–21.

2. Speroff L, Glass RH, Kase, NG. Amenorrhea. In Mitchell C, ed., *Clinical Gynecologic Endocrinology and Infertility*, 5th edn. Williams & Wilkins, Baltimore, MD, 1994, pp. 401–56.

3. Warren MP, Biller BMK, Shangold MM. A new clinical option for hormone replacement therapy in women with secondary amenorrhea: Effects of cyclic administration of progesterone from the sustained release vaginal gel Crinone (4 percent and 8 percent) on endometrial morphologic features and withdrawal bleeding. *Am J Obstet Gynecol* 1999;**180**:42–8.

4. Fraser IS, Baird DT. Endometrial cystic glandular hyperplasia in adolescent girls. *J Obstet Gynecol* 1972;**79**:1009–13.

5. WHO Task Force on Method for the Natural Regulation of Fertility. The World Health Organization multinational study of breast feeding and lactational amenorrhea. I. Description of infant feeding patterns and of the return of menses. *Fertil Steril* 1998;**70**:448–60.

6. Szreter S. *Fertility, Class and Gender in Britain, 1860–1940*. Cambridge University Press, Cambridge, 1996.

7. WHO Task Force on Method for the Natural Regulation of Fertility. The World Health Organization multinational study of breast feeding and lactational amenorrhea. II. Factors associated with the length of amenorrhea. *Fertil Steril* 1998;**70**:461–70.

8. Beckvid-Henrikkson G, Schnell C, Linden-Hirschberg A. Women endurance runners with menstrual dysfunction have prolonged interruption of training due to injury. *Gynecol Obstet Investig* 2000;**49**:41–6.

9. Edge D, Segatore M. Assessment and management of galactorrhea. *Nurse Pract* 1993;**18**(6):35–6, 43–4, 49.

10. Battinno S, Ben-Ami M, Geslevich Y, Weiner E, Shalev E. Factors associated with withdrawal bleeding after administration of oral dydrogesterone or medroxyprogesterone acetate in women with secondary amenorrhea. *Gynecol Obstet Investig* 1996;**42**:113–16.

11. Genazzani AD, Gastaldi M, Petraglia F et al. Naltrexone administration modulates the neuroendocrine control of luteinizing hormone secretion in hypothalamic amenorrhoea. *Human Reprod* 1995;**10**:2870–1.

12. Glueck CJ, Wang P, Fonataine R, Tracy T, Sieve-Smith L. Metformin induced resumption of normal menses in 39 of 42 (91%) previously amenorrheic women with the polycystic ovary syndrome. *Metabolism* 1999;**48**:511–19.

13. Guzick D. Polycystic ovary syndrome. Symptomatology, pathophysiology and epidemiology. *Am J Obstet Gynecol* 1998;**179**:S89–S93.

14. Schneider LG. Causes of abnormal vaginal bleeding in a family practice center. *J Fam Pract* 1983;**16**:281–3.

15. Hertweck SP. Dysfunctional uterine bleeding. *Obstet Gynecol Clin North Am* 1992;**19**:129–49.

16. Emanuel MH, Verdel MJ, Wamstenea K, Lames FB. A prospective comparison of transvaginal ultrasonography and diagnostic hysteroscopy in the evaluation of patients with abnormal uterine bleeding: Clinical implications. *Am J Obstet Gynecol* 1995;**172**:547–52.

17. Indman PD. Abnormal uterine bleeding. Accuracy of vaginal probe ultrasound in predicting abnormal hysteroscopic findings. *J Reprod Med* 1995;**40**:545–8.

18. Emanuel MH, Wamsteker K, Lammes FB. Is dilatation and curettage obsolete for diagnosing intrauterine disorders in premenopausal patients with persistent abnormal uterine bleeding? *Acta Obstet Gynecol Scand* 1997;**76**:65–8.

19. Gull B, Carlsson S, Karlsson B. Transvaginal ultrasonography of the endometrium in women with postmenopausal bleeding: Is it always necessary to perform an endometrial biopsy? *Am J Obstet Gynecol* 2000;**182**:509–15.

20. Chuong CJ, Brenner PF. Management of abnormal uterine bleeding. *Am J Obstet Gynecol* 1996;**175**:787–92.

15 Sexually transmitted diseases

Kay Bauman, MD, MPH

STDs are common and many are easily treatable. However, close follow-up and public health evaluation to treat contacts are very important.

Gonococcal (GC) infections

Etiology

Neisseria gonorrhea, a Gram-negative diplococcus.

Epidemiology

1. This infection is limited to humans. Secretions from infected mucus membranes usually from intimate contact transmit it, either in sexual activity or from the mother to her newborn during delivery.
2. The incubation period for this infection is two to seven days.
3. In the USA, the rate per 100 000 population has consistently fallen from 298.7 in 1988 to 121.4 in 1997, the last year for which reporting is complete (Figure 15.1).[1]
4. In the USA, the age range with the greatest incidence is 15 to 24 years, with a 1997 rate of 513.3/100 000 population. Rates are approximately the same for men (125.4) and women (119.3).[1]
5. In one population in the UK, the incidence of GC in 1990 was 61/100 000. Men had a higher infection rate than women (54/100 000) while women had an average of 38.5 cases/100 000. Peak incidences occurred in men aged 20 to 24 and women aged 15 to 19 (Figure 15.1).[2]
6. Fifty-nine percent of the reported cases in the USA were identified in African-American individuals, 11 percent in white individuals, 29 percent did not designate race and fewer than 1 percent were either Asian/Pacific Islander or American Indian/Alaskan Native. In the African-American population, the rate has dropped markedly over the past decade from 2000 infections/100 000 population in 1986 to approximately 600/100 000 in 1997 (Figure 15.2).[1]

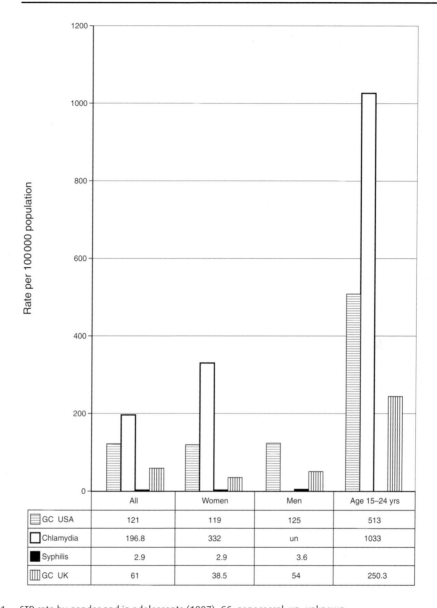

Figure 15.1.   STD rate by gender and in adolescents (1997). GC, gonococcal; un, unknown.

	All	Women	Men	Age 15–24 yrs
GC USA	121	119	125	513
Chlamydia	196.8	332	un	1033
Syphilis	2.9	2.9	3.6	
GC UK	61	38.5	54	250.3

7.   In the USA, GC has become an inner city disease, with a very high prevalence in lower socioeconomic, inner city populations contrasted with middle class populations. However, behavioral risk factors for STDs, including rates of condom use, seem to be similar in populations with and without infection.

8.   In the UK, the incidence of GC in inner city south London was eight to nine times higher in nonwhites than in whites in all age and sex strata and these ethnic differences persisted after adjustment for socioeconomic status.[3]

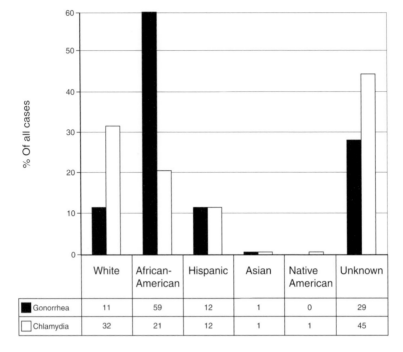

% Of all cases

	White	African-American	Hispanic	Asian	Native American	Unknown
■ Gonorrhea	11	59	12	1	0	29
☐ Chlamydia	32	21	12	1	1	45

% Of all cases

Figure 15.2.   Incidence of gonorrhea and chlamydia by race (1997).

Increased rates of GC were also reported for Afro-Caribbean people living in Leeds; rates were 12 times higher for Afro-Caribbean women and 54 times higher for Afro-Caribbean men than among white individuals.[2]

The incubation period for gonorrhea is two to seven days.

Clinical presentation

1. Signs and symptoms: The disease may be asymptomatic in both men and women, but is frequently so in women (approximately 80 percent). If symptomatic, women usually present with purulent vaginal discharge that is endocervical or urethral. Infection of the rectum or pharynx can occur. Dysuria, spotting with intercourse, or localized pain such as from an abscess may be described. If infection has already spread to upper levels of the genitourinary (GU) system, the women may experience lower abdominal pain and tenderness, fever, and/or dysmenorrhea. A chronic infection can present as chronic pelvic pain, infertility, or an ectopic pregnancy.

Table 15.1. Differential diagnosis of gonorrhea infections

- Chlamydia infections
- Urinary tract infection
- Vaginitis from other causes such as trichomonas, bacterial vaginosis or others
- Culture-negative mucopurulant cervicitis

2. Physical findings include: vaginal, urethral or endocervical discharge; lower abdominal tenderness; Bartholin's gland abscess; and if the woman has PID, then she may have cervical motion tenderness, palpable, tender fallopian tubes or ovaries, and/or lower abdominal tenderness with rebound.

3. Diagnosis:
   a. If a woman presents with the symptoms given in (2) above, the physician can choose to treat presumptively. A known positive intimate partner also warrants presumptive treatment (Table 15.1).
   b. Because mucopurulant cervicitis can also exist with negative diagnostic testing for both chlamydia and gonorrhea, other clinicians may wish to document infection prior to treating. Clinicians must also be attentive to screening high risk women for asymptomatic infection. Sexually active teenagers and women aged 20 to 25 are at highest risk.
   c. Attention to the incidence of gonorrhea in one's own community is important for a physician to add other risk groups to one's screening protocols.
   d. Commercial sex workers, illicit drug users, and women with a history of incarceration are at high risk for sexually transmitted infections and may warrant presumptive treatment.

4. Laboratory testing:
   a. A diagnosis of gonorrhea can be established by direct culturing on special media, (e.g. Thayer–Martin). A culture requires three to seven days. A Gram stain of the discharge from the vaginal pool or cervix is not diagnostic in women even if it shows clumps of Gram-negative diplococci together with polymorphonucleocytes, although it can be used for men and children.
   b. Nonculture tests are rapid, highly specific and moderately to highly sensitive. They include (i) enzyme immunoassay (EIA), (ii) DNA probe, and (iii) first voided urine screen by ligase chain reaction (LCR).

5. Imaging: Pelvic ultrasound or CT scan may demonstrate tuboovarian abscess or thickened tubes.

Because mucopurulant cervicitis can also exist with negative diagnostic testing for both chlamydia and gonorrhea, clinicians may wish to document infection prior to treating.

Table 15.2. Treatment of gonorrhea

- Cephalosporins
  125 mg ceftriaxone i.m.,
  OR
  400 mg cefixime p.o.,
  OR
- Fluoroquinolones (not in pregnancy)
  500 mg ciprofloxacin p.o.,
  OR
  400 mg ofloxacin p.o.
- To also cover frequently associated chlamydia, it is recommended to add either:
  azithromycin 1 g p.o. (single dose), or doxycycline 100 mg p.o. twice a day for 7 days
- Alternative treatments
  - Spectinomycin 2 g i.m.
  - Other cephalosporins can be used, although there is less clinical experience with their
    use: (a) ceftizoxime 500 i.m., (b) cefotaxine 500 mg i.m., (c) cefotetan 1 g i.m., or (d)
    cefoxitin 2 g i.m. with probencid 1 g orally
  - Other quinolones also with limited clinical experience: (a) enoxacin 400 mg p.o., (b)
    lomefloxacin 400 mg p.o., or (c) norfloxacin 800 mg p.o.

Data from Centers for Disease Control and Prevention. 1998 Guidelines for treatment of
sexually transmitted diseases. *MMWR Morb Mortal Wkly Rep* 1998;**47**:11–17, 28–40, 46–9,
53–6, 59–61,79–86, 101–2.

Treatment and follow-up[4]

1. Treatment must cover both chlamydia, the more common of the two infections, and gonorrhea.
2. Some treatment options cost less than the cost of testing, so treating presumptively may also be cost effective (Table 15.2).
3. Follow-up: Test of cure is not recommended for patients who become asymptomatic after treatment. However, symptomatic women after treatment require a repeat culture and antimicrobial sensitivity testing. Sexual partners need to be referred for evaluation and treatment. Patients with GC need to be evaluated for other STDs including chlamydia, HIV, hepatitis B, and/or syphilis when appropriate.

Prevention

Condom use offers a high degree of protection in heterosexual and anal intercourse.

Patient education

Community education among adolescents to control sexually transmitted infection is a worthwhile investment.

Special considerations

Occasionally gonorrheal infections can become blood borne, causing other systemic problems such as arthralgias, septic arthritis, skin lesions, or even endocarditis. All pregnant women should be screened for sexually transmitted infections.

Patients with gonococcal infections need to be evaluated for other sexually transmitted diseases including chlamydia, HIV, hepatitis B, and/or syphilis when appropriate.

Chlamydia infections

Etiology

Chlamydia trachomatis genital infections.

Epidemiology

1. Transmission is overwhelmingly sexual, but can occur from one mucous membrane to another.[1] Incubation period is approximately one week.
2. Over half a million cases of chlamydia were reported in the USA in 1997, surpassing gonorrheal infection rates. Estimates are that for every reported case there may be seven or more unreported cases. Thus, annually in the USA, there may be more than four million cases.[1]
3. *Chlamydia trachomatis* is also the most common sexually transmitted bacterial pathogen in Britain.[5]
4. The rate for women in 1997 in the USA was 322.1/100 000 population (Figure 15.1). There is not adequate CDC data for a comparison with the rates for men. Most men are treated presumptively without culture.
5. Because chlamydia only became a reportable disease in all US states in 1995, there is less historical data for comparison of rates over time than for other STDs. Rates for 1995 to 1997 are given in Figure 15.3.[1] The slight increases noted may be attributed to either improved reporting of this infection or increased rates in our local communities.
6. Chlamydia rates in the USA are highest in the 15 to 24 year age group (rate 1033.34/100 000) (Figure 15.1), followed by ages 25 to 39 years at a fraction of

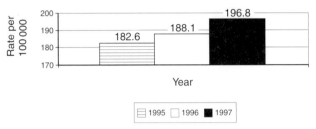

Figure 15.3.   Rates of chlamydial infection in women.

the rate: 167.46 (Figure 15.1).[1]

7. Chlamydial rates in the USA reported by race show 32 percent African-American, 21 percent white, 45 percent race not stated, and 1 percent each for American Indian/Alaska Native and Asian/Pacific Islander. Twelve percent are reported as Hispanic. Rates are also higher for persons who live in inner cities and have lower socioeconomic status.[1]

8. Because the infection is more often asymptomatic than symptomatic, transmission occurs effectively. Screening programs in high risk populations (often determined solely by age) is an important way to decrease the prevalence of this infection.

Cost

The costly sequelae of this infection occur primarily in women and include PID, infertility and ectopic pregnancy. In the USA, chlamydia costs range from $2 billion to $3 billion annually.[6]

Clinical presentation

1. Signs and symptoms: Approximately 70 percent of cases in women are asymptomatic, and many of these are undetected and untreated.[6] If symptomatic, a typical presentation is a mucopurulant cervicitis that cannot be differentiated clinically from gonorrhea or other infections. Other presentations include the urethral syndrome, Bartholin's gland abscesses, and as upper levels of the GU tract become involved, endometritis, salpingitis/PID, and Fitz-Hugh–Curtis perihepatitis syndrome.

2. Physical findings include a mucopurulant cervical discharge, cervical motion tenderness, tenderness of tubes, ovaries and/or uterus, and/or abdominal findings such as generalized or rebound tenderness.

3. Diagnosis:
   a. If a women presents with the above, the clinician may opt to treat presumptively, covering for both gonorrhea and chlamydia. This may be cost

effective, because some treatment options are less expensive than the cost of testing.

b. Some women have a mucopurulant cervicitis that is culture negative for GC and chlamydia testing. Thus some providers prefer to document infection prior to treating. Most often, the diagnosis of chlamydia is established when the clinician is attentive to screening high risk women, such as sexually active teenagers and women aged 20 to 25 years.

c. Knowing the infection rates in one's own community to be able to expand screening efforts to other high risk groups is important. Commercial sex workers, illicit drug users and women with a history of incarceration are at higher risk for chlamydia infection.

4. Laboratory testing:

a. *Chlamydia* culture requires three to seven days and is 70 to 90 percent sensitive. It remains the gold standard and must be used when noncervical sites are cultured (eye, urethra, nasopharynx, rectum).

b. DNA probes (nucleic acid hybridization), monoclonal antibody, direct fluorescent antibody and enzyme-linked immunosorbent assay (ELISA) determinations are available, with wide ranges of sensitivities and costs.

c. All screening specimens should be collected from the endocervix. A urethral specimen may increase culture sensitivity significantly, but has not been shown to aid in nonculture tests. The appropriate swab (with plastic or wire shaft, not wood) should be maintained 1 to 2 cm into the endocervical canal for 10–30 seconds, rotating it against the wall to collect an endocervical specimen, which is then directly placed in the transport medium.[4]

d. The differential diagnosis includes gonorrhea, *Ureoplasma urealyticum* infection, and UTIs.

5. Imaging: Pelvic ultrasound or CT scan may demonstrate tuboovarian abscess or thickened tubes.

Treatment

This is listed in Table 15.3.

Follow-up

For first infections, test of cure is not recommended unless the woman remains symptomatic. If erythromycin was given, a test of cure is appropriate at approximately three weeks, because this treatment is less effective. Sexual partners should be referred for evaluation and treatment. Abstinence from intercourse for one week or until treatment is complete is recommended.

Table 15.3. Treatment for chlamydial infections[4]

- Azithromycin 1 g p.o. once,
  OR
- Doxycycline 100 mg p.o. twice a day for 7 days
  Azithromycin is more expensive than doxycycline, but if given at the site and time of clinical presentation with directly observed therapy, compliance is nearly 100 percent
- Alternative treatments
  - Erythromycin base 500 mg p.o. q.i.d. for 7 days,
    OR
  - Erythromycin ethylsuccinate 800 mg p.o. q.i.d. for 7 days,
    OR
  - Ofloxacin 300 mg p.o. b.i.d. for 7 days (not in pregnancy)
    OR
  - Erythromycin base 250 mg p.o. q.i.d. for 14 days,
    OR
  - Erythromycin ethylsuccinate 800 mg p.o. q.i.d. for 7 days,
    OR
  - Erythromycin ethylsuccinate 400 mg p.o. q.i.d. for 14 days
    Doxycycline is contraindicated in pregnancy and to date there are few studies supporting routine use of azithromycin in pregnancy. Thus recommended regimens include erythromycin base (just use CDC guidelines) as above or amoxicillin 500 mg t.i.d. for 7 days
    Erythomycin estolate is also contraindicated in pregnancy

Data from Centers for Disease Control and Prevention. 1998 Guidelines for treatment of sexually transmitted diseases. *MMWR Morb Mortal Wkly Rep* 1998;**47**:11–17, 28–40, 46–9, 53–6, 59–61, 79–86, 101–2.

Prevention

Consistent use of condoms will prevent chlamydial infections. Other behavioral changes that can decrease the incidence of chlamydia include delaying the age of first intercourse and decreasing the number of sexual partners.

Consistent use of condoms will prevent chlamydial infections.

Patient education

Explaining the etiology of infection (i.e., sexual transmission), and the importance of completing treatment is important. The woman should abstain from intercourse for one week or until treatment is completed and sexual partners should be seen or referred for evaluation and treatment.

Special considerations

All sexually active teenage women should be screened because the prevalence is very high in that age group, and most often chlamydia is asymptomatic. Treating infected young women may prevent the sequelae of PID, infertility, or ectopic pregnancies. All pregnant women should be screened.

> All sexually active teenage women should be screened because the prevalence is very high in that age group.

Syphilis

Etiology

Treponema pallidum, a spirochete.

Epidemiology

1. The USA experienced an increase in syphilis cases in the second half of the 1980s, reaching a peak of 20.3 cases/100 000 population in 1990. There has since been a decline and the 1998 rate was a record low of 2.6/100 000, below the Healthy People 2000 Guidelines of 4/100 000 (Figure 15.1). Rates are higher in the south (5.1/100 000) than in all other geographical areas.[1] Rates for men (1997 data), 3.6/100 000, exceed those for women, 2.9/100 000.[1]

2. Rates by race and ethnicity are (per 100 000 individuals), African-Americans, 17.1; American Indians/Alaska Natives, 2.8; Hispanics, 1.5; non-Hispanic whites, 0.5; and Asian/Pacific Islanders, 0.4. The ratio of primary and secondary syphilis for African-Americans: whites fell from 53:1 in 1990, to 44:1 in 1997 to 34:1 in 1998.[1]

3. Rates are highest among women aged 20 to 24 years and men aged 30 to 39 years.[7]

4. In the USA, congenital syphilis increased during the same years and reached a peak in 1991 of 110 cases/100 000 live births. It has abruptly declined and in 1998 was 20.6 cases/100 000 live births. It still exists because women with syphilis often receive no prenatal care (36 percent). Testing may be performed too late in pregnancy or tested mothers receive late or no follow-up.[7]

5. In the UK, the incidence of congenital syphilis has decreased since 1980.[8]

6. Incubation period is typically three weeks after sexual contact for primary infections.

Costs

The estimated national annual direct and indirect costs of syphilis in the USA are an estimated $966 million.[9]

Clinical presentation

1. Symptoms: Women may seek care for a painless indurated ulcer (chancre) usually on the genitalia, but if the ulcer is intravaginal or cervical the woman would not be aware of its presence.

    Half of untreated patients progress to secondary syphilis two months after the chancre has healed. At this time, women may present for care with a generalized rash or with new lesions on the vulva. Tertiary syphilis can occur 5 to 10 years after primary infection, but clinical presentation is often for other problems such as cardiovascular lesions or central nervous system (CNS) involvement, where syphilis may be low on a differential list and only discovered with astute laboratory evaluation.

2. Physical findings:

    a. Primary syphilis: This is evident as a single, nontender 0.5 to 2 cm indurated ulcer with a clean, yellow base, usually genital, which, if it has existed for a few days may be accompanied by painless regional adenopathy. The ulcer heals over three to six weeks with scarring and is infectious during this time.

    b. Secondary syphilis: Two to six weeks after exposure, patients may have a maculopopular generalized nonpruritic, symmetrical rash that includes palms and soles. Patchy alopecia can occur. Less commonly, condyloma lata, which are moist, flat, pink lobular papules of the vulvar area, can develop. During this time, the woman remains infectious. These clinical findings can resolve without treatment.

    c. Latent syphilis: There are no physical findings and diagnosis is made on laboratory screening.

        i. Early latent: Less than one year.

        ii. Late latent: More than one year or of unknown duration.

    d. Tertiary syphilis: The patient presents with mucocutaneous nodules and gummas, cardiovascular lesions such as aortitis, ophthalmic problems such as uveitis or optic neuritis, cranial nerve palsies, or meningitis. Neurosyphilis can occur, with symptoms of CNS changes such as tabes dorsalis or dementia. Note: neurological findings necessitate a cerebrosppinal fluid (CSF) examination.

3. Diagnosis: Laboratory tests.[4,10]

    a. Dark-field microscopy to visualize the spirochete in the serous exudate from suspicious genital lesions is the only method of diagnosis in primary syphilis, because it is too early for serological testing to be accurate.

Women may seek care for a painless indurated ulcer (chancre) usually on the genitalia, but if the ulcer were intravaginal or cervical, the woman would not be aware of its presence.

b. Nontreponemal tests are the most common and inexpensive screening tests. VDRL (Venereal Disease Research Laboratory) and RPR (Rapid Plasma Reagin) are equally sensitive, can be used both qualitatively and quantitatively, but do not become positive until four to six weeks after infection. These tests may revert to negative after treatment of primary or secondary syphilis, but it may take one to two years. Neither test is sufficient for diagnosis without a confirmatory treponemal test.

c. Either VDRL or RPR titers can monitor the disease activity, but once one is used, the caregiver should use it consistently, and preferably from the same laboratory.

d. Treponemal tests include FTA-ABS (fluorescent treponemal antibody absorbed) and MHA-TP (microhemagglutination assay for *T. pallidum* antibody). These are confirmatory tests after a positive VDRL or RPR, and are not used quantitatively.

e. For neurosyphilis, a reactive VDRL-CSF is considered diagnostic.

f. Differential diagnosis of the primary ulcer includes herpes, chancroid, lymphogranuloma venereum, granuloma inguinale. Differential diagnosis of the secondary rash includes pityriasis rosea (no herald patch), guttate psoriasis, drug eruption.

Nontreponemal tests are the most common and inexpensive for the diagnosis of syphilis.

Treatment

See Table 15.4.

Follow-up

Regular appointments to monitor success of antibiotic therapy is important, with use of quantitative tests, usually repeated at 6, 12, and 24 months. Titers should fall at least two dilutions (fourfold) within 12 to 24 months. Contacting all previous sexual partners so that they, too, can be evaluated and treated is essential.

Prevention

Condom use.

Patient education

Sexual intercourse should be avoided until the disease is cured. All sexual contacts should be referred for evaluation and, if needed, treatment. The

Table 15.4. Treatment for syphilis

- Parenteral penicillin G has been used effectively for over 40 years to treat syphilis, but without comparative trials to select the optimal regimen. Even fewer data support nonpenicillin regimens
- Primary, secondary and early latent disease (known to be of < 1 year duration): benzathine penicillin G, 2.4 million units i.m. for 1 dose
- Late latent disease (> 1 year) or tertiary syphilis (no neurological involvement): benzathine penicillin G, 2.4 million units i.m. weekly for 3 weeks
- Neurosyphilis: aqueous crystalline penicillin G, 18 to 24 million units per day, given as 3 to 4 million units i.v. every 4 hours for 10 to 14 days
- Alternative regimen (must have compliance): procaine penicillin 2.4 million units i.m. per day plus probenecid 500 mg p.o. q.i.d., both for 10 to 14 days
- Penicillin allergy
  - Primary, secondary, early latent (nonpregnant women)
    Doxycycline 100 mg b.i.d. for 2 weeks,
    OR
    Tetracycline 500 mg q.i.d. for 2 weeks
  - Late latent
    Doxycycline 100 m.g. b.i.d. for 4 weeks,
    OR
    Tetracycline 500 mg q.i.d. for 4 weeks
- Pregnancy: all patients allergic to penicillin should be desensitized and treated with penicillin

Data from Centers for Disease Control and Prevention. 1998 Guidelines for treatment of sexually transmitted diseases. *MMWR Morb Mortal Wkly Rep* 1998;**47**:11–17, 28–40, 46–9, 53–6, 59–61, 79–86, 101–2.

importance of regular follow-up to monitor success of therapy should be explained.

Special considerations

1. All patients with syphilis should be tested for hepatitis B and HIV infections.
2. The Jarisch–Herxheimer reaction is an acute febrile reaction that may be accompanied by headache or myalgia. It can occur in the first 24 hours of treatment for syphilis, more commonly in early syphilis. Treatment is only antipyretics.[4]
3. Syphilis during pregnancy: All women should be screened upon entering care. In high risk areas, women should be screened again at 28 weeks and at delivery. A woman delivering a stillborn after 20 weeks of gestation should be

tested for syphilis. Women treated during the second half of pregnancy are at risk for premature labor/fetal distress if treatment precipitates the Jarisch–Herxheimer reaction described above.

Genital herpes

Etiology

Herpes simplex virus (HSV) type 1 (10 to 30 percent) and 2 (70 to 90 percent), a double-stranded DNA virus.

Epidemiology

1. Genital herpes is a chronic infection, most often asymptomatic, whose course can include long periods of latency and occasional to frequent exacerbations of painful genital ulcers.
2. The virus can be shed when asymptomatic, thus transmission can occur at unknown times.
3. Treatment can shorten symptomatic outbreaks, but does not eradicate the virus.
4. On the basis of serological studies, it is estimated that 45 million persons in the USA are infected or approximately one in five persons. Seroprevalence is dependent on age from fewer than 1 percent at age younger than 15 years to over 20 percent in 30 to 44-year-olds.[4]
5. Women have higher reported rates than men; rates vary considerably by country.
6. The highest rated risk behavior for seropositivity to HSV2 is number of sexual partners.

> The highest rated risk behavior of seropositivity to herpes simplex virus type 2 is number of sexual partners.

Clinical presentation

1. The initial infection occurs by exposure through mucosal surfaces. The average incubation period is five to seven days, but it can be 1 to 45 days. After infection, virus particles are transported along peripheral nerves to the dorsal root ganglia where they remain latent and can cause recurrent disease.

2. The woman may present to the clinician with vulvar or vaginal ulcers that might be accompanied by systemic symptoms such as fever and malaise, and/or perhaps inguinal adenopathy. Shedding of the virus lasts two to three days but vesicles take one to three weeks to heal. Primary infection may be more extensive and longer lasting than recurrent herpes.

3. Recurrence rates are extremely variable. In one study of 457 persons with active herpes, 89 percent experienced a recurrence during the first year of follow-up. The average recurrence was once every three months and 20 percent had more than 10 recurrences in the first year.[11] Consideration can be given to suppressive treatment if frequency of recurrence is every one to two months or if recurrences are disabling. Women may note a prodrome of paresthesias, or itching can occur prior to vesicle outbreak.

4. Physical findings include multiple vesicles that become shallow, tender ulcers on an erythematous base that occur on the inner thighs, vulva, vaginal walls or cervix; can be accompanied by inguinal adenopathy or fever.

5. Diagnosis: The clinical presentation is specific to HSV. Often cultures or other diagnostic work-ups are unnecessary.

6. Laboratory testing:
   a. The viral culture remains the gold standard. It takes approximately five days, and it is most likely to be positive in earlier stage lesions. Thus cultures can be falsely negative 20 to 30 percent of the time.
   b. ELISAs for viral antigen: low sensitivity.
   c. DNA detection by polymerase chain reaction.
   d. Tzanck preparation for multinucleated giant cells: specific but only 40 to 50 percent sensitive. It can also be present in zoster.
   e. Serology: HSV can be detected by ELISA, complement fixation, radio-immunoassay (RIA) or direct fluorescent assay (DFA).

7. The differential diagnosis includes primary syphilis, chancroid, lympho-granuloma venereum, allergic contact dermatitis, trauma, zoster.

The woman with herpes simplex virus infection may present to the clinician with vulvar or vaginal ulcers that might be accompanied by systemic symptoms such as fever and malaise, and/or perhaps inguinal adenopathy.

Treatment

See Table 15.5.

Prevention

Condom use will prevent viral transmission.

Table 15.5. Treatment of herpes simplex virus

- Primary herpes
  - Acyclovir 200 mg 5 times a day, or 400 mg t.i.d. for 7 to 10 days
    OR
  - Famciclovir 125 mg b.i.d. for 7 to 10 days,
    OR
  - Valacyclovir 500 mg b.i.d. for 7 to 10 days
- Recurrent infection (if treated very early): Same medications and doses as above but for a 5-day course
- Suppression of infection
  - Acyclovir 200 mg b.i.d. or 400 mg once per day
  - Famciclovir 125 mg t.i.d., or 250 mg b.i.d.
  - Valacyclovir 500 mg once per day
- Drug resistance to acyclovir has been reported, particularly in women coinfected with HIV. Foscarnet can be used in these women

Patient education

1. Natural history of this disease including:
   a. Transmissibility even when no lesions are present.
   b. Possibility of transmission to a newborn.
   c. Potential for recurrent episodes.
2. Regular use of condoms to prevent transmission.

Special considerations

1. Pregnancy: The virus can be transmitted from mother to newborn even if no lesions are present. However, only women with active lesions should be considered for operative delivery. Approximate neonatal infection rate is 10 to 20/100 000 live births in the USA. Transmission is highest among women who are experiencing their first herpes infection at or near delivery. The safety of acyclovir and related drugs in pregnancy has not been established, but to date there has been no increase in major birth defects in women treated with acyclovir in pregnancy.

2. Vaccine trials: Multiple centers are working on vaccines to prevent HSV2 infection. A recent publication described two randomized, double blind, placebo-controlled multicenter trials of a recombinant vaccine of two major HSV2 surface glycoproteins. A series of immunizations were given at zero, one, and six months to HSV2 seronegative persons. The overall efficiency of the vaccine at one year follow-up was only 9 percent, with no significant difference between vaccine and control groups of HSV2 infection, and no

influence on duration of first infection or frequencies of reactivation. High levels of neutralizing antibiotics were produced, but this vaccine was not efficacious in preventing disease.[12]

3. HIV coinfection: Immunocompromised women can have prolonged or severe episodes of genital herpes. Intermittent or suppressive treatment is often beneficial. These women may require increased doses of acyclovir and like medications and in severe infections may require intravenous administration.

> Herpes simplex virus can be transmitted from pregnant mother to newborn at delivery even if no lesions are present. However, only women with active lesions should be considered for operative delivery.

Pelvic inflammatory disease

Definition

PID is a spectrum of pelvic infections of the upper genital tract that include endometritis, salpingitis, tuboovarian abscess and pelvic peritonitis.

Etiology

PID is usually polymicrobial and may include one or more of chlamydia and gonorrhea (either present in two-thirds of cases), anaerobes such as *Bacteroides* sp., *Peptostreptococcus* sp., *Prevotella* sp., *Mycoplasma hominis*, and *Ureoplasma urealyticum*, and facultative bacteria such as *Gardnerella*, *Streptococcus* sp., and coliforms.

Epidemiology

1. Each year in the USA one million women experience an episode of PID.[13] Approximately one-quarter go on to longer term sequelae that can include recurrent PID, chronic pelvic pain, ectopic pregnancy, and infertility.
2. Approximately one in five may be hospitalized and half of those need surgical intervention.
3. PID is more highly prevalent in younger (i.e. age < 25 years) and more sexually active women with either multiple partners, a new partner or increased frequency of intercourse.[4]

> PID is usually polymicrobial.

Clinical presentation

1. Women can present acutely ill with fever and severe abdominal pain but

Table 15.6. Criteria for diagnosis of pelvic inflammatory disease

- Minimal criteria include
  - Lower abdominal tenderness
  - Adnexal tenderness
  - Cervical motion tenderness
- Additional supportive clinical criteria include: (1) fever > 38.4 °C (101 °F) and (2) cervical or vaginal discharge

perhaps the majority have lesser symptoms. They may have several days of pelvic pain, irregular menses, vaginal discharge, and/or dyspareunia. Because unrecognized and untreated PID can have severe consequences, a low index of suspicion is appropriate.

2. Physical findings can include lower abdominal or adnexal tenderness, cervical motion tenderness, fever, vaginal discharge, and palpation or ultrasound designation of a pelvic mass.

3. Diagnosis: There is no gold standard for clinical diagnosis; even laparoscopy can miss 20 percent of confirmed cases. Thus most PID is diagnosed and treated presumptively (Table 15.6).

4. Laboratory testing: Findings for any of the following provide additional criteria to support a diagnosis of PID.
   a. Positive cultures for gonorrhea and/or chlamydia.
   b. Elevated erythrocyte sedimentation rate.
   c. Elevated C-reactive protein.

5. Imaging: Transvaginal sonography (or other imaging technique) may show thick and fluid-filled tubes with or without free pelvic fluid. Surgical diagnostic techniques include biopsy evidence of endometriosis or laparoscopic abnormalities consistent with PID.

Differential diagnosis

Appendicitis, ovarian cyst (rupture, torsion, hemorrhage), UTI, gastroenteritis, diverticulitis.

Treatment

1. All regimens must include coverage for chlamydia and gonorrhea, even if cultures are negative, because negative endocervical cultures do not preclude upper tract infection. Anaerobic coverage is also important. Treatment should begin as soon as a presumptive diagnosis is made, because administration of antibiotics prevents long-term sequelae.

2. Hospitalization should occur when surgical emergencies such as appendicitis

have not been ruled out, when the woman is pregnant, if the woman does not respond to or is unable to tolerate outpatient management, if the women is severely ill with high fever or nausea and vomiting, if there is a tuboovarian abscess, or in a woman who is immunodeficient. There are many outpatient and inpatient (intravenous) regimens (Table 15.7).

Follow-up

Substantial clinical improvement.

Prevention

1. Primary prevention of STDs can decrease PID. Clinicians must therefore counsel women effectively; this means taking an adequate sexual history and emphasizing risk reduction approaches such as consistent use of condoms and approaching sexual involvement in a relationship slowly.
2. Practitioners must screen target populations routinely for chlamydia and gonorrhea.

Patient education

Thorough discussion of the nature of this disease and the need for completely taking all medications, even after the symptoms disappear, is important. Other priorities include:
1. Abstinence from sex until well.
2. Early access to health care if symptoms of PID recur.
3. Treatment of sexual partners.

Special considerations

1. All pregnant women should be screened for STDs because PID in pregnancy can cause adverse outcomes.
2. IUD use: IUD use increases the relative risk of PID in the range of 1.5 to 2.6, but this risk is transient and only for certain at-risk women. Risk for IUD-associated PID is primarily at the time of insertion and within the first four months of use. Administration of doxycycline 200 mg one hour prior to IUD insertion and then daily for two days reduces PID risk.[14]
3. Oral contraceptives: Studies are contradictory; some show a significant decrease in serious PID events and others show an increase in *Chlamydia* infection, a leading cause of PID.[14]
4. Douching: More women with PID have a history of douching, but this can only be considered an association.[14]

Table 15.7. Treatment for pelvic inflammatory disease

Outpatient therapy (in order of lesser to more expensive)

- Cefoxitin 2 g i.m. plus probenecid 1 g single dose plus doxycycline 100 mg b.i.d. for 14 days

  OR
- Can substitute ceftriaxone 250 mg i.m. once or another third-generation cephalosporin, for the cefoxitin and probenecid
- Ofloxacin 400 mg and metronidazole 500 mg both p.o. b.i.d. for 14 days
- Ofloxacin 400 mg and clindamycin 300 mg both p.o. b.i.d. for 14 days. (Dose of clindamycin has been recommended over a range of 300 mg b.i.d. to 450 mg q.i.d.; studies are under way to further support the lower dose)

Inpatient regimens (from lesser to more costly)

- Cefotetan 2 g i.v. every 12 hours plus doxycycline 100 mg i.v. or p.o. every 12 hours (oral is preferred). Doxycycline must be given for 14 days. An oral regimen can be substituted within 24 hours of clinical improvement
- Clindamycin 900 mg i.v. every 8 hours plus gentamycin 2 mg/kg i.v. or i.m. loading dose followed by 1.5 mg/kg every 8 hours. When improved, can switch to oral doxycycline 100 mg b.i.d. to a total of 14 days
- Clindamycin as above but followed by oral clindamycin 450 q.i.d. to a total of 14 days
- Cefoxitin 2 g i.v. every 6 hours until improved plus doxycycline 100 mg i.v. or p.o. for 14 days

Follow-up

- Substantial clinical improvement should be demonstrated within 3 days of therapy or further work-up is warranted. Sex partners of women with PID should be treated, especially to cover chlamydia and gonorrhea

---

Data from Centers for Disease Control and Prevention. 1998 Guidelines for treatment of sexually transmitted diseases. *MMWR Morb Mortal Wkly Rep* 1998;**47**:11–17, 28–40, 46–9, 53–6, 59–61, 79–86, 101–2. Washington E and Berg AO. Preventing and managing pelvic inflammatory disease: Key questions, practices and evidence. *J Fam Pract* 1996;**43**:283–93.

5. Menses: The onset of PID symptoms more often begins within seven days of onset of menses than later in the cycle.

HIV/AIDS

Etiology

HIV belongs to a subgroup of retroviruses called lentiviruses. These viruses are cytopathic (they destroy their host cells).

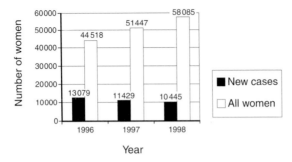

Figure 15.4. Number of women with AIDS in USA.

Epidemiology

1. In the USA through June 1999 the cumulative percentage of AIDS cases that were women was 16.7 percent. In 1998 alone, the percentage of AIDS in women was 24 percent, a striking increase. New AIDS cases are decreasing in numbers across both genders, all races/ethnicities, all ages including pediatric, and for both sexual and injecting drug use risk behaviors (Figure 15.4).[15]

2. Deaths from AIDS in the USA have dropped dramatically because potent antiretroviral therapy has been instituted, from a peak in 1995 of 48 895 to 17 171 in 1998 (both sexes).[15]

3. The epidemiological trends are important to change the consideration of HIV/AIDS as a highly mortal disease to a chronic disease. Prevalence in the USA has never been higher.

4. HIV/AIDS has disproportionately affected African-American and Hispanic women, 57 percent and 20 percent of cases, respectively. Thus pediatric AIDS is also disproportionately affected: 58.4 percent are African-American and 23.2 percent Hispanic.[15]

5. The world burden for HIV/AIDS continues to be mindboggling. It is now the world's deadliest infectious disease – 1.5 times as many people die of AIDS as of malaria. Estimates of persons living with HIV/AIDS are approximately 33.4 million, including 22.7 million in Africa, nearly 7 million in Eastern Europe, Central, South and Southeast Asia, 1.4 million in Latin America, 0.89 million in North America, 0.56 million in East Asia and the Pacific, 0.5 million in Europe, and 0.33 million in the Caribbean. Of note is that 96 percent of cases are in developing countries (Figure 15.5).

6. Worldwide, women represent 43 percent of cases. Life expectancy has dropped sharply in many countries to preimmunization and prepublic health program levels. Child survival has deteriorated: for example, in South Africa, pre AIDS infant mortality rate was 38/1000 live births; current estimate is 61/1000. South African rate increases are now exceeding those of East and

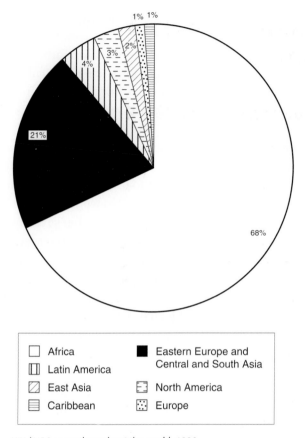

Figure 15.5.   HIV/AIDS cases throughout the world, 1999.

West Africa. In some areas, seroprevalence exceeds 30 percent in prenatal clinic populations. In countries such as Botswana, Zimbabwe, Malawi, Rwanda, Burundi, and Zambia, more than 25 percent of women and men in their 20s are infected.[16,17]

Ninety-six percent of cases of HIV are in developing countries.

Clinical presentation

1. Because HIV/AIDS has an incubation period that can last from two (or fewer) years to 12 or more, many women are diagnosed with population screening while still asymptomatic. This is an advantage for early access to potent antiretroviral drug therapy, for decreasing risk of transmission to sexual

partners and newborns, and for early practice of healthier life behaviors that may affect disease progression.

2. Once the immune system has been threatened, any number of clinical pictures can represent AIDS, such as rapidly advancing cervical cancer, *Pneumocystis carinii* pneumonia (PCP), bacterial pneumonia, refractory vaginal candidiasis, or wasting. A complete discussion of HIV/AIDS is beyond the scope of this text.

3. Diagnosis: Testing for HIV should be offered to all women whose behaviors may put them at risk of transmission (intravenous drug use, drug user as sexual partner), and it should be more broadly offered to women at lesser perceived risk. A large proportion of HIV-infected women cannot immediately identify risky behavior, yet may have a history of other sexually transmitted infections such as chlamydia or cervical dysplasia on Pap screening, diagnostic of human papillomavirus infection.

4. The standard of care is to offer HIV screening as a routine part of prenatal care. Highly debated pending federal legislation is to make this mandatory, because antiretroviral therapy to infected women and their newborns can drastically reduce rates of infection to the babies. At present, pretest and posttest counselling are an integral part of HIV testing and informed consent must be obtained.

5. Laboratory testing:

    a. Antibody tests: EIA is a sensitive screening test but must be confirmed with a supplemental test with high specificity such as the Western blot or immunofluorescence assay (IFA). HIV antibody is detectable within six months of infection 95 percent of the time.

    b. Antigen tests: HIV RNA viral load testing has generally replaced p24 and other antigen testing. Both can be used in infants and children under 18 months because maternal antibody crosses the placenta and obscures the use of antibody test for detection of infection in infants. Viral load testing is used with CD4 counts to monitor the effectiveness of therapy.

    c. Other laboratory tests: A wide range of laboratory tests is used to help the clinician manage the HIV-infected woman. This can include measures of immune function such as CD4 and CD8 counts, serologies for infection that can become life-threatening such as toxoplasmosis and cytomegalovirus, and screening for infections such as hepatitis A and B, which if the test is negative, can be immunized against.

Testing for HIV should be offered to all women whose behaviors may put them at risk of transmission (intravenous drug use, drug user as sexual partner), and it should be more broadly offered to women at lesser perceived risk.

The standard of care is to offer HIV screening as a routine part of prenatal care.

Treatment

1. The clinician and woman together may decide when to begin treatment for HIV infection on the basis of most recent guidelines. If the initial HIV illness can be identified (often precedes seroconversion), treatment with potent antiretroviral therapy has been shown to lower the viral set point and thus probably to increase the natural latency period before severe immunosuppression occurs.

2. Women who are identified during the multiyear latency period can be offered potent antiretroviral therapy at many stages: early disease, mid-disease or when severe immunosuppression has occurred. Measures of both CD4 count and viral load are useful to determine when to begin therapy. The highest-level goal is to achieve or maintain a normal CD4 count and a nondetectable viral load. The approach to potent antiretroviral therapy is beyond the scope of this text. There are currently 14 or 15 drugs approved for therapy in categories including six nucleoside reverse transcriptase inhibitors, three nonnucleoside reverse transcriptase inhibitors, and five or six protease inhibitors.

3. Others under investigation include nucleotide analogs, fusion and integrase inhibitors and known cancer drugs such as hydroxyurea and cyclophosphamide.

Prophylaxis and prevention

1. Vaccines:
   a. Screen for hepatitis A virus (HAV) and hepatitis B virus (HBV) and offer immunization to those with negative HAV or HBV markers.
   b. Annual influenza shot.
   c. Pneumococcal vaccine at first presentation for care.

2. Avoid use of live oral polio vaccine for anyone in household.

Special consideration

Pregnancy:

1. As noted above, to be able to offer prophylactic treatment to infected pregnant women to decrease infection rates to their newborns, HIV-positive women must be identified. Thus the current standard of obstetric care is to offer HIV testing to all pregnant women. Pending legislation suggests that this HIV testing should be made mandatory.

2. Zidovudine monotherapy to infected mothers and their newborns decreases infection rates in newborns from an average of 25 percent to 8 percent. Potent antiretroviral therapy in the mothers has decreased this even further, in some studies to 2 percent.
3. Elective cesarian section prior to rupture of the amniotic fluid sac also has been shown to lower the transmission rate to about 2 percent.
4. Clinicians caring for HIV-positive pregnant women in the USA should avoid the use of scalp electrodes in labor, should wash newborns immediately, and should counsel against breast feeding.

Hepatitis B

Etiology

Hepatitis B virus.

Epidemiology

1. HBV is a sexually transmitted infection. Transmission of this virus occurs (1992–3 data) 50 percent sexually (41 percent heterosexually and 9 percent homosexually), 31 percent unknown, 15 percent injection drug user, 2 percent from household contact, 1 percent in the workplace, and 1 percent other places and ways.[4,18]
2. Carrier rates increase with decreasing age of acquisition. If a child older than age 5 years or an adult becomes infected, 1 to 6 percent become chronically infected. However, if the newborn child is exposed, 10 to 85 percent become infected, depending on the mother's e antigen (HBe Ag) status, and, if infected, 90 percent develop chronic HBV infection. If the exposed child is vaccinated at birth, only 10 percent become chronically infected.
3. Worldwide carrier rates of hepatitis B vary widely.[19]
   a. USA and developed world, < 2 percent.
   b. Eastern and Southern Europe, Japan, former Soviet Union, 2 to 7 percent.
   c. Most of Asia, Africa, Pacific Islands, Amazon region of South America, 8 to 15 percent.
4. The USA has an estimated 1.25 million carriers. Approximately 6000 deaths occur annually from HBV.[4,18]

Clinical disease

This predominately sexually transmitted infection has the serious sequelae of fulminant hepatitis, chronic active hepatitis, cirrhosis of the liver and hepatocellular cancer. Half of adults become ill when infected with HBV; only 5 percent of preschoolers become symptomatic.

Treatment

Protocols for use of alpha-2b interferon are beyond the scope of this text; some studies show 40 percent effectiveness in eliminating the chronic HBV infection. Antiretroviral agents such as lamivudine are showing effectiveness; these and others are currently under study.[4]

Prevention

Condom use will prevent the large portion of disease that is sexually transmitted. Fewer infected women will result in fewer infected newborns. Screening of all pregnant women can identify newborns at risk of transmission and they can be treated with immunoglobulin and vaccination. Routine immunization of all infants, children, and teenagers will increase the herd immunity of any population and so eventually susceptibility to HBV will decrease when individuals reach the ages where behaviors that transmit the virus are common. Women with a history of commercial sex work, other STDs, illicit drug use or on hemodialysis should be considered for vaccination.

Conclusions

A wide variety of STDs exists and specific recommendations for their treatments have been established. Prevention is possible, diagnosis is usually easy and treatment effective, but close follow-up and treatment of sexual contacts is important.

REFERENCES

1. Centers for Disease Control and Prevention. Summary of notifiable disease, United States, *MMWR Morb Mortal Wkly Rep* 1997;**46**:5, 10–13, 60, 62, 73.
2. Lacey CJN, Merrick DW, Bensley DC, Fairley I. Analysis of the sociodemography of gonorrhoea in Leeds, 1989–93. *BMJ* 1997;**314**:1715–20.
3. Low N, Molokwu B, Daker-White G, Barlow D, Pozniak A. Gonorrhoea in inner London: The hidden epidemic. The Medical Society for the Study of Venereal Diseases. Spring Meeting 1996, Edinburgh, 9–11 May. *Genitorurin Med* 1996;**72**:305.

4. Centers for Disease Control and Prevention. 1998 Guidelines for treatment of sexually transmitted diseases. *MMWR Morb Mortal Wkly Rep* 1998;**47**:11–17, 28–40, 46–9, 53–6, 59–61, 79–86, 101–2.

5. Grun L, Tassano-Smith J, Carder C et al. Comparison of two methods of screening for genital chlamydial infection in women attending in general practice: Cross-sectional survey. *BMJ* 1997;**315**:226–30.

6. Centers for Disease Control and Prevention. Recommendations for the prevention and management of *Chlamydia trachomatis* infections, 1993. *MMWR Morb Mortal Wkly Rep* 1993;**42**:1–2.

7. Centers for Disease Control and Prevention. Congenital syphilis – United States, 1998. *MMWR Morb Mortal Wkly Rep* 1999;**48**:757–61.

8. Hurtig AK, Nicoll A, Carne C et al. Syphilis in pregnant women and their children in the United Kingdom: Results from national clinician reporting surveys 1994–7. *BMJ* 1998;**317**:1617–19.

9. Centers for Disease Control and Prevention. Primary and secondary syphilis – United States, 1998. *MMWR Morb Mortal Wkly Rep* 1999;**48**:873–8.

10. Rudy D, Kurowski K, eds. *Family Medicine*. Williams & Wilkins, Baltimore, MD, 1997, pp. 308–17.

11. Benedetti J, Corey L, Ashley R. Recurrent rates in genital herpes after symptomatic first-episode infection. *Ann Intern Med* 1994;**122**:847–54.

12. Cory L, Langenberg AGM, Ashley R et al. Recombinant glycoprotein vaccine for the prevention of genital HSV-2 infection. *JAMA* 1999;**280**:887–92.

13. Washington AE, Katz P. Cost of and payment source for pelvic inflammatory disease. *JAMA* 1991;**266**:2565–9.

14. Washington E, Berg AO. Preventing and managing pelvic inflammatory disease: Key questions, practices and evidence. *J Fam Pract* 1996;**43**:283–93.

15. Centers for Disease Control and Prevention. HIV/AIDS surveillance report. *Obstet Gynecol Clin North Am* 1999;**11**:5–37.

16. International AIDS Society – USA. HIV in Africa: Epicenter of the global pandemic. *Am J Obstet Gynecol* 1999;**7**:20–4.

17. Stickel A. Facing the global AIDS crisis. *HIV: Issues in Patient Care*, 1999;**2**:1, 9–12.

18. Zimmerman RK, Reuban FL, Ahwesh ER. Hepatitis B virus infection, hepatitis B vaccine, and hepatitis B immune globulin. *J Fam Pract* 1997;**45**:295–315.

19. Douglas RG. The heritage of hepatitis B vaccine. *JAMA* 1996;**276**:1796–8.

16 Vaginitis

Mari Egan, MD

Vaginitis is an extremely common infection or complaint. With recent over-the-counter medications, evaluation and treatment of women who present with vaginal complaints is even more important.

Definition

1. Inflammation of the vagina is the most common gynecological problem encountered by primary care physicians.[1] Approximately 5 million to 10 million women yearly visit the medical office for vaginitis.[2]
2. The symptoms of vaginitis may include itching, irritation, purulent discharge, and a bad odor. Many women, however, are asymptomatic.

> Inflammation of the vagina is the most common gynecological problem encountered by primary care physicians.

3. Symptoms of vaginitis may result from fungal, bacterial, or protozoan infections, atrophic vaginitis, cervicitis, genital ulcers, desquamative vaginitis, lichen sclerosis, vulvar intraepithelial neoplasia, lactobacillosis, vestibulitis, and allergic reactions. Yeast infections, bacterial vaginosis, and trichomoniasis are the three most common causes of vaginitis.[3]

> Yeast infections, bacterial vaginosis, and trichomoniasis are the three most common causes of vaginitis.

Epidemiology

Bacterial vaginosis

1. Bacterial vaginosis (BV) is the most common cause of vaginitis in the USA, accounting for 40 to 50 percent of cases of vaginitis in women of childbearing

Table 16.1. Complications of bacterial vaginosis

In pregnant women
- Premature labor
- Premature rupture of membranes
- Choriamnionitis
- Postpartum endometritis
- Postabortion infections

In all women
- Increased rates of abnormal pap smears
- Endometritis
- Increased morbidity following gynecological surgery

age,[4] and the second most common cause of vaginitis in Europe with a prevalence of 30 percent.[5]

2. BV represents a disruption in the vaginal ecosystem. A reduction in the normal vaginal flora results in fewer hydrogen peroxide-producing lactobacilli and an overgrowth of *Gardnerella vaginalis*, *Mobiluncus* sp., *Mycoplasma hominis* and other anaerobic Gram-negative rods. The pathology behind the disruption is complex and not completely understood.[6]

3. BV can be transferred sexually but most studies agree that BV is more likely to be caused by the disruption of the vaginal flora with sexual activity rather than through transmission of microorganisms.[7] Women describe having increased symptoms after sexual intercourse.

4. Risk factors for bacterial vaginosis include use of an IUD, douching, orogenital sex, nonwhite race and prior pregnancy.[8]

5. BV has been associated with a number of complications (Table 16.1). In pregnant women, bacterial vaginosis has been associated with premature labor, premature rupture of membranes, choriamnionitis, postpartum endometritis and postabortion infections.[9] Gynecological complications include increased rates of abnormal Pap smears, endometritis and increased morbidity following gynecological surgery.[9]

Bacterial vaginosis is the most common cause of vaginitis in the USA, accounting for 40 to 50 percent of cases of vaginitis in women of childbearing age, and the second most common cause of vaginitis with a prevalence of 30 percent.

Vulvovaginal candidiasis

1. Epidemiological data on vulvovaginal candidiasis (VVC) are difficult to determine because of many factors including self-diagnosis and self-treatment.

Table 16.2. Risk factors for candidal vulvovaginitis

- Initiation of sexual activity
- Increased frequency of sexual intercourse
- Orogenital sex
- Use of oral contraceptives, diaphragms, vaginal sponges and IUDs
- Use of antibiotics
- Pregnancy
- Uncontrolled or poorly controlled diabetes

2. VVC is the second most common vaginal infection in North America and the primary vaginal infection in Europe.[6]
3. Approximately 75 percent of sexually active women have experienced at least one episode of symptomatic VVC in their life.[10]
4. *Candida albicans* causes approximately 92 percent of cases of VVC.[11] Other *Candida* sp., such as *C. glabrata* are becoming more prevalent causes of VVC.[12]
5. *Candida* sp. can be found in the vagina of asymptomatic healthy females and the difference between asymptomatic colonization and symptomatic disease can be difficult to define.
6. The incidence of VVC starts to increase after menarche with more than half of women experiencing an infection by age 25 years.[13]
7. Although it is not traditionally considered an STD, the risk of infection with VVC rises with initiation of sexually activity, frequency of sexual intercourse, and orogenital sex.[14]
8. Other risk factors are listed in Table 16.2.[15] Some risk factors such as diet or tight clothes have less research to support them.
9. Complications of CVV can include vulvar vestibulitis syndrome and reported cases of chorioamnionitis in pregnancy.[16,17]

The incidence of candidal vulvovaginitis starts to increase after menarche with more than half of women experiencing an infection by age 25 years.

Trichomoniasis

1. Trichomoniasis is an STD that is caused by the protozoan *Trichomonas vaginalis.*
2. Trichomoniasis has an annual incidence of approximately 180 million cases worldwide. In North America, eight million new cases are reported yearly.[18]
3. Trichomonas infection is an STD. The protozoan can be identified in the male

sexual partners of infected women, although infection in men is largely asymptomatic.[19]

4. Trichomoniasis infection can increase the transmission of HIV.[20] Spermicide and condoms can reduce the transmission of trichomonads.[21]

5. Additional risk factors for developing trichomoniasis include using an IUD, cigarette smoking, and having multiple sex partners.[19]

6. Complications of trichomoniasis are atypical PID, endometritis, and abnormal Pap smears. During pregnancy, trichomoniasis is associated with preterm labor and premature rupture of membranes.[19]

> Trichomoniasis infection can increase the transmission of HIV.

Signs and symptoms

Presentation

Women infected with these three organisms can be asymptomatic. Each of the infectious causes of vaginitis has a classic description of the signs and symptoms associated with it. However, women with these three types of infection have no significant differences in their vaginal or urinary symptoms.[19]

Bacterial vaginosis

1. In symptomatic women with BV, the vaginal discharge is typically the most noticeable symptom. The discharge has been described as thin, homogeneous, gray to white in color and having a bad, fishy, or amine odor. The odor is more noticeable after sexual intercourse.

2. Approximately 50 percent of women with BV will have no appreciable symptoms. If asymptomatic patients are followed, only 20 percent will develop symptoms if not treated.[18]

3. Physical examination may reveal the typical vaginal discharge with normal vaginal mucosa.

> Approximately 50 percent of women with bacterial vaginosis will have no appreciable symptoms.

Vulvovaginal candidiasis

1. The symptoms of vulvovaginal candidiasis (VVC) may include vulvovaginal itching, irritation, dyspareunia, and burning and frequency of urination. The

discharge of VVC has been described as being increased in amount, with a thick, white, and "cottage-cheese" consistency. Lack of odor is consistent with VVC.[22]

2. On physical examination, the vulva may be erythematous and edematous with scaling and fissures. The vaginal mucosa is inflamed, with thrush-like white patches of discharge adherent to it, and satellite lesions can occur.

Trichomoniasis

1. Symptoms of trichomoniasis may present in a wide range of clinical patterns from asymptomatic to flagrant vaginitis. Approximately 60 percent of infected women are asymptomatic. One third of asymptomatic women become symptomatic within six months.[19]

2. The classical clinical symptoms of an acute infection include a copious, frothy, yellow to green vaginal discharge that may have a foul odor. Infected women may complain of vaginal itching and burning, dysuria and dyspareunia. In chronic infections, the symptoms are mild with vaginal itching and soreness.

3. Vaginal discharge maybe scanty or absent. Symptoms usually are exacerbated around the time of menses.

4. On physical examination, the vulvar area may be spared. Examination findings are typically described as diffuse vaginal erythema and edema, with the described vaginal discharge. There may be punctate, hemorrhagic spots on the cervix and vagina giving it the classical "strawberry" appearance.

Diagnosis (see Table 16.3)

Bacterial vaginosis

1. In clinical practice, BV is diagnosed by identifying three out of four criteria defined by R. Amsel and colleagues (Table 16.4).[21]

2. The Spiegel or Nugent criteria may be used to evaluate a Gram stain of vaginal secretions; this increases the sensitivity and specificity of BV diagnosis.[22] The criteria use a scoring system to count both bacterial morphotypes associated with BV and the number of lactobacilli seen on a slide per oil immersion field (1000 ×). A higher score indicates an increased likelihood of BV.

3. Additional tests such as gas–liquid chromotography, the proline aminopeptidase test and DNA probes have been used to diagnosis BV.[18] The use of a vaginal culture to diagnose BV is not recommended.

Table 16.3. Differential diagnosis of vaginal infection

	Normal	Bacterial vaginosis	Candidiasis	Trichomoniasis
Symptoms	No symptoms	Unpleasant, "fishy" odor Increased odor after intercourse Thin, off-white, discharge	Pruritus Thick, white "cottage cheese" discharge Nonmalodorous Dysuria	Copious, malodorous, yellow-green or discolored discharge Pruritus Vaginal irritation 20 to 50 percent are asymptomatic
Physical exam.	No findings	Usually normal appearance of tissue Homogeneous discharge that adheres to vaginal walls Discolored discharge with abnormal odor	Vulvar and vaginal erythema, edema and fissures Thick, white discharge adherent to vaginal walls	Vulvar and vaginal edema and erythema Frothy, purulent discharge "Strawberry" cervix (up to 25 percent of cases)
pH	<4.5	Elevated (>4.5)	Normal	Elevated (>4.5)
Saline/KOH microscopy	Vaginal cells only, no WBCs	Presence of clue cells Few lactobacilli Occ. motile, curved rods (mobiluncus)	Presence of pseudohyphae, "mycelial tangles", or budding yeast cells	Presence of motile trichomonads Many PMN
Whiff test	Negative	Positive	Negative	Can be positive
Additional tests		1. Amsel's criteria, 3 out of 4 diagnosed 90 percent correctly (Table 16.4) 2. Spiegel's criteria for Gram stain (a scoring criteria to count bacteria associated with BV and the number of lactobacillus) 3. Sensitivity 93 percent; specificity 70 percent Other tests are controversial	KOH microscopy Gram stain Culture	1. DNA probe sensitivity 90 percent, specificity 99.8 percent 2. Culture sensitivity 98 percent, specificity 100 percent

WBC, white blood cell; BV, bacterial vaginosis; occ., occasional; PMN, polymorphonucleocytes.

Table 16.4. Amsel's diagnostic criteria for bacterial vaginosis (BV)

- Presence of clue cells – epithelial cells whose borders are obscured by organisms associated with BV
- Vaginal discharge with pH > 4.3
- A thin homogeneous gray vaginal discharge
- An amine or fishy smell released on mixing vaginal secretion with 10 percent KOH solution (positive Whiff test)

Vulvovaginal candidiasis

1. Demonstration of the presence of yeast blastospores or pseudohyphae in saline/potassium hydroxide solution using microscopy confirms the diagnosis. The vaginal fluid in women with VVC will also have a normal pH.
2. One-third of women with symptomatic VVC will have negative results on microscopy.[5] In these patients, when VVC is suspected, a vaginal culture for yeast should be obtained. A culture may also help to diagnose suspected recurrent or resistant VVC.

Trichomoniasis

1. Classically the diagnosis of trichomoniasis depends on microscopically observing motile protozoa in vaginal secretions. The sensitivity of microscopy for diagnosing trichomoniasis ranges from 40 to 80 percent.[19]
2. Additional tests used for diagnosing trichomoniasis include cultures, Pap smears, polymerase chain reaction (PCR) tests, direct antibody tests and DNA probes. These tests should be considered in women with symptoms suggestive of trichomoniasis but with negative microscopy.[19]

Treatment (Table 16.5)

1. Table 16.5 reviews the 1998 CDC guidelines for treating vaginitis.[23]
2. Among the causes of acute infectious vaginitis, only trichomoniasis requires treating the male sexual partner.
3. The use of alternative medicine for treating vaginitis is becoming more prevalent and the use of boric acid for treating recurrent VVC has been added to the table.[5]

Irritative or allergic vaginitis

1. Women can develop irritative vaginitis in response to excessive or increased

Table 16.5. Treatment of vaginal infections

Disease	Treatment

Trichomoniasis	Metronidazole 2 gm p.o. in a single dose (for acute therapy cure, rate is 90 to 95 percent. Single-dose therapy is associated with better compliance)
	Alternative regimen
	  Metronidazole 500 mg p.o. b.i.d. for 7 days
	Pregnancy
	  Metronidazole 2 g p.o. in a single dose (most consultants avoid use in first trimester)
	Recurrence
	  Metronidazole 2 to 4 g daily for 10 to 14 days
	Notes:
	1. Ensuring treatment of sex partners will improve the cure rate.
	2. No follow up is necessary if symptoms resolve.
	3. Do not use topical therapy because there are not therapeutic levels in urethra/perivaginal glands.
	4. Avoid alcohol use during treatment with metronidazole and 24 hours after.

Bacterial vaginosis	Metronidazole 500 mg p.o. b.i.d. for 7 days
	Clindamycin cream 2 percent one applicatorful (5 g) intravaginally q.h.s. for 7 days (clindamycin cream is oil based and might weaken latex condoms and diaphragms)
	Metronidazole gel 0.75 percent one applicatorful intravaginally b.i.d. for 5 days (all three regimens for BV have cure rates of 74 to 85 percent)
	Alternative regimen
	  Metronidazole 2 g p.o. in a single dose
	  Clindamycin 300 mg p.o. b.i.d. for 7 days
	Pregnancy
	Low risk patients (women who have not had a premature delivery in the second trimester)
	  Metronidazole 250 mg p.o. t.i.d. for 7 days (lower doses of medication are recommended during pregnancy, avoid use in first trimester and clindamycin cream not recommended during pregnancy)
	  Metronidazole 2 g p.o. in a single dose
	  Clindamycin 300 mg p.o. b.i.d.
	Recurrence
	  Metronidazole 500 mg p.o. b.i.d. for 10 to 14 days

Candidiasis	*Primary acute*
	  Topical antifungals (all topical creams are oil based and might weaken latex condoms and diaphragms)
	  Cure rate
	    Polyene 75 to 80 percent
	    Imidazole 85 to 90 percent
	    Terconazole 85 to 90 percent

Table 16.5. (*cont.*)

Disease	Treatment
	Fluconazole 150 mg orally one time (only oral antifungal approved by the FDA for yeast vaginitis; side effects include gastrointestinal intolerance, rash, headaches and rarely liver abnormalities)
	Pregnancy
	Only topical imidazole agents intravaginally for 7 to 10 days
	Recurrence (4 or more episodes of symptomatic VVC annually)
	Initial intensive intravaginal regimen for 10 to 14 days followed immediately by maintenance regimen for at least 6 months (i.e., ketoconazole 100 mg p.o. per day)
	Alternative
	Boric acid topical in size 0 gelatin capsules intravaginally once to twice daily for two weeks – 98 percent cure rate for patients previously failing commonly used treatments

BV, bacterial vaginosis; FDA, Food and Drug Administration.

Data extracted from Centers for Disease Control and Prevention. 1998 Guidelines for treatment of sexually transmitted diseases. *MMWR Morb Mortal Wkly Rep* 1998;**47**:1–118.

friction from sexual or other activity, or allergic vaginitis in response to soaps, detergents, vaginal contraceptive, or other preparations or medications.

2. Symptoms may include swelling, redness, heat and/or itching of the vagina and perineal areas.

3. Examination may show erythema, swelling, discharge, nodules or even urticaria.

4. Laboratory examination will not reveal any infective agent, and may show white blood cells.

5. Treatment:

    a. Treatment for irritative vaginitis will include warm baths and hydrocortisone cream either as cream or foam, topically and/or intravaginally.

    b. Treatment for allergic vaginitis will include the above and possibility oral antihistamines.

Women can develop irritative vaginitis in response to excessive or increased friction from sexual or other activity, or allergic vaginitis in response to soaps, detergents, vaginal contraceptive, or other preparations or medications.

Conclusion

When diagnosing women with vaginal irritation, it is important to keep your mind open to all diagnostic possibilities and use additional laboratory tests if the diagnosis is not clear.

REFERENCES

1. American College of Obstetricians and Gynecologists. Vaginitis. *Int J Gynecol Obstet* 1996;**54**:293–302.
2. Haefner HK. Current evaluation and management of vulvovaginitis. *Clin Obstet Gynecol* 1999;**42**:184–95.
3. Carr PL, Felsenstein D, Friedman RH. Evaluation and management of vaginitis. *J Gen Intern Med* 1998;**13**:335–46.
4. Hill GB. The microbiology of bacterial vaginosis. *Am J Obstet Gynecol* 1993;**169**:450–4.
5. Kent HL. Epidemiology of vaginitis. *Am J Obstet Gynecol* 1991;**165**:1168–76.
6. Sobel JD, Faro S, Force RW et al. Vulvovaginal candidiasis: Epidemiologic, diagnostic, and therapeutic considerations. *Am J Obstet Gynecol* 1998;**178**:203–11.
7. Bump RC, Buesching WJ. Bacterial vaginosis in virginal and sexually active females: evidence against exclusive sexual transmission. *Am J Obstet Gynecol* 1988;**158**:935–9.
8. Hay PE. Recurrent bacterial vaginosis. *Dermatol Clin* 1998;**16**:769–73.
9. Hillier SL, Nugent RP, Eschenbach DA et al. Associations between bacterial vaginosis and preterm delivery of a low birth weight infant. *N Engl J Med* 1995;**333**:1737–42.
10. Eckert LO, Hawes SE, Stevens CE et al. Vulvovaginal candidiasis: Clinical manifestations, risk factors, management algorithm. *Obstet Gynecol* 1998;**92**:757–65.
11. Sobel JD. Vaginitis. *N Engl J Med* 1997;**337**:1896–903.
12. Horowitz BJ, Giaquinta D, Ito S. Evolving pathogens in vulvovaginal candidiasis: Implications for patient care. *J Clin Pharmacol* 1992;**32**:248–55.
13. Geiger AM, Foxman B. Risk factors in vulvovaginal candidiasis: A case-control study among university students. *Epidemiology* 1996;**7**:182–7.
14. Foxman B. The epidemiology of vulvovaginal candidiasis: risk factors. *Am J Public Health* 1990;**80**:329–31.
15. Spinillo A, Capuzzo E, Accianao S, De Santolo A, Zara F. Effect of antibiotic use on the prevalence of symptomatic vulvovaginal candidiasis. *Am J Obstet Gynecol* 1999;**180**:14–17.
16. Pagano R. Vulvar vestibulitis syndrome: An often unrecognized cause of dyspareunia. *Aust NZ J Obstet Gynaecol* 1999;**39**:79–83.
17. Cotch MF, Hillier SL, Gibbs RS, Eschenback DA. Epidemiology and outcomes associated with moderate to heavy *Candida* colonization during pregnancy. *Am J Obstet Gynecol* 1998;**178**:374–80.
18. Petrin D, Delgaty K, Bhatt R, Garber G. Clinical and microbiological aspects of *Trichomonas vaginalis*. *Clin Microbiol Rev* 1998;**11**:300–17.
19. Berg AO, Heidrich FE, Fihn SD et al. Establishing the cause of genitourinary symptoms in

women in a family practice: Comparison of clinical examination and comprehensive microbiology. *JAMA* 1984;**251**:620–5.

20. Laga M, Alary M, Nzila N et al. Condom promotion, sexually transmitted disease treatment, and declining incidence of HIV-1 infection in female Zairian sex workers. *Lancet* 1994;**344**:246–8.

21. Amsel R, Totten PA, Spiegel CA et al. Nonspecific vaginitis: Diagnostic criteria and microbial and epidemiological associations. *Am J Med* 1983;**74**:14–22.

22. Mazzulli T, Simor AE, Low DE. Reproducibility of interpretation of Gram-stained vaginal smears for the diagnosis of bacterial vaginosis. *J Clin Microbiol* 1990;**28**:1506–8.

23. Centers for Disease Control and Prevention. 1998 Guidelines for Treatment of Sexually Transmitted Diseases. *Morb Mortal Wkly Rep* 1998;**47**:1–118.

17 Chronic pelvic pain, dysmenorrhea, and dyspareunia

Jo Ann Rosenfeld, MD

Pain related to menstrual disorders is very common. Frustrating to the patient and the physician because of their subjective nature, with a sensible plan, the symptoms of these disorders can be lessened with collaborative care.

CHRONIC PELVIC PAIN

Definition

Chronic pelvic pain (CPP) occurs for more than six months, affects social and physical functioning and is usually noncyclic and unrelated to the menstrual cycle.

Epidemiology

1. CPP may affect up to one in seven women. However, its actual incidence is difficult to determine because prevalence data has been taken from skewed populations: gynecological referral clinics, CPP clinics, or STD clinics. What percentage of ambulatory women have CPP is unclear.
2. One study in the UK found no community-based study from which to deduce prevalences. CPP occurred in 39 percent of women undergoing laparoscopy for sterilization or infertility.[1] Another US population-based study suggested that 15 percent of more than 5000 women aged 18 to 50 years suffered CPP.[2] Another US study of women in gynecology or family practice offices, found that 39 percent of women reported CPP.[3]
3. However, CPP is responsible for one-third of all laparoscopies and more than 80 000 (or 12 percent of all) hysterectomies in the USA.[4]

4.   Pelvic pain is more common in low income women and women aged 26 to 30 years.[3]

Chronic pelvic pain occurs for more than six months, affects social and physical functioning and is usually noncyclic and unrelated to the menstrual cycle.

Approach

1.   The approach to CPP cannot be purely biomedical. There is seldom just one cause for the pain.
2.   The pain may not be related to gynecological organs. Many women who come to a chronic pain clinic have already had a hysterectomy, and 40 percent of women who have hysterectomy for CPP still have pain after the operation.
3.   The approach to the woman with CPP must be:
     a. Nonemergent.
     b. The history, physical examination, and treatment take time over many visits.
     c. The physician and patient must realize that there is seldom one curable cause and that the illness is neither totally physical nor totally psychiatric.
4.   The physician and patient must accept partial gains and improvement.

One etiology is seldom the cause for the pain in chronic pelvic pain.

5.   As well, even when a contributing cause is determined, there is little evidence that the presence of pathology causes the pain, or that there is a correlation between the presence and/or degree of pain and the pathology.[5] In women with CPP, there is very little correlation between clinical evidence, the extent of disease, and the quality, quantity, or appearance of the pain.[6]
     For example, endometriosis may be found in one-third of patients with CPP, but it was also found in 15 percent of the 50 pain-free women who underwent laparoscopy for tubal ligation.[7] Pelvic adhesions were found in 14 percent of pain-free women and in other studies found in 15 to 20 percent of women with CPP. Fibroids, a common cause of hysterectomy, have never been proven to cause CPP.[8]
6.   CPP must be approached in a cooperative interactive multidisciplinary style, incorporating lifestyle modification, therapeutic relationships, and psychiatric and personal counselling.

The physician and patient must accept partial gains and improvement.

LIVERPOOL JOHN MOORES UNIVERSITY
LEARNING SERVICES

Table 17.1. Causes of chronic pelvic pain

• Gastrointestinal	• Musculoskeletal pain
• Irritable bowel syndrome	• Lumbosacral pain
• Constipation	• Myofascial pain
• Diverticulitis	• Urological
• Cholelithiasis	• Bladder spasms
• Gynecological	• Cystitis
• Ovarian cysts	• Kidney or bladder stones
• Endometriosis	• Urethritis/urethral syndrome
• Chronic pelvic inflammatory disease	• Urinary tract infections
• Adhesions	• Chronic pain syndrome
• Dysmenorrhea	

Etiology (Table 17.1)

1. Gastrointestinal causes may be the most common. Irritable bowel syndrome (IBS), constipation and diverticulitis can all cause chronic pelvic pain. History should reveal an abnormal stooling pattern.

2. IBS is a functional bowel disorder in which abdominal pain "is associated with defecation or changes in bowel habit, . . . ",[9] and it may be responsible for as much as one-half of all CPP.[10] The pain is usually colicky, relieved with defecation, and associated with change in frequency of consistence of stool for more than three months. The pain may be more intense during menses. IBS is associated with CPP, urinary irritability, dyspareunia, alternating constipation, and diarrhea. Many women with IBS also have a history of sexual abuse and women with IBS are more likely to have significant anxiety and depression.[9]

3. Gynecological organ diseases cause CPP. Chronic or recurrent ovarian cysts, endometriosis, chronic PID, adhesions, and dysmenorrhea have been associated with CPP. As mentioned above, the degree of disease found on laparoscopy and the degree or duration of pain does not correlate well. Disease has been found in symptom-free women, and women with severe pain may be found to have little pathological evidence of disease.

4. Musculoskeletal pain.

5. Urological pain: Bladder spasms, cystitis, kidney or bladder stones, urethritis and urethral syndrome can all cause CPP.

Pain syndromes

1. A proportion of women who have CPP resemble women and men with other pain syndromes. These individuals have other chronic pain syndromes, chronic headaches, and/or chronic abdominal and back pain. Chronicity of pain, several concurrent pain syndromes, inability to respond to standard primary treatments, multiple providers, frequent visits to the physician and often narcotics dependence, all occur in individuals with chronic pain syndromes.
2. Up to 40 percent of women in CPP clinics have had a history of childhood abuse and sexual abuse and/or have had traumatic sexual experiences.[11]

> Chronicity of pain, several concurrent pain syndromes, inability to respond to standard primary treatments, multiple providers, frequent visits to the physicians, and often narcotics dependence, all occur in individuals with chronic pain syndromes.

Symptoms

1. Pain: The pain can be sharp, dull, piercing, or colicky. It is usually persistent and recurrent. The symptoms may worsen with menses, but should be present at times other than menses.
2. Associated symptoms: Often, there are other complaints that span several organ systems, including dyspareunia, dysmenorrhea, anorgasmy, postcoital pain, disturbances in the menstrual cycle, backache, nausea, malaise, diarrhea, headaches, and vertigo (Figure 17.1).[12]

Evaluation

1. A complete history and physical examination including pelvic and rectal examination is sufficient.
2. A complete blood count, erythrocyte sedimentation rate, and urine analysis (U/A) are recommended. A urine culture can be obtained if the U/A is abnormal, and thyroid functions can be tested if there are associated menstruation abnormalities.
3. Further studies are not indicated, unless history or physical examination indicate other conditions that may contribute to the pain. These studies should be initiated while treatment is begun.

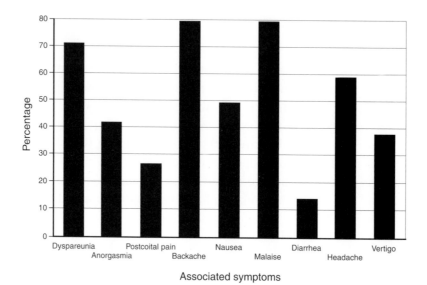

Figure 17.1.   Frequency of associated symptoms in women with chronic pelvic pain.

4. Laparoscopy: Laparoscopy has been a tool for diagnosis and treatment of CPP.
    a. However, from 10 to 69 percent of laparoscopies in women with CPP are normal[13] and 15 to 20 percent of laparoscopies in women without pain show endometriosis or adhesions.[4]
    b. Thus laparoscopy is unlikely to be needed in every woman unless history or physical suggests an indication.
    c. Laparoscopy alone relieves CPP, perhaps through a psychological mechanism, in some women.[14]
5. Ultrasonography: Although less invasive, ultrasound scans similarly are often negative in individuals with pain. Unless physical examination or history indicates abnormalities, ultrasound scans are not universally needed.
6. Other studies such as intravenous pyelograms, barium enemas and CT scans are rarely needed.

Laparoscopy is not needed in every woman with chronic pelvic pain.

7. Psychological evaluation and counselling are often a supplementary part of the evaluation. Some women have long-term psychological needs, including depression for which treatment, either psychotherapy or pharmacotherapy, is helpful. As well, all women with CPP have had chronic psychological effects

Table 17.2. Treatment of chronic pelvic pain

- Pain relief
  Nonsteroidal antiinflammatory drugs and lifestyle methods – heat, baths, showers, tea, massage, etc. Tricyclic antidepressants and SSRIs may be used additionally
- No narcotics
- Pain diary
- Exercise
- High bulk diet
- Counselling or psychotherapy
- Frequent visits to physician's office

SSRI, selective serotonin reuptake inhibitor.

from the pain and its effects on their lives and relationships that could benefit from evaluation and therapy.

Psychological evaluation and counselling are often a supplementary part of the evaluation.

Treatment (Table 17.2)

A multidisciplinary, integrated approach to the biological, nutritional and psychological causes is important and will produce results. Using the following procedures, 75 percent of women will have good or better improvement.[13]

1. Pain relief: The patient and physician should decide on what has helped to relieve pain in the past. Nonnarcotic NSAIDs often work, as do heat, baths, showers, sleeping, or exercise. Tricyclic antidepressants including amitriptyline and the SSRIs may be helpful adjuncts.
   a. The patient and physician should create a "pain prescription". They should decide what to try first, second, and when the patient should call the physician.
   b. The patient should keep a diary with the levels of pain (ranked 1 to 10, slight to worst), and what she did to help the pain and bring this to office visits for discussion.
   c. No narcotics should be given.
2. An exercise prescription should be developed and started.
3. A low fat, high bulk diet should be advised and initiated. A consultation with a dietician may help.
4. Simultaneous counselling and appropriate psychotherapy should be started.

Table 17.3. Treatment of endometriosis

Drug		Method
Leuprolide		
Lupron	5 mg/mL	i.m.
Lupron-Depot	3.75 mg monthly	i.m.
Lupron-Depot–3	11.25 mg every 3 months	i.m.
Goserelin		
Zoladex	3.6 mg monthly	i.m.
Gestrionone	2.5 mg twice a week	p.o.
Danazol		
Danocrine	800 mg daily in divided doses	p.o.

5. There should be regular frequent appointments during the first three months. These can be made less frequent as pain improves.

Specific therapy

1. Endometriosis: Endometriosis is disease in which implants of endometrial tissue occur ectopically, and by their swelling and sometimes rupture cause pain, infertility, and bleeding. It is the most common diagnosis at laparoscopy in women with CPP.
   a. Diagnosis is made by clinical symptoms, findings of tender masses on pelvic examination, and laparoscopy.
   b. Treatment is menstrual suppression, if the woman does not desire immediate pregnancy. OCPs, Danocrine (danazol) or gonadotropin-releasing hormone analogs (see Table 17.3), can accomplish this.
   c. Use of Danocrine in high or low doses reduces the pain of endometriosis. In high doses, it is associated with gastrointestinal distress and diarrhea. It does not reliably inhibit ovulation and another barrier method of contraception must be used in addition.
   d. Leuprolide and gonadotropin analogs are effective. For example, in a RCT of more than 100 women, leuprolide (3.75 mg/mo-depot) gave significant improvement in pain in women with CPP and endometriosis.[15] However, leuprolide is associated with gastrointestinal side effects and irregular menses and breakthrough bleeding. It is not a contraceptive, and another contraceptive method should be used simultaneously.
2. Constipation or irritable bowel: Treatment with high bulk diet, fiber and

antispasmodic medications, and exercise will help. Laxatives may be needed for constipation. Anxiolytic and antidepressants may be adjunctive therapy.

Indications for referral

1. Drug addiction or dependence may require referral to a chronic pain center.
2. Indications for surgery are disputed.
    a. Whether surgical treatment for endometriosis and adhesions is appropriate is argued.
    b. Hysterectomy has been performed as last resort, but 21 to 40 percent of women who had hysterectomy for CPP continue to have pain after the procedure.[16]
    c. Women who had chronic PID, were poorer, or had not identified pelvic pathology were more likely to have continued CPP after hysterectomy.

DYSMENORRHEA

Definition and impact

1. Dysmenorrhea is painful menses.
2. Dysmenorrhea may be a major cause of absenteeism in women workers.
3. Dysmenorrhea is more common in the years just after menarche and approaching menopause, when irregular and heavier periods are more likely.
4. Dysmenorrhea occurred in 45 to 97 percent of women in community-based studies in the UK, but definitions varied, making prevalence data unreliable.[1]

Dysmenorrhea, painful periods, is more common in the years just after menarche and approaching menopause.

Diagnosis

Diagnosis is made clinically.
1. A history and physical examination may uncover other gynecological conditions that contribute to dysmenorrhea, including leiomyomas, uterine masses, or menorrhagia.

Table 17.4. Treatments of dysmenorrhea studied for efficacy

Drug or treatment	Dose	Duration	Type of study
NSAIDs			
Bromfenac	10 or 50 mg	3 days	RCT (dp)
Diclofenac	50 mg q.i.d.	3 days	RCT (dp)
Ibuprofen	400 mg q.i.d.	3 days	RCT (dp)
Ketoprofen	50 mg q.i.d.	3 days	RCT (dp)
Dexketoprofen	12.5–25 mg q.i.d.	3 days	RCT (dp)
Mefenamic acid	500 mg t.i.d.	3 days	RCT (dp)
Naproxen sodium	275 mg	3 days	RCT (dp)
Tolfenamic acid	200 mg t.i.d.	3 days	RCT (dp)
Transdermal nitroglycerine	0.1–0.2 mg/hour	3 days	Observational
Herbal/diet/alternative medicines			
1. "Toki-shakuyau-san" TSS Chinese herbal medicine		3 days	RCT (dp)
2. Oral vit. B1 (thiamine)	100 mg	Daily for 90 days	RCT (dp)
3. Omega-3 polyunsaturated fatty acids with vit. E		Daily	RCT

NSAID, nonsteroidal antiinflammatory drug; RCT (dp), randomized controlled trial, double blind, versus placebo; vit., vitamin.

2. After a history, physical examination, and Pap test, a complete blood count is probably sufficient evaluation.
3. Thyroid function tests and a pelvic ultrasound scan are indicated for abnormal menses and/or enlarged uterus, masses or tenderness on examination. Cultures for gonorrhea and chlamydia are indicated if pelvic tenderness, cervicitis or a discharge is discovered.

Treatment

There have been many studies, anecdotal, observational, and many RCTs, double and single blind, investigating the treatment for dysmenorrhea (Table 17.4).

1. NSAIDs are the first-line treatment. Various NSAIDs have been investigated

against placebo and each other and most are superior to placebo. No one NSAID is inherently more effective than any other.

2. OCPs and depot MPA, because they reduce the amount of menstrual bleeding and incidence of clots and heavy bleeding, can improve dysmenorrhea.

3. Various alternative and herbal treatments have been proposed. Spinal manipulation has not been shown to improve dysmenorrhea.

4. Hysterectomy will cure dysmenorrhea, and of course, fibroids (leiomyomata). Hysterectomy may be a reasonable treatment for leiomyomata that cause severe bleeding, after medical treatment has failed. Hysterectomy for dysmenorrhea alone is seldom suggested.

> NSAIDs are the first-line treatment for dysmenorrhea.

DYSPAREUNIA

Definition and impact

1. Dyspareunia is painful intercourse.
2. In community-based studies in the UK, dyspareunia occurred in 8 percent of women.[1] One study of more than 300 women interviewed at random found that 28 percent complained of short-term dyspareunia and 16 percent of chronic dyspareunia.[17] Another study in gynecology clinics found 8 to 48 percent of women presented with dyspareunia.[18]

Associated symptoms

1. Dyspareunia is associated with higher pain scores and psychological distress, lower levels of marital adjustment and more problems with sexual function. Which is the cause and which the result is difficult to determine.
2. Women with dyspareunia are more likely to report a history of traumatic sexual assaults,[19] and unlubricated, unaroused, and undesired sexual experiences.[20]
3. A history of PID increases the risk of dyspareunia (OR = 3.87).[21]

> Women with dyspareunia are more likely to have higher total pain scores, psychological distress, and a history of traumatic sexual assaults.

Table 17.5. Causes of dyspareunia

- Insertional dyspareunia
  - Lubrication difficulties
    Lack of knowledge of sexual response
    Lack of arousal
    Postmenopausal atrophy
  - Vulvitis – infectious or irritative
  - Vaginitis – infectious or irritative
  - Vaginismus
  - Psychological concerns
- Pain in a specific area of vulva or vagina
  - Hymenal ring difficulty
  - Old scars, lesions, abscesses, gland enlargement
  - Vulvitis – infectious or irritative
  - Vaginitis – infectious or irritative
- Pain with deep penetration
  - Masses or uterine enlargement
  - Endometriosis
  - Adhesions
  - Vaginismus
  - Condyloma accuminata
  - Psychological concerns

Diagnosis

1. History is most important. When the pain started, under what circumstances it occurs and how long has it occurred are important concerns. A history of abuse or sexual trauma must be inquired into, as is a sexual history and a history of relationships and past sexual experiences.
2. The physical examination is important but often totally normal. However, it can be a stressful and painful process. Small or Peterson specula may be needed, or the examination may have to be postponed. Examination of the vulva, vagina, and cervix is essential. A rectal examination is not needed unless endometriosis is suggested by history.
3. No routine laboratory or X-ray studies are needed.

Treatment

Treatment is based on defining one of three types of dyspareunia: insertional dyspareunia, pain in a specific area of vulva or vagina, and pain with deep penetration (Table 17.5).

Insertional dyspareunia

1. Insertional dyspareunia may be most commonly caused by lubrication problems. Education into normal sexual functioning and the need and time for lubrication may help. Helping the woman to discover how she becomes aroused and how long it takes her to lubricate naturally can help her with expectations. Exogenous addition of lubricants, such as KY® jelly, can help. Difficulties in arousal may increase the time to adequate lubrication.

2. Postmenopausal vaginal atrophy can cause difficulties with lubrication and pain. The use of estrogen creams, if not contraindicated, or Estring (an estrogen-imbedded vaginal ring with no systemic absorption of estrogen), if contraindications to systemic estrogen exist, will help. The patient or physician places Estring every three months.

3. Infectious or irritative vulvitis or vaginitis, especially from *Candida* or herpes simplex virus infections can cause significant insertional dyspareunia.
   a. The vulva and vagina will be red and irritated with satellite lesions in candidal infections. Treatment is usually topical.
   b. Chemicals, perfumes or dyes or scents in bath products or contraceptives can cause irritations. These would be treated with hydrocortisone creams and foams. Vulvitis occurring without *Candida* infection may be improved by use of antidepressants.[22]
   c. Occasionally women with dyspareunia who also have musculoskeletal and dermatological complaints may have Sjögren's syndrome. Dyspareunia may occur up to seven years before the other symptoms.[23]

4. Vaginismus is a psychological reaction to a variety of traumatic and psychological sexual stresses. Treatment must include education, counselling and "sensate" exercises. The physician must teach the woman that she can control sex and her vagina, and that she can learn how to keep her pelvic muscles relaxed through a variety of exercises, first alone and then with her partner.

Pain in a specific area of vulva or vagina

Occasionally, pain occurs in one spot, either in the vagina or the vulva. This may be a site of a scar, hymenal thickening, or chronic gland enlargement. In this case, physical examination should discover the area. Vulvitis or vaginitis as described above can cause local pain.

Pain with deep penetration

1. The vagina has no light touch sensation. Pain with deep penetration may have a structural or psychological cause. Masses or uterine enlargement may cause this. Although retrograde uteruses have been said to cause dyspareunia, no proof supports this. Endometriosis implants, especially in the retrovaginal pouch could cause pain with deep penetration, as could adhesions.

2. If pain is reproduced with bimanual examination, ultrasound may help to diagnose a cause.

3. Trying different sexual positions, side-to-side or with the woman on top, or using a pillow under the buttocks may improve the pain.

A couples' approach

While the above causes are being investigated, the physician can discuss the woman's present and past relationships. Sexual dysfunction can be both the cause and the result of dysfunctional relationships. Inadequacy of communication about sexual intercourse needs can contribute or be the result of dyspareunia. Marital and personal counselling may be needed. The physician may want to offer crisis counselling for both members of the partnership, or offer referral to psychological or marital counselling.

Conclusions

Pain associated with menstrual disorders and sexual relations are common and often the presenting complaint to the physician. CPP is seldom caused by one etiology and needs a comprehensive, organized approach to treatment that can produce effective results. Dysmenorrhea is common and although the exact etiology is unknown a variety of effective therapies exist. The case of dyspareunia may be difficult to discover but an organized approach including psychological expectations may produce improvement.

REFERENCES

1. Zondervan KT, Yukin PL, Vessey MP, Dawes MG, Barlow DH, Kennedy SH. The prevalence of chronic pelvic pain in women in the United Kingdom: A systematic review. *Br J Obstet Gynecol* 1998;**105**:93–9.

2. Mathias SD, Kupperman M, Liberman RF, Lipschutz RC, Steege JF. Chronic pelvic pain. Prevalence, heatlh related quality of life and economic correlates. *Obstet Gynecol*

1996;**87**:321–7.

3. Jamieson DJ, Steege JF. The prevalence of dysmenorrhea, dyspareunia, pelvic pain and irritable bowel syndrome in primary care practices. *Obstet Gynecol* 1996;**87**:55–8.

4. Walling MK, Reiter RC, O'Hara MW et al. Abuse history and chronic pain in women: I. Prevalences of sexual abuse and physical abuse. *Obstet Gynecol* 1994;**84**:193–9.

5. Roseff SJ, Murphy AA. Laparoscopy in the diagnosis and therapy of chronic pelvic pain. *Clin Obstet Gynecol* 1990;**33**:137–44.

6. Rosenfeld JA. Chronic pelvic pain: An integrated approach. *Am Fam Physician* 1996;**54**:2187–9.

7. Kresch AJ, Seifer DB, Sachs LB, Barrese I. Laparoscopy in 100 women with chronic pelvic pain. *Obstet Gynecol* 1984;**64**:672–4.

8. Carlson KJ, Miller BA, Fowler FJ Jr. The Maine Women's Health Study: II. Outcomes of nonsurgical management of leiomyomas, abnormal bleeding and chronic pelvic pain. *Obstet Gynecol* 1994;**83**:566–72.

9. Farthing MJG. Irritable bowel, irritable body or irritable brain? *BMJ* 1995;**310**:171–5.

10. American College of Obstetricians and Gynecologists. Chronic pelvic pain. Technical Bulletin. *Int J Gynecol Obstet* 1996;**54**:59–68.

11. Walling MK, O'Hara MW, Reiter RC, Milburn AK, Lilly G, Vincent SD. Abuse history and chronic pain in women: II. A multivariate analysis of abuse and psychological morbidity. *Obstet Gynecol* 1994;**84**:200–6.

12. Peters AA, van Dorst E, Jellis B, van Zuuren E, Hermans J, Trimbos JB. A randomized clinical trial to compare two different approaches in women with chronic pelvic pain. *Obstet Gynecol* 1991;**77**:740–4.

13. Steege JF, Stout AL, Somkuti SG. Chronic pelvic pain in women: Toward an integrative model. *Obstet Gynecol Surv* 1993;**48**:95–110.

14. Elcome S, Gath D, Day A. The psychological effects of laparoscopy on women with chronic pelvic pain. *Psychol Med* 1997;**27**:1041–50.

15. Ling FW. Pelvic pain study group. Leuprolide in patients with chronic pelvic pain and clinically suspected endometriosis. *Obstet Gynecol* 1999;**93**:51–8.

16. Hillis SD, Marchbanks PA, Peterson HB. The effectiveness of hysterectomy for chronic pelvic pain. *Obstet Gynecol* 1995;**86**:941–5.

17. Glatt AE, Zinner SH, McCormack WM. The prevalence of dyspareunia. *Obstet Gynecol* 1990;**75**:433–66.

18. Phillips NA. The clinical evalution of dyspareunia. *Int J Impot Res* 1998;**10S2**:S117–S120.

19. Meana M, Binik YM, Khalife S, Cohen D. Psychosocial correlates of pain attributions in women with dyspareunia. *Psychosomatics* 1999;**40**:497–502.

20. Marin MG, King R, Dennerstein GJ, Sfameni S. Dyspareunia and vulvar disease. *J Reprod Med* 1998;**43**:952–8.

21. Heisterberg L. Factors influencing spontaneous abortion, dyspareunia and pelvic pain. *Obstet Gynecol* 1993;**81**:594–7.

22. Pagano R. Vulvar vestibulitis syndrome. *Aust NZ J Obstet Gynecol* 1999;**39**:79–83.

23. Mulherin DM, Shereran TP, Kumararatne DS et al. Sjögren's syndrome in women presenting with chronic dyspareunia. *Br J Obstet Gynecol* 1997;**104**:1019–23.

The Papanicolaou smear and cervical cancer

Barbara S. Apgar, MD, MS

The Papanicolaou (Pap) test remains the mainstay of cervical cancer prevention. While accounting for fewer than 2 percent of all cancer deaths, carcinoma of the cervix is one of the most common malignancies in women. Cervical
cancer is an important public health problem and is one of the most treatable
cancers if detected early.

Cervical cancer

1. There are about 4500 cervical cancer deaths yearly in the USA and approximately 14 500 new cases per year.
2. The rate for diagnosis of cervical cancer in African-Americans is 15/100 000,
   white Americans 8/100 000 and for the UK approximately 10/100 000.[1] The
   rate has declined in the USA from 15 to 8 per 100 000 from 1970 to 1990, and in
   the UK from 15 to 10/100 000 (Figure 18.1).
3. Risk factors include never having had a Pap test, being nonwhite (Table 18.1),
   or factors that correlate with increased and risky sexual activity – increased
   numbers of sexual partners, and having had human papilloma virus infection.
   The risks of developing cervical cancer and dying of cervical cancer declined
   in African-Americans, although it was still higher than that of whites.[2]

The effectiveness of Pap test and access problems

1. The goal of cervical cytological screening is to detect precancerous and
   cancerous lesions and to initiate further evaluation based on the cytological
   diagnosis.

Table 18.1. Risk factors for cervical cancer

Risky sexual behavior
- Early first intercourse
- Human papilloma virus infections
- Cigarette smoking and passive smoking
- Never having a Pap test (this is the greatest risk factor for cervical cancer)
- Long-term use of oral contraceptive pills

Factors that reduce the risk of cervical cancer
- Avoidance of high risk sexual activity
- Quitting smoking

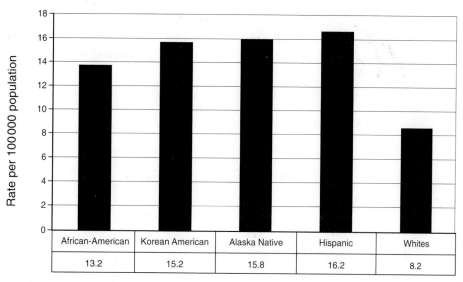

	African-American	Korean American	Alaska Native	Hispanic	Whites
	13.2	15.2	15.8	16.2	8.2

Figure 18.1.   Rate of cervical cancer in US women by race.

2. Most women with cervical cancer have never had a Pap smear. Cervical cytological testing has been successful in preventing cervical cancer in women who present for screening, with reduction of the cervical cancer rate by 70 percent over the past 50 years. More women develop cervical cancer because of a failure to get regular Pap screening than because of errors in cytopathological diagnosis.[3]

The goal of cervical cytological screening is to detect precancerous and cancerous lesions.

3. Some women do not have easy access to health care or view health care as an obstacle rather than a benefit. Even in Finland, where Pap tests are free and reminders are mailed yearly, only 75 percent of women have had regular screening. Two populations of women, adolescents and the elderly, may be at risk for not receiving Pap smears at appropriate intervals.

4. The US Breast and Cervical Cancer Mortality Prevention Act of 1990 established a nationwide public health program for increasing access to screening for breast and cervical cancer to underserved populations.[4] The target group included older women, low income women, and uninsured or underinsured women and ethnic/racial minority women. One goal was to increase to at least 80 percent the proportion of low income women and women aged 18 years or older who have received a Pap smear within the preceding three years.

Adolescents and the elderly are less likely to receive appropriate Pap test screening.

Etiology – the role of the human papillomavirus

1. The human papillomavirus (HPV) is the etiological agent of most of the lower genital tract carcinomas and intraepithelial neoplasias.[5] About 90 percent of cervical carcinomas are caused by infection with one of about 15 oncogenic HPV types.[6]

2. Infection with oncogenic types of HPV confers high risk of developing cervical and other lower genital cancers, including vulvar and vaginal cancers.[7]

3. Cervical cancer is preceded by HPV infection; in some women, this infection causes a progression to a high grade squamous intraepithelial lesion (HGSIL) and then to invasion. About 10 to 20 percent of women after the cytological diagnosis of low grade squamous intraepithelial lesion (LGSIL) or atypical squamous cells of undetermined significance (ASCUS) will progress to HGSIL.[8]

4. Whether HPV infection requires synergism with cofactors such as cigarette smoking, early sexual debut or multiple sexual partners in order to produce intraepithelial and invasive lesions is a subject of intense investigation.[9]

5. A percentage of women who have a Pap diagnosis of ASCUS are actually found to have HGSIL. Approximately one-half of those women who are HPV-positive but have no cytological abnormality, develop detectable cytologic abnormalities within four years.[6]

6. Most clinical spectrum of HPV-associated disease is highly variable and

screening and treatment guidelines have focused on preventing or modulating the oncogenic potential of the virus expression.

Most of the epithelial abnormalities of the Pap smear are directly or indirectly related to the presence of human papillomavirus.

The Pap smear

1. The conventional Pap smear has been widely used for nearly 50 years and is considered to be one of the most effective screening tests developed for the commonly known cancers. Since being introduced by Georg Papanicolaou and Herbert Traut in 1942, the Pap smear is the most widely used cancer screening test in the USA and until recently has remained basically unchanged during this time.

2. The effectiveness of a screening program is proportional to the number of screening tests a woman has had in her life. The degree to which cervical cancer incidence rates are decreased in a particular population is related to the percentage of the population screened and the length of the screening interval. In highly screened populations, routine testing can significantly decrease the cancer rate. Screening for cervical cancer, however, has not eradicated the disease in any population studied to date, regardless of screening intervals. The relative protection against developing cervical cancer decreases steadily with the increasing interval since the last Pap smear, especially if the woman remains HPV-positive.

The effectiveness of a screening program is proportional to the number of screening tests a woman has had in her life.

The false-negative rate of the conventional Pap smear

The vast majority of Pap smears are adequately sampled and correctly interpreted. Results of large studies indicate that the combined screening error and inadequate sample rate ranges from 0.14 to 9.4 percent. Laboratory interpretive error rates in competent laboratories with a low prevalence of SIL are usually less than 0.01 percent. A metaanalysis found that the conventional Pap smear sensitivity was 0.51 (95 percent confidence interval 0.37 to 0.66) and the specificity of Pap smear screening was 0.98 (95 percent confidence intervals 0.97 to 0.99).[10]

Limitations

A conventionally prepared Pap smear is not a perfect test. Multiple factors can affect the accuracy of the smear, including patient preparation, sampling technique, fixation and staining of the smear, screening by the cytotechnologist and the interpretation of potential cellular abnormalities by the cytopathologist. There is wide agreement that most (60 to 90 percent) of false-negative Pap smears result from sampling errors and the remaining from laboratory errors.

New methods

Although the conventional Pap smear has resulted in a significant reduction in cervical cancer, there are new screening techniques with reported greater sensitivity. Although some of these have resulted in a reduction of screening errors, it should be emphasized that none of the new technologies will completely eliminate the false-negative rate of the Pap smear. The main advantages of the new screening methods, including liquid-based technology, are the ability to diagnose increased abnormalities including HGSIL and to decrease the percentage of unsatisfactory or satisfactory although limited by the quality of the smears.

The need for screening

Initiation

1. The initiation of sexual activity is a marker for the appearance of HPV DNA in the host tissue and the necessity of introducing cytological screening. The American Academy of Pediatrics Recommendations for Preventive Pediatric Health Care state that a pelvic examination and Pap smear be offered as part of preventive health maintenance at the time of sexual debut.[11] The American College of Obstetricians and Gynecologists, the American Academy of Family Practice and the American Cancer Society promote Pap smear screening of all sexually active adolescents. The CDC has shown that rates of HGSIL are increasing in young women in the USA.[4] Adolescents are exposed to cofactors that may increase the risk of progression of preinvasive lesions.

2. In a study of 888 sexually active adolescents, 13.4 percent had an abnormal Pap smear over a 12-month study period.[12] Thirteen percent of these young women had cervical intraepithelial neoplasia (CIN), grades 2 to 3, at the time of initial screening. Because only 10 percent of these adolescents had a history

of a previous STD, a targeted screening of only sexually active adolescents who present to STD clinics would miss most adolescents with abnormal Pap smears.[13]

Because sexually active teenagers are more likely to have HPV infections and 13 percent had cervical intraepithelial neoplasia in one study, all sexually active teenagers should have yearly Pap tests or cytological screening.

Cessation

1. The recommendation on when to stop performing Pap smears on elderly women is not based on strong evidence. Because fewer women are infected with HPV later in life, older women, especially if widowed or monogamous and who have had previous normal screenings, may not need to obtain Pap smears on a yearly basis once they reach age 65 years.

2. However, the importance of performing Pap smears on older women who have been infrequently or never screened in the past cannot be overemphasized.

3. However, the rates of squamous cell carcinoma of the cervix increase with age, representing a 17-fold increase in women over the age of 40 years compared with women at age 20 years.

4. Pap smear adequacy is a concern in elderly women. Rates of false-positive smears can increase with age because of atrophic epithelial changes. False-negative smears can occur as the transformation zone becomes less accessible to cytological sampling and cellular exfoliation is reduced.

Older women who have had normal previous Pap tests may not need regular screening after age 65 years.

The Bethesda system

1. The Bethesda System (TBS) was introduced in the late 1980s because of the recognized need to redefine the cytological interpretation categories on the basis of current knowledge of cytopathology, reflective of what was known about HPV.[14] TBS attempted to standardize the reporting of cervical smears by recommending the use of nonepithelial and epithelial cell abnormalities for squamous and glandular cells.[15]

2. Approximately 10 percent of the 50 million Pap smears performed annually in the USA will show some type of abnormality and 5 percent of the abnormal smears will demonstrate findings of LGSIL or worse.[16]

> Under the Bethesda System, approximately 10 percent of Pap smears performed annually will show some abnormality.

Inflammatory cells

1. Many Pap smear reports will indicate the presence of inflammatory cells, which to some implies that an "infection" should be treated. Although extensive infiltration of the cervix by leukocytes is indicative of an STD, the significance of this inflammation is not well defined.[17] Leukocytes are often quantified on the report and the clinician has to determine whether they are of clinical significance. Inflammation is usually classified as mild, moderate, severe, or profuse.

2. Some studies ascribe the inflammatory cells to chemical irritants, douching, or local trauma such as occurs during sexual activity. Leukocytes are present throughout the fallopian tubes, endometrium, and the lower genital system during all stages of the menstrual cycle and after menopause,[18] without the presence of demonstrable infection and regardless of the diagnosis of cervicitis.

3. The percentage of cervical leukocytes was approximately 10 to 15 percent of the total number of cervical cells isolated. The diagnosis of cervicitis should be reserved for cases of extensive leukocytic infiltration accompanied by other evidence of pathology.[19] Leukocytes should be considered a part of "normal" cervical histology. This avoids the needless time spent tracking down the source of the "inflammation".

Atypical squamous cells of undetermined significance

1. Under the Papanicolaou system, atypical cells were listed as a component of the class 2 category along with inflammation and koilocytosis (perinuclear clearing of the cytoplasm). When TBS was devised, the atypical cells were given their own category.[17]

2. The ASCUS category incorporates cellular changes that are abnormal but not

definitely SIL but that cannot be classified as benign cellular changes or normal. ASCUS is a cytological diagnosis and there is no exact histological correlate. Histologically, ASCUS can represent normal, CIN or invasive disease. Realistically, an ASCUS interpretation implies that it is up to the clinician to determine the source of the atypical cells.

3. Lack of reproducibility of cytological criteria of ASCUS has been a significant impediment to the ability to make consistent management decisions. Inter-observer variability of ASCUS can lead to an overdiagnosis of cells that are actually normal or an underdiagnosis of SIL, and even HGSIL.[20]

4. Achieving an ASCUS rate of less than 5 percent may not be possible. However, ASCUS rates of 20 percent cannot be justified either. There will continue to be cytological smears that cannot be specifically interpreted as anything but ASCUS. In the National Cancer Institute (NCI) Interim Guidelines (1994), it was stated that the rate of atypical slides should not exceed two to three times the rate of SIL.[19]

5. According to the NCI Interim Guidelines, cytological smears with an ASCUS diagnosis can be managed by one of four options (Figure 18.2).

6. Ideally, all patients with ASCUS should receive colposcopic evaluation. Practically, this is an unreasonable approach. Since the publication of the Interim Guidelines, there continues to be great variability in how patients with ASCUS are triaged. Recent data demonstrating the risk of histological CIN in ASCUS might encourage more clinicians to triage all patients with ASCUS to colposcopy and cause some reconsideration of management by repeat cytology. Although data are beginning to emerge that more specifically define the best management approach, until the results of the NCI ASCUS/LGSIL Triage Study (ALTS) trial are completed, the optimal path will not be known. The American Society of Colposcopy and Cervical Pathology (ASCCP) has published a series of Practice Guidelines based on recent clinical and scientific data.

7. A prospective important study of women in the Kaiser–Permanente health system stressed that the ASCUS does not imply a totally benign histological diagnosis. The results of Pap smears of more than 46 000 women revealed that ASCUS was the most common diagnosis (3.6 percent); this rate was similar to the 50th percentile of the rates of other major laboratories. Of the total number of cases of histologically confirmed HGSIL, 85 percent occurred in women younger than age 40 years and the largest proportion (38.8 percent) was in women with a diagnosis of ASCUS. This study, the largest to date, stressed the importance of the minimally abnormal Pap smear in the subsequent diagnosis of HGSIL.[21]

8. In another study of patients presenting with ASCUS or LGSIL, a significant

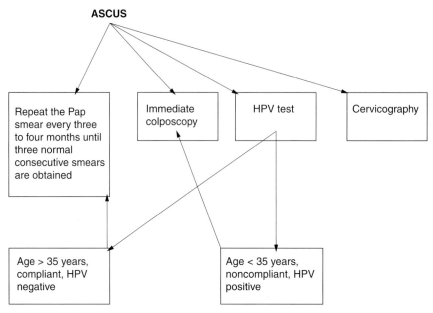

Figure 18.2. Options for evaluation of atypical squamous cells of undetermined significance (ASCUS) readings. HPV, human papillomavirus.

incidence of histologic SIL was observed.[22] When patient outcomes were analyzed by age (under 35 versus 35 years or above), those women age 35 years or older with ASCUS had lower incidences of histological SIL (14 percent) and HGSIL (1 percent) than in younger women. In this group of women over age 35 years, few cases of HGSIL would be missed if the women were triaged to repeat Pap smears.

9. Twenty-eight percent of the women under age 35 years with ASCUS, however, had histological SIL. The authors[22] suggested immediate colposcopy to avoid delay of treatment and potential for progression to invasive disease in this age group. A total of 6.1 percent of women with ASCUS specifically harbored histological HGSIL.

Realistically, an interpretation of atypical squamous cells of undetermined significance implies that it is up to the clinician to determine the source of the atypical cells.

10. Because of this underestimation of significant disease, colposcopy may be recommended.

11. On the other hand, because up to 63 percent of women have either normal findings or inflammatory changes, repeat cytological testing might be recommended.[23] It is not an all-or-none strategy.

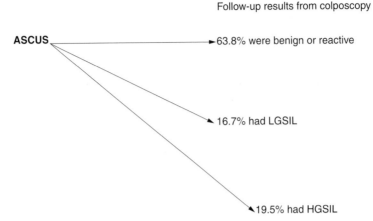

Follow-up results from colposcopy

ASCUS ————————————→ 63.8% were benign or reactive

◄ 16.7% had LGSIL

◄ 19.5% had HGSIL

Figure 18.3.   Evaluation of women with atypical squamous cells of undetermined significance (ASCUS). LGSIL, low grade squamous intraepithelial lesion; HGSIL, high grade squamous intraepithelial lesion. (Data from Suh-Burgmann E, Darragh T, Smith-McCune K. Atypical squamous cells of undetermined significance: Management patterns at an academic medical center. *Am J Obstet Gynecol* 1998;**178**:991–5.

12.   About 75 percent of those triaged to colposcopy will have no abnormalities. Of those triaged to cytological follow-up (repeat Pap test), some may develop invasive disease if they do not return for further work-up.

13.   In a large study of cytological/histological correlation, after biopsies were obtained from 560 patients with ASCUS, 357 (63.8 percent) were benign or reactive, 109 (19.5 percent) had HGSIL and 94 (16.7 percent) had LGSIL (Figure 18.3).[23]

14.   The NCI Interim Guidelines emphasize that if patient compliance is an issue, colposcopy should be performed on women with ASCUS. Compared with more aggressive strategies such as immediate colposcopy, triaging to repeat Pap testing is less expensive and incurs fewer complications but lower life expectancies per patient and more cancers result.

15.   The dilemma of ASCUS is that it may represent an undetected HGSIL or greater, and if the patient does not return for cytological screening, the disease could progress. This has to be balanced against the morbidity and cost of aggressive intervention versus the spontaneous regression of some lesions. In a published review of management options for ASCUS at an academic center, initial follow-up consisted of repeat Pap smears alone in 94 percent of the cases.[24] Of these, 29 percent were retested within two months and 68 percent within four months. This study demonstrates that about a third of the patients with ASCUS were returning sooner than is recommended by the NCI or ACOG. The relevant data indicated that 16 percent of patients did not return for follow-up until 18 months after the initial smear.

Women under age 35 with ASCUS were more likely than those older than age 35 to progress to low grade or high grade intraepithelial lesions.

Adjunctive testing

1. It would be helpful to have an intermediate triage test that would decrease the chance of missing significant lesions for those patients triaged to repeat cytological screening (Pap or other tests) and increase the probability that those who are triaged to colposcopy.[25]
2. The availability of a nonintrusive method for detecting those women most likely to have CIN, particularly high grade, would make the decision to follow ASCUS by repeat Pap smear a more reasonable option. The NCI Interim Guidelines included HPV testing as an option for management of ASCUS for physicians who understand its use. At the time the Interim Guidelines were published, there was no clinical HPV test that was sensitive enough to detect serious disease. Since that time, new technology (Hybrid Capture (HC) – Digene) has been introduced into the clinical setting; it has good interobserver correlation and is relatively easy to perform. HPV testing must be sensitive enough to identify the presence of high grade disease.[26]
3. Combined use of HC and a repeat Pap smear would detect 100 percent of HGSIL, thus limiting unnecessary colposcopy in those women who have no disease.[27] HPV-positive women with negative cytology and/or ASCUS are at a greatly increased likelihood of harboring histological CIN $(p < 0.001)$.[28] In another study, HPV-negative women were also much more likely to have no visible lesion at colposcopy or, if a biopsy of an abnormally appearing area was performed, to have normal histology.
4. If the woman tested twice negatively for oncogenic HPV, then it was almost impossible that she could have CIN.[27]
5. Other studies suggested that use of a repeat Pap smear combined with HC would correctly identify 96 percent of women with high grade CIN.[29] Most women who are HPV negative for a significant length of time do not develop significant cervical disease.[30] This combination protocol could be especially effective where colposcopy resources are scarce, prevalence of HGSIL is low, or if patients desire to avoid colposcopy.[28] The combined negative predictive

Combined use of HPV testing and a repeat Pap smear would detect 100 percent of high grade intraepithelial lesions in women with atypical squamous cells of undetermined significance.

value of the two tests would mean that a woman is at extremely low risk of developing CIN.

The combined negative predictive value of the two tests would reassure the clinician and patient that a significant cellular abnormality is not being missed, and may allow Pap smears to be performed at less frequent intervals.[31]

> Use of a repeat Pap smear combined with HPV would correctly identify 96 percent of women with high grade cervical intraepithelial neoplasia.

Low grade squamous intraepithelial lesion

1. Definition: In TBS, cytopathic changes consistent with HPV (LGSIL, mild dysplasia and CIN-1) are included under the category of low grade squamous intraepithelial lesions.
2. Management: Options for management according to the NIC Interim Guidelines include repeating the cytology every four to six months until three consecutive normal smears are obtained or immediate colposcopy.
3. Pathological correlation: Strict pathological interpretation should be done to decrease the chance of overdiagnosing koilocytosis unrelated to HPV.[32] Perinuclear clearing can be seen in nonneoplastic cells such as squamous metaplasia and reparative states. The most specific diagnosis of LGSIL requires the documentation of at least two, and preferably three, of the following cellular changes: multinucleation, nuclear atypia with enlargement, and koilocytosis.
4. Progression: SIL can exhibit variable biological behavior. CIN incorporates two different entities.
   a. One is reflective of the HPV infection (CIN-1, koilocytosis).
   b. The other (CIN-2 or 3) is the true cancer precursor.
5. Most LGSILs either persist or spontaneously regress and rarely progress. Approximately 50 percent of the LGSILs behave as nonneoplastic, productive viral infections that exhibit a high regression rate, but the other half behaves as a neoplasm and either persist or progress to a more serious abnormality (Figure 18.4).
6. Because of this variable rate of progression, some experts recommend that all women with LGSIL be referred for colposcopic evaluation because of the high rate of noncompliance, especially adolescents, who may not return for successive visits for repeat Pap sampling.
7. However, because of the high rate of regression of LGSIL, repeat cytology is an

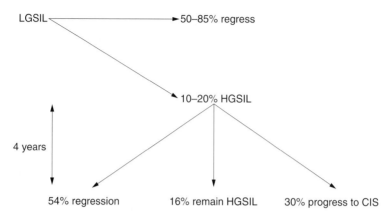

Figure 18.4.   Evolution of precancerous lesion. LGSIL, low grade squamous intraepithelial lesion; HGSIL, high grade squamous intraepithelial lesion; CIS, carcinoma in situ.

option if compliance is not an issue. The success of repeat cytology for not missing any significant disease rests with the validity of cytological interpretation. Many of the repeat cytological smears will be abnormal and, at that point, a referral to colposcopy should be made.[33]

8. Repeating cytology following a LGSIL diagnosis is based on the transient nature of most LGSILs, especially in young women. A total of 618 young women of 13 to 22 years who presented for routine gynecological care were HPV DNA tested using RNA–DNA dot–blot hybridization and followed every four months for 24 months.[34] Women with low-risk HPV types were more likely to show HPV regression compared with women with high risk HPV types. Of the initial cohort, 207 were found to have LGSIL. Seventy-four women had the diagnosis of LGSIL at the first visit. The remaining women had development of the diagnosis over time. Eleven of the 22 women with histological high grade disease had LGSIL on initial cytological evaluation. The development of HGSIL occurred only in approximately 5 percent of the cohort over the two-year study period. Only 7 percent of the women with documented high risk HPV types developed histological high grade disease. These results suggest that studies that rely on cytological diagnosis only for the diagnosis of HGSIL in HPV-positive women would initially misclassify approximately 17 percent of women with LGSIL and 9 percent of women with abnormal colposcopic findings yet normal cytology. Almost all low risk HPV infections and two-thirds of high risk HPV infections are eradicated over a two-year period, as demonstrated by repeatedly negative tests for HPV.

9. Persistently positive HPV tests for oncogenic types represented a significant risk for the development of HGSIL. HPV-related lesions are relatively uncommon in the older-aged woman.[8]

10. Adjunctive testing to delineate SIL: The first analysis of results of 642 women (mean age 24.9 years) with LGSIL who underwent HPV testing (Hybrid Capture II), found that HPV was detected in cervical samples from 532 (82.9 percent) of the women who had LGSIL. A total of 81.4 percent were positive by both Hybrid Capture II and the polymerase chain reaction (PCR). Because a very high percentage of women with a LGSIL diagnosis are positive for HPV, there is limited potential for HPV testing to direct decision about the triage of women with LGSIL.[35]

11. Older women with LGSIL may benefit from HPV testing. Misclassification of LGSIL lesions can lead to an overdiagnosis of CIN that is more likely in the older the woman.[36] Given the high positive predictive value of HPV detection with increasing age, HPV testing may clarify the true significance of LGSIL in this age group. This approach has not been tested in prospective studies.

Almost all low risk human papillomavirus (HPV) infections and two-thirds of high risk HPV infections are eradicated over a two-year period, as demonstrated by repeatedly negative tests for HPV.

Atypical glandular cells of undetermined significance

1. Recognition of glandular neoplasia presents a challenging problem for colposcopists and pathologists. Unlike squamous disease of the cervix, glandular lesions are subtler in appearance and cytological and histological differentiation of preinvasive and invasive glandular lesions of the cervix is more difficult.

2. Definition: According to TBS, AGUS are defined as glandular cells that show nuclear atypia that exceeds that of reactive or reparative changes but lack the degree of atypia needed to make a diagnosis of adenocarcinoma. The cytological diagnosis of AGUS includes the spectrum from benign to invasive disease and it is not always clear to the pathologist what is the absolute origin of the abnormal glandular cells.[37]

3. The cytological diagnosis differentiating AGUS, adenocarcinoma in situ (AIS), or invasive adenocarcinoma is very difficult. Cytological criteria for glandular abnormalities are not as specific as they are for squamous lesions. Cytology indicating AIS should be confirmed by review of the pathologist. The cytological diagnosis of AIS is easily confused with tubal metaplasia or invasive disease.

4. The specificity and sensitivity of cervical cytological testing for glandular neoplasia suffers from the challenge of differentiating benign conditions from premalignant and malignant disease. Cytological sampling can be hampered

if glandular lesions occupy the deep recesses of endocervical clefts, if they are covered by metaplastic epithelium, or if they are located deep within the endocervical canal.

5. Because there are no gradations of atypical, low grade or high grade glandular lesions, AGUS represents the full spectrum from benign to malignancy. If the cytology indicates a glandular lesion, a histological specimen is required.

6. Although the morphological criteria are poorly defined, many studies have detected significant CIN, AIS or cancer in 30 to 50 percent of women with AGUS. Any AGUS report deserves careful evaluation.

7. Unlike ASCUS, there are relatively few clinical guidelines established for AGUS smears. Laboratories reporting AGUS may report the results as unspecified changes or "favor reactive" or "favor neoplasia or AIS". Regardless of the designation, AGUS requires a colposcopic evaluation.

8. The practice of repeating AGUS-favor reactive or unspecified smears has not been studied prospectively.

9. Colposcopic evaluation with biopsy and endocervical curettage (ECC) is recommended for women with cytological reports of AGUS "favor neoplasia or AIS".[38]

Atypical squamous cells of undetermined significance represent the full spectrum from benign to malignancy.

---

10. Negative colposcopic findings are not totally reassuring. The proximal gland crypts are very difficult to access with endocervical sampling. The source of the atypical glandular cells must be determined. Cervical coninzation is the only way to reliably obtain histological data. If the cone biopsy is negative, other sources such as endometrium, tubes or ovaries should be considered and appropriately evaluated.

11. Excisional coninzation is mandatory if AIS is suspected from cytology or histology. AIS may be focal, multicentric, or located deep in the canal. Coninzation is necessary to determine the extent of the disease, confirm the diagnosis, exclude, or confirm the presence of adenocarcinoma and serve as possible therapy. Aggressive therapy is recommended because a third of women with glandular neoplasia on cytology will have adenocarcinomas.[39] A negative colposcopic examination of patients with AIS requires a coninzation to determine the location of the abnormal cells. A colposcopic examination is useful also in excluding the presence of squamous disease.

One-third of women with glandular neoplasia on cytology will have adenocarcinoma.

High-grade squamous intraepithelial lesion

1. Definition: HGSIL encompasses the categories of moderate dysplasia (CIN-2) and severe dysplasia/carcinoma in situ (CIN-3). Unlike LGSIL, HGSIL is an intraepithelial neoplasia with significant potential to progress to invasive cervical neoplasia if left untreated. High grade cervical lesions are the immediate precursors to nearly all cervical carcinomas.

2. The best opportunity for prevention of invasive squamous carcinoma lies in screening women aged 20 to 39 years when the incidence of CIN-3 in the screened population is highest.[40]

3. Among women who are appropriately screened, the rate of histologically verified CIN-2 or 3 or higher is practically nonexistent after the age of 60 years. Some cytological smears previously diagnosed as normal in women with current HGSIL are found to contain abnormal cells on retrospective review.[41]

4. Approximately 10 to 20 percent of women may progress to CIN-2 to 3 after a cytological diagnosis of LGSIL.[8]

5. A natural history study of 894 women with CIN-2 for 50 to 78 months found that the regression rate was 54 percent, persistence rate was 16 percent and the progression rate was 30 percent.[42] In another study, where the follow-up period was 18 months, a total of 14 percent of the CIN developed into a more severe grade of CIN.[43] The regression rate was demonstrated to be inversely related and the progression rate directly related to the grade of CIN.

6. The significant rate of progression of HGSIL to microinvasive or invasive disease has led to the recommendation that these lesions be definitively treated rather than observed. There is a strong argument of the necessity of careful follow-up and the importance of active surveillance of abnormal findings following treatment of high grade lesions to ensure that any failures will be detected early and that adequate eradication be accomplished.

7. Because nearly all women with cytologically proven HGSIL harbor HPV, HPV testing is not of value in women with HGSIL.

   a. HPV can be detected in over 95 percent of HGSIL. There is a significant association of histological grade of severity with oncogenic HPV types (16, 18, 31, 33).[44] HGSIL is characterized by the presence of oncogenic HPV types that are the same as those found in invasive cancer. Harboring a high risk HPV type is associated with a two- to threefold increased risk of CIN-3.[45]

   b. Although lower risk HPV types (6, 11) can be found in HGSIL, most of the HPV types are HPV 16, 18, and 33. One study demonstrated that 84 percent of histological CIN-3 contained high levels of at least one of the following HPV types: 16, 18, 31, 33, and 35.[46]

c. Only a few women with HGSIL have multiple HPV types.

d. The persistence of HPV infection is higher among women infected with oncogenic HPV types than among women with low risk HPV types.[47] Comparing women prospectively who were positive for HPV 16 but had normal cytology, significantly more women in the persistently positive group subsequently developed CIN.[50] Lesions in women with persistent HPV 16 were more severe than those in women infected for a short time. Based on this two-year study, the probability of CIN developing in women with persistent HPV 16 infection and normal cytology was 44 percent. There was a cumulative incidence of 28 percent of developing CIN in cytologically normal women in a two-year period.[48] However, both studies demonstrated that high grade CIN develops quickly in women with persistent HPV 16 infection.

e. Older women may have fewer sexual partners and be exposed to fewer HPV types, although older women may harbor oncogenic HPV types. Women with HGSIL tend to be older than those with LGSIL. The peak incidence of cervical cancer in women over 40 years of age may be a combination of older age and persistence of high risk HPV types.[49]

f. Untreated women with cervical epithelial abnormalities exhibit a significantly increased risk of subsequent disease progression if they harbor HPV 16 or 18.[50] The prevalence of HPV 16 increases from 24.5 percent to 50.2 percent corresponding to the increasing degree of severity of CIN.[51] The frequency of detection of high risk HPV among women with all grades of CIN was age dependent. However, the prevalence of histological CIN-2 or 3 significantly increased with increasing age.

Cervical cancer

1. Because so many cancers are found at stage 0 (carcinoma in situ) or early, the prognosis is excellent.

2. The five-year relative survival rate for stage I cervical cancer is 79 percent, reducing to 7 percent for stage IV disease. Survival for precancerous lesions is almost 100 percent, which provides the incentive for screening.

3. The treatment for stage O (less than 3 mm invasion) is simple hysterectomy. Radiation and chemotherapy are often not needed, although local radiation has been used. A hysterectomy is not curative for women with stage I or higher, although it may be done for hemorrhage.

4. Radiation is often used for higher stage cancers. Patients with stages I and IIA disease have a 70 to 85 percent cure rate with either radical surgery or radiation.

Conclusions

Cervical cancer is preventable and often curable if discovered early. Proper diagnosis, evaluation and treatment of abnormal Pap tests will allow the prevention of cervical cancer.

REFERENCES

1. Quinn M, Babb P, Jones J, Allen E. Effect of screening on incidence of and mortality from cancer of cervix in England: Evaluation based on routinely collected statistics. *BMJ* 1999;**318**:904.
2. Parazzini F, La Vecchia C, Negri E et al. Case-control study of oestrogen replacement therapy and risk of cervical cancer. *BMJ* 1997;**315**:85–8.
3. Boronow RC. Death of the Papanicolaou smear? A tale of three reasons. *Am J Obstet Gynecol* 1998;**179**:391–6.
4. Centers for Disease Control and Prevention. CDC update. National Breast and Cervical Cancer Early Detection Program – July 1991–September 1995. *MMWR Morb Mortal Wkly Rep* 1996;**45**:484–7.
5. Schiffman MH, Bauer HM, Hoover RN et al. Epidemiologic evidence showing that human papillomavirus infection causes most cervical intraepithelial neoplasia. *J Natl Cancer Inst* 1993:**85**:958–64.
6. Bosch FX, Manos MM, Munoz N et al. Human papillomavirus in cervical cancer: A worldwide perspective. *J Natl Cancer Inst* 1995;**87**:796–802.
7. Bjørge T, Dillner J, Anttila T. Prospective seroepidemiological study of role of human papillomavirus in non-cervical anogenital cancers. *BMJ* 1997;**315**:646–9.
8. Ostor AG. Natural history of cervical intraepithelial neoplasia: A critical review. *Int J Gynecol Pathol* 1993;**12**:186–92.
9. Schiffman MH, Brinton LA. The epidemiology of cervical carcinogenesis. *Cancer* 1995;**76**(Suppl):1888–901.
10. Agency of Health Care Policy and Research. Pap test still best bet, but new technologies show promise of improving screening outcomes. Press release 21 January 1999. (http://www.ahrq.gov/news/press/pr1999/cytopr.htm).
11. American Academy of Pediatrics. Recommendations for preventive pediatric health care. *Pediatrics* 1995;**96**:712.
12. Lavin C, Goodman E, Perlman S et al. Follow-up of abnormal Pap smears in a hospital based adolescent clinic. *J Pediatr Adolesc Gynecol* 1997;**10**:141–5.
13. Perlman SE, Kahn JA, Emans SJ. Should pelvic examinations and Papanicolaou cervical screening be part of preventive health care for sexually active adolescent girls? *J Adolesc Health* 1998;**23**:62–9.

14. National Cancer Institute Workshop. The 1988 Bethesda System for reporting cervical/vaginal cytologic diagnosis. *JAMA* 1989;**262**:931–4.

15. The Bethesda Committee. *The Bethesda System for Reporting Cervical/Vaginal Diagnoses.* Springer-Verlag, New York, 1994.

16. Kurman RJ, Henson DE, Herbst AL et al. Interim guidelines for management of abnormal cervical cytology. *JAMA* 1994;**271**:1866–9.

17. Dimian C, Nayagam M, Bradbeer C. The association between sexually transmitted diseases and inflammatory cervical cytology. *Genitourin Med* 1992;**68**:305–6.

18. Stern JE, Givan AL, Gonzalez JL et al. Leukocytes in the cervix: A quantitative evaluation of Cervicitis. *Obstet Gynecol* 1998;**91**:9987–92.

19. Ecert LO, Koutsky LA, Kiviat NB et al. The inflammatory Papanicolaou smear: What does it mean? *Obstet Gynecol* 1995;**86**:360–6.

20. Sherman ME, Schiffman MH, Lorincz AT et al. Towards objective quality assurance in cervical cytopathology: Correlation of cytopathologic diagnosis with detection of high risk HPV types. *Am J Clin Pathol* 1994;**102**:182–7.

21. Kinney WK, Manos MM, Hurley LB, Ransley JE. Where's the high-grade cervical neoplasia? The importance of minimally abnormal Papanicolaou diagnoses. *Obstet Gynecol* 1998;**91**:973–6.

22. Kobelin MH, Kobelin CG, Burke L et al. Incidence and predictors of cervical dysplasia in patients. With minimally abnormal Papanicolaou smears. *Obstet Gynecol* 1998;**92**:356–9.

23. Lachman MF, Cavallo-Calvanese C. Qualification of atypical squamous cells of undetermined significance in an independent laboratory: Is it useful or significant? *Am J Obstet Gynecol* 1998;**179**:421–9.

24. Suh-Burgmann E, Darragh T, Smith-McCune K. Atypical squamous cells of undetermined signficance: Management patterns at an academic medical center. *Am J Obstet Gynecol* 1998;**178**:991–5.

25. Cox JT, Wilkinson EJ, Lonky N et al. ASCCP practice guidelines management guidelines for follow-up of atypical squamous cells of undetermined significance (ASCUS). *J Lower Genital Tract Dis* 2000;**4**:99–105.

26. Shen LH, Rushing L, McLachlin CM, Sheets EE, Crum CP. Prevalence and histologic significance of cervical human papillomavirus DNA detected in women at low and high risk for cervical neoplasia. *Obstet Gynecol* 1995;**86**:499–503.

27. Cox JT, Lorincz AT, Schiffman MH et al. HPV testing by hybrid capture appears to be useful in triaging women with a cytologic diagnosis of ASCUS. *Am J Obstet Gynecol* 1995;**172**:946.

28. Cox TJ, Schiffman MH, Winzelberg AJ, Patterson JM. The evaluation of human papillomavirus testing as part of referral to colposcopy clinics. *Obstet Gynecol* 1992;**80**:389–95.

29. Wright TC, Sun XW, Koulos J. Comparison of management algorithms for the evaluation of women with low-grade cytologic abnormalities. *Obstet Gynecol* 1995;**85**:202–10.

30. Moscicki B, Palefshy J, Smith G, Siboshski S, Schoolnik G. Variability of human papillomavirus DNA testing in a longitudinal cohort of young women. *Obstet Gynecol* 1993;**82**:578–85.

31. Remmink A, Helmerhorst T, Walboomers JM et al. HPV in follow-up of patients with cytomorphologically abnormal cervical smears: A prospective nonintervention study. *Int J Cancer* 1995;**61**:1–5.

32. Cox JT, Massad S, Lonky N et al. ASCCP practice guidelines management guidelines for the follow-up of cytology read as low grade squamous intraepithelial lesion. *J Lower Genital Tract Dis* 2000;**4**:83–92.

33. Ferris DG, Wright TC, Litaker MS et al. Triage of women with ASCUS and LGSIL Pap smear reports: Management by repeat Pap smear, HPV testing or colposcopy? *J Fam Pract* 1998;**46**:125–34.

34. Moscicki AB, Shiboski S, Broering J et al. The natural history of human papillomavirus infection as measured by repeated DNA testing in adolescent and young women. *J Pediatr* 1998;**132**:277–84.

35. Koutsky LA. Human papillomavirus testing for triage of women with cytologic evidence of low-grade squamous intraepithelial lesions: Baseline data from a randomized trial. *J Natl Cancer Inst* 2000;**92**:397–402.

36. Schiffman MH, Manos MM, Sherman ME et al. Response: Human papillomavirus and cervical intraepithelial neoplasia. *J Natl Cancer Inst* 1993;**85**:1868–70.

37. Raab SS, Issacson D, Layfield LJ et al. Atypical glandular cells of undetermined significance. Cytologic criteria to separate clinically significant from benign lesions. *Am J Clin Pathol* 1995;**104**:574–82.

38. Taylor RR, Guerrieri JP, Nash JD et al. Atypical cervical cytology: Colposcopic follow-up using the Bethesda System. *J Reprod Med* 1993;**38**:443–7.

39. Laverty CR, Farnsworth A, Thurloe J, Bowditch R. The reliability of a cytologic prediction of cervical adenocarcinoma in situ. *Aust NZ J Obstet Gynaecol* 1988;**28**:307–11.

40. Smith HA. Cervical intraepithelial neoplasia grade III (CIN III) and invasive cervical carcinoma: The yawning gap revisited and the treatment of risk. *Cytopathology* 1999;**10**:161–79.

41. Montes MA, Cibas ES, DiNisco SA, Lee KR. Cytologic characteristics of abnormal cells in prior "normal" cervical/vaginal Papanicolaou smears form women with a high-grade squamous intraepithelial lesion. *Cancer* 1999;**87**:45–7.

42. Nasiell K, Roger V, Nasiell M. Behavior of mild cervical dysplasia during long-term follow-up. *Obstet Gynecol* 1986;**67**:665–8.

43. Syrjanen K, Vayrynen M, Saarikoski S et al. Natural history of cervical human papillomavirus (HPV) infections based on prospective follow-up. *Br J Obstet Gynaecol* 1985;**92**:1086–92.

44. Monsonego J, Valensi P, Zerat L, Clavel C, Birembaut P. Simultaneous effects of aneuploidy and oncogenic human papillomavirus on histological grade of cervical intraepithelial neoplasia. *Br J Obstet Gynaecol* 1997;**104**:723–7.

45. Kjellberg L, Wang Z, Wiklund F et al. Sexual behavior and papillomavirus exposure in cervical intraepithelial neoplasia: A population-based case-control study. *J Gen Virol* 1999;**80**:391–8.

46. Cuzick K, Terry G, Ho L, Hollingworth T, Anderson M. Type-specific human papillomavirus DNA in abnormal smears as a predictor of high-grade cervical intraepithelial neoplasia. *Br J Cancer* 1994;**69**:167–71.

47. Hildesheim A, Schiffman MH, Gravitt PE et al. Persistence of type specific human papillomavirus infection among cytologically normal women. *J Infect Dis* 1994;**169**:234–40.

48. Koutsky LA, Holmes KK, Critchlow CW et al. A cohort study of the risk of cervical intraepithelial neoplasia grade 2 or 3 in relation to papillomavirus infection. *N Engl J Med* 1992;**327**:1272–8.

49. Romney SL, Ho GYF, Palan PR et al. Effects of β-carotene and other factors on outcome of cervical dysplasia and human papillomavirus infection. *Gynecol Oncol* 1997;**65**:483–92.

50. Woodman CB, Rollason T, Ellis J et al. Human papillomavirus infection and risk of progression of epithelial abnormalities of the cervix. *Br J Cancer* 1996;**73**:553–6.

51. Adam E, Berkova Z, Daxnerova Z et al. Papillomavirus detection: Demographic and behavioral characteristics influencing the identification of cervical disease. *Am J Obstet Gynecol* 2000;**182**:257–64.

Endometrial cancer and postmenopausal bleeding

Jo Ann Rosenfeld, MD

Endometrial cancer is the most common pelvic cancer but, luckily, it is usually discovered early and is often curable. Postmenopausal bleeding is worrisome because as many as one-quarter may be caused by cancer.

Epidemiology

1. Endometrial cancer (ECa)(cancer of the body or corpus of the uterus) is the fourth most common malignancy in women in the USA and ranks seventh in cancer deaths in women. Since 1972, ECa has been the most common female pelvic malignancy. In the USA, 36 000 new cases are identified yearly and ECa caused 6300 deaths in 1998.[1] In Europe, 5 percent of cancer in women is endometrial cancer.[2]

2. Seventy-five percent of ECa occur in postmenopausal women, although 5 percent occur in women younger than age 40 years.

3. Because the primary symptom is postmenopausal bleeding, which is noteworthy and dramatic, most ECa cases are found at an early stage, have a good prognosis, and are usually curable by surgery.

4. Risk factors (Table 19.1) include use of unopposed estrogen, hyperestrogen states, and tamoxifen use. Other risk factors include obesity, nulliparity, diabetes, hypertension, chronic anovulation, PCOS, and estrogen-producing tumors. ECa is associated with early menarche and late menopause.

5. Use of tamoxifen for breast cancer therapy produces a sixfold increased risk in developing ECa at doses of 40 mg daily. Nonetheless, tamoxifen continues to be used, because the risk of ECa is much smaller than the risk of recurrent breast cancer.[3]

6. Administration of unopposed estrogen in postmenopausal women who still have their uteruses, the way estrogen was used for HRT in the past, is asso-

Table 19.1. Risk factors for most endometrial cancers

- Post menopausal
- Obesity
- Diabetes
- Hypertension
- Chronic anovulatory states – polycystic ovary syndrome, etc.
- High estrogen states
  - Estrogen-producing tumors
  - Administration of unopposed estrogen

    ciated with a four- to eightfold increase in endometrial cancer. Progesterone was added to HRT regimens to reduce the risk of ECa.

7. ECa has a higher prevalence in whites, though it is also among the top five cancers in women in incidence in many US ethnic groups including African-Americans, Chinese-Americans, Japanese-Americans, Native Americans, and Hispanic Americans (Figure 19.1).[4]

8. Even though white Americans have a higher incidence of ECa than African-Americans, for every stage of ECa, white women's survival rates exceed that of African-Americans by 15 percent. White women are more likely to have ECa identified at an earlier stage. African-American women present with more advanced disease. Of African-Americans diagnosed with ECa, 22 percent had grade 3 or 4 cancer, as compared with 13 percent of white women.[5] Nonetheless, even though African-Americans usually had more advanced disease, even within the same stage of disease, African-American women received less treatment and less surgery.[5]

9. Use of OCPs and pregnancy reduce the risk of ECa.

Most endometrial cancer cases are found at an early stage, have a good prognosis, and are usually curable by surgery.

Symptoms and diagnosis and evaluation of postmenopausal bleeding

1. The primary symptom of ECa is postmenopausal bleeding (PMB).
2. Women who have been on HRT and still have withdrawal bleeding or intermittent bleeding do not need an evaluation for ECa. However, if they have become amenorrheic for at least six months while on HRT, especially if on continuous combined estrogen and progesterone therapy, and then have vaginal bleeding, they need an evaluation to eliminate ECa as a cause of PMB.

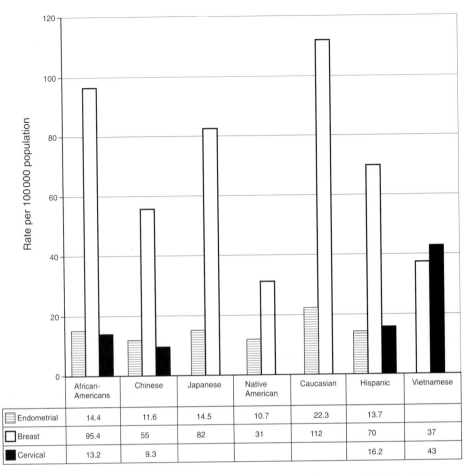

	African-Americans	Chinese	Japanese	Native American	Caucasian	Hispanic	Vietnamese
Endometrial	14.4	11.6	14.5	10.7	22.3	13.7	
Breast	95.4	55	82	31	112	70	37
Cervical	13.2	9.3				16.2	43

Figure 19.1.   Gynecological cancer incidence in the USA by ethnicity. (Data from Parker SL, Davis KJ, Wingo PA, Ries LA, Heath CW. Cancer statistics by race and ethnicity. *CA Cancer J Clin* 1998;**48**:31–48.)

3.   PMB can be caused by vaginal, cervical, uterine or ovarian causes (Table 19.2).

4.   Evaluation: The evaluation of the woman with PMB has changed remarkably in the past 10 years. Previously, because up to 25 percent of women with PMB might have ECa, all women had a dilatation and curettage (D&C). Now that is not universally necessary (Figure 19.2).

   a. A physical examination should look for vaginal and cervical abnormalities, uterine size, masses and asymmetries, or ovarian masses. Trauma or abuse can appear as vaginal or uterine bleeding.

   b. A Pap test should be performed. It is not sensitive but may be specific for endometrial cancer. It will discover any cervical cancers that may be causing PMB.

Table 19.2. Causes of postmenopausal vaginal bleeding

- Vaginal
  - Cancer
  - Polyps
  - Condylomata
  - Trauma
  - Vaginitis – irritative or infectious
- Cervical
  - Cervicitis – infectious – chlamydia, gonorrhea, yeast, *Trichomonas*, other
  - Cervical polyps
  - Trauma
  - Cancer
- Uterine
  - Fibroids
  - Withdrawal bleeding from HRT
  - Cancer
- Ovarian/fallopian tubes
  - Cysts
  - Cancer

   c. A transvaginal ultrasound is necessary. A retrospective study of more than 1100 women with PMB in several centers in Scandinavia found that no woman with an endometrial thickness less than 5 mm was found to have ECa. Women with atrophic vaginitis had a mean endometrial thickness of 3.9 mm. The 95 percent confidence limit for excluding endometrial abnormality was an endometrium thickness of 4 mm or less.[6] Several subsequent prospective studies have confirmed that, in women with PMB, an endometrial thickness of less than 5 mm and perhaps even 10 mm may nearly eliminate ECa as a cause.[7]

5. An in-office endometrial biopsy performed on the woman with PMB, in addition to the transvaginal ultrasound, has been found, in a prospective study, to further increase the accuracy of diagnosis.[8] If both are normal, ECa is very unlikely.

6. Any positive findings or cytology would necessitate a D&C or surgery.

7. Any mass, uterine enlargement or continued bleeding may need a referral for D&C, hysteroscopy, laparoscopy, or other surgery.

> In women with postmenopausal bleeding, an endometrial thickness of less than 5 mm and perhaps even 10 mm may nearly eliminate ECa as a cause.

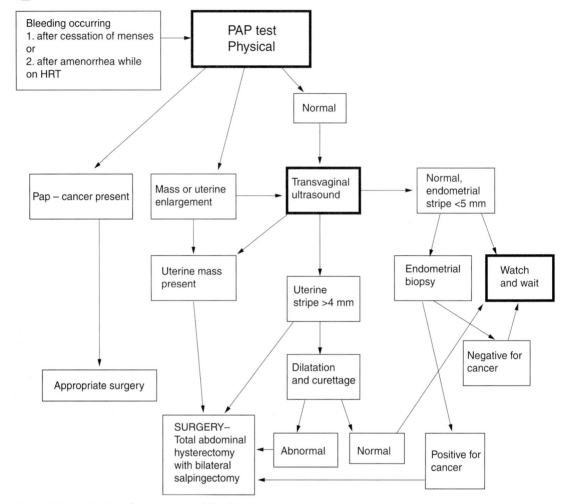

Figure 19.2.   Evaluation of postmenopausal bleeding.

Staging and treatment

Staging

Staging has been standardized. Staging helps to determine treatment and is predictive of prognosis (Table 19.3). Seventy-five percent of women present in stage I.

Prognostic factors

1. Prognostic factors are related to age, race, endocrine status, histological cell type, tumor grade, depth of myometrial invasion, extension beyond the

Table 19.3. Staging of endometrial cancer

- Stage I – confined to body of uterus
  - IA – uterine cavity $< 8\,cm$
  - IB – uterine cavity $> 8\,cm$
  - Grade I – highly differentiated to grade 3 – undifferentiated
- Stage II – cancer confined to the corpus and cervix
- Stage III – cancer extends outside uterus but not into the true pelvis
- Stage IV – cancer extends into the true pelvis or into the mucosa of bladder and rectum

   uterus, adnexal metastases, extrauterine and peritoneal spread.

2. Elevated levels of the tumor-associated antigen CA 125 are associated with ECa and the levels reflect the course of the disease, rising with metastatic and recurrent disease.

Treatment

1. The treatment for stage I cancer is surgical and is a total abdominal hysterectomy with bilateral salpingoophorectomy.
2. The need for postoperative adjunctive chemotherapy depends on the stage and grade of the tumor. Stage I or IA tumors do not benefit from postoperative radiation. Stage IB or IC cancers have shown no improvement in mortality with radiation unless more than half of myometrial walls was involved. Higher risk disease including women with pelvic nodes positive for cancer need radiation.
3. Those women with abdominal metastases or recurrence may also need chemotherapy.

Follow-up

1. Use of HRT post cancer: Whether, in women who have had endometrial cancer and then total abdominal hysterectomy with bilateral salpingoophorectomy, HRT will adversely affect recurrence and mortality rates is not known. Studies have not proven the safety of HRT in women with ECa, but a large prospective trial is needed.
2. Postoperative surveillance guidelines suggest clinical visits alone are sufficient. If the woman has no evidence of disease, an interval history and physical every three months for two years, then every six months for three years should be sufficient. Repeat chest X-rays do not improve survival.
3. Fourteen percent of women develop recurrent disease. Ninety-three percent

of endometrial cancer patients survive for one-year and 95 percent survive for five years, if the disease is discovered at an early stage. With more advanced disease, 66 percent survive for five years.

Conclusions

Endometrial cancer is often discovered at an early stage and is usually a disease of postmenopausal women. Postmenopausal bleeding is the most common presentation of endometrial cancer, but only one-quarter of women with postmenopausal bleeding have cancer. An office-based evaluation with minimal invasive testing is adequate for diagnosis.

REFERENCES

1. Barakat RR. Contemporary issues in the management of endometrial cancer. *CA Cancer J Clin* 1998;**48**:299–314.
2. Black RJ, Bray F, Ferlay J, Parkin DM. Cancer incidence and mortality in the European Union. *Eur J Cancer* 1997;**33**:1075–107.
3. Fisher B, Costatino JP, Redmond CK et al. Endometrial cancer in tamoxifen-treated breast cancer patients. Findings from the National Surgical adjuvant breast and bowel project B-14. *J Natl Cancer Inst* 1994;**86**:527–37.
4. Parker SL, Davis KJ, Wingo PA, Ries LA, Heath CW. Cancer statistics by race and ethnicity. *CA Cancer J Clin* 1998;**48**:31–48.
5. Fremgen AM, Cland KI, McGinnis LMS et al. Clinical highlights from the National Cancer Database 1999. *CA Cancer J Clin* 1999;**49**:145–58.
6. Karlsson B, Granberg S, Wilkand M et al. Transvaginal ultrasonography of the endometrium in women with postmenopausal bleeding – a Nordic multicenter study. *Am J Obstet Gynecol* 1995;**172**:1488–94.
7. Mateos F, Zaranz R, Seco C et al. Assessment with transvaginal ultrasonography of endometrial thickness in women with postmenopausal bleeding. *Eur J Gynecol Oncol* 1997;**18**:504–7.
8. Gull B, Carlsson S, Karlsson B et al. Transvaginal ultrasonography of the endometrium in women with postmenopausal bleeding: Is it always necessary to perform an endometrial biopsy? *Am J Obstet Gynecol* 2000;**182**:509–15.

20 Ovarian cancer and ovarian masses

Jo Ann Rosenfeld, MD

Ovarian cancer is rare, but unfortunately has a high mortality rate because it is usually discovered at an advanced stage. There are few risk factors amenable to prevention, and the most appropriate and sensitive screening methods have not been discovered.

Epidemiology

1. Ovarian cancer is the leading cause of death from gynecological malignancy. Other gynecological malignancies are usually discovered early, treated, and cured.[1] In the USA in 1999, there were 25 000 new cases and 14 500 deaths from ovarian cancer. About 1 woman in 70 in the USA will have a lifetime chance of developing ovarian cancer.
2. During the period 1994–1999 in the UK 21 241 deaths were caused by ovarian cancer.[2]
3. The number of women with ovarian cancer in the USA has increased 30 percent and the number of ovarian cancer deaths has increased 18 percent in the last few years.[3]
4. The rate of ovarian cancer in Native Americans at 17.5/100 000 is higher than that of the white population at 15.8/100 000.[3]

Risk factors

1. Age: The number 1 risk factor is advancing age. The rate rises with age from 15.7 to 54/100 000 from age 40 to 79 years. The mean age is 59 years.[1]
2. Family history: Genetic disposition or a family history of ovarian cancer is the second most important risk factor. There are three hereditary syndromes. Most breast and ovarian cancer genetic syndrome patients have the *BRCA1* or

BRCA2 gene. The penetration of this gene mutation is 95 percent, giving a cumulative risk of 63 percent for developing breast cancer by age 70 years.

3. Other risk factors include nulliparity, early menarche and late menopause. Each pregnancy reduces risk of ovarian cancer by 10 percent.[1]
4. Use of OCPs reduces the risk of ovarian cancer by 30 to 60 percent. Women using oral contraceptives for five years or more decrease their risk of ovarian cancer by 50 percent.[4] Having a tubal ligation or a hysterectomy reduces the risk as well.[5]

Signs and diagnosis

1. Ovarian cancer is usually a disease of postmenopausal women and is silent. There are few symptoms until it is advanced. An ovarian or pelvic mass may be seen incidentally on an ultrasound or felt on a pelvic examination. There may be signs of an ovarian or pelvic mass – frequent UTIs, vaginitis or constipation. There may be pelvic pain from invasion into nerves or bone. Finally, ovarian cancer usually spreads locally and, then, into the peritoneum where it causes ascites, an enlarging abdomen, and shortness of breath, and usually, by this point, weight loss.
2. Difficult to diagnose early, most ovarian cancers are diagnosed at advance stage histologically. The diagnosis can be suspected by pelvic examination, elevated levels of CA 125 (a tumor-associated antigen), or findings on an ultrasound or ovarian duplex scanning, but can only be definitely made by laparoscopy or surgery.

Ovarian masses

1. Incidence and importance: Most ovarian masses are benign or functional, but the specter and risk of ovarian cancer rises with age. Ovarian cysts are common. Six percent of asymptomatic postmenopausal women have adnexal masses and 90 percent of these are cysts.

Most ovarian masses are benign or functional.

2. An accurate diagnosis is difficult, although essential.
    a. Clinical examination is poor. Thirty to 65 percent of tumors, especially those less than 5 cm, are overlooked on physical examination.

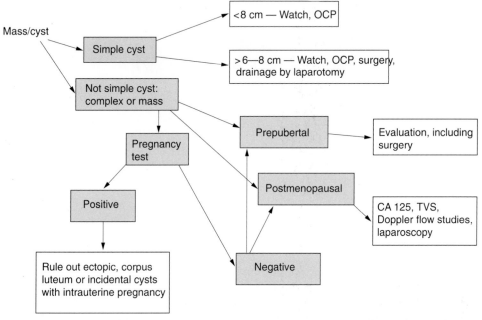

Figure 20.1.   Evalution of ovarian mass/cysts. TVS, transvaginal sonography; OCP, oral contraceptive pill.

    b. Transvaginal sonography (TVS) is better at establishing a correct diagnosis. TVS can predict an ovarian tumor in 96 percent of cases – up to 71 percent negative predictive value.[6]

    c. CA 125 serum levels are normal in 97 percent of women with benign cysts. Eighty percent of women older than age 50 years with malignant lesions have a level greater than 35 IU/mL. However, only 50 percent of women with stage I ovarian cancer have an elevated CA 125 level.[7]

    d. Ovarian cytology (needle aspiration of cysts with immediate fixation) is reliable for diagnosis.

  3. The evaluation must be based on age (Figure 20.1).

    a. In prepubertal adolescents, pelvic or ovarian masses and cysts are very worrisome and a complete evaluation including ultrasound and surgery or laparoscopy is recommended. Germ cell tumors are a possibility.

    b. In menstruating women, pregnancy, pregnancy complications, and functional cysts are the most common causes.

      i. First, a urine or blood human chorionic gonadotropin test should be

In prepubertal adolescents, pelvic or ovarian masses and cysts are very worrisome and a complete evaluation including ultrasound and surgery or laparoscopy is recommended.

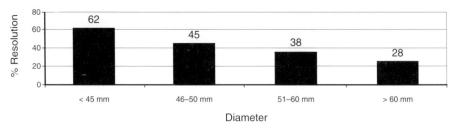

Figure 20.2.   Percentage of ovarian cysts that resolved within six months, by size. (Data from Zanetta G, Lissoni A, Torri V et al. Role of puncture and aspiration in expectant management of simple ovarian cysts: A randomised study. *BMJ* 1996;**313**:1110–13.)

carried out to eliminate most pregnancies, ectopic pregnancy, and pregnancy complications such as a molar pregnancy.

ii. Then a TVS should be done to determine whether the mass is ovarian and simple cystic, complex or solid.

iii. The CA 125 level should be ascertained. If it is elevated, a consultation for surgery may be indicated.

iv. If the mass is cystic and smaller than 8 cm and the CA 125 level is less than 35 IU/mL, the woman and the physician can wait and watch or use hormonal suppression including OCPs. The smaller the cyst, the more likely it is to resolve without treatment (Figure 20.2). A RCT followed 278 women with simple ovarian cysts for six months, either by watching or with a fine needle biopsy directed by ultrasound. Forty-six percent resolved with aspiration and 45 percent with observation. Only the diameter of the cyst was a significant independent prognostic factor.[8] The mean size of cysts was 52 mm. The larger the cysts, the less likely were they to resolve.

v. If the mass is cystic and larger than 8 cm or the woman has an elevated CA 125 level, a gynecological surgery consultation is indicated, although the treatment may be waiting, hormones, or surgery.

vi. If the mass is a complex cyst or solid, the woman should have an ovarian duplex scan for better definition. However, she will probably need a laparoscopy or surgery.

c. Postmenopausal women with any ovarian masses should be considered to have cancer until proven otherwise. Some experts believe that if the physician can feel the ovary in a postmenopausal woman, she needs an evaluation for cancer. The woman will need surgery unless the TVS shows a simple cyst less than 5 cm *and* she has a normal CA 125 level.

In menstruating women, pregnancy, pregnancy complications, and functional cysts are the most common causes of ovarian masses.

Postmenopausal women should be considered to have cancer until proven otherwise.

Prevention

1. Prevention is not possible for the general population.
2. However, with women with two or more first-degree relatives with epithelial ovarian cancer, a pedigree of multiple occurrences of nonpolyposis colon cancer endometrial cancer, and ovarian cancer, or a pedigree of multiple cases of ovarian and breast cancer, and who have finished childbearing, a prophylactic oophorectomy may be considered to prevent ovarian cancer.

Screening

1. There is no acceptable method of screening, although CA 125 levels and TVS have been used.
2. Computer models predict that universal screening for ovarian cancer might save three years of life per case.[9] However, even with a test that was 99 percent specific in women aged 45 to 75 years, the positive predictive value would be only 4 percent. This kind of test would cause 24 normal women to have laparoscopy for each one positive for cancer.
3. Pelvic examination has a limited value because of poor sensitivity. Its sensitivity for detecting a mass that is 4 cm × 6 cm is only 67 percent. A 15-year retrospective study evaluating pelvic examination found only six ovarian cancers in 1319 women who had 18 753 pelvic examinations, showing the inadequacy of this method.[10]
4. CA 125 levels may be a better indicator, but they still lack the sensitivity and specificity of a good screening test.
   a. A RCT of ovarian cancer screening followed 22 000 postmenopausal women who were randomized to three annual screens or control using CA 125 as the tumor marker. The women were referred to TVS if their CA 125 level was greater than 30 IU/ml. If the TVS found a mass, they were sent to surgery.[11] Although this was a pilot study and too small to show efficacy in terms of mortality reduction, it did show that an acceptable positive predictive value can be obtained by selecting women on the basis of CA 125 levels.

      Forty-nine cancers were found in this study. The cumulative risk of

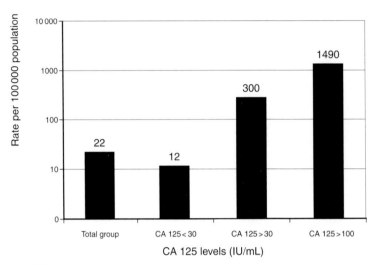

Figure 20.3.   Risk of developing ovarian cancer in one study by CA 125 levels. (Data from Jacobs IJ, Skates S, Davies AP et al. Risk of diagnosis of ovarian cancer after raised serum CA concentration: A prospective cohort study. *BMJ* 1996;**313**:1355–8.)

developing cancer was 0.0022 for the total population (22/10 000), 0.0012 for those with CA 125 levels less than 30 IU/mL, 0.030 for those with CA 125 levels greater than 30 IU/mL, and 0.149 for levels greater than 100 IU/mL (Figure 20.3).[12] The RR was 35.9 for developing ovarian cancer within one year, if the woman's CA 125 level was greater than 30 IU/mL, and 204, if her level was greater than 100 IU/mL.

   b. The CA 125 level is also elevated in endometriosis, PID, adenomyosis, liver disease, pancreatitis, peritonitis and other benign processes, and other malignant processes including endometrial cancer, biliary tract tumors, and liver, pancreas, breast, and colon cancer.

5. TVS has been proposed as a screening test because it images the ovary well, but it has insufficient specificity. However, when combined with color Doppler, the combined sensitivity is 94 percent and specificity is 97 percent.

6. Even for women at high risk, studies have not decided whether systematic screening will reduce mortality and morbidity.

7. In one study, although neither TVS nor CA 125 was specific enough when used alone,[13] when both tests were positive, the positive predictive value approaches 20 percent. Nonetheless, this would mean five surgeries performed for each malignant cancer found, four done with negative results.

8. The newest research shows a growth factor called lysophosphatidic acid (LPA) produced in hematopoietic cells. LPA was highly elevated in 48 women with ovarian cancer as compared with healthy women.

There is no acceptable method of screening for ovarian cancer, although CA 125 levels and transvaginal sonography have been used.

Treatment and survival

1. Survival: Survival from ovarian cancer is based on the stage, and ranges from 87.8 percent five-year survival for women with stage IA to 18 percent for women with stage IV.
2. Treatment: Treatment is surgery, and staging is very important – whether one or both ovaries are involved and degree of extension. If fertility is not an issue a total abdominal hysterectomy and bilateral salpingoophorectomy should be done with biopsies of right and left pelvic peritoneum and bladder.
3. In advanced disease, debulking surgical resection is done. Debulking the tumor mass to less than 2 cm will improve survival.
4. Chemotherapy is used as an adjuvant, often cisplatin and doxyrubicin, and now paclitaxel, especially for recurrence.
5. The use of radiation of women with ovarian cancer is controversial in the USA.

Conclusions

Ovarian cancer is a disease that so far lacks adequate screening tests and is most often lethal and already metastatic when discovered. Thus any ovarian or pelvic mass in a woman of any age is suspect for ovarian cancer. Except in menstruating women with completely cystic masses smaller than 6 to 7 cm, most evaluations of women with pelvic masses will require surgical exploration.

REFERENCES

1. Partridge EE, Barnes MN. Epithelial ovarian cancer: Prevention, diagnosis and treatment. *CA Cancer J Clin* 1999;**49**:297–320.
2. Richards MA, Stockton D, Babb P, Coleman MP. How many deaths have been avoided through improvements in cancer survival? *BMJ* 2000;**320**:895–8.
3. Parker SL, Davis KJ, Wingo PA, Ries LA, Heath CW. Cancer statistics by race and ethnicity. *CA Cancer J Clin* 1998;**48**:31–48.

4. WHO. Collaborative study of neoplasia and steroid contraceptives: Epithelial ovarian cancer and combined oral contraceptives. In *J Epidemiol* 1989;**18**:538–45.

5. Hankinson SE, Hunter DJ, Colditz GA et al. Tubal ligation, hysterectomy and risk of ovarian cancer: A prospective study. *JAMA* 1993;**270**:2813–18.

6. Salat-Baroux J, Merviel PH, Kuttenn F. Management of ovarian cysts. *BMJ* 1996;**313**:1098.

7. Jacobs I, Bast R. The CA-125 tumor associated antigen: A review of literature. *Hum Reprod* 1989;**4**:1–12.

8. Zanetta G, Lissoni A, Torri V et al. Role of puncture and aspiration in expectant management of simple ovarian cysts: A randomised study. *BMJ* 1996;**313**:1110–13.

9. Skates SJ, Singer DE. Quantifying the potential benefit of CA-125 screening for ovarian cancer. *Clin Epidemiol* 1991;**44**:365–80.

10. McFarlane C, Sturgis MD, Fetterman FC. Results of an experience in the control of cancer of the female pelvic organs: A report of a 15 year research. *Am J Obstet Gynecol* 1956;**294**:301–6.

11. Jacobs I, Skates SJ, MacDonald N et al. Outcome of a pilot randomised controlled trial of ovarian cancer screening. *Lancet* 1999;**253**:1207–10.

12. Jacobs IJ, Skates S, Davies AP et al. Risk of diagnosis of ovarian cancer after raised serum CA concentration: A prospective cohort study. *BMJ* 1996;**313**:1355–8.

13. Urban N. Screening for ovarian cancer. *BMJ* 1999;**319**:1317–18.

Urinary incontinence and infections

Jo Ann Rosenfeld, MD

URINARY INCONTINENCE

Urinary incontinence (UI) is a problem for many women and at least half of women never mention the problem to their health care professionals.

Importance and epidemiology

1. The prevalence is difficult to determine and varies with the population surveyed. Approximately 38 percent of community-dwelling older women have significant incontinence.[1] The incidence varies from 1 percent of all patients to 51 percent of all women sometime in their lives.[2] Approximately 5 to 10 percent of women, 13 million persons in the USA, have clinically significant UI.[3] In the Hormone and Estrogen Replacement Study (HERS) of 2763 older women with heart disease, 56 percent reported at least weekly incontinence.[4]

2. UI has a large social and financial toll. It predisposes the woman to depression, social isolation, and dependency. It is a major factor in admissions to long-term health care facilities and in long-term morbidity including catheterization, pressure sores, infection, chronic infections, immobility, and falls. It costs the USA approximately $16 billion yearly.

> Approximately 38 percent of community-dwelling older women have clinically significant incontinence.

3. UI occurs more often in institutionalized women. One-half of homebound and institutionalized elderly and 25 to 30 percent of those that leave the hospital are incontinent. In Sweden in 1985, 34 percent of community-dwelling women and 86.9 percent of women in residential care were incontinent.[5]

Table 21.1. Risk factors for urinary incontinence

Medical history
- Older age
- Stroke
- Immobility from chronic neurological or degenerative disease
- Dementia/delirium
- Medication use (see Table 21.2)
- Diabetes
- Pelvic muscle weakness
- ?Pregnancy
- Increased parity
- Vaginal delivery
- History of episiotomy
- More than two UTIs

Social history
- Smoking
- White race

Physical findings
- Fecal impaction
- Obesity

However, in a population of women in residential care in Leicester, UK, only 40 percent were incontinent.[6]

Urinary incontinence occurs more often in institutionalized women.

Risk factors (Table 21.1)

1. Gender: Being a woman is a risk factor for UI. The female : male ratio is 4 : 1 at age 60 years and 2 : 1 after age 60.[7]
2. Age: Five to 6 percent of women less than age 60 years and 10 percent more than age 60 report UI.[2]
3. Exercise: Approximately one-half of postmenopausal women develop UI while exercising.[8]
4. Obstetrical history: Parity, vaginal delivery, episiotomy and traumatic or surgical vaginal delivery are factors for UI.[7] Although having had a hysterectomy was not found to be a factor in prospective study, cross-sectional epidemiological studies have found it increased risk.

Table 21.2. Medications that affect bladder functioning

Medication	Usual type of UI caused
Alcohol	Urge
Alpha-adrenergic antagonists	Stress, overflow
Anticholinergics	
Antidepressants, antipsychotics	Overflow
Antihistamines	Overflow
Beta-blockers	Stress, urge
CNS depressants	
Narcotics	Overflow
Caffeine	Urge
Calcium channel antagonists	Overflow
Diuretics	Urge
Sedatives	Overflow, urge

UI, urinary incontinence; CNS, central nervous system.

5. The HERS study[4] found the following factors increased the risk of UI: white race (RR = 2.8), BMI (increased risk of 1.1 per 5 units) and higher waist to hip ratio (increased risk = 1.2 per 0.1 unit), diabetes (OR = 1.5) and a history of more than two UTIs (OR = 2.0).
6. The major predictors of urge incontinence were age, diabetes and UTIs. The major predictors of stress urinary incontinence (SUI) were white race, high BMI, and high waist to hip ratio.[4] There was no association with parity.
7. Other risk factors include strokes, immobility, chronic neurological or degenerative disease, dementia, delirium, and medication use (Table 21.2).

Definitions

There are four major causes of UI. The approximate incidences from the women of the HERS[4] study are shown in Figure 21.1.

Urge incontinence

Urge incontinence, also called irritable bladder or detrusor instability, is defined differently by different clinicians.

1. Urge UI is the sudden involuntary loss associated with a strong sensation to void. This leads to sudden large-volume urinary accidents.
2. It may be caused by uncontrollable contractions from the bladder that

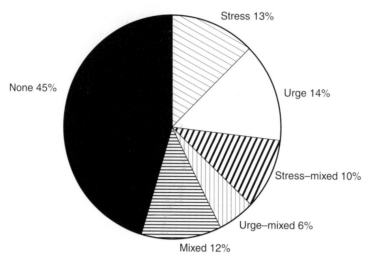

Figure 21.1.   Incidence of types of urinary incontinence in women from HERS study. (Data from Brown JS, Grady D, Ouslander JG et al. Prevalence of urinary incontinence and associated risk factors in postmenopausal women. *Obstet Gynecol* 1999;**94**:66–70.)

overwhelm the ability of cerebral centers to inhibit them. These contractions may be caused by:

   a. Inflammation or irritation resulting from malignancy, infection, calculi, urethritis or atrophic vaginitis.

   b. The central nervous system (CNS) centers inhibiting bladder contractions impaired by neurological conditions such as stroke, Parkinson's disease or dementia.

   c. A sudden large volume of urine introduced rapidly with diuretic therapy, or glucosuria from diabetes.

3. However, the degree of detrusor instability found on cystometric testing does not correlate completely with symptoms.[1]

4. Urge incontinence accounts for 12 to 14 percent of UI in community-dwelling women[4] to 60 percent in outpatient UI clinics and women in residential care.[2]

Urge urinary incontinence is the sudden involuntary loss associated with strong sensation to void.

Stress incontinence

1. SUI is loss of urine with coughing, sneezing or increased abdominal pressure. It often occurs during exercise.

2. It is caused by malfunction of the urethral sphincter that causes urine to leak with increased intraabdominal pressure. It is also associated with pelvic organ

prolapse, or denervation from alpha-adrenergic blocking drugs, surgical trauma, or radiation damage.

3. SUI is the most common type of UI.

Stress is loss of urine with coughing, sneezing or increased abdominal pressure.

Overflow bladder

1. This form of incontinence usually is associated with neurological dysfunction, such as from diabetes and neurological and muscular problems impairing mobility such as strokes. The bladder fills completely and UI occurs from the overflow.

2. It can be caused by medicines (anticholinergic agents, calcium channel blockers) (Table 21.2) or outflow obstruction from fecal impaction, stricture or urethral constriction.

Functional incontinence

This is UI caused by inability to reach the toilet in time or inability to sense the need to urinate. Strokes, arthritis, casts, immobility from any cause or altered mental states such as dementia, coma, or delirium can cause this form of UI.

Mixed

Many women have combinations of types of incontinence.

Diagnosis (Table 21.3)

1. Family and general physicians can diagnose and help the patient with UI. Evaluation by history, physical examination, urine analysis and postvoid residual is usually sufficient to identify many causes of UI. The type of UI is usually discernable by history and physical examination. Then treatment can be started. Sophisticated tests are not usually needed to evaluate and treat incontinence.[3]

   a. Identify if any cause of transient incontinence is present (Table 21.4); many of these occur while a patient is in hospital. Transient causes occur in one-half of hospitalized patients with UI, and one-third of community-dwelling individuals with UI. Reducing fecal impactions, improving glucose control, decreasing i.v. and p.o. fluids, treating UTIs or obstructions, determining whether unnecessary or new medications are causing UI,

Table 21.3. Historical evaluation of urinary incontinence

- History of incontinence – duration and characteristics, frequency, onset, precipitants
- Other urinary symptoms
- Obstetrical/gynecological history – deliveries, surgeries, symptoms, pain
- Bowel habits
- Medications
- Other medical illnesses
- Mental status and CNS function
- Gait and muscular function
- Social factors – living arrangements, effect of incontinence, self-treatments

CNS, central nervous system.

Table 21.4. Transient causes of urinary incontinence

- Medication use
- Delirium/hypoxia
- Acute change in mobility
- Fecal impaction
- UTI
- Acute change in diabetic control/glucosuria
- Excessive fluid intake (p.o. or i.v.)

UTI, urinary tract infection.

improving mental status and access to toileting facilities will reverse many causes of UI.

b. Identify conditions that may require evaluation or referral.

c. Analyze a urine sample to evaluate for infection.

d. Perform a postvoid residual with an intermittent catheter to evaluate for overflow incontinence. Postvoid residuals are normally less than 50 mL after urination. Volumes greater than 200 mL are abnormal.

e. Decide the type of UI, and start treatment.

f. If the treatment does not work, a specialized evaluation with a urologist or urogynecologist may be necessary. In the UK, there are "continence specialists" available for consultation. Conditions requiring specialized evaluations are uncommon.

2. Even when specialized cystometric tests are used, there is poor correlation

Evaluation by history, physical examination, urine analysis and postvoid residual is usually sufficient to identify many causes of urinary incontinence.

Table 21.5. Treatment of urinary incontinence

	Behavioral	Drug
Stress	Supertampon in special situations (or pessary) Pelvic floor exercises (Kegel) Pads	Estrogen (oral or topical) in HRT program Imipramine (5–50 mg b.i.d.)
Urge	Electrostimulation Bladder and breathing training (see Table 21.6)	Estrogen (oral or topical) in HRT program Imipramine (5–50 mg b.i.d.) or other antidepressants Oxybutynin 2.5–5.0 mg/day to q.i.d. Calcium channel antagonist Nifedipine 30 mg SR/day
Overflow	Bladder/abdominal wall exercise Electrostimulation	Bethanecol 525 mg b.i.d. to q.i.d.
Functional	Treat mechanically – move bed, add beside commode Correct constipation	
Mixed	Pelvic floor exercises Electrostimulation	

SR, sustained release; HRT, hormone replacement therapy.

between symptoms and urodynamic findings. In one study, cystometric testing was predictive of only 55 to 64 percent of patients with UI. There were many false negatives and false positives.

> There is poor correlation between symptoms and urodynamic findings.

Treatment (Tables 21.5 and 21.6)

Success

There are medical, behavioral, electrostimulatory, and surgical treatments of UI. Any type of treatment has a greater than 50 percent success rate (Figure 21.2). Physicians can help patients using a wide variety of methods simultaneously or sequentially. Placebo treatment in many studies had a greater than 50 percent success rate, making statements about the efficacy of all treatments difficult (Figure 21.2).[9] Also many studies defined the types and outcome measures differently, making evidenced-based decisions more difficult.

Table 21.6. Medical treatment of urinary incontinence

	Drug	Dose	Type of study	Effectiveness	Adverse effects
Urge incontinence	Propantheline	15–30 mg q.i.d.	CT	None to only 17 percent more effective than placebo	53 percent (placebo = 33 percent) nausea, vomiting, urinary retention and syncope
	Oxybutynin	5 mg t.i.d. to q.i.d. to 20 mg q.d.	Double blind RCT (n = 31) 5 mg q.i.d.	50–62 percent, 20 percent more than placebo	66 percent to 82 percent; 1/3 withdrew because of dry mouth and blurred vision
	Tropium chloride[a]	20 mg b.i.d.	RCT placebo controlled (n = 61)	Significant improvement	Less than placebo, 4 to 25 percent dry mouth
	Doxepin	50–75 mg q.h.s.	RCT – 20 patients	Improvement at night	73 percent fatigue and 42 percent dry mouth
	Imipramine	25–100 mg q.h.s.	CT vs. placebo (n = 33)	70 percent became continent but not significantly more than placebo	Dry mouth, constipation
	Calcium channel blocker – flunarizine	20 mg q.d.	CT (n = 14)	Some improvement	1 patient with atonic bladder
Stress incontinence	Imipramine	5–50 mg b.i.d.	Several small RCT vs. placebo, cross-over	Clinical improvement in 60–75 percent	23 percent dry mouth

CT, controlled trial.

[a]Not Available in USA.

Data from Owens RG, Karram MM. Comparative tolerability of drug therapies used to treat incontinence and enuresis. *Drug Safety* 1998;**19**:123–39.

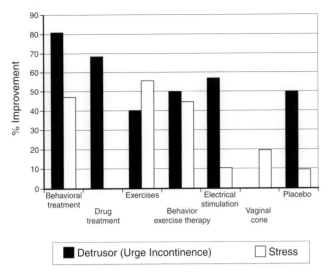

Figure 21.2. Comparative efficacies of treatments of urinary incontinence. (Data from Seim A, Sivertsen B, Ericksen BC, Hunskaar S. Treatment of urinary incontinence in women in general practice: Observational study. *BMJ* 1996;**312**:1459–62. Burgio KL, Locher JL, Goode PS et al. Behavioral vs. drug treatment for urge urinary incontinence in older women. *JAMA* 1998;**280**:1995–2001. Wyman JF, Fantl JA, McClish DK et al. Comparative efficacy of behavioral interventions in the management of female urinary incontinence. *Obstet Gynecol* 1998;**179**:999–1006.)

Almost any type of treatment for urinary incontinence has a greater than 50 percent success rate.

In observational studies UI has been treated successfully by general practitioners using pelvic floor exercises, electrostimulation, estrogen, anticholinergic drugs, bladder training and pads, with a 62 percent improvement. Severe incontinence decreased from 64 percent to 28 percent. Only 16 percent of women needed referral to a specialist.[10]

Stress incontinence

1. Treatment of SUI includes pelvic or Kegel exercises, and medication (Tables 21.5 and 21.6).
2. A randomized and small study teaching women to contract pelvic floor muscles before coughing to reduce stress found that women, with one week's training, could reduce urine loss by 98.3 percent with medium coughs.[11] Pelvic floor exercises are effective treatment.[12]
3. Exercise SUI: Women with exercise SUI do well with a supertampon placed vaginally during exercise. A randomized single blind efficacy study of two mechanical devices – the Hodge pessary and supertampon – found that

tampons achieved continence more frequently than a pessary and were one-third as expensive.[8]

Women with exercise stress urinary incontinence do well with a supertampon placed vaginally during exercise.

Urge incontinence

Treatment for urge incontinence includes behavioral therapy, electrostimulation, and medications (Table 21.6).

1. Behavioral therapy includes bladder retraining, increased frequency of urination, and teaching women not to run immediately to the toilet, but stop, relax, reduce intraabdominal pressure and, when pain and pressure decrease, then go. All of these methods improve urge incontinence.
2. Electrical stimulation of vagina, anus, and suprapubic areas for 20 to 30 minutes once to three times a day improved urge incontinence in some studies.[13,14]
3. Medication has a significant place in the treatment of urge incontinence (Table 21.6). No medication is specific for UI, and all have significant and sometimes distressing side effects.
4. Oxybutynin has had the greatest use and has good efficacy over placebo and some but tolerable side effects. In one study, women who used oxybutynin (2.5 to 5.0 mg daily to twice daily) showed 86 percent improvement as compared to 55 percent of women in the placebo group.[2]
5. Tricyclic antidepressants, trospium, propantheline, and calcium channel blockers have also been used, but their success is less significant and side effects may be more distressing.

Medication has a significant place in the treatment of urge incontinence.

Mixed types

1. A variety of treatments can work for mixed UI, with good results. In a RCT of 197 community-dwelling women older than age 55 years, behavioral therapy (four sessions of biofeedback-assisted behavioral treatment) and drug treatment (oxybutynin 2.5 mg to 5.0 mg twice daily) were compared with placebo. All the women in treatment groups had reduction of incontinence. Behavioral therapy alone had 80 percent reduction, more than drug treatment (68.5 percent), and both therapies were significantly more effective than placebo

(39.4 percent). Behavioral therapy included learning anorectal feedback, relaxing pelvic muscles, learning not to rush to the toilet but instead pause, sit down, relax and contract the pelvic muscles.[1]

2. For mixed types of UI, a variety of methods should be started simultaneously – behavioral and medication.

> For treatment of mixed types of urinary incontinence, a variety of methods should be started simultaneously – behavioral and medication.

Hormonal therapy

Although estrogen lack and vaginal atrophy have been implicated as causes of UI, especially stress UI, and observational studies have suggested the efficacy of hormonal therapy, few RCTs have shown that estrogen use significantly affects UI. Most of the observational and uncontrolled studies have had small numbers of participants and used a wide variety of estrogens, orally and topically.[7] In a metaanalysis of 166 articles examining the effect of estrogen on women with postmenopausal UI, only six were RCTs. Estrogen showed a small amount of selective improvement but no efficacy based on significant objective outcomes.[15]

One RCT using topical estradiol found significant improvement in stress and urge incontinence.[3] Estrogen definitely returns the vaginal pH to its acidic premenopausal state but whether this reduces UI has not been proven.[16]

Surgical treatment

1. When to refer: When a variety of behavioral, medical, and/or electrical treatment does not improve stress incontinence, when women have a greater than grade II pelvic prolapse (prolapse beyond introitus), or in a woman with recurrent UTIs, surgical treatment may be considered.

2. The efficacies of a variety of surgical treatments have been touted from 50 to 85 percent (Figure 21.3). The studies, however, seldom compared medical to surgical treatment, rather comparing types of surgical treatment, and the definitions and outcome measures were different, making comparisons difficult. However, surgical therapy can be very effective.

3. For stress incontinence there are three kinds of surgical procedures:
   a. Vaginal plication of bladder neck with sutures through the pubocervical fascis (Kelly plication).
   b. Needle suspension of the bladder neck (Pereyra and others).
   c. Retropubic urthroplexy (Marshall–Marquetti–Krantz and others).

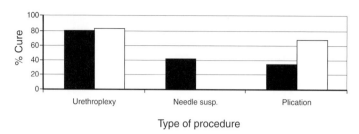

Figure 21.3.   "Cure" rate of surgical procedures at five years. Susp., suspension. (Data from (■) Bergman A, Elia G. Three surgical procedures for genuine stress incontinence: Data from five year follow-up of prospective randomized study. *Am J Obstet Gynecol* 1995;**173**:66–71. (□) Leach GE, Dmochowski RR, Appell RA et al. Female stress urinary incontinence clinical guidelines panel summary report on surgical management of female stress urinary incontinence. *J Urol* 1997;**158**:875–80.)

A five-year prospective study of 127 women who had surgery for SUI found that 64 were "cured" postoperatively. Twenty-nine women were documented failures one year after surgery.[17] Another study of 442 women followed prospectively after surgery for SUI over one year in North Thames, UK, found that 87 percent reported improvement in severity of UI and 71 percent had improvement of mental health, although only 28 percent were cured.[18]

The American Urologic Association reviewed studies, finding that after 48 months retropubic suspensions and slings were more efficacious than transvaginal suspension and anterior repairs, but have higher complication rates with synthetic materials. Surgical treatment of female SUI is effective and offers a long-term cure in a significant proportion of women, both as primary and secondary treatment.[19]

Conclusion

Family and general physicians can diagnose and treat UI in women with a great deal of efficacy using a history, physical examination, simple tests in the physician's office, and a variety of methods including behavioral therapy and medication.

URINARY TRACT INFECTIONS

UTIs are a nearly universal experience for women. Although usually benign and easily treated, recurrent and persistent infections can lead to serious disease.

Table 21.7. Risk factors for urinary tract infections

- Being a woman
- Stenosis or obstruction of urinary tract
- Abnormal urinary tract
- Kidney stones
- Pregnancy
- Menopause
- Catheterization
- Sexual intercourse
- Diaphragm use

Impact

1. UTIs are very common in women. UTIs account for more than 6 million visits to physicians in the USA yearly.[20]
2. Twenty to 80 percent of women will have a UTI at some time during their life, and approximately 35 percent of women aged 20 to 40 years have had UTIs.[21]
3. Approximately 20 percent of women will have recurrent UTIs.[22]
4. UTIs are the most common hospital-acquired infection, causing more than 40 percent of all nosocomial infections.[22]
5. Chronic UTIs are responsible for 11 to 13 percent of all causes of renal failure.[23]

Risk factors (Table 21.7)

1. Being a woman is a significant risk factor for UTIs.
2. Obstruction, stasis, or stenosis of any part of the urinary system will predispose to UTIs. Women with abnormal urinary tracts – those with double ureters, horseshoe kidney or other abnormalities – are more likely to develop UTIs. Pregnancy causes urinary stasis and hydroureter and predisposes to UTIs. Uterine or ovarian enlargement, or any mass pressuring the urinary tract can predispose to UTIs.
3. Pregnancy results in right-sided hydroureter and, often, left hydroureter and hydronephrosis. These usually clear up postpartum. If a pregnant woman has significant bacteriuria (greater than 10^6 organisms/mL), even if she is asymptomatic, she has a 60 percent chance of developing pyelonephritis during pregnancy. If treated, cured, followed closely and given prophylactic

treatment if necessary, her risk of developing pyelonephritis drops to 20 percent.[23]

4. Extrarenal obstruction including congenital abnormalities, kidney stones, uterine or other pelvic masses will increase the likelihood of UTIs.

5. Urinary incontinence increases the risk of UTIs.

6. Diaphragm use and use of spermicidal-coated condoms has been linked to an increased incidence of UTIs. Use of spermicide-coated condoms was responsible for 42 percent of UTIs caused by *Escherichia coli* in a case-controlled study (OR = 3.4 to 5.6).[24]

7. Sickle cell anemia and sickle cell trait in pregnant women has been correlated to an increased incidence of UTIs.

Obstruction, stasis, or stenosis of any part of the urinary system will predispose to urinary tract infections.

Symptoms

1. Common symptoms include dysuria, polyuria, urgency and nocturia. The woman may have trouble starting to urinate or stopping.

2. Constant suprapubic, flank, costovertebral angle (CVA) or back pain can occur with lower UTIs. Upper tract UTIs or pyelonephritis often have CVA pain. Colicky pain is more consistent with kidney stones.

3. Fever, chills, nausea, and vomiting are usually symptoms of pyelonephritis.

4. Hematuria can occur, from microscopic to frank gross hematuria. However, when a patient has hematuria, especially if she has concurrent pain, kidney stones should be part of the differential diagnosis. Painless hematuria may be consistent with bladder polyps and cancer.

Fever, chills, nausea, and vomiting are usually symptoms of pyelonephritis.

Diagnosis

1. Diagnosis is made by history, physical examination, and urine analysis and confirmed by urine culture. Some experts believe that a dipstick test of urine consistent with infection in a woman with infrequent UTIs is sufficient.

2. The physical examination may be normal. CVA tenderness or suprapubic pain may be elicited. Fever would suggest pyelonephritis.

Table 21.8. Urine analysis

	Normal	UTI
pH	7.3–7.4	Often low
Specific gravity	1.010	Unchanged
Glucose	None	None
Protein	None	Often 1 to 2+ on dipstix, more with significant pyuria
Urobilinogen	None	None
Ketones	None	None, unless vomiting
Blood	None	None to positive
Nitrites	None	Positive
Leukocyte esterase	None	Positive
White blood cells	0 to 1 cell	1 cell per HPF unspun, 10 to 20 per HPF spun
Red blood cells	0 to 1 cell	None to TNTC
Bacteria	Occasional	10 to 20 per HPF spun to TNTC
Yeast	None	None
Casts	None	None; WBC casts indicate pyelonephritis
Vaginal cells	None	None

HPF, high power (40 power) field; TNTC, too numerous to count; WBC, white blood cell.

3. Urine analysis (Table 21.8).
   a. A urine analysis positive for nitrites, protein and leukocyte esterase, with pyuria and bacteruria is suggestive of a UTI.
   b. White blood cells (WBC) may be present in the urine (pyuria), if the woman also has vaginitis or cervicitis. Pyuria by itself may not indicate a UTI.
   c. The presence of vaginal cells may indicate that the specimen is not a clean catch and bacteria and WBCs present may be from the vagina, not the urinary tract.
   d. A positive leukocyte esterase test is 75 to 95 percent sensitive and 95 percent specific in detecting more than 10 WBCs/mL, consistent with a UTI.
   e. Nitrites are produced by Gram-negative bacilli, and if the test is positive, it has a specificity of more than 92 percent for UTI.
   f. A positive urine analysis is a presumptive diagnosis of UTI and treatment can be started, especially if this is a first UTI, or the first in a long time.
4. Urine culture:
   a. Growth of more than 10^5 colonies of a single organism is diagnostic of a UTI.

A urine analysis positive for nitrites, protein and leukocyte esterase, with pyuria and bacteruria is suggestive of a urinary tract infection.

b. However, more than half of women with UTIs will not have a culture with this many organisms.[25] Lower colony counts of a single organism (10^3 to 10^4) in urine specimens not taken as first morning specimens, in women with typical symptoms or in those who have been partially treated, may be significant of early UTIs.

c. In approximately 15 percent of women with UTI symptoms, cultures are negative and a diagnosis of *Chlamydia*, *Ureoplasma* or *Mycoplasma* urethritis should be considered.

d. Polymicrobial UTIs may occur in women with indwelling catheters, diabetes or obstruction.

5. Organisms:

a. The predominant organisms are *E. coli*, occurring in approximately 85 to 90 percent of UTIs.

b. Other Gram-negative bacteria such as *Proteus*, *Serratia*, *Citrobacter*, *Pseudomonas* and *Klebsiella* occur in fewer than 1 percent of uncomplicated UTIs, but in up to 5 percent of complicated UTIs or UTIs in women with other illnesses.

c. Gram-positive organisms such as *Staphylococcus epidermidis* and *Staph. saphrophyticus* occur in 5 to 10 percent of uncomplicated UTIs. *Staph. aureus* is an occasional pathogen.

The predominant organism is *E. coli* occurring in approximately 85 to 90 percent of urinary tract infections.

Treatment

Acute uncomplicated UTI or acute cystitis

1. This would be a UTI in an otherwise healthy woman, with typical symptoms and a single organism, usually *E. coli* (see Table 21.9).

2. Amoxicillin, trimethoprim/sulfa or a quinolone may be a good first choice. The latter two should *not* be used in women at risk for pregnancy or pregnant.

3. How long to treat is under investigation. Many acute UTIs caused by *E. coli* respond to one or three days' treatment with a wide variety of antibiotics. UTIs caused by *Staph. saphrophyticus* usually need longer treatment.[26]

a. Several studies have proven that one dose of medication is sufficient to treat many uncomplicated UTIs, although it is significantly less effective than longer courses (Table 21.10).[27,28,29]

Table 21.9. Antibiotics for first or uncomplicated urinary tract infection or cystitis

Drug	Dose	Acceptable in pregnancy	Note
Amoxicillin	250–500 mg t.i.d.	Yes	*E. coli* resistance rates of 25 have been reported
Cephalexein	250–500 mg t.i.d.	Yes	
Nitrofuradatoin	50–100 mg b.i.d. to q.i.d.	Yes	Good for penicillin allergic
Ciprofloxacin	250–500 mg b.i.d.	No	
Norfloxacin	400 mg every 12 hours or 800 mg q.d.	No	
Trimethoprim	100 mg every 12 hours	No	
Trimethoprim/sulfa	One DS b.i.d.	No	

DS, double strength.

Table 21.10. Some single-dose antibiotics for uncomplicated urinary tract infections

Drug	Dose
Amoxicillin	3 g
Cefuroxime	1000 mg
Cephalexein	3 g
Fosfomycin	3 g
Nitrofuradantoin	400 mg
Norfloxacin	400–800 mg
Ciprofloxacin	1 g
Ofloxacin	800 mg
Sparfloxacin	400 mg
Trimethoprim/sulfa	2 double strength tablets
Sulfisoxazole	2 g
Trimethoprim	400–600 mg

b. However, test of cure is important. Ten to 20 percent of women will continue to have significant bacteriuria and infection after one or three days' treatment; these women may need a full 7 to 10 days of antibiotics or have upper tract disease.

c. Several RCTs of various antibiotics have proven that three days of the following medications is sufficient to treat uncomplicated UTIs, and is as effective as longer courses: cefuroxime 125 mg twice daily, ciprofloxacin 100 mg, trimethoprim/sulfa one double strength twice daily, trimethoprim

Table 21.11. Intravenous antibiotics for complicated urinary tract infections and pyelonephritis

Drug	Dose	Note
Ampicillin	150–250 mg/kg per day divided every 3–4 hours	
Ticarcillin/clavulanate	3.1 g every 4–6 hours	
Ampicillin/sulbactam	1.5–3.0 g every 6 hours	
Ceftriaxone	1–2 g q.d. or divided b.i.d. i.v.	
Ciprofloxacin	400 mg i.v. every 12 hours	Not in pregnant women
Gentamycin	1–5 mg/kg per day	Change dose with renal insufficiency. Monitor levels

100 mg twice daily, ofloxacin 200 mg twice daily.[30,31] More than 90 percent of women remained without infection at six weeks with all drugs.

Ten to 20 percent of women will continue to have significant bacteriuria and infection after one or three days' treatment; these women may need a full 7 to 10 days of antibiotics or have upper tract disease.

Recurrent or complicated UTI

1. A repeat UTI in a woman who has just or recently finished UTI treatment may require a different antibiotic or one with greater coverage. A full 7- to 10-day course of antibiotics is probably needed.
2. A pregnant woman or a woman with diabetes or some urinary obstruction must have a full 7- to 10-day course of antibiotics.
3. Some *E. coli* strains are not sensitive to first-line medication. Hospital and community outpatient sensitivities should be checked.

Pyelonephritis

1. Pyelonephritis or upper tract UTIs may present just like a lower tract UTI, may be evident by systemic signs such as fever, chills, nausea, vomiting, and high WBC count, or appear as an infection that does not respond to a short course of antibiotics.
2. Treatment may require hospitalization and i.v. antibiotics and hydration, including a third-generation cephalosporin or aminoglycoside. If i.v. therapy is needed, a parenteral fluoroquinolone, an aminoglycoside, or an extended coverage cephalosporin with an aminoglycoside is suggested (see Table 21.11).[27]
3. Indications for hospitalization and i.v. antibiotics would include dehydration,

pregnancy, severe vomiting, diabetes, elderly or immunocompromised women, severe pain or uncertainty about diagnosis. Women who develop infections with organisms insensitive to outpatient oral medication, especially *Proteus* infections, may need i.v. antibiotics.

4. Treatment has traditionally been for six weeks, with two weeks of i.v. therapy. Recent studies have suggested that even seven days of therapy may be sufficient, especially in mild cases. In cases requiring i.v. antibiotics, after clinical response and after three days of i.v. antibiotics, an oral regimen can be followed.[27]

Follow-up

Acute cystitis

Follow-up would include a repeat culture to prove sterility.

Recurrent cystitis or pyelonephritis

1. Follow-up would include a repeat negative culture to prove sterility.
2. Repeat UTIs may indicate the need for prophylaxis. Prophylaxis can be given intermittently (such as before each sexual intercourse) or chronically (Table 21.12).
3. An evaluation for causes of obstruction such as kidney stones or an abnormal urinary tract including an intravenous pyelogram or ultrasound scan is indicated. Ten to 20 percent of women admitted with pyelonephritis, in one observational study, were found to have kidney stones or an abnormal urinary tract.[32]

Secondary prevention

1. Some women have recurrent or persistent UTIs. An evaluation to discover diabetes, immunosuppression or causes of urinary obstruction should be started. If the test is positive, the woman may need diabetic treatment, or surgical therapy such as removal of secondary collecting systems. Chronic antibiotic prophylaxis is treatment or adjunct treatment for these women. Taking antibiotics nightly or every other night has been found to decrease the incidence of recurrent UTIs (Table 21.12).[33,34]
2. Some women with persistent or recurrent UTIs have no demonstrable cause.

Table 21.12. Antibiotics for prophylaxis

Drug	Dose
Postcoital single-dose prophylaxis	
Trimethoprim/sulfa	$\frac{1}{2}$ DS or one regular strength tablet
Sulfamethoxazole	500 mg
Cephalexein	250 mg
Nitrofuradantoin	50 mg
Chronic prophylaxis – taken q.h.s. or every other night	
Trimethoprim/sulfa[a]	$\frac{1}{2}$ DS or one regular strength tablet
Sulfamethoxazole	500 mg
Cephalexein	250 mg
Nitrofuradantoin	50–100 mg
Norfloxacin[b]	200 mg
Ciprofloxacin[b]	250 mg

DS, double strength.
[a]Not indicated in pregnant or unprotected fertile women.
[b]Contraindicated in pregnant women and should not be used in fertile women who are not using an effective method of contraception.

These women may relate the development of UTIs to coitus. Single postcoital doses of antibiotics, including trimethoprim/sulfa, sulfamethoxisole or ciprofloxacin or other quinolone has been shown to decrease the recurrence of UTIs, with less antibiotic use than daily dosing (Table 12.12).[35,36]

3. Another suggestion is that because women can accurately self-diagnose UTI from their symptoms, they can start antibiotics when they feel a UTI coming on. One study of 34 women who took norfloxacin (six tablets of 400 mg – take one twice daily for three days) at the beginning of urinary tract symptoms found that self-start therapy was effective and economical.[37]

4. Other adjunctive methods such as cranberry juice ingestion,[38] and use of high dose vitamin C have been suggested to reduce the recurrence of UTIs.

5. Postmenopausal vaginal and urethral atrophy caused by estrogen deficiency has been linked to an increase in UTIs. Many observational studies have suggested that use of estrogen decreases the incidence of UTIs. One RCT of intravaginal estradiol in approximately 50 women found that eight months' treatment reduced the number of episodes of UTI per patient year by 5.5.[39]

Because women can accurately self-diagnose a urinary tract infection from their symptoms, they can start antibiotics when they feel a UTI coming on.

In women who cannot use estrogen because of contraindications, an Estring, a estradiol-releasing vaginal ring (Pharmacia) with no systemic absorption, that is placed intravaginally every three months reduced by half the number of UTIs in women with recurrent UTIs.[40]

Topical estrogen vaginal treatment in postmenopausal women with UTIs may decrease recurrence.

> Topical estrogen vaginal treatment in postmenopausal women with UTIs may decrease recurrence.

Conclusions

UI is very common. Fortunately, if the woman and physician work together there are a variety of treatments, mechanical and medical, that can help to improve the situation. UTIs are common, but must be identified and treated, and sterility proven. Recurrent UTIs should be treated rigorously and may be able to be prevented.

REFERENCES

1. Burgio, KL, Locher JL, Goode PS et al. Behavioral vs. drug treatment for urge urinary incontinence in older women. *JAMA* 1998;**280**:1995–2001.
2. Gorton E, Stanton S. Urinary incontinence in elderly women. *Eur Urol* 1998;**33**:241–7.
3. Weiss BD. Diagnostic evaluation of urinary incontinence in geriatric patients. *Am Fam Physician* 1998;**57**:2675–84, 2688–90.
4. Brown JS, Grady D, Ouslander JG et al. Prevalence of urinary incontinence and associated risk factors in postmenopausal women. *Obstet Gynecol* 1999;**94**:66–70.
5. Helstrom L, Ekelund P, Milson I, Mellstrom D. The prevalence of urinary incontinence and use of incontinence aids in 85 year old men and women. *Age Ageing* 1990;**19**:383–9.
6. Peet SM, Castleden CM, McGrother CW. Prevalence of urinary and faecal incontinence in hospitals and residential nursing homes for older people. *BMJ* 1995;**311**:1063–4.
7. Thomas DH, Brown JS. Reproductive and hormonal risk factors for urinary incontinence in later life: A review of the clinical and epidemiological features. *J Am Geriat Soc* 1998;**46**:1411–17.
8. Nygaard I. Prevention of exercise incontinence with mechanical devices. *J Reprod Med* 1995;**40**:90–5.
9. Wyman JF, Fantl JA, McClish DK et al. Comparative efficacy of behavioral interventions in the management of female urinary incontinence. *Obstet Gynecol* 1998;**179**:999–1006.
10. Seim A, Sivertsen B, Ericksen BC, Hunskaar S. Treatment of urinary incontinence in women in general practice: Observational study. *BMJ* 1996;**312**:1459–62.

11. Miller JM, Ashton-Miller JA, DeLancey JOL. A pelvic muscle precontraction can reduce cough-related urine loss in selected women with mild SUI. *J Am Geriat Soc* 1998;**46**:870–4.

12. Bo K, Talseth T, Holme I. Single blind randomized controlled trial of pelvic floor exercise, electrical stimulation, vaginal cones and no treatment in management of genuine stress incontinence in women. *BMJ* 1999;**318**:487–93.

13. Brubaker L, Benson JT, Bent A, Clark A, Shott S. Transvaginal electrical stimulation for female urinary incontinence. *Am J Obstet Gynecol* 1997;**177**:536–40.

14. Bower WF, Moore KH, Adams RD, Shepherd R. A urodynamic study of surface neuromodulation versus sham in detrusor instability and sensory urgency. *J Urol* 1998;**60**:2133–6.

15. Fantl JA, Cordozo L, McClish DK. Estrogen therapy in the management of urinary incontinence in postmenopausal women: A meta-analysis. First report of the Hormones and Urogenital Therapy Committee. *Obstet Gynecol* 1994;**83**:12–18.

16. Mikkelsen AL, Felding C, Clausen HV. Clinical effects of preoperative oestradiol treatment before vaginal repair operation. *Gynecol Obstet Invest* 1995;**40**:125–8.

17. Bergman A, Elia G. Three surgical procedures for genuine stress incontinence: Five year follow-up of prospective randomized study. *Am J Obstet Gynecol* 1995;**173**:66–71.

18. Black N, Griffiths J, Pope C, Bowling A, Abel P. Impact of surgery for stress incontinence on morbidity: Cohort study. *BMJ* 1997;**315**:1493–8.

19. Leach GE, Dmochowski RR, Appell RA et al. Female stress urinary incontinence clinical guidelines panel summary report on surgical management of female stress urinary incontinence. *J Urol* 1997;**158**:875–80.

20. Kovar M. *Data Systems of the National Center for Health Statistics Through the 1980s.* National Center for Health Statistics, United States Department of Health and Human Services. DHHS publication no. PHS 89-1325. GPO no. 89016133. Hyattsville, MD, 1994.

21. Stamm WE, Hooton TM, Johns JR et al. Urinary tract infections from pathogenesis to treatment. *J Infect Dis* 1989;**159**:400–6.

22. Meares EM. Current patterns in nosocomial urinary tract infections. *Urology* 1991;**37**:S9–S12.

23. Rosenfeld JA. Renal disease in pregnancy. *Am Fam Physician* 1989;**39**:209–12.

24. Fihn SD, Boyko EJ, Normand EH et al. Association between use of spermicide-coated condoms and *Escherichia coli* urinary tract infections in young women. *Am J Epidemiol* 1996;**144**:512–20.

25. Stamm WE, Counts GW, Running KR et al. Diagnosis of coliform infection in acutely dysuric women. *N Engl J Med* 1982;**307**:463–8.

26. Saginur R, Nicolle LE. Single dose compared with 3 day norfloxacin treatment of uncomplicated urinary tract infection in women. *Arch Intern Med* 1993;**152**:1233–7.

27. Warren JW, Abrutyn E, Hebel JR et al. Guidelines for antimicrobial treatment of uncomplicated acute bacterial cystitis and acute pyelonephritis in women. *Clin Infect Dis* 1999;**29**:745–54.

28. Pfau A. Sacks TG. Single dose quinolone treatment in acute uncomplicated urinary tract infection in women. *J Urol* 1993;**149**:532–4.

29. Henry DC, Nenad RC, Iravani A et al. Comparison of sparfloaxacin and ciproflaxacin in the treatment of community-acquired acute uncomplicated urinary tract infection in women. *Clin Therapeut* 1999;**21**:966–80.

30. McCary JM, Richard G, Huck W. A randomized trial of short course ciprofloxacin, ofloxacin or trimethoprim/sulfamethoxazole for the treatment of acute urinary tract infections in women. *Am J Med* 1999;**106**:293–8.

31. Naber KG, Koch EM. Cefuroxime axetil versus ofloxacin for short term therapy of acute uncomplicated lower urinary tract infection. *Infection* 1993;**21**:34–9.

32. Rosenfeld JA. Radiological abnormalities in women admitted with pyelonephritis. *Del Med J* 1987;**59**:717–19.

33. Raz R, Boger S. Long-term prophylaxis with norfloxacin versus nitrofurantoin in women with recurrent urinary tract infection. *Antimicrob Agents Chemother* 1991;**35**:1241–2.

34. Brumfitt W, Hamilton-Miller JM, Smith GW, al-Wali W. Comparative trial of norfloxacin and macrocrystalline nitrofuradantoin in the prophylaxis of recurrent urinary tract infection in women. *Q J Med* 1991;**81**:811–20.

35. Pfau A, Sacks TG. Effective postcoital quinolone prophylaxis of recurrent UTIs in women. *J Urol* 1994;**152**:136–8.

36. Melekos MD, Asbach HW, Gerharz E et al. Post-intercourse versus daily ciprofloxacin prophylaxis for recurrent urinary tract infection in premenopausal women. *J Urol* 1997;**157**:935–9.

37. Schaeffer AJ, Stuppy BA. Efficacy and safety of self-start therapy in women with recurrent urinary tract infections. *J Urol* 1999;**161**:207–11.

38. Fleet JC. New support for a folk remedy. Cranberry juice reduces bacteriuria and pyuria in elderly women. *Nutr Rev* 1994;**52**:168–70.

39. Raz R, Stamm WE. A controlled trial of intravaginal estriol in postmenopausal women with recurrent urinary tract infection. *N Engl J Med* 1993;**329**:802–3.

40. Eriksen BC. A randomized open parallel-group study on the preventive effect of an estradiol-releasing vaginal ring (ESTRING) on recurrent urinary tract infection in postmenopausal women. *Am J Obstet Gynecol* 1999;**180**:1072–9.

Breast disorders

Jo Ann Rosenfeld, MD, and Kris Pena, MD

This chapter discusses breast pain, fibrocystic breast disease, infections, galactorrhea and other nipple discharges.

Breast pain

Breast pain (mastalgia) may be unilateral (75 percent) or bilateral, continuous or intermittent, related to menstrual cycle (40 percent)[1] or associated with a mass. Breast pain alone was the presenting complaint in 15 to 50 percent of women attending breast clinics.[2,3] Breast pain is the presenting complaint of operable breast cancer in 5 to 24 percent of patients in breast clinics.[4,5] In one case-controlled study of French women with cancer, a previous history of cyclic mastalgia was associated with an increased risk of developing breast cancer.[6]

Noncyclic pain without a mass

1. If the pain occurs without a mass, malignant disease is very unlikely. Noncyclic pain accounted for 27 percent of women with mastalgia in a breast clinic.[1]
2. Mammography of women who have breast pain but do not have a mass is usually normal and reassuring. In one large observational study of more than 6500 women with mastalgia alone, 85 percent had normal mammography, 9 percent had benign findings and only 1.2 percent had suspicious or malignant mammographic findings.[7]
3. Biopsy of a tender or painful area is not needed, if there are no mass and no suspicious mammographic findings.
4. Treatment of noncyclic pain includes wearing a firm bra, and NSAIDs.[3] If these symptoms do not improve, treatment with drugs for cyclic pain (see below) is suggested.[1]

In the evaluation of noncyclic breast pain, biopsy of a tender or painful area is not needed, if there is no mass and no suspicious mammographic findings.

Cyclic pain

1. Cyclic premenopausal pain usually improves after menses occurs and is relieved by menopause. It is often hormonally caused and often associated with fibrocystic breast disease (FBD) (see below). It is often bilateral and associated with modularity on physical examination.

2. Pregnancy and OCPs do not affect its course. OCPs can increase or relieve the pain.

3. Treatment: Only a few clinical trials have examined drugs for cyclic breast pain. All treatments may take three to four months before a definite improvement is seen. In some clinical trials, treatment resolved the pain in as many as 77 to 80 percent of the patients.[8]

   a. OCPs have been used to reduce pain and nodularity. No one OCP is more likely to cure cyclic mastalgia than any other.[1] Approximately 53 percent of women, in a small study, found relief of pain but not nodularity when placed on OCPs.[9] Concerns about adversely affecting an occult breast cancer may keep OCPs from being used.

   b. Neither progestins nor diuretics have been proven to relieve pain.[1]

   c. One medication suggested (but not approved by the US FDA) and used in the UK is evening primrose oil (gamolenic or gamma linolenic acid 40 mg, six to eight pills a day in divided doses). A diet rich in primrose oil or added evening primrose oil may elevate levels of dihomo-gamma-linolenic acid (DGLA; 20: n-6), which leads to elevation of prostaglandin 1, and is thought to suppress inflammation.[10] Several trials have suggested that it is effective in reducing pain. It has few side effects.[11]

   d. Danazol (200 to 300 mg daily and reduced later to 100 mg daily) can be tried; women on this drug should not be taking OCPs and should use other nonhormonal mechanical contraceptives.[3] There are significant nausea and other gastrointestinal side effects, amenorrhea, weight gain, acne, and hirsutism in up to 30 percent of patients. Danazol must be used for three months to assess for effect.

   e. Bromocriptine has been used and has proven effective in a double blind placebo-controlled small trial in the Cardiff Mastalgia Clinic,[12] and other trials. The FDA does not approve it for this indication. The dose is titrated from 1.25 mg nightly in 1.25 mg increments twice daily and slowly increased to maximum of 2.5 mg twice daily. Advised for use of mastalgia in

Table 22.1. Percentages of types of breast masses by age

Age	Abscesses	Fibroadenomas	Localized benign masses	Cysts	Cancer
<20	10	60	30	<1	<1
21–30	8	30	60	1	1
31–40	1	15	60	15	9
41–50	<1	10	40	30	20
>51	<1	5	10	20	70

Data from Dixon JM, Mansel RE. ABC of breast diseases: Symptoms assessment and guidelines for referral. *BMJ* 1994;**309**:722–6.

the UK, bromocriptine use has been approved only for specific syndromes in the USA. Because of side effects of nausea and headache and severe reactions including hypertension, and myocardial infarctions, its use should probably be reserved for women with proven hyperprolactinemia.

f. Tamoxifen: Tamoxifen, used for and approved only for breast cancer treatment in the USA, has been shown to be effective in reducing pain in 98 percent of women with cyclic mastalgia at 10 mg daily.[13] Even use for 11 days per month (day 15 to 25) for three months may give pain relief. Long-term use is not suggested.

Breast pain with mass

Breast pain with an accompanying mass needs evaluation of a mass, first with mammography and possible ultrasonography and fine needle or other biopsy (see Chapter 23). Breast masses in women younger than age 50 years are usually benign, but need evaluation (Table 22.1).

Fibrocystic breast disease

Impact

FBD is the most common benign breast disease. As many as 19 percent of women may have cysts of 1 to 2 mm diameter.[1]

Symptoms

FBD can be asymptomatic and discovered on routine mammography or may present as symptomatic cyclic mastalgia occurring in the last half of the menstrual cycle and during menses.

Fibrocystic breast disease is the most common benign breast disease.

Etiology

1. The pain may be related to edema and increase in breast volume.
2. FBD appears as microcysts and fibrosis in 65 percent of patients.[14] The cysts become larger as the woman ages and can reach 3 to 4 cm and be bilateral. There may be chronic inflammation, ductal ectasia, and nipple discharge.
3. Cysts usually start in women at age 35 years, and occur more frequently in women between ages 40 and 50 years.
4. The pain usually subsides after menstruation and cysts disappear postmenopause. They are rare in the postmenopausal woman.

Diagnosis

Diagnosis is made by a typical history and mammographic findings.

Treatment

1. A variety of treatments has been suggested, many dietary. Elimination of caffeine, chocolate, cigarette smoking, and alcohol, and additional vitamins A and E have all been suggested to treat FBD. Although many observational studies suggest improvement of pain with caffeine elimination, case-controlled studies of caffeine elimination have not shown significant improvement in pain or nodularity.[15] Some of the other dietary modifications, especially vitamin treatments, have only observational evidence to suggest their use.[16]
2. Diuretics have often been prescribed, but studies have shown no significant improvement in pain with their use.[16]
3. Use of OCPs can help, but only after 12 to 24 months use. OCPs with higher progesterone levels may have a more beneficial effect.[14]
4. Danazol and gonadotropin-releasing hormone analogs have been used (see doses above), but are not approved and have significant side effects.
5. Bromocriptine use has not been shown to be effective.[16]
6. Needle aspiration of large cysts and excision of masses may be needed.

Elimination of caffeine, chocolate, cigarette smoking and alcohol, and additional vitamins A and E have all been suggested to treat fibrocystic breast disease.

Infection – mastitis and abscess

Symptoms

1. Breast infections are much less common now. Mastitis (breast cellulitis) occurs in approximately 2 percent of breast-feeding women.[17]
2. Breast infections can affect the skin, a primary cellulitis, or may be secondary to an infection of a sebaceous gland or axillary gland, such as in hidradenitis suppurativa.
3. Most mastitis occurs in women who are breast feeding.
4. The symptoms of breast infections are the same as cellulitis elsewhere, just more dramatic. The woman's breast becomes hot, bright red, exquisitely tender, and swollen. She may have a green or pus-like nipple discharge. The area of redness extends quickly.
5. The woman may have a fever, chills and an elevated white blood cell count.
6. If she has an abscess, there may be a fluctuant localized enlarged area. Abscesses, sometimes multiple and usually small, often occur in the sweat glands in the axillae, and these do not involve breast tissue.

Treatment

1. The organisms causing mastitis are usually Gram-positive bacteria, either *Streptococcus* or *Staphylococcus aureus*. In breast-feeding women, the most common organism is *Staph. aureus*. In nonlactating women, the most common organisms are *Staph. aureus*, enterococci and anerobic streptococcus.[18]
2. Treatment must start quickly with a bactericidal Gram-positive-covering antibiotic to decrease abscess formation. However, treatment can be started orally. Amoxicillin/clavulanate (Augmentin – 375 to 500 mg three times daily), cephalexein (500 mg four times daily), or dicloxacillin orally would be good choices. For penicillin-allergic breast-feeding patients, cephalexein or erythromycin (500 mg twice daily) can be used. Metronidazole (200 mg three times daily) should be added in penicillin-allergic women who have a breast infection and are not breast feeding (Table 22.2). Treatment should be continued for 7 to 10 days. Tetracyclines and sulphonamides should be avoided in breast-feeding women.
3. If the woman is dehydrated or vomiting, has diabetes or an immunosuppressive disease, or becomes worse on oral medications, intravenous antibiotics should be started. Ampicillin/sulbactam (Unisyn), a first- or third-generation cephalosporin, or nafcillin would be an appropriate choice. Vancomycin might be needed if the patient is penicillin allergic, or there are high levels of methicillin-resistant *Staph. aureus* in the community.

Table 22.2. Treatment for breast infections

Lactating	Amoxicillin/clavulanate (Augmentin – 375–500 mg t.i.d.)
	Cephalexein (500 mg q.i.d.)
	Dicloxacillin (250–500 mg q.i.d.)
Penicillin allergic	Erythromycin (500 mg b.i.d.)
Nonlactating	Amoxicillin/Clavulanate (Augmentin – 375–500 mg t.i.d.)
	Cephalexein (500 mg q.i.d.)
	Dicloxacillin (250–500 mg q.i.d.)
Penicillin allergic	Erythromycin (500 mg b.i.d.) or cephalexein (500 mg q.i.d.), with metronidazole 500 mg b.i.d.

4. Heat should be used 20 minutes four times a day.
5. Pain medicine may be needed.
6. Whether the woman should stop breast feeding is disputed. Definitely, she should pump her breasts, and many experts suggest discarding the milk from the infected breast.
7. If there is an associated breast mass, it should be investigated by biopsy after the infection resolves.

The organisms causing mastitis are usually Gram-positive bacteria, either *Streptococcus* or *Staphylococcus aureus*.

Abscess

1. Most abscesses occur in breast-feeding women within the first month postpartum or at weaning.
2. Patients with abscesses should have them drained. Draining may be needed more than once. The woman should be placed on oral antibiotics that cover *Streptococcus* and *Staphylococcus* as above. The infant should not nurse on the breast with the abscess, although breasts should be pumped.

Nonlactational infections or abscess

1. If infection occurs in someone who is neither breast feeding nor having pathological or physiological galactorrhea, the suspicion of ductal or inflammatory must be entertained.
2. Subareolar abscesses are related most often to ductal ectasia, caused by a variety of organisms and related to cigarette smoking. Peripheral abscesses are usually caused by *Staphylococcus*, are in older women, and are treated by drainage.[1]

3.   Mammography and biopsy are needed for evaluation, after the infection is cleared.

Galactorrhea

Impact and symptoms

1.   Galactorrhea is a relatively common symptom, reported by 15 to 40 percent of women.
2.   The woman may be completely unaware of the discharge or anxiety ridden and concerned about malignancy.
3.   The woman may also have menstrual disorders, such as amenorrhea or oligomenorrhea, or symptoms of an intracranial mass, visual disturbance or headache.

Galactorrhea is a relatively common symptom, reported by 15 to 40 percent of women.

Etiology

1.   Fourteen percent of galactorrhea has physiological causes, including pregnancy, being postpartum, hormone use, and breast stimulation.[19,20] Prolactin production is inhibited by prolactin-inhibiting factor from the pituitary and has an involved feedback system (Figure 22.1).
2.   Twenty percent of galactorrhea is caused by medication use (Table 22.3). Approximately 15 percent of women starting antipsychotic medications report galactorrhea.[21]
3.   Systemic diseases, such as chronic renal failure, hypothyroidism, Cushing's disease, and acromegaly cause fewer than 10 percent of all cases of galactorrhea.
4.   Tumors such as prolactinomas of the pituitary and nonpituitary nonprolactinomas such as craniopharyngiomas cause about 18 percent. These tumors cause hyperprolactinemia, and thus, galactorrhea.
     a.   Approximately 20 percent of galactorrheic women have radiologically evident brain tumors, and the incidence increases to 34 percent in women who also have amenorrhea.[22]
     b.   The most common tumor causing hyperprolactinemia is the pituitary prolactinoma.
     c.   Woman with prolactin levels higher than 200 ng/mL and amenorrhea are more likely to have prolactinomas.

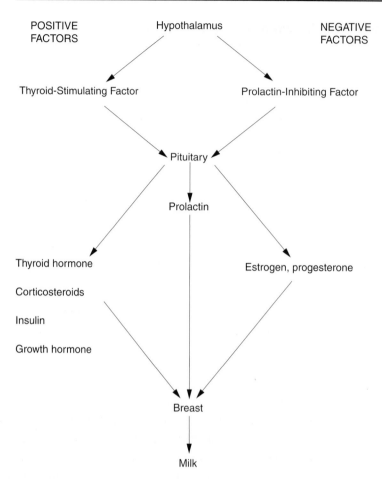

Figure 22.1. Milk production.

    d. Most women with the tumors, nonetheless, do well. Either the tumors regress or remain stable for many years.

    e. Nonpituitary malignancies such as bronchogenic carcinomas, renal adenocarcinomas, Hodgkin's and T-cell lymphomas, may also release prolactin.

5. Diseases that affect the hypothalamic and pituitary areas, such as sarcoidosis, tuberculosis histiocytosis, and multiple sclerosis can also cause galactorrhea.

6. Chest wall irritation including burns and herpes zoster can cause galactorrhea, although no reason or "idiopathic" reasons are found in 35 percent of women.

Women with prolactin levels higher than 200 ng/mL and amenorrhea are more likely to have prolactinomas.

Table 22.3. Medications that can cause galactorrhea

- CNS drugs
- Amphetamines
- Anesthetics
- Antidepressants: MAO inhibitors, SSRIs, tricyclics
- Antipsychotics: clozapine, molindone, risperidone
- Benzodiazepines
- Butyrophenones: haloperidol
- Cannabis
- Opiates
- Phenothiazines: prochlorperazine, chlorpromazine, thioxanthenes
- Antihypertensives: methyl-dopa, atenolol, reserpine, verapamil
- H2 receptor blockers: cimetidine, famotidine, ranitidine
- Hormones: Oral contraceptives, depomedroxyprogesterone, danazol
- Herbs: fenugreek seed, blessed thistle, fennel, nettle, marshmallow, red clover, red raspberry
- Metoclopromide

CNS, central nervous system; MAO, monoamine oxidase; SSRI, selective serotonin reuptake inhibitor.

Diagnosis

1. Physical examination includes evaluation of the visual fields, thyroid, breasts, and skin, and evaluation for the presence of a nipple discharge.
2. Laboratory studies include serum pregnancy test, prolactin level, and thyroid-stimulating hormone (TSH) and free T4.
3. Because stresses and breast stimulation influence prolactin levels, the blood should not be drawn within one hour after a breast examination.
4. If the initial prolactin level is borderline, the level should be repeated one to two times because of the great fluctuation of prolactin levels throughout the day.
5. A level of prolactin over 200 ng/mL is almost always associated with a prolactinoma or other prolactin-secreting tumor. CT or MRI of the head is indicated.
6. If a patient has amenorrhea or oligomenorrhea, even with a normal prolactin level, CT or MRI is necessary.[23]
7. If a patient has normal menses and a normal prolactin, the likelihood she has a pituitary adenoma is very low, and CT or MRI is not necessary.
8. A mammogram is not necessary in the work-up of galactorrhea unless there are other findings on examination suggestive of breast pathology.

If a patient with galactorrhea also has amenorrhea or oligomenorrhea, even with a normal prolactin level, computed tomography or magnetic resonance imaging is necessary.

Treatment

1. If a primary disease, such as hyperthyroidism is discovered, it should be treated first.
2. If the woman is on a medication that can cause galactorrhea, and it can be changed, this should be attempted.
3. Patients with idiopathic or physiological galactorrhea and normal prolactin levels should be reassured. All patients with galactorrhea should be advised to avoid excessive breast stimulation, including repeated breast examinations.
4. Because hyperprolactinemia can decrease bone density, patients with high prolactin levels *and* normal MRI scans should be treated with bromocriptine. This will reduce the risk of osteoporosis. Bromocriptine use will improve fertility and reduce galactorrhea as well. The dose is 1.25 to 2.5 mg/day. The dose is slowly increased to a goal of 2.5 mg two or three times per day. Side effects include nausea, vomiting, postural hypotension, headache, and nasal congestion.
5. Patients with prolactinomas may need surgery, if they have headaches or visual changes, symptoms of intracranial mass or a tumor is greater than 1 cm in size.
   a. Medical treatments for prolactinoma include dopamine agonists such as bromocriptine, and the newer agents pergolide and cabergoline.
   b. Surgery cure rates are poor, ranging from 10 to 40 percent, with a recurrence rate up to 80 percent. Radiation is also an option if a patient cannot tolerate medications and is not a surgical candidate.

Because hyperprolactinemia can decrease bone density, patients with high prolactin levels *and* normal magnetic resonance imaging should be treated with bromocriptine.

Nipple discharges

Impact

1. The importance of evaluating nipple discharges is that between 10 to 25 percent of nongalactorrhea nipple discharges are caused by cancer, specifically ductal carcinomas. The prevalence of cancer with nipple discharges is hard to discover, because most studies were retrospective and had preselec-

ted populations, but retrospective studies suggest that approximately 9 percent of women with nipple discharges have cancer with a range of from 1 to 72 percent.[24,25]

2.   The traditional conservative treatment for a nipple discharge that was not galactorrhea was mastectomy or biopsy and excision of tissue below the nipple. To reduce the need for surgical excision, attempts have been made to determine which nipple discharges might be considered more or less likely to be cancer. Lack of research, partially caused by the infrequence of nipple discharge, has hampered this research, so that definitive guidelines are difficult to develop.

3.   Nipple discharges are the third most common complaint concerning breasts. It was the primary complaint of only 5 percent of women attending breast clinics.[2,24]

Symptoms and importance

1.   Nipple discharge may be from one breast or both, from one duct or more, intermittent, spontaneous or continuous, or related to a mass or soreness.

2.   Discharges from one breast or one duct are more likely to be caused by cancer than discharges that come from both breasts or are multiductal.

3.   Discharges associated with a breast mass are more likely to be pathological than those without a mass.

4.   Discharges that are spontaneous and not provoked are more likely to be pathological. In one large retrospective study of 243 women with spontaneous nipple discharges, 30 percent had carcinoma, whereas only 3 percent of those with a provoked discharge had carcinoma.[24]

5.   Nipple discharges can be classified as one of seven colors: yellow, bloody (red), pink, multicolored (or gray, black or brown), clear, purulent or white (Table 22.4).

   a.   Yellow or green-black discharges may be from ductal ectasia, a form of blocked lymphatics and are rarely caused by cancer. Ectasia usually produces spontaneous multiple ductal discharge. This is a noninflammatory self-limited condition.

   b.   Bloody or serosanguinis discharges are pathological. Up to 25 percent may be cancerous, although some are associated with trauma.

   c.   Bilateral, multiductal white discharges are usually milk and the woman may need evaluation for galactorrhea.

   d.   Purulent discharges are consistent with an infection.

   e.   Clear discharges are rare, serious, pathological and may be associated with

Table 22.4. Characteristics of nipple discharges

Color	More or less likely to be caused by cancer
Bloody	More
Serous	More
Serosanguinis	More
Clear	More
Grey	Less
Black	Less
Brown	Less
Green	Much less – often an infection
Milky	Much less – usually galactorrhea

ductal carcinoma in situ. Between one-third and one-half of these are caused by cancer.

6. Nipple discharges in postmenopausal women are more serious. Nipple discharges in women older than age 60 years are more than twice as likely to be cancerous.[26] In a study of more than 7000 Chinese women with breast problems, older age was significantly more likely to be associated with cancer. (Figure 22.2).[27]

> Bloody or serosanguinis discharges are pathological. Up to 25 percent may be cancerous, although some are associated with trauma.

Diagnosis

1. There are no guidelines that give a definite method to investigate a woman's nipple discharge.
2. The discharge may be caused by cancer even with normal mammography, ultrasonography and cytology. Some studies have stated that cytology is useless.
3. Ductography, or galactography, injection of dye into a duct, does not reliably exclude cancerous lesions and is painful. It adds little to the evaluation of a nipple discharge.[28]
4. Thus diagnosis is not linear (Figure 22.3).
   a. In a woman with a nipple discharge, examination should first decide whether a mass is present.
   b. Then mammography is suggested in all patients.

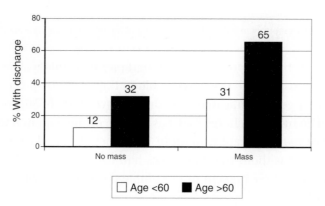

Figure 22.2.   Percent of women with nipple discharge who have cancer, by age and presence of palpable mass. (Data from Fiorica JV. Nipple discharge. *Obstet Gynecol Clin North Am* 1994;**21**:453–60.)

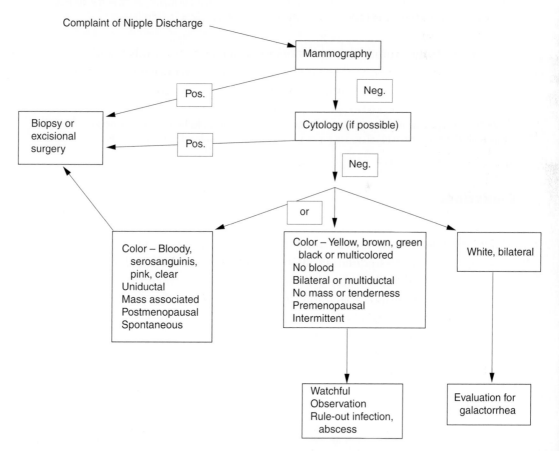

Figure 22.3.   Evaluation of a woman with a nipple discharge. Pos., positive; Neg., negative.

> The discharge may be caused by cancer even with normal mammography, ultrasonography and cytology.

c. If there is a mass, a positive mammography or cytology, the woman is postmenopausal or the discharge is blood tinged, heme positive or clear, biopsy or surgery is indicated. One prospective study of 56 women found that 17 of 56 had a discharge that was bloody, or the patient had a positive cytology or mammography. In these 17 women, five had cancer, whereas none of those without these positives had cancer in the subsequent five years. Seventy-three percent of the nipple discharges disappeared within five years.[29]

d. In women with spontaneous, continuous and unilateral discharges, biopsy or surgery should be considered.

> If there is a mass, a positive mammography or cytology, the woman is postmenopausal or the discharge is blood tinged, heme positive or clear, biopsy or surgery is indicated.

e. If the woman is premenopausal, has negative studies and a nonbloody, heme-negative discharge, especially if it is provoked or related to trauma, then cautious waiting without biopsy may be considered.

> If the woman is premenopausal, has negative studies and a nonbloody, heme-negative nipple discharge, especially if it is provoked or related to trauma, then cautious waiting without biopsy may be considered.

Conclusions

Breast disorders are common. However, little rigorous research has offered solutions to frequent problems. Hormones are the usual treatment for many breast disorders after the possibility of breast cancers has been removed by evaluation and radiographic evaluation. Galactorrhea is often physiological or caused by medication or treatable endocrine abnormalities; a rational evaluation can produce significant response.

REFERENCES

1. Hughes LE, Mansel RE, Webster DJT. *Benign Disorders and Diseases of the Breast*, 2nd edn. Saunders, London, 2000, pp. 94–121.
2. Dixon JM, Mansel RE. ABC of breast diseases: Symptoms assessment and guidelines for

referral. *BMJ* 1994;**309**:722–6.

3. Mansel RE. ABC of breast diseases: Breast pain. *BMJ* 1994;**309**:866–8.

4. River L, Silverstien J, Grout J et al. Carcinoma of the breast: The diagnostic significance of pain. *Am J Surg* 1951;**82**:213–15.

5. The Yorkshire Breast Cancer Group. Symptoms and signs of operable breast cancer. *Br J Surg* 1983;**70**:350–1.

6. Plu-Bureau G, Thalabard JC, Sitruk-Ware R, Asselain B, Mauvais-Jarvis P. Cyclic mastalgia as a marker of breast cancer susceptibility: Results of a case-control study among French women. *Br J Cancer* 1992;**65**:945–9.

7. Duijm LE, Guit GL, Hendriks JC, Zaat JO, Mali WP. Value of breast imaging in women with painful breasts: Observational follow-up study. *BMJ* 1998;**317**:1492–5.

8. Gateley CA, Miers M, Mansel RE, Hughes LE. Drug treatments for mastalgia: 17 years experience in the Cardiff Mastalgia Clinic. *J R Soc Med* 1992;**85**:12–15.

9. Dileito A, De Rosa G, Albano G et al. Desogestrel versus gestodine in oral contraceptives. *Eur J. Obstet Gynaecol Reprod Biol* 1994;**55**:71–83.

10. Belch JJ, Hill A. Evening primrose oil and borage oil in rheumatologic conditions. *Am J Clin Nutr* 2000;**71**:352S–356S.

11. Cheung KL. Management of cyclic mastalgia in oriental women. Pioneer experience of using gamolenic acid in Asia. *Aust NZ J Surg* 1999;**69**:492–4.

12. Mansel RE, Preece TE, Hughes LE. A double blind trial of the prolactin inhibitor bromocriptine in painful benign breast disease. *Br J Surg* 1978;**65**:724–7.

13. Fentiman IS, Caleffi M, Brame K et al. Double blind controlled trial of tamoxifen therapy for mastalgia. *Lancet* 1986;**1**:287–8.

14. Drukker BH. Breast disease: A primer on diagnosis and management. *Int J Fertil* 1997;**43**:278–87.

15. Lubin F, Ron E, Wax Y et al. A case control study of caffeine and methyl xanthines in benign breast disease. *JAMA* 1985;**253**:2388–92.

16. Marchant DJ. Controversies in benign breast disease. *Surg Oncol Clin North Am* 1998;**7**:285–98.

17. Scott-Conner CE, Schoor SJ. The diagnosis and management of breast problems during pregnancy and lactation. *Am J Surg* 1995;**170**:401–6.

18. Dixon JM. ABC of breast diseases: Breast infection. *BMJ* 1994;**309**:946–9.

19. Tolis G, Somma M, van Campenhout J, Friesen H. Prolactin secretion in sixty-five patients with galactorrhea. *Am J Obstet Gynecol* 1974;**188**:91–101.

20. Kleinberg D, Noel G, Frantz A. Galactorrhea: A study of 235 cases, including 48 with pituitary tumors. *New Engl J Med* 1977;**296**:589–99.

21. Windgassen K, Wesselmann U, Schulze H. Galactorrhea and hyperprolactinemia in schizophrenic patients on neuroleptics: Frequency and etiology. *Neuropsychobiology* 1996;**33**:142–6.

22. Edge D, Segatore M. Assessment and management of galactorrhea. *Nurse Pract* 1993;**18**:6,35–49.

23. Davajan V, Kletzky O, March C, Roy S, Mishell D. The significance of galactorrhea in patients with normal menses, oligomenorrhea, and secondary amenorrhea. *Am J Obstet Gynecol* 1978;**130**:894–904.

24. Hughes, LE. Nipple discharges. In Hughes LE, Mansel RE, Webstyer DJT. *Benign Disorders and Diseases of the Breast*. WB Saunders Co, Philadelphia, 2000, pp. 171–86.

25. Donnegan WL, Gren FL, Love SM. Nipple discharge: Is it cancer? *Patient Care* 1990;**24**:79–96.

26. Fiorica JV. Nipple discharge. *Obstet Gynecol Clin North Am* 1994;**21**:453–60.

27. Cheung KL, Alagaratnam TT. A review of nipple discharge in Chinese women. *J R Coll Surg Edinb* 1997;**42**:179–81.

28. Dawes LG, Bowen C, Venta LA, Morrow M. Ductography for nipple discharge: No replacement for ductal excision. *Surgery* 1998;**124**:685–91.

29. Carty NJ, Royule GT, Mudan SS, Taylor I, Ravichandran D. Prospective study of outcome in women presenting with nipple discharge. *Ann R Coll Surg Engl* 1994;**76**:387–9.

23 Breast cancer screening

Abenaa Brewster, MD, and Nancy Davidson, MD

Breast cancer is the second leading cause of cancer deaths for women in the USA. Screening and prevention are important tasks in primary care.

Impact

1. In the year 2001, it is estimated that 192 000 women will be diagnosed with breast cancer and 40 200 women will die from the disease.[1]
2. The risk of being diagnosed with breast cancer increases with age.
3. A woman's lifetime risk of being diagnosed with breast cancer is 13 percent and her lifetime risk of dying from breast cancer is 3.39 percent.[1]

Risk factors

Several risk factors are associated with an increased risk of developing breast cancer (Table 23.1). None is modifiable.

Familial breast cancer
1. Familial breast cancer accounts for fewer than 10 percent of all breast cancers and is associated with multiple affected family members, an early age at diagnosis and bilateral breast cancer.
2. The major genes that increase breast cancer susceptibility are *BRCA1* and *BRCA2*. In the group of women diagnosed with breast cancer in the general population, 3 percent of women will have mutations in the breast cancer susceptibility gene *BRCA1*.[2]
3. In women with breast cancer and a family history of the disease, the frequency of a *BRCA1* mutation is much more likely. Women who are carriers

Table 23.1. Risk factors for breast cancer

- Young age at menarche
- Family history of breast cancer, nulliparity
- Age greater than 55 years at menopause
- History of breast atypical hyperplasia
- Radiation exposure
- A previous history of breast cancer

of mutations in *BRCA1* or *BRCA2* have a lifetime risk of 56 to 87 percent for breast cancer and an elevated risk for ovarian cancer.

4. Genetic testing for *BRCA1* and *BRCA2* is now available for women with a strong genetic predisposition for breast cancer. Identification of these higher risk women has significant implications for cancer surveillance methods. Currently, secondary prevention through screening procedures is the most effective measure for reducing the morbidity and mortality of breast cancer.

Screening for breast cancer – secondary prevention

Purpose

The high incidence and mortality from breast cancer represents a significant public health burden and makes it a disease appropriate for screening. The goal of screening women for breast cancer is to detect cancer in its earliest stage when surgery and medical treatment can be most effective in reducing mortality. Screening is only beneficial when an earlier diagnosis results in a reduction in mortality and morbidity and when the risks of the screening test are low. Criteria for screening a disease require it to be detectable in the preclinical phase and likely to progress to clinical symptoms if left untreated.

Screening is only beneficial when an earlier diagnosis results in a reduction in mortality and morbidity and when the risks of the screening test are low.

Impact

Screening for breast cancer can lead to the detection of preinvasive lesions such as ductal carcinoma in situ (DCIS) and small node-negative invasive cancers. Treatment of these early lesions carries a good prognosis and accounts for most of the reduction in mortality.

Methods

Mammography, clinical breast examination (CBE) and breast self-examination (BSE) are three modalities currently available for screening for breast cancer.

Screening mammography

Importance

The first randomized clinical trial to demonstrate an improved survival in women screened for breast cancer was the Health Insurance Plan (HIP) Breast Cancer Screening Project conducted in 1963. In this study, 60 696 women aged 40 to 64 years were randomly assigned either to undergo breast cancer screening with four annual mammograms and CBE or to receive usual care. After 10 years of follow-up, women in the screened group had a statistically significant 30 percent reduction in breast cancer mortality.[3]

Efficacy

Seven subsequent randomized clinical trials have evaluated the efficacy of screening mammography in reducing breast cancer mortality.[4–10] The studies differ in important features pertaining to their conduct and this has led to the challenge in comparing their results. The HIP, Edinburgh and Canadian National Screening Studies 1 and 2 included CBE by a trained professional as part of the screening protocol whereas the four Swedish studies did not. The method of randomization, the ages of the women at entry into the study, the interval of mammography screening, the quality of mammography and the length of follow-up time also vary considerably among the studies. Nonetheless, with an average follow-up time of 10 years, all but one of these studies have shown a significant reduction in breast cancer mortality among the women assigned to undergo screening (Table 23.2). Indeed, the controversy regarding recommendations for screening mammography is focused largely on the age of the women at which screening mammography should be initiated.

With an average follow-up time of 10 years, studies have shown a significant reduction in breast cancer mortality among the women assigned to undergo screening.

Table 23.2. Controlled randomized trials of breast cancer screening

Controlled randomized trial (start date)	Age at entry (years)	Screening modality	Screening interval (months)	Follow-up time (years)	All ages RR (95 percent CI)
Health Insurance Plan (1963)[a]	40–64	2 view MM and CBE	12	18	0.77 (0.61–0.97)*
Malmö (1976)[b]	45–69	1 or 2 view MM	18–24	12	0.81 (0.62–1.07)
Swedish Two-County (1977)[c]	40–74	1 view MM	24 for ages 40–49 33 for ages 50–74	13	0.69 (0.57–0.84)*
Edinburgh (1979)[d]	45–64	1 or 2 view MM	24	10	0.82 (0.61–1.11)
Canadian NBSS-1 (1980)[e]	40–49	2 view MM and CBE	12	10.5	1.14 (0.83–1.56)
Canadian NBSS-2 (1980)[f]	50–59	2 view MM and CBE vs. CBE alone	12	8.3	0.97 (0.62–1.52)
Stockholm (1981)[g]	40–64	1 view MM	28	11.4	0.74 (0.50–1.10)
Gothenburg (1982)[h]	40–59	2 view MM	18	7	0.86 (0.34–1.37)

RR, relative risk; CI, confidence intervals; MM, mammograms; CBE, clinical breast examination.

* Statistically significant ($p < 0.05$).

[a]Shapiro Venet W, Strax P et al. Ten to fourteen year effect of screening on breast cancer mortality. *J Natl Cancer Inst* 1982;**69**:349–55.

[b]Andersson I, Aspegren K, Janzon L et al. Mammographic screening and mortality from breast cancer: The Malmö mammographic screening trial. *BMJ* 1988;**297**:943–8.

[c]Tabar L, Fagreberg G, Day NE et al. Efficacy of breast cancer screening by age: New results from the Swedish Two-County Trial. *Cancer* 1995;**75**:2507–17.

[d]Alexander FE, Anderson TJ, Brown HK et al. The Edinburgh randomized trial of breast cancer screening: Results after 10 years of follow-up. *Br J Cancer* 1994;**70**:542–8.

[e]Miller AB, To T, Baines CJ et al. Canadian National Breast Screening Study: Update on breast cancer mortality. *Monogr Natl Cancer Inst* 1997;**22**:37–41.

[f]Miller AB, To T, Baines CJ et al. Canadian National Breast Screening Study: 2. Breast cancer detection and death rates among women age 50–59 years. *Can Med Assoc J* 1992;**147**:1477–88.

[g]Frisell J, Lidbrink E, Hellstrom L et al. Follow up after 11 years: Update of mortality results in the Stockholm mammography screening trial. *Breast Cancer Res Treat* 1997;**45**:263–70.

[h]Bjurstam N, Bjorneld L, Duffy SW et al. The Gothenburg Breast Screening Trial: First results on mortality, incidence, and mode of detection for women aged 39–49 years at randomization. *Cancer* 1997;**80**:2091–9.

Screening mammography in women aged 50 years and older

1. There is a clear benefit of screening mammography in women aged 50 years and older. Several RCTs and case-controlled studies have demonstrated a 20 to 30 percent reduction in breast cancer mortality for women in this age group who undergo regular mammography. A metaanalysis of mammography studies showed a statistically significant 26 percent reduction in breast cancer mortality at seven to nine years of follow-up in women age 50 to 74 years.[11]

2. The benefit of mammography in women older than age 70 years is less clear because of the small number of women in this age category enrolled in mammography screening trials. An analysis of the four Swedish RCTs showed a nonsignificant reduction in mortality in the small number of women aged 70 to 74 years undergoing screening with mammography.[12]

3. Recommendations for screening women older than age 70 years are vague and unsubstantiated by scientific evidence of benefit. Investigators have used cost–benefit analysis with varying results to address the question of whether screening mammography should be recommended to women older than age 70 years. In a decision model, it was cost-effective to screen women over the age of 70 only if they were at a higher than age-predicted risk for breast cancer.[13]

4. Elderly women with several comorbidities and a limited life expectancy may not experience the benefit of mammography screening.[14] Proponents for continuing mammography screening in women older than age 75 years emphasize that the physician and patient must consider these factors individually.

There is a clear benefit of screening mammography in women aged 50 years and older.

Mammography screening in women aged 40 to 49 years

1. The efficacy of screening mammography in reducing breast cancer mortality for women aged 40 to 49 years is controversial. Retrospective subgroup analysis of data from the randomized trials of screening mammography of women aged 40 to 49 years has been used to determine the magnitude of benefit of screening mammography in this age group. The Canadian National Breast Screening Study 1 is the only RCT specifically conducted to evaluate the efficacy of combined screening mammography and CBE in women aged 40 to 49 years. During an average follow up time of 10 years, the study failed to find a benefit from screening in women entering into the study at age 40 to 49.[6] This study has been criticized because of its study design, although an independent review showed no bias in the randomization.

2. In 1997, the National Institutes of Health (NIH) convened a Consensus Development Conference to address breast cancer screening in women aged 40 to 49 years. The panel of experts concluded that the scientific data available did not warrant a universal recommendation for mammography for all women in their 40s.[14]

3. Updated results from the Malmö and Gothenburg RCTs have since shown a statistically significant reduction in breast cancer mortality of 36 percent and 44 percent, respectively, in women first screened in their 40s.

4. A metaanalysis that included the latest follow-up data from each of the seven RCTs indicates a statistically significant 18 percent mortality reduction among women aged 40 to 49 years assigned to screening.[15] A longer follow-up time of greater than 10 years was needed to show a statistically significant benefit from screening mammography in women aged 40 to 49 years compared with women aged 50 and older.

5. Much of the debate on the utilization of screening mammography in women in their 40s versus 50s focuses on the artificial cut-off at age 49 years. Women in their late 40s are biologically similar to women in their 50s and therefore would be expected to experience similar benefits of mammography. The delayed benefit of screening mammography has led some investigators to propose that the benefit of screening is observed when women entered in the studies in their 40s are diagnosed with breast cancer in their 50s. Other factors that may contribute to the delayed benefit of screening mammography are the lower incidence of breast cancer in the 40s compared to women aged 50 years and older and the higher incidence of diagnosis of earlier stage cancers (e.g., DCIS) with good prognosis. Conflicting guidelines for mammography screening for women aged 40 to 49 years reflect the uncertainty about benefit.

> Studies have shown a statistically significant 18 percent mortality reduction among women aged 40 to 49 years assigned to mammographic screening.

Accuracy of mammography

1. The sensitivity of mammography ranges from 75 to 88 percent and specificity from 83 to 98 percent.[16]

2. The sensitivity of mammography is lower in younger women and depends on additional factors such as the breast and cancer characteristics.

3. The positive predictive value (PPV) of the test increases with age and family history of breast cancer. The PPV of first screening mammography increases from 4 percent in women aged 40 to 49 years to 9 percent for women aged 50 to 69 years to 19 percent for women aged 70 or older.[17] The PPV for screening mammography in women aged 40 to 49 and 50 to 59 with at least one

first-degree relative with breast cancer is almost three times higher than similarly age women without a family history of breast cancer.

> The sensitivity of mammography is lower in younger women and depends on additional factors such as the breast and cancer characteristics.

Risks of mammography

1. The risks of any screening intervention need to be evaluated as closely as the benefits. The risks associated with screening mammography for breast cancer include radiation exposure, false positives, and overdiagnosis. The decision to undergo mammography should be an informed decision based on the woman's understanding of the risks versus benefits.

2. The risk of radiation-induced breast cancer from screening mammography is estimated to be minimal. Information obtained from the atomic bomb survivors has been used to approximate the age-specific radiation risk for women undergoing screening mammography. Approximately eight radiation-induced breast cancer deaths might occur for every 100 000 women receiving yearly mammograms over 10 years starting at age 40 years.[18]

3. The excess risk for breast cancer caused by radiation is increased with a younger age of the woman at exposure and increasing cumulative radiation dose. Although the risk of radiation-induced breast cancer is higher in women younger than age 50 years, the benefits of mammography still significantly outweigh the risk of radiation-induced breast cancer.

> The benefits of mammography still significantly outweigh the risk of radiation-induced breast cancer.

4. A false positive is defined as a positive test that does not result in the diagnosis of cancer within one year of the test. As the specificity of the screening intervention decreases, the risk of a false positive result increases. The risk of a false positive mammogram is therefore higher in younger women, who have lower mammogram specificity than older women. In a retrospective cohort study of Health Maintenance Organization participants screened over 10 years, the false positive mammography rate was 7.8 percent in women aged 40 to 49 years, 7.4 percent in women aged 50 to 59 years and 4.4 percent in women aged 70 to 79 years. The cumulative risk of a false positive result was 49 percent after 10 mammograms.[19] False positives from mammography lead to additional procedures such as breast biopsies, ultrasound scans and mammograms. These additional procedures increase the cost and morbidity

associated with screening. In retrospective studies, false positive mammo-grams have been demonstrated to cause increased anxiety and to elevate a woman's perceived risk of developing breast cancer.[20]

> The cumulative risk of a false positive result was 49 percent after 10 mammograms.

Overdiagnosis

1. The detection of DCIS, which is classified as a noninvasive carcinoma, has increased significantly since the advent of population-based screening mam-mography. DCIS represents the highest proportion of breast cancers detected through mammography in women aged 40 to 49 years.
2. The incidence of DCIS increases with age and approximately 25 percent of cases occur in elderly women. Although the natural history of DCIS is unclear, retrospective case-controlled and autopsy studies provide evidence that the majority of DCIS lesions do not progress to invasive carcinoma.
3. Despite this evidence, the majority of women diagnosed with DCIS receive treatment because prognostic factors are unavailable to accurately predict which DCIS cases will undergo progression to invasive disease.[21] For many women, especially the elderly, the detection and treatment of DCIS may result in minimal clinical benefit.

> Ductal carcinoma in situ represents the highest proportion of breast cancers detected through mammography in women aged 40 to 49 years.

Clinical breast examination

Efficacy

1. The efficacy of CBE alone in screening for breast cancer is uncertain. No studies have evaluated the benefit of CBE versus no screening in reducing breast cancer mortality. Evidence of the benefit of CBE is derived from clinical trials that randomized women to undergo dual-modality screening with CBE and mammography versus no screening or CBE alone.
2. In the HIP study,[3] women were randomized to receive CBE and annual mammography versus no screening. Forty-five percent of breast cancers were detected by CBE alone and the proportion detected by CBE was higher in women aged 40 to 49 years than in women aged 50 to 64 years. The Edinburgh study,[5] which also randomized women to combined screening or no screen-

ing, detected 3 percent of cancers by CBE alone. In both of these studies, CBE was clearly effective in diagnosing a percentage of breast cancer cases missed by screening mammography.

3. In the NBSS-2 clinical trial,[7] women aged 50 to 59 years were randomized to receive five annual mammograms with CBE versus annual CBE alone. At seven years of follow-up there was no statistically significant difference in breast cancer mortality between the two groups. In this study, CBE was comparable to screening mammography in reducing breast cancer mortality.

4. Although mortality rates are similar between studies that utilized dual screening versus mammography alone, CBE remains an important part of the screening process, since it can detect cancers missed by mammography.

Clinical breast examination was comparable to screening mammography in reducing breast cancer mortality.

Accuracy of clinical breast examination

A pooled analysis of data from human studies on the accuracy of CBE in detecting breast cancer showed a sensitivity of 54 percent and a specificity of 94 percent.[22] In this metaanalysis, the accuracy of CBE was dependent on a longer duration of CBE and a higher number of specific techniques used while the patient was examined. Additional factors affecting accuracy included older age of the patient, breast characteristics such as "lumpiness", and size and cancer characteristics. The low sensitivity of CBE limits its use as a single screening modality for breast cancer.

Breast self-examination

1. BSE is advocated as a complementary screening modality for the early detection of breast cancer. RCTs have not shown that BSE, performed as a single screening intervention, reduces breast cancer mortality. Two RCTs conducted in Russia and the People's Republic of China, with an average follow-up time of seven years, showed that women who received instruction on BSE had a similar breast cancer mortality to the unscreened group.[23,24]

2. The number of breast cancers detected and the size and stage of the tumors were also similar between the women instructed in BSE and the unscreened group.[23] There were, however, an increased number of breast biopsies for benign breast disease performed in the women instructed in BSE. Generalization of the results of the Chinese study to women in the USA is limited because China has an almost three times lower breast cancer mortality rate.

3. The UK, which has breast cancer mortality similar to that of the USA, conducted a nonrandomized trial of early detection of breast cancer. This study included women educated about BSE without physical instruction. A combined analysis of the screening groups educated about BSE showed no reduction in the 10-year mortality from breast cancer.[25]

4. Although BSE is publicized as an effective breast cancer screening modality, there is little scientific evidence to support its benefit. Routine BSE may have the disadvantage of resulting in unnecessary breast biopsies especially in women at low risk for breast cancer.

> Randomized controlled trials have not shown that breast self-examination, performed as a single screening intervention, reduces breast cancer mortality.

Guidelines

Several professional organizations have provided evidence-based recommendations for mammographic screening, CBE and BSE. Some of the recommendations for screening women at an age-appropriate risk for breast cancer are shown in Table 23.3.

Primary prevention of breast cancer

1. The goal of breast cancer primary prevention is to prevent the development of breast cancer in the otherwise healthy woman. The multistep process of carcinogenesis allows several opportunities for introducing interventions to prevent cancer formation.

2. Chemopreventive agents such as tamoxifen and raloxifene act to prevent the development of breast cancer by interrupting the process of initiation and promotion of tumors. The antiestrogenic effect of these agents appears also to lead to growth inhibition of malignant cells.[26,27] Chemoprevention is the most promising intervention for achieving primary prevention of breast cancer at this time.

   a. Tamoxifen:

      i. Tamoxifen is a nonsteroidal antiestrogen with a partial estrogen agonist effect. It is FDA-approved for use in women at an increased risk for breast cancer. A study of its efficacy in reducing the incidence of breast

Table 23.3. Selected breast cancer screening guidelines

Organization	Screening guidelines Age 40–49 years	Screening guidelines Age > 50 years	Routine BSE teaching
American Cancer Society	Annual mammography. Annual CBE	Annual mammography. Annual CBE. No age limit	Yes
National Cancer Institute	Mammography every 1–2 years. Annual CBE	Mammography every 1–2 years. Annual CBE. No age limit	Yes
US Preventative Services Task Force	Insufficient evidence (C)[a]	Mammography every 1–2 years OR mammography + CBE every 1–2 years. Age limit 69 years	Insufficient evidence (C)[a]
American College of Obstetricians and Gynecologists	Mammography every 1–2 years. Annual CBE	Annual mammography. Annual CBE	Yes
American College of Physicians	Counsel. Individual decision	Mammography every 2 years. Annual CBE. Age limit 74 years	No
American Academy of Family Physicians	Counsel. Individual decision	Mammography + CBE every 1–2 years. Age limit 69 years	No
Canadian Task Force on The Periodic Health Examination	Not recommended	Annual mammography. Annual CBE. Age limit 69 years	Insufficient evidence (C)[a]

CBE, clinical breast examination; BSE, breast self-examination.

[a](C) There is insufficient evidence to recommend for or against this clinical practice as part of the periodic health examination.

cancer found a lower incidence of contralateral breast cancer in women receiving tamoxifen as adjuvant therapy for breast cancer.

ii. Three placebo RCTs have been conducted to investigate whether tamoxifen can prevent the development of breast cancer in healthy women at risk for this disease. The Breast Cancer Prevention Trial (BCPT) conducted in the USA enrolled 13 388 women who were either age 60 years or older, age 35 to 39 years with a five-year predicted risk for breast cancer of at least 1.66 percent or had a history of lobular carcinoma in situ. At 69 months of follow-up time, the study showed an approximate 50 percent reduction in the incidence of estrogen receptor positive invasive and noninvasive breast cancers in the study group receiving 20 mg of tamoxifen daily.[26]

iii. The side effects of tamoxifen were increased in the study group particularly among women older than age 50 years. Among the women who received tamoxifen there was a 2.5 times greater risk of developing stage I endometrial cancer and an increased rate of thromboembolic disease.

iv. Two other smaller randomized studies conducted in the UK and Italy failed to show a benefit of tamoxifen in reducing the incidence of breast cancer.[28,29] Explanations for this inconsistency have included smaller sample size, differences in the study population and differences in drug compliance. The UK study enrolled a greater percentage of women with a first-degree relative with breast cancer than the BCPT.[26] Tamoxifen may be a less effective as a preventive agent in women with a strong family of breast cancer. In addition, unlike the BCPT, the other two studies included women on HRT. This difference in study population makes it difficult to exclude HRT as a confounder in the relationship between tamoxifen and breast cancer reduction. Although the BCPT demonstrated that tamoxifen reduces breast cancer incidence, which women experience the greatest benefit : risk ratio from the drug is still unclear. The decision to initiate tamoxifen in a woman should carefully consider her individual risk of breast cancer weighed against the long- and short-term risk of adverse complications.

b. Raloxifene:

i. Raloxifene hydrochloride is a selective estrogen receptor modulator (SERM) that blocks the action of estrogen in the breast and endometrial tissue. Information regarding the efficacy of raloxifene in reducing the development of breast cancer was obtained from the Multiple Outcomes of Raloxifene Evaluation (MORE) trial.[30] This study was conducted primarily to investigate the efficacy of raloxifene in reducing the risk of fracture among postmenopausal women with osteoporosis. A total of 7705 post-menopausal women with osteoporosis were randomized to receive raloxifene 60 mg daily or 60 mg twice a day versus placebo.

ii. The incidence of estrogen receptor positive invasive breast cancer was reduced by 76 percent among women treated with either dose of raloxifene at 40 months of follow-up time.[27]

Table 23.4. Trials of primary prevention for breast cancer

Trials	Chemoprevention agent	Number of participants	Breast cancer events	Median follow-up (months)	Eligibility criteria	Results
NSABP P-1	Tamoxifen	13 388	358	55	Age > 60 years or > 1.66 percent 5-year risk of developing breast cancer or history of lobular carcinoma in situ. No concurrent HRT	49 percent reduction in breast cancer in tamoxifen vs. placebo group
Italian	Tamoxifen	5408	41	46	Hysterectomized women aged 35–70 years at low to normal risk of breast cancer. Concurrent HRT allowed	No difference in breast cancer except in tamoxifen + HRT group
UK	Tamoxifen	2471	70	70	Women aged 30–70 years at increased risk because of a family history. Concurrent HRT allowed	No difference in breast cancer

iii. The side effects of raloxifene included an increased risk of thromboembolic disease, but not an increased risk of endometrial cancer.

iv. Limitations of this study include the evaluation of breast cancer incidence as a secondary end point and the short follow-up time. It is possible that the reduction in breast cancer may have been secondary to raloxifene's treatment effect on occult breast cancers among the women.

v. The Study of Tamoxifen and Raloxifene (STAR) trial, which randomizes postmenopausal women at increased risk for breast cancer to receive raloxifene versus tamoxifen, is currently being conducted. Results from this study will provide additional information regarding the benefit and risk profile of tamoxifen (Table 23.4) and raloxifene.

> There was an approximate 50 percent reduction in the incidence of estrogen receptor positive invasive and noninvasive breast cancers in a study group of women at high risk for developing breast cancer who received 20 mg of tamoxifen daily.

Conclusions

Breast cancer is one of the most common cancers in women. Screening and prevention are possible, and breast cancer can be cured if detected early enough.

REFERENCES

1. Greenlee RT, Harmon M, Murray T et al. Cancer statistics 2001. *CA Cancer J Clin* 2001;**51**:15–36.
2. Newman B, Mu H, Butler L et al. Frequency of breast cancer attributable to *BRCA1* in a population-based series of American women. *JAMA* 1998;**279**:915–21.
3. Shapiro S, Venet W, Strax P et al. Ten to fourteen year effect of screening on breast cancer mortality. *J Natl Cancer Inst* 1982;**69**:349–55.
4. Tabar L, Fagerberg G, Day NE et al. Efficacy of breast cancer screening by age: New results from the Swedish Two-County Trial. *Cancer* 1995;**75**:2507–17.
5. Alexander FE, Anderson TJ, Brown HK et al. The Edinburgh randomized trial of breast cancer screening: Results after 10 years of follow-up. *Br J Cancer* 1994;**70**:542–8.
6. Miller AB, To T, Baines CJ et al. The Canadian National Breast Screening Study: Update on breast cancer mortality. *Monogr Natl Cancer Inst* 1997;**22**:37–41.
7. Miller AB, To T, Baines CJ et al. Canadian National Breast Screening Study: 2. Breast cancer detection and death rates among women age 50–59 years. *Can Med Assoc J* 1992;**147**:1477–88.

8. Frisell J, Lidbrink E, Hellstrom L et al. Follow up after 11 years: Update of mortality results in the Stockholm mammography screening trial. *Breast Cancer Res Treat* 1997;**45**:263–70.

9. Andersson I, Aspegren K, Janzon L et al. Mammographic screening and mortality from breast cancer: The Malmö mammographic screening trial. *BMJ* 1988;**297**:943–8.

10. Bjurstam N, Bjorneld L, Duffy SW et al., The Gothenburg Breast Cancer Screening Trial: First results on mortality, incidence, and mode of detection for women ages 39–49 years at randomization. *Cancer* 1997;**80**:2091–9.

11. Kerlikowske K, Grady D, Rubin S et al. Efficacy of screening mammography: a meta-analysis. *JAMA* 1995;**273**:149–54.

12. Larsson LG, Nyström L, Wall S et al. The Swedish randomized mammography screening trials: analysis of their effect on the breast cancer related excess mortality. *J Med Screen* 1996;**3**:129–32.

13. Kerlikowske K, Salzman P, Phillips KA et al. Continuing screening mammography in women aged 70 to 79 years: Impact on life expectancy and cost effectiveness. *JAMA* 1999;**282**:2156–63.

14. Satariano W, Ragland D. The effect of comorbidity on 3-year survival of women with primary breast cancer. *Ann Intern Med* 1994;**120**:104–10.

15. Hendrick ER, Smith R, Rutledge JH et al. Benefit of screening mammography in women age 40–49: A new meta-analysis of randomized controlled trials. *Monogr Natl Cancer Inst* 1997;**22**:87–92.

16. Fletcher SW, Black W, Harris R et al. Report of the International Workshop on Screening for Breast Cancer. *J Natl Cancer Inst* 1993;**85**:1644–56.

17. Kerlikowske K, Grady D, Barclay J. Positive predictive value of screening mammography by age and family history of breast cancer. *JAMA* 1993;**270**:2444–50.

18. Feig SA, Hendrick RE. Radiation risk from screening mammography of women aged 40–49 years. *Monogr Natl Cancer Inst* 1997;**22**:119–24.

19. Elmore J, Barton M, Moceri V et al. Ten-year risk of false positive screening mammograms and clinical breast examinations. *N Engl J Med* 1998;**338**:1089–96.

20. McCaul KD, Branstetter AD, Schroeder DM et al. What is the relationship between breast cancer risk and mammography screening? A meta-analytic review. *Health Psychol* 1996;**15**:423–9.

21. Ernester V, Barclay J. Increases in ductal carcinoma in situ (DCIS) of the breast in relation to mammography: A dilemma. *Monogr Natl Cancer Inst* 1997;**22**:151–6.

22. Barton M, Harris R, Fletcher S. Does this patient have breast cancer? The screening clinical breast examination: Should it be done? How? *JAMA* 1999;**282**:1270–80.

23. Semiglazov VF, Moiseyenko VM, Bavli JL et al. The role of breast self-examination in early breast cancer detection (results of the 5-year USSR/WHO randomized study in Leningrad). *Eur J Epidemiol* 1992;**8**:498–502.

24. Thomas DB, Gao DL, Self SG et al. Randomized trial of breast self examination in Shangai: Methodology and preliminary results. *J Natl Cancer Inst.* 1997;**89**:355–65.

25. UK Trial of Early Detection of Breast Cancer Group. 16-year mortality from breast cancer in the UK trial of early detection of breast cancer. *Lancet* 1999;**353**:1909–14.

26. Fisher B, Costantino J, Wickerham L et al. Tamoxifen for prevention of breast cancer: Report of the National Surgical Adjuvant Breast and Bowel Project P-1 study. *J Natl Cancer Inst* 1998;**90**:1371–88.

27. Cummings R, Eckert D, Kreuger KA et al. The effect of raloxifene on risk of breast cancer in postmenopausal women. *JAMA* 1999;**281**:2189–97.

28. Powles T, Eeles R, Ashley S et al. Interim analysis of the incidence of breast cancer in the Royal Marsden Hospital tamoxifen randomized chemoprevention trial. *Lancet* 1998;**352**:98–101.

29. Veronesi U, Maisonneuve P, Costa A et al. Prevention of breast cancer with tamoxifen: Preliminary findings from the Italian randomized trial among hysterectomised women. *Lancet* 1998;**352**:93–7.

30. Ettinger B, Black DM, Mitlak BH et al. Reduction of vertebral fracture risk in postmenopausal women with osteoporosis treated with raloxifene. Multiple Outcomes of Raloxifene Evaluation (MORE) investigators. *JAMA* 1999;**282**:637–46.

Psychological disorders

24 Woman battering

Sandra K. Burge, PhD

Case   A 55-year-old woman came to see her family physician for a routine follow-up of her hypertension. After a brief conversation about symptoms, medications, and side effects, the physician stood to retest her blood pressure. As he placed the cuff around her arm, she sighed and said, "I know it's going to be high today. I didn't get much sleep last night." She paused. "We had a misunderstanding." The physician asked, "What do you mean by 'a misunderstanding'?" and she described her husband's rampage of the night before: after a night of heavy drinking, he stormed into the house at 2:00 a.m., yelling, demanding dinner, and smashing dishes against the wall when his wife did not move fast enough to suit him. The physician learned that the woman's husband had a pattern of terrorizing her, usually after drinking. Last Christmas, he had threatened her with a shotgun. Recently, her adult son had joined his father in drinking and abusing her.

Introduction

1. Violence against women is widely prevalent, causes serious psychological and physical damage, and brings women to the attention of the health care system on a daily basis.
2. Women account for 70 percent of all murdered spouses in the USA, and are 10 times more likely than men to be assaulted by an intimate other.[1] Present or former partners kill 40 to 45 percent of female homicide victims in the UK as compared with only 6 percent of male homicide victims.[2]
3. Among the 572 000 women assaulted by intimate partners each year, 27 percent receive medical care and 15 percent require hospitalization.[1] Victimized women are more likely to seek medical help than any other type of help – even more than legal or psychological help.[3,4] In the UK, 36 percent of battered women seek help from their general practitioners, while only 25 percent ask for help from the police.[5]

4. Primary care providers are ideally positioned to intervene in woman battering. Throughout their lives, women make frequent visits to primary care providers – two or three visits per year, on the average – for help with acute and chronic health problems, for annual prevention examinations, and for prenatal care.[6]

5. Women also frequently accompany other family members for health care visits. When women and health care providers establish sustained, continuity relationships, providers have the opportunity to understand the context of women's lives and to discover patterns of symptoms, behaviors, and social situations that indicate the potential for or existence of abuse. Given frequent, sustained access to women, primary care providers can contribute to violence prevention and intervention efforts through screening, patient education, counselling, support, and referral.

Primary care providers are ideally positioned to intervene in woman battering.

Definitions

1. Interpersonal violence refers to aggressive behavior intended to cause harm.[7]
2. The frequency and severity of interpersonal violence varies widely, and is inflicted by women and men, homosexuals and heterosexuals, and people of all ethnic groups and income levels.
3. Woman battering refers to the infliction of harm by a man toward a woman who is his intimate partner, with the intention of causing her pain or controlling her behavior (for female–female violence see Chapter 12). Some authors call this act partner violence, spouse abuse, wife abuse, or domestic violence.

Woman battering refers to the infliction of harm by a man toward a woman who is his intimate partner, with the intention of causing her pain or controlling her behavior.

Incidence and prevalence

Incidence

1. Moderate levels of violence: Population-based surveys find that the rate of man-to-woman violence among couples in the USA is 11 to 12 percent yearly.[8]

A man is considered "moderately" violent if he grabs, pushes, or slaps a woman, or throws things with the intention of hitting his partner.

2. Severe levels of violence: Severe violence occurs in about 3 percent of American couples each year.[8] "Severe" violence includes punching, kicking, choking, or beating up a woman, or threatening her with a knife or gun, or using weapons to harm her.

Prevalence

1. In the population: According to population surveys, the lifetime prevalence of moderate or severe violence among American couples is approximately 21 percent.[9] Authors believe that these findings are a low estimate, and that the true prevalence could be twice as high.

2. In ambulatory clinics: The prevalence of man-to-woman violence is similar or higher in outpatient clinical settings, ranging from 10 to 54 percent.[10]

The nature of violent relationships

1. Why do some men hurt women? Several theories explain the etiology of violent relationships. Research indicates that many factors operate to incite and reinforce man-to-woman aggression.

    a. Psychological theories posit that men who hurt their partners have a psychopathology that explains why they act in violent ways. For example, one author found batterers' behavior to be consistent with borderline personality disorder.[11] Others have found that men who batter have higher rates of alcoholism and drug dependence, antisocial personality disorder, and depression.[12]

    b. Sociological theories posit that Western society implicitly condones woman battering and contains structures that support men who hit, but suppress women who try to escape violent relationships. One sociologist found systematic differences in woman battering in the USA, in states where women's status was lowest (as defined by political and socioeconomic indicators and state laws that protect women), the rate of husband-to-wife violence was highest.[13]

    c. Social psychological theories:

        i. Social learning theory states that children model behaviors seen in adult family members and test them in their relationships with others. Researchers have found the most consistent risk marker of becoming a batterer (for men) or a victim of battering (for women) is the childhood experience of witnessing one's father hurting one's mother.[14]

    ii. Social exchange theory posits that violence occurs when the rewards of violence outweigh the consequences. When violence "works", i.e., it stops an argument or brings about another reward, that outcome reinforces the violent behavior, beginning a cycle of interactions that is very difficult to break.[15]

2. Two types of relationship: Research on woman battering comes from varying sources: from women who are victims of violence, men who are perpetrators, and community-based samples. Each source portrays very different patterns of violence in intimate relationships. For example, findings from population surveys indicate that women are just as likely as men to hit their partners, while findings from battered women's shelters, emergency rooms, and law enforcement agencies show that couple violence is primarily men's aggression toward women. One author has concluded that two types of violent relationship exist.[16]

    a. "Common couple violence" is characterized by occasional outbursts for the purpose of winning an argument, or controlling an immediate situation, but not for exerting complete domination over the partner. In this type of relationship, where the hitting may be mutual, violent behaviors tend to be of low severity and low frequency; one study showed an average of six assaults per year. The hitting does not escalate over time, but remains stable. Women in this type of relationship are generally not afraid of their partners. To date, research on common couple violence is extremely limited and there is little information about the exact nature of these relationships, or about etiology, risk factors, health consequences, or effective interventions.

    b. "Patriarchal terrorism" is well researched and documented. In this type of relationship, women flee to battered women's shelters. In contrast to common couple violence, this aggression is unidirectional, man-to-woman violence that escalates in severity and frequency over time. A husband who is extremely dangerous and controlling characterizes patriarchal terrorism. In addition to physical assaults, these men tend to use a pattern of strategies that function to control their partners' behaviors and to keep them in the relationship. For some, the hitting may be sporadic; however, the control is a constant force in a battering relationship. Even when infrequent, hitting reinforces the power of the following strategies.[17]

"Common couple violence" is characterized by occasional outbursts for the purpose of winning an argument, or controlling an immediate situation, but not for exerting complete domination over the partner.

A husband who is extremely dangerous and controlling characterizes "patriarchal terrorism".

    i. Physical harm is only part of the picture.

    ii. Intimidation: A man who batters will use threatening looks or gestures. He may destroy his partners' property or pets, or display weapons. All these behaviors serve to send the woman a message of danger.

    iii. Coercion and threats: He will threaten to hurt his partner, to leave her, to report her to welfare, or to commit suicide. He will coerce her to drop charges against him. Some force their partners to do illegal things.

    iv. Emotional abuse: A man who batters will insult his partner, call her names, embarrass or humiliate her in public, and make her feel guilty or stupid or ugly or unlovable. He may treat her like a child, doling out punishment when she "misbehaves".

    v. Isolation: He may control what his partner does, who she talks to, what she reads, and where she goes. He will use jealousy or guilt to limit her interactions with others, and he may create public scenes to alienate her family or friends.

    vi. Minimizing, denying, and blaming: A man who batters will shift responsibility for the abusive behavior, most often blaming the victim. He may say she is clumsy or deserves to be hit. He may believe his behavior is less harmful than it really is. Some will make light of the violence, or pretend it did not happen.

    vii. Using children: A man who batters may make his partner feel guilty about her care of the children. If separated, he will use visitation to harass her, and may threaten to take the children away or to harm them unless she cooperates with his wishes.

    viii. Male privilege: A man who batters acts like "king of the castle", treating his partner like a servant, and making all the big decisions. He will insist that family schedules and activities revolve around his priorities, and will expect everyone in the family to know (and meet) his needs, even if he has not spoken them. Male privilege is enforced through fear.

    ix. Economic abuse: A man who batters will limit his partner's employment outside the home. He will take her money, restrict her spending, make her ask him for money, and hide information about family finances from her.

3. Who are the victims? Can one predict who is at risk for becoming a battered woman? In general, there is no "typical victim profile" that predicts

A man who batters will shift responsibility for the abusive behavior, most often blaming the victim.

victimization. Before the abuse, battered women differ from nonvictims in only a few variables:

a. Age: In a large population study, women under age 25 years were more likely to experience abuse within the past year than women aged 25 years and older (27 percent versus 11 percent).[18]

b. Marital status: Unmarried, cohabiting women are more likely to be abused.[15]

c. Pregnancy: Many have proposed that pregnant women are at particularly high risk for battering; however, studies indicate that it is not pregnancy per se that puts women at risk for abuse, rather, the risk is due to their young age.[18] However, for those who are already in battering relationships, the violence may escalate during pregnancy.[19] Approximately 20 percent of pregnant women in the UK may have experienced severe abuse.[20]

d. Witnesses of parental violence: One finding is consistent across several studies: battered women are far more likely than nonvictims to have witnessed parental violence during their childhood.

> Younger women are more likely to be battered.

4. Who are the perpetrators?

a. Demographic characteristics: Compared with nonviolent men, men who batter are more likely to have lower income, lower education, and fewer socioeconomic resources.[21] Several studies found such men had low levels of assertiveness.[14]

b. Psychopathology: Men who batter tend to use higher quantities of alcohol than nonviolent men. Batterers have higher scores on anxiety, depression and negativity scales.[22] Many are diagnosed with personality disorders.[11]

> Men who batter differ from nonviolent men in intimacy, impulsivity and problem-solving skills.

c. Generally aggressive: In addition to physical abuse of women, men who batter are likely to be sexually violent and to be aggressive toward their children.[14]

d. Witnesses of parental violence.

> Like women who are battered, men who batter are very likely to have witnessed parental violence during their childhoods.

Table 24.1. Psychological consequences of battering in the woman

- More difficulty coping with anger or aggression
- Lower self-esteem
- Impaired ability to trust important others
- Higher scores on the depression, anger, confusion, fearfulness, paranoia, and social introversion scales of the Minnesota Multiphasic Personality Inventory (MMPI)
- Higher risk for chemical abuse
- Higher risk for suicide

Data from Carmen EH, Rieker PP, Mills T. Victims of violence and psychiatric illness. *Am J Psychiatry* 1984;**141**:378–83. Rosewater LB. Battered or schizophrenic? Psychological tests can't tell. In Yllo K, Bograd M, eds., *Feminist Perspectives on Wife Abuse*. Sage Publications, Newbury Park, CA, 1988, pp. 200–16.

Consequences of violence

Psychological consequences

1. Symptoms: Compared to nonvictims, battered women have many problems (Table 24.1).[23]
2. Diagnosis: Posttraumatic stress disorder (PTSD):
   a. Diagnostic criteria include elements of depression, anxiety, intrusive thoughts about victimization and avoidance of reminders of the abuse.
   b. Predictors of symptom severity include:
      i. Severity and the recentness of the violence.
      ii. Life threats within the relationship.
      iii. Few personal resources such as education, employment.
      iv. Low levels of social support.[24]

Acute medical consequences

1. Death: In 1992, more than 2000 people in the USA were known to be murdered by intimate others – spouses, ex-spouses, boyfriends or girlfriends.[1]
2. Physical trauma: Each year, 27 percent of battered women receive medical care and 15 percent require hospitalization.[1] In one study, battering accounted for one-half of all serious injuries women brought to the emergency room.[19] Compared to other female victims of accidents who visit the emergency department, battered women:
   a. make three times more visits to the emergency department,
   b. are more likely to have facial injuries,
   c. are 13 times more likely to have injuries in the chest, breasts, or abdomen,

d. are more likely to have multiple injuries, and to have injuries in various stages of healing.[19]

In 1992, more than 2000 people in the USA were known to be murdered by intimate others – spouses, ex-spouses, boyfriends or girlfriends.

Long-term medical consequences

Battered women often see their physicians for relief from vague, unremitting symptoms.[25]

1. Utilization: Female victims of assault visit primary care providers significantly more often than nonvictims, sustaining high utilization for years following the original assault.[3]

2. Health care costs for severely assaulted women are 2.5 times greater than for nonvictims.[3]

3. Common somatic symptoms of battered women include insomnia, fatigue, gastrointestinal symptoms, premenstrual symptoms, chronic pain, and anemia.[25]

4. Negative pregnancy outcomes include higher rates of abortion, stillbirths, and low birth-weight newborns.[26]

5. Negative health behaviors are more prevalent in battered women: eating disorders, substance abuse, risk for STDs and HIV.[25]

In addition to acute injuries, women who have been battered develop long-term health problems that appear to be unrelated to physical trauma.

Effects on children

The impact of violence in intimate relationships extends beyond the battered woman; children are also at risk.

1. Victims of violence: Men who batter their wives are also likely to be violent with their children.[14]

2. Infants who witness violence exhibit poor health, poor sleeping habits, and excessive screaming.[27]

3. Preschoolers show signs of terror exhibited as yelling, irritable behavior, hiding, shaking, and stuttering.[27]

4. School-age children experience more somatic complaints and regress to earlier stages of functioning.[27]

5. Adolescents may use aggression as a predominant form of problem solving, may project blame onto others, and may exhibit a high degree of anxiety (e.g., bite nails, pull hair, somatize feelings).[27]

6.   Adults: Adult children of battered women are likely to have violent relationships. The single most consistent predictor of becoming a batterer or a
battered wife is witnessing parental violence as a child.

The impact of violence in intimate relationships extends beyond the battered woman; children are also at
risk.

Screening for violence

1.   Many health care providers feel awkward asking women about emotionally
painful experiences. However, most women are accepting of such inquiries
and, in fact, often expect them. In a brief survey about family conflict, 261
family practice patients – including battered women and nonvictims – from
six private practices were asked "Do you think doctors should ask patients
about family stress or conflict?". Only 3 percent said, "No, never," while the
remainder – 97 percent – responded, "Yes, sometimes," or "Yes, often".[28]

2.   With some battered women, it may take several visits for her to develop
enough trust and confidence to reveal abuse. However, routinely asking about
abuse sends several positive messages: "This is legitimate medical business; I
am concerned about your safety and the stress in your life. I am willing to hear
about violence – it is not too shameful, deviant, or insignificant for us to
discuss. Furthermore, the situation is not hopeless, but can be changed."

3.   When should I ask about violence?
   a.   First visit: Primary care providers can ask about violence during an initial
getting-to-know-you visit in the context of a trauma, hospitalization, social
or sexual history.
   b.   Prevention visits: One can ask during annual or general examinations,
preemployment physical examinations, prenatal visits, well-baby visits,
premarital examinations, and adolescent general examinations and sports
physical examinations.
   c.   Signs of injury: One should get a good history of the cause of physical
trauma when injuries are present. Many battered women will have evidence of multiple injuries, in various stages of healing.
   d.   "Red flag" somatic complaints: When a woman presents with chronic pain
syndromes, gastrointestinal symptoms, sleep disturbances, signs of depression, problems in pregnancy, STDs, or substance abuse, the provider
should ask about violence.
   e.   Verbal clues: In the story presented at the beginning of this chapter, the

woman dropped a clue to her physician, referring to a misunderstanding with her husband. A woman's reference to marital conflict or controlling behaviors on the part of her partner is a signal to ask about violence.

f. Direct statements: When a woman states directly, "My husband hits me", the physician should gather a good history of the relationship, discuss local resources for assistance and support, and help the woman to formulate a plan for ending the violence.

4. How should I ask about violence?

a. Avoid abstract concepts. Do not use these words unless the woman uses them first: "violence", "abuse", "assault" or "rape". These abstract terms are subject to a variety of interpretations, but most individuals understand them to mean immoral, illegal, or abnormal behavior.

b. Many women with violent partners do not apply the term "abuse" to their relationships until the violence has progressed to very severe levels. To discover aggressive patterns *early*, a physician must use other terms. Women may be hesitant to apply the term "abuse" because of the following:

i. His behavior seems normal. For women who were raised by aggressive, controlling men, violent behavior may appear to be a normal male behavior.

ii. The term seems too severe. Many women may be hesitant to apply immoral, illegal, or abnormal terms to their husbands, especially if the violence has not yet progressed to severe levels.

iii. The progression of violence over time can delay her realization that the aggression is "abuse". A pattern of abuse generally begins with a minor aggressive event that is distressing but does not cause the couple to separate. A violent husband's impulse is to apologize deeply, then to justify his behavior so that he and his partner maintain the belief that he is a moral man. Over time, an abused woman will learn to tolerate and forgive more and more severe aggression. If she is isolated from those who might criticize his behavior, she is likely to tolerate even more violence. However, most abused women have a limit: if the children witness violence, if injuries occur, if her life is threatened, then she will recognize the behavior as dangerous or unreasonable and seek help.

c. Set the context for the screening questions, especially if the previous discussion seems unrelated to abuse. Professionals from the Family Peace

The single most important thing a physician can do for a battered woman is to ask about violence.

Project in Milwaukee use this approach: "In my practice I am concerned about prevention and safety, especially in the family."[29]

d. Do not assume the husband is the perpetrator. Ex-husbands and ex-boyfriends may be involved. Often, in abusive relationships, the violence does not end when the abuser moves out of the house. Men who are very possessive and controlling may in fact escalate their violent behaviors when they fear their control over the woman is threatened – as when she moves away.

e. Focus on behaviors. The screening question should focus on behaviors, such as hitting, hurting, or threatening.

f. Sample questions:

i. Does anyone in your life ever hit you or hurt you?

ii. Are you in a relationship now where you are afraid for your personal safety, or where someone is threatening you, hurting you, forcing you to have sex, or trying to control your life?

Do not use these words unless the woman uses them first: "violence", "abuse", "assault" or "rape".

Clinical interventions

The impact of violence on a woman's health and family life demands a comprehensive response from health care providers. Episodic treatment of acute injuries, while important, is not enough. In fact, some claim that ignoring violence works to enable men to keep hitting.[30] Effective interventions require a safe, collaborative, accepting patient–provider relationship, and a longitudinal approach.

Effective interventions require a safe, collaborative, accepting patient–provider relationship, and a longitudinal approach.

The clinical environment

1. Safety is addressed by protecting women's confidentiality. As with all patients, primary care providers should talk in private and assure confidentiality of their conversations. Some male partners may try to stay in the room during an office visit. The provider can respectfully address a partner's concerns about the woman's medical problems, then invite him to wait outside during the physical examination. At that time, confidential discussions may occur.

No information should be shared with the woman's partner without her permission. The present method of obstetrical care, with husband involvement, may reduce the chance for a battered woman to speak to the provider confidentially.

2. Collaboration: When a health care provider is working with battered women, a collaborative position provides the greatest benefit to the woman. Rather than using a directive and controlling approach – like a batterer – providers should model collaborative decision-making and encourage battered women to think independently of powerful others. The provider must recognize that the responsibility for change belongs to the woman, and that she knows best when a particular strategy, such as escape, will be safe or effective. The provider's role should be that of consultant and supporter, presenting intervention options to the woman and encouraging all steps toward safety.

3. Acceptance: A nonjudgmental approach is necessary, but not always easy. One study found that health care workers were sympathetic toward battered women who were taking action to change their life situation, but irritated with others whom they described as "passive", "evasive", or "uncooperative". These providers made more inappropriate referrals and discharge plans for battered women than other women. What the health care workers encountered in some women were behaviors that were adaptive in a violent environment – passivity, evasiveness, mistrust – but frustrating in the emergency room, where self-motivation and cooperation are expected. Understanding the source of troublesome behaviors will help the health care provider to maintain the objectivity needed to avoid mismanagement of battered women.

When a health care provider is working with battered women, a collaborative position provides the greatest benefit to the woman.

The intervention process

1. Assess "readiness for change": Battered women who are unwilling to change their living situations can be very frustrating for primary care providers. Before dispensing advice, the provider should assess the woman's readiness for change. J. O. Prochaska and colleagues have developed a model that describes an individual's progression through several steps of behavior change.[31] When working with battered women, consider one of six stages:

    a. Precontemplation is characterized by the statement, "My relationship is not a problem." In these relationships, the frequency and severity of violence may be low, and/or the women may believe their partners' aggression is normal or justified.

b. Contemplation is characterized by ambivalence: "I know the violence is a problem, but I need to stay in the marriage." Some women believe that the benefits of staying with their partners outweigh the costs of enduring the abuse. For others, low self-esteem, depression, or lack of support may render them incapable of making any change in the situation.

c. Preparation is characterized by, "I know the violence is a problem, and I'm planning changes." Women who change or leave violent relationships need preparation time. Some have to save money to move; some need to find employment; some must think through how they will explain the separation to family, friends, children and spouse; some must plan a very careful escape.

d. Action is characterized by "I am making changes to end the violence", and generally describes the early phase of the new lifestyle. This is an unstable period, when women discover the costs of change. Women who leave their partners will discover loneliness, uncertainty, poorer finances, and the entire burden of childrearing. Many partners will work very hard to get the women back into the relationship using seduction, or threats, or both. This phase is the most dangerous for women; partners who are extremely controlling will exaggerate their measures of coercion when challenged by separation. Most women will find the change too difficult and go back into the relationship. However, when violence reemerges, most women will try to leave again.

e. Maintenance is characterized by "I have adapted to the changes I have made". This stage begins about six months after the change.

f. Relapse is a normal occurrence when making major life changes such as leaving a violent marriage. As mentioned above, leaving is a challenge of authority, and many ex-husbands will work very hard to bring their wives back into the relationship, using both seductive and coercive techniques.

2. Tailor conversations to the stage of change: Health care providers can best enable a woman to change violent relationships when they begin "where the woman is", help her to assess her situation, and nudge her along the continuum of readiness to change. A continuity-of-care practice, where providers see patients several times over long periods, is an ideal setting to encourage the next step. Table 24.2 lists some "nudging strategies" to help women to develop the motivation to move to the next stage. In these discussions, the provider should express concern for the patient's safety and health, and willingness to discuss relationship issues at any time. Even if the woman is reluctant to change her relationship now, she should know that the physician is a source of support and information when she is ready.

3. Assess danger: Primary care providers should help battered women to assess

Table 24.2. "Stages of change" for battered women

Stages of change	Patient's belief	Physician "nudging" strategies
Precontemplation	"My relationship is not a problem."	Learn about the relationship: "Tell me how you and your partner handle conflict in your relationship." "What kinds of arguments are problematic for you?"
Contemplation or ambivalence	"I know the violence is a problem, but I need to stay in the marriage."	Discuss the ambivalence: "What are the good things about your relationship? What are the not-so-good things?" "How would you change things in your relationship if you could?"
Preparation	"The violence is a problem, and I'm planning some changes."	Offer support and encouragement Clarify plans List community resources Provide anticipatory guidance
Action	"I am making changes to end the violence."	Offer support and encouragement List community resources Provide anticipatory guidance Review coping strategies
Maintenance	"I have adapted to the changes."	Offer support Review need for community resources Discuss coping strategies
Relapse	"I cannot maintain this change."	Remain positive and encouraging Discuss the lessons learned from the effort Review "safe plan" Remain open for future discussions about the relationship

Data from Prochaska JO, Velicer WF, Rossi JS et al. Stages of change and decisional balance for 12 problem behaviors. *Health Psychol* 1994;**13**:39–46.

the danger that the violent partner presents. Prior to discharging a woman from care, the provider can ask, "Do you feel safe going home?" If the answer is negative, providers can present and discuss other options. Other signs of danger and lethality are listed in Table 24.3.

4. Inquiry about child safety: Providers should inquire about the safety of the

Table 24.3. Indications of danger or lethality in a battering relationship

- Severity of past violence
- Increasing severity over time
- Extreme controlling behaviors
- Life transitions such as pregnancy, separation or divorce
- Drug and alcohol abuse
- Availability of weapons
- History of violence/suicide attempts in partner

Data from American Medical Association. *Diagnostic and Treatment Guidelines on Domestic Violence.* AMA, Chicago IL, 1992.

children. If child abuse has occurred, the physician is obligated to report the situation to Child Protective Services.

5. Develop an emergency "safe-plan": If the physician determines that a woman is in danger of serious harm from her partner, but she is not yet ready to leave the relationship, the physician should encourage her to develop a "safe-plan" that can be implemented in an emergency. The physician can begin with a statement of concern, then assess the woman's preparedness to escape: "I am concerned that your husband will hurt you badly next time he gets angry. Can you recognize his potential for danger before he actually hurts you? Do you have a plan to get away from him quickly?" Discussion should address predicting the next episode of violence, whether to leave the house, when to leave, where to go, how to arrange transportation, how long to stay away, what to take (clothes, money, important papers), and whether to get legal protection. Most women have resources that allow them some respite and protection, such as a relative who will temporarily shelter them, but others will need public assistance. For this reason, the physician needs to be acquainted with local agencies who can provide shelter and services to battered women.

6. Describe community resources: Another important service health care providers can offer to battered women is a description of community resources that may help to change violent relationships.

   a. Resources for battered women: Table 24.4 lists a variety of resources that may help battered women. These agencies guide women to basic resources such as food, shelter, jobs, and legal assistance, and offer emotional support.

Prior to discharging a woman from care, the provider can ask, "Do you feel safe going home?"

Table 24.4. Referrals and community resources to help battered women

- Battered women's shelters
- Treatment programs for men who batter
- Women's centers
- Mental health centers
- Private psychotherapist or psychiatrist
- Clergy
- Support groups for battered women
- Family counselling clinics
- Alcoholics Anonymous, if appropriate
- Narcotics Anonymous, if appropriate
- Al-Anon groups
- Legal advocacy
- Police
- Emergency services telephone number

Data from American Medical Association. *Diagnostic and Treatment Guidelines on Domestic Violence.* AMA, Chicago, IL, 1992.

b. Resources for men who batter: Many communities have treatment programs for men who batter. Many batterers' programs involve several weeks of group therapy, followed by individual therapy. Most men who attend batterer's programs are mandated into treatment by the courts; however, therapists generally welcome self-referrals and physician-referrals as well.

c. Resources for couples: Couples therapy is *not* recommended for violent relationships. Women who are battered are not free to speak their minds in therapy where the abuser is present; women may be physically punished for things they say to a couples therapist. Instead, the health care provider may want to recommend individual psychotherapy for each partner. While there is no research on interventions for men at early stages of violent relationships, or on men exhibiting common couple violence, individual psychotherapy will certainly benefit the woman in the relationship. If the male partner is both controlling and physically aggressive, batterers' programs, described above, may be a more appropriate referral.

If the physician determines that a woman is in danger of serious harm from her partner, but she is not yet ready to leave the relationship, the physician should encourage her to develop a "safe plan".

7. Documentation: Well-documented medical records are important for any health problem, but are especially useful when the health care provider is following conditions with long-term effects, such as victimization. For bat-

Table 24.5. Guidelines for photographs

- Take photos before medical treatment (if possible)
- Use color film with a color standard
- Photograph from different angles, full body and close-up
- Hold up a coin, ruler, or other object to illustrate the size of an injury
- Include the woman's face in at least one picture
- Take two pictures of each major trauma area
- Mark photographs precisely, including the woman's name, location of injury, names of the photographer, and others present

tered women, the medical record also represents legal evidence about the violence. The American Medical Association recommends inclusion of the following, especially for women seen soon after a violent event.[32]

a. Subjective description: Document the chief complaint and an objective description of the violent event, using the woman's own words whenever possible. The health care provider's interpretations (e.g., "patient was abused") should not be included. The record should contain a complete medical history and a relevant social history.

b. Objective description of injuries: The health care provider should provide a detailed description of injuries, including type, number, size, location, resolution, and possible causes. Use of a body-map is recommended. The woman's explanations of the injuries and the provider's opinion about the adequacy of those explanations should be recorded.

c. Photographs: Color photographs are useful only if they clearly portray an injury. Photographs with subtle or unidentifiable findings can be used against a woman in court as evidence that the injuries were not very serious (Table 24.5).

d. Laboratory findings: The documentation must include results from all pertinent laboratory tests and diagnostic procedures. Imaging studies can be particularly useful as legal evidence.

e. Police involvement: If the police are called, record the name of the officer, the actions taken, and the case number.

f. Follow-up is necessary: Options discussed in the physician's office require contemplation, planning, and time on the part of the woman. Physicians should use regular appointments or phone conversations to monitor safety and the decision-making process. One discussion does not "cure" violence in relationships, but continuing communication, support, and exploration of options will empower women to make changes that eliminate violence from their lives.

Couples therapy is *not* recommended for violent relationships.

Violence prevention in primary care settings

Primary prevention

Good education of parents may prevent violence before it happens. Teach parents what to expect from their children at every level of development, reviewing cognitive as well as physical and motor expectations. Offer parents nonviolent options for disciplining their children. Allow them to ventilate about the frustrations of parenting, and to discuss the impact of parenthood on their intimate relationship. If partner/spousal conflict becomes serious, remind them that they are the models for their children's future relationships, and guide them to appropriate therapy. Avoiding violence in this generation should also influence relationships in the next generation.

Secondary prevention

1. Especially with young men and women, ask about the quality of their relationships. If they describe "fights" or "problems with temper", ask them about hitting or hurting each other, and ask about their parents' relationships. People in the early stages of aggressive relationships may not identify violent behaviors as an ongoing problem.
2. Men who hit are very remorseful, and women who are hurt are convinced that these events are rare. Both believe the violence will never happen again.
3. Express concern about physical fights. Describe negative consequences for couples where deliberate harm is inflicted: injuries, divorce, arrest, emotional distress in their children, and adult children who become batterers or victims.
4. Offer to refer them to psychotherapists, or to groups for batterers and victims of violence. At this point, it may be difficult to determine whether the hitting is an early stage of patriarchal terrorism, or the pattern described as common couple violence.
5. Close follow-up will help determine the exact nature of the relationship and provide more opportunities for intervention.

Tertiary prevention

1. Currently, tertiary prevention is our country's most common violence prevention strategy. Action is taken when professionals identify a chronic and dangerous pattern of behaviors. At this late stage, it is difficult to save the

marriage, and the "treatment of choice" for many professionals is to get the woman out of the relationship before further harm is done.

2. When speaking to the battered woman, acknowledge the strength it requires to endure the stress inherent in her daily life. Assess current levels of danger and her readiness to change.

3. Label the violence as a problem, and inform her that there are options she can consider. In a collaborative fashion, list those options with her input.

4. Ask her to devise an escape plan in the event that the batterer becomes dangerous again. Document injuries.

5. Follow-up frequently in order to assess ongoing levels of danger, and to provide her with a place of safety and support.

Conclusions

Primary care providers are in an ideal position to contribute significantly to violence prevention in America. In the context of sustained patient–provider relationships, where all aspects of health are addressed – biomedical, psychological, and social – primary care providers are able to identify life patterns that indicate risk for victimization. Battered women are well served by providers who routinely ask about victimization, treat health consequences of battering, provide information and encouragement, guide women to effective community resources, and offer emotional support through the long journey to end violence.

REFERENCES

1. United States Department of Justice. *Violence between intimates.* Bureau of Justice Statistics: Selected Findings. ncj-149259. 94. Bureau of Justice, Washington, DC.
2. Richardson J, Feder G. Domestic violence against women. *BMJ* 1995;**311**:964–5.
3. Koss MP, Woodruff WJ, Koss PG. Relation of criminal victimization to health perceptions among women medical patients. *J Consult Clin Psychol* 1990;**58**:147–52.
4. Golding JM, Siegel JM, Sorenson SB, Burnam MA, Stein JA. Social support sources following sexual assault. *J Commun Psychol* 1989;**17**:92–107.
5. Gottlieb S. Doctors could have greater role in spotting domestic violence. *BMJ* 1998;**317**:99.
6. Donaldson MS, Yordy KD, Lohr KN, Vanselow NA, eds. *Primary Care: America's Health in a New Era.* National Academy Press, Washington, DC, 1996.
7. Englander EK. Understanding Violence. Lawrence Erlbaum Associates, Mahwah, NJ, 1997.

8. Straus MA, Gelles RJ. Societal change and change in family violence from 1975 to 1985 as revealed by two national surveys. *J Marriage Fam* 1986;**48**:465–79.

9. Straus MA, Gelles RJ, Steinmetz SK. *Behind Closed Doors: Violence in the American Family.* Doubleday, Garden City, NY, 1980.

10. Elliott BA, Johnson MM. Domestic violence in a primary care setting. Patterns and prevalence. *Arch Fam Med* 1995;**4**:113–19.

11. Dutton DG. *The Abusive Personality: Violence and Control in Intimate Relationships.* Guilford Press, New York, 1998.

12. Lee WV, Weinstein SP. How far have we come? A critical review of the research on men who batter. *Rec Dev Alcohol* 1997;**13**:337–56.

13. Yllo K. Sexual equality and violence against wives in American states. *J Comp Family Studies* 1983;**14**:67–86.

14. Hotaling GR, Sugarman DB. An analysis of risk markers in husband-to-wife violence: The current state of knowledge. *Violence Vict* 1986;**1**:101–24.

15. Giles-Sims J. *Wife Battering: A Systems Theory Approach.* Guilford Press, New York, 1983.

16. Johnson MP. Patriarchal terrorism and common couple violence: Two forms of violence against women. *J Marriage Fam* 1995;**57**:283–94.

17. Pence E, Paymar M. *Education Groups for Men Who Batter: The Duluth Model.* Springer-Verlag, New York, 1993.

18. Gelles RJ. Violence and pregnancy: Are pregnant women at greater risk of abuse? In Straus MA, Gelles RJ, ed., *Physical Violence in American Families: Risk Factors and Adaptations to Violence in 8,145 Families.* Transaction Publishers, New Brunswick, NJ, 1995, pp. 279–86.

19. Stark E, Flitcraft A. *Women at Risk: Domestic Violence and Women's Health.* Sage Publications, Thousand Oaks, 1996.

20. Abbasi K. Obstetricians must ask about domestic violence. *BMJ* 1998;**316**:7.

21. Barnett OW, Hamberger LK. The assessment of maritally violent men on the California Psychological Inventory. *Violence Vict* 1992;**7**:15–28.

22. Hastings JE, Hamberger LK. Psychosocial modifiers of psychopathology for domestically violent and nonviolent men. *Psychol Rep* 1994;**74**:112–14.

23. Carmen EH, Rieker PP, Mills T. Victims of violence and psychiatric illness. *Am J Psychiatry* 1984;**141**:378–83.

24. Houskamp BM, Foy DW. The assessment of posttraumatic stress disorder in battered women. *J Interpersonal Violence* 1991;**6**:367–75.

25. Koss MP, Heslet L. Somatic consequences of violence against women. *Arch Fam Med* 1992;**1**:53–59.

26. Helton AS, McFarlane J, Anderson ET. Battered and pregnant: A prevalence study. *Am J Public Health* 1987;**77**:1337–9.

27. Jaffe PG, Wolfe DA, Wilson SK. *Children of Battered Women.* Sage Publications, Newbury Park, CA, 1990.

28. Burge SK, Schneider FD, Ivy L. Patients' advice to physicians about working with family conflict, 1995. Unpublished report.

29. Ambuel B, Brownell EE, Hamberger LK. Implementing a community model for training medical students and physicians to diagnose, treat, and prevent family violence, 1994. Milwaukee. Personal communication.

30. Stark E, Flitcraft A, Frazier W. Medicine and patriarchal violence: The social construction of a "private" event. *Int J Health Serv* 1979;**9**:461–93.

31. Prochaska JO, Velicer WF, Rossi JS et al. Stages of change and decisional balance for 12 problem behaviors. *Health Psychol* 1994;**13**:39–46.

32. American Medical Association. *Diagnostic and Treatment Guidelines on Domestic Violence.* American Medical Association, Chicago, 1992.

25 Rape and the consequences of sexual assault

Jo Ann Rosenfeld, MD, Amy Ellwood, MSW, and Patricia Lenahan, MA

Sexual assault is the fastest growing crime in America. Women are the targets of rape, the most underreported violent crime. Conviction rates for rape are poor. Sexual assault induces a life crisis, which inflicts major psychological and physiological trauma upon the victim. Health care providers must understand the horrific nature of this violent crime. Understanding the context of the assault, the type of rapist, as well as the sexual and violent acts forced on the victim will help physicians in providing appropriate care. Family physicians uniquely can monitor and provide care in the postassault period because many women do not report rapes or utilize rape crisis centers.

Definitions

1. "A sex offender is a person who has been legally convicted as a result of an overt act, committed by him for his own immediate sexual gratification, which is contrary to the prevailing sexual mores of the society in which he lives and/or is legally punishable."[1]
2. Sexual crimes may be perpetrated by mentally disordered individuals or may be part of a person's underlying personality disorder. Some sexually deviant acts arise in the context of traumatic brain injury, psychoses or mental retardation. Some authors believe that rapists meet criteria for having a paraphilia.
3. Rape is the nonconsensual oral, anal, or vaginal penetration obtained by force, with threat of bodily harm, or when the victim is incapable of giving consent. The legal definition in the USA varies from state to state. Most definitions include the use of threat, duress, physical force, intimidation, or deception, sexual contact, and nonconsent of the victim.[2]

4.   Feminists describe rape as a hostile, forcible act aimed at dominating, degrading, and humiliating the victim.[3]
5.   Sexual assault is a crime of violence but includes a wide range of sexual acts. Some sexual assaults occur quickly, while others take hours or occasionally days.[4]
6.   The predominant fear of most rape victims is death.[5]
7.   The majority of victims are women and most assailants are men. Male rape including gay rape has become increasingly recognized. This chapter focuses on the female victims of sexual assault.

Incidence

1.   Rape is vastly underreported. Yet in 1996, for every 1000 individuals aged 12 years or older, there occurred one rape or sexual assault, two assaults with serious injury, and five robberies.[6]
2.   Attempted rape is more common than completed rape and more victims are familiar with their assailants.
3.   The assailants rape a victim of the same race in 69 percent of cases.[7]
4.   Women, regardless of their age, health status or physical attractiveness are all potential rape victims.
5.   The Federal Bureau of Investigation (FBI) speculates that one in five murders of women are sex related.[8]

Attempted rape is more common than complete rape and more victims are familiar with their assailants.

Types of sexual assault

1.   The context of the assault is important in understanding the stress experienced by the victim. There are many myths about rape.
2.   One major myth is that sexual assault is a spur of the moment event, perpetrated by a stranger lurking in a dark place.
     a. Actually, stranger rape is less common than acquaintance or marital rape but is more likely to be reported. Sexual assault occurs more frequently in a woman's home, workplace or car and is usually well planned.[9]
     b. In confidence rape, the victim knows the offender and the victim's realization of the danger is gradual. The victim has spent time with the offender, who was nonviolent, but she is more likely to resist.

c. Resistance may not always result in injury but a lack of physical injury should not imply consent. Through deceit, the offender gains the victim's trust then betrays that trust.

d. Confidence rape victims and assailants may have used alcohol or drugs before the assault. Confidence assaults are more prolonged, sometimes taking more than five hours.

e. Self-blame is common in the confidence rape victim because of the non-violent interaction that existed prior to the assault. This type of rape may have delayed reporting because of the victim's feelings of shame for somehow having "caused" the attack.

3. Delayed reporting may also occur because of impaired cognitive processing, altered states of consciousness and cognitive dissonance.[10] Examples include the following: rape by health care providers during medical procedures while the patient is under anesthesia, rape of a comatose person or those with head injury, rape while being asleep or rape of a demented person. If a woman is choked during the assault there may be a loss of oxygen to the brain resulting in hypoxia.[10] Hypoxia can produce diminished memory and result in delayed reporting.

4. Victimization by authority figures may result in confusion. The victim may not know what is a legitimate physical procedure. She may fear retaliation by the clinician or fear that authorities will take the clinician's word over hers. The victim may be too ashamed to report the assault or may feel that she is responsible.

5. Recently, flunitrazepam or Rohypnol has gained notoriety as the "date rape drug".[11] Street names for this drug include: Rochies, Roofies, Ruffies, Roches, Mexican Valium, R-2 and Roach-2.[12] This drug is legally available in Mexico and Central and South America, and its use has been reported in Florida, Texas, and Southern California. The drug dissolves readily and is colorless, odorless, and tasteless. The unsuspecting woman is not able to detect the drug placed in her drink by the rapist. The victim may have a drink at a bar or someone's home and wake up partially clothed or nude in a strange bed with no recollection of the previous events. Rohypnol is also sold at special "techno" dance parties that teenagers and young adults call "raves". Physicians should consider testing for flunitrazepam when women present with altered mental status, amnesia for recent events in association with clinical suspicion for sexual assault. Physicians and counsellors must educate them-

Resistance may not always result in injury but a lack of physical injury should not imply consent.

selves and their students about the use of drugs in association with date or acquaintance rape.

6. Acquaintance or date rape is the most common type of sexual assault. Of victims who contact rape crisis centers, 70 to 80 percent are victims of acquaintance rape.[13] A survey of 32 college campuses by the US National Institute of Mental Health indicated that one in four women were victims of rape or attempted rape. However, date rape usually goes unreported due to victims' feelings of shame and self-blame.

7. Blitz rape is a sudden surprise attack by a stranger.
   a. Blitz rape victims are more likely to be confronted with a weapon, abducted, and threatened with murder.
   b. These assaults tend to occur in the victim's home or familiar outdoor location.
   c. Blitz victims may be exposed to greater threats to life and experience more subjective terror.
   d. The survivor of a blitz attack may suffer from problems of autonomically based posttraumatic symptoms such as nightmares, flashback, panic episodes, and a heightened startle response.[14]

8. Gang rapes with multiple assailants are more common among adolescents and college students.[15]
   a. More alcohol, drugs, fewer weapons, more night attacks, less victim resistance, and more severe sexual assault outcomes characterize gang rapes as compared with individual rapes.
   b. Most gang rapes are completed and the victims experience more forced sexual acts.
   c. Gang rape victims are more likely to report the incident to police and to have contemplated suicide in the postassault period.[16]

9. Marital rape is often an act in the continuum of violence in domestic abuse. Until recently it was not considered a crime.
   a. Victims of marital rape suffer the additional burdens of legal and attitudinal discrimination as compared with victims of stranger rape.[17]
   b. Historically, women were viewed as possessions. This view has influenced attitudes toward spousal rape because it may be assumed that a married woman has given consent for sexual intercourse in the marriage contract.
   c. This type of assault is often repetitive and more violent. It is less commonly reported because of economic considerations, fear of violence being directed toward the children or pets, or fear of death.

Physicians should consider testing for flunitrazepam when women present with altered mental status, amnesia for recent events in association with clinical suspicion for sexual assault.

    d. Some women agree to marital rape to minimize the amount of abuse they have to suffer. Physicians assessing their women patients for abuse should consider spousal rape.

> Marital rape is often an act in the continuum of violence in domestic abuse.

Victim responses

Initial response

1. Sexual assault is a crime of violence and inflicts major psychological and physiological trauma on the victim.
2. During the attack, the victim has to decide whether to fight back or to cooperate to stay alive.
3. The feelings of terror and helplessness may impair the ability to think clearly resulting in confusion and disorientation. Some victims experience disassociation during the attack and feel as if they are outside of their body.
4. A. W. Burgess first coined the term "rape trauma syndrome".[18] She found victims during the immediate response phase to have either controlled or expressed emotions. Immediately after a sexual assault, a victim may experience a wide range of emotions: crying, shock, disbelief, fear, anxiety, anger, restlessness, guilt, shame, and fear associated with a life-threatening event. The world is no longer seen as a safe place.[19]
5. In the controlled style, the feelings of the victim may be masked in a calm, composed or subdued affect. Immediate physical reactions may include overall soreness, abdominal and genital pain, headache and nausea. Realization of the assault and brush with death may not occur while in the health care setting.[5]

> Sexual assault is a crime of violence and inflicts major psychological and physiological trauma on the victim.

Intermediate phase

1. The intermediate or recoil phase begins several days or weeks after the attack and has components of denial, symptom formation, and anger.[20] The victim may fear to be alone and exhibit hypervigilance. Denial is the victim's attempt to gain anonymity. A woman may change her telephone number, residence, the lock on her front door or her job. Some women take up karate or weight lifting to be better able to defend themselves against men.[21]
2. In the anger phase, the woman may direct anger at the assailant, all men, the therapist, the physician and/or the legal system. Prosecution provides a focus

for the anger and restoring a sense of control. Some victims may have an exacerbation of symptoms during the trial or sentencing.

3. The final phase of resolution occurs when the assault becomes part of the past in a meaningful way and when the woman can discuss the rape without undue emotion. At this point the woman becomes more independent and self-reliant, and has a more positive view of herself. This phase depends on the individual and may take from six months to two years.

> In the anger phase, the woman may direct anger at the assailant, all men, the therapist, the physician and/or the legal system.

Long-term psychological sequelae

1. Long-term follow-up and research on the psychological sequelae has been difficult. Many studies are limited to one year due to difficulty in maintaining victim samples. Retrospective studies are difficult due to the victims' symptoms of shame, fear, depression, and their hesitation to seek psychological treatment.

2. Those who do come for follow-up see their primary care physicians and have physical complaints that are related to the assault, but most have normal physical findings.[7]

Long-term effects

1. Trauma, whether it is rape or a series of events such as incestuous abuse of a child, has permanent effects on the survivor. The psychobiology of an overwhelming experience is stored in the visceral sensations instead of being stored in the declarative memory.[22] The visceral sensations may be anxiety, nightmares, or flashbacks.

2. For some survivors, the posttraumatic stress response fades over time.

3. However, for others the response can elicit feelings that are as vivid as the original event happening again. The body's emotional response cannot be relied on to give signals and indicate how to act. A woman may have an intense response to stimuli that are reminders of the rape. It might be a certain odor, a location similar to the site of the original sexual assault, or music that was played during the assault.

   These stimuli can trigger vivid recollections of the event. For example, if a physician is going to do an invasive procedure such as a Pap smear or rectal examination the woman may respond with an aversive reaction to penetration.[23]

   For women who have experienced forced anal penetration, a sense of re-victimization may occur during invasive procedures such as flexible sig-moidoscopy. Women patients may integrate their experiences of distressing treatment if they know what to expect and have some control in the treatment setting.

4. Many researchers have found survivors of rape to have depression, anxiety, sadness, anhedonia, sexual dysfunction, and sleep disruption in the first two years after sexual assault.[20,24] Those who perceived that they had higher levels of control in their lives had lower rates of depression, while those with low perceived levels of control had increased rates of depression.

5. Women who had been previously raped or experienced child sexual abuse had high rates of depression. One study reported that 22 percent of sexual assault victims made a suicide attempt or seriously began to abuse drugs or alcohol after the assault.[10] Many survivors have haunting intrusive recollec-tions of the rape. Some have revenge obsessions while others experience a paradoxical gratitude for the gift of life if they were threatened with death during the assault.

Victims

Adolescent women, married women, elderly women, and lesbian women are also targets of sex offenders.

1. Adolescent women and girls often know the assailant. Alcohol or drugs are often used prior to the assault. Adolescent victims are less likely to sustain physical injury and weapons are infrequently used to subdue the adoles-cent.[25]

2. Elderly rape victims tend to live alone and allow the strangers into their homes. Most of these rapes occur during daylight hours and are associated with theft. Physical force is frequently involved and the severity of the injury is high.[3] P. S. Cartwright and R. A. Moore's study of elderly rape victims found that the victim was more often white and the assailant black than in younger victims. Their data suggested that the rapists of elderly women are of a serial nature and these rapists are motivated by racially generated anger to express power.[26]

3. Lesbian women, as members of a stigmatized group, are often targeted for attack because of their sexual orientation by antigay attackers. Humiliation and degradation are common components of sexual victimization. Anti-lesbian rape may include attempts by the perpetrator to degrade lesbian sexuality. When behaviors that were formerly expressions of love are asso-

ciated with humiliation and violence, lesbian partners, as heterosexual women do, may experience problems defining their sexuality in a positive manner. When a woman is attacked because she is lesbian, the negative psychological consequences converge with those resulting from societal heterosexism to create additional challenges for the lesbian survivor of sexual assault.[27]

Elderly rape victims tend to live alone and allow the strangers into their homes.

Social support following sexual assault

Significant others reactions

1. The woman's family, husband, intimate partner and friends share the impact of rape. Social support is the single most important factor influencing recovery in the post assault period.[20]
2. Those close to the victim suffer distress and have often been termed "secondary victims" of the sexual assault.[19] Clinicians working with rape victims should be aware that there is a strong probability that female family and friends may experience a heightened fear of crime. They may also have secondary posttraumatic stress symptoms including intrusive thoughts of the rape.
3. The intimate partner's response has a significant impact on the victim's recovery. Unsupportive behavior, including emotional withdrawal and blaming the victim, may be detrimental to a woman's self-esteem. Often a romantic partner may not be aware of the negative impact of his/her behavior and may need help from the clinician in understanding the role he/she plays in the victim's recovery. The social support network provides a context for feeling loved, valued, secure, and esteemed.

Social support is the single most important factor influencing recovery in the post assault period.

Family reactions

1. Sexual assault has a rippling effect on the family system. Following the assault, the family homeostasis may be disrupted. Each member begins a process of healing. This can be a complex process, since the victim and family members may be at different stages of recovery at different times in the family life cycle.
2. Family members may feel guilt for not having prevented the rape. They

may not know what to do or say to help the victim. They may become overprotective or intrusive in the victim's life. Family anxiety about the victim's safety may prolong the recovery process.

3. Coping style of families, cultural views of the meaning of rape, and prior functioning are factors influencing recovery. Families with chronically disturbed relationships, role inflexibility, few resources, externalized blaming, and poor communication will have a negative impact on the victim's recovery.[28]

4. Families with healthy relationships are better able to recover from any crisis. Supportive friends and family members must be able to adapt to the changed behavior and mood of the victim following sexual assault. The victim who is able to integrate and resolve sexual trauma usually has a strong social support system.

Families with healthy relationships are better able to recover from any crisis.

Implications

1. Emotional support from friends and family is highly related to better recovery than emotional support from other sources. Police and physicians appear to be the least helpful in the long-term recovery process.[29]

2. However, victims are more likely to seek treatment from primary care physicians than from mental health clinicians or victim assistance.[30] Primary care physicians may be the initial point of contact for traumatized persons who have high levels of health care utilization postassault.

3. As a group, crime victims perceive their health to be poor.[31] Sexual assault by strangers and spouses has a significant positive association with poor subjective health.[32] As a result, somatic complaints are common among those victims who utilize the health care system. Somatic complaints are the ticket of admission to the medical system, which is not associated with the criminal justice or mental health system. The medical system may be more accessible to many victims who are reluctant to use victim compensation resources.

4. There is a significant relationship between sexual and/or physical abuse and the use of outpatient health care and pain medication in patients with fibromyalgia.[33] With increased utilization of the health care system by assault and crime victims, physicians' education needs to be expanded.

5. Material on rape should be integrated into medical, dental, and nursing education. Obtaining a sexual trauma history should be included in the history and physical examinations of all women patients. Physicians should provide the rape survivor with sensitive, compassionate care that includes

close-focused follow-up and preservation of the physical evidence should the victim choose to prosecute.[34]

6. Mental health professionals should be cognizant of the physical as well as behavioral sequelae in their postsexual assault clients. Health care professionals working collaboratively can play a major role in healing the physical and psychological wounds of sexual trauma.

Medical evaluation of rape victims

Place

This can occur in the emergency room, although many women come to their family or primary care physician. The family physician must be involved in the follow-up care and coordination of psychological and trauma counselling.

Providers

Sensitive and direct questioning and examination is necessary. A team approach can facilitate the necessary examination.

History

1. A complete history of the assault, in the words of the patient, is needed.
2. A complete discussion is necessary of sites of trauma, including those not in the genitalia, possibility of ejaculation, and the areas of penetration. Oral and anal penetration occurs in 20 to 35 percent of rapes.[35]
3. Inquiring into the family situation, safety and where the woman can go to stay after the visit is important.
4. A menstrual, medical, and gynecological history and details of contraceptive use must be obtained.

Examination

1. This must be done in a sensitive and respectful manner. If the rape was recent, evidence for legal prosecution will have to be obtained. If the rape was remote (> 24 hours), this may be impossible. In either case, pictures of lesions and trauma are important.
2. A complete physical examination with documentation of all injuries and state of areas of trauma is important. The physician should look for bruises, lacerations, and bite marks. A complete gynecological examination is mandatory, although the experience may be difficult for the patient. The physician should

Table 25.1. Laboratory studies of a rape victim

Immediately
- Legal
  - Pubic hair scrapings
  - Vaginal vault content sampling for semen determination of acid phosphatase
  - Ejaculate collection
- STD
  - Cultures of samples from cervix, throat, and anus for gonorrhea, *Chlamydia*, herpes simplex virus
  - Wet preparation for *Trichomonas*, *Candida*, *Gardnerella*
  - Blood tests for syphilis, HIV, hepatitis B and frozen serum for future testing
- Pregnancy test

Postrape
- At 2–3 weeks: Pregnancy test
- At 6 weeks: Syphilis, HIV, hepatitis B, gonorrhea and *Chlamydia*
- At 3–6 months: HIV test

explain the importance and move through the procedure slowly and sensitively. Examination for trauma, pregnancy, or infection is important. An anal examination for cultures, signs of trauma, fissures or bleeding is also important.

3. An estimation of emotional state and need for immediate psychological support should be considered.

Laboratory evaluation (Table 25.1)

1. Laboratory examination is performed to document rape legally and medically, determine preexisting pregnancy or STD, and discover acquired STDs or pregnancy.

2. Legal evidence should be obtained as soon as possible. A rape "kit" should be available in emergency rooms. Scrapings of hair, semen, wet preparation for sperm, any clothing fibers, and vaginal vault content analysis (for semen and acid phosphatase) should be properly obtained in sterile containers and marked.

3. Serological tests for syphilis, HIV, and hepatitis B should be obtained immediately. Samples from the cervix, pharynx, and anus should be cultured for gonorrhea, *Chlamydia* and herpes simplex virus. A wet preparation should be examined for *Trichomonas*, *Gardnerella* and *Candida*.

4. A pregnancy test should be obtained immediately.

Table 25.2. Medical treatment immediately postrape

- STD prophylaxis
  Ceftriaxone 250 mg i.m. or 3.0 g amoxicillin (with 1.0 g probenecid), or ciprofloxacin
  500 mg p.o. or cefixime 400 mg p.o.
  PLUS
  doxycycline (100 mg b.i.d. for 7–10 days) or erythromycin (EES 800 m.g. q.i.d. for 7 days)
  or amoxicillin 500 mg b.i.d. for 7 days
- HIV prophylaxis
  Zidovudine (retrovir) 200 mg p.o. t.i.d. for 4 weeks
  PLUS
  lamivudine 150 mg p.o. b.i.d. for 4 weeks
- Hepatitus B virus vaccine
  1 mL i.m. at 0, 1, and 6 months
  AND/OR
  hepatitis B immunoglobulin (0.06 mL/kg i.m. single dose)
- Tetanus toxoid
- Offer postcoital contraception (if not on an effective continuous contraceptive)
  Various preparations of OCPs
    Ovral 2 immediately and 2 in 12 hours
    Lo Ovral 4 immediately and 4 in 12 hours
    Levonorgestrel
    Prevens[R]
  Immediate placement of IUD

Medical treatment

Repair

Trauma with rape is common. After lesions are examined, documented, and photographed, suturing and even surgery may be needed. Four percent of rape victims need surgery for repair of genital trauma.[36] Pain relief, analgesia, and antibiotic orally and topically may be needed.

Infection (Table 25.2)

1. Pregnancy: Emergency contraception should be offered (see Table 25.2 and Chapter 10).
2. Prophylactic therapy (see Table 25.2).
   a. Prophylactic treatment against gonorrhea and chlamydia is indicated, as is HIV prophylaxis.
   b. Hepatitis B prophylaxis should be given, if the woman has not had hepatitis B vaccine or the disease previously.
   c. Tetanus prophylaxis may be needed if there are lacerations.

Tetanus prophylaxis

Provide if needed.

Immediate psychotropic drugs

The need for this must be evaluated individually. Most experts do not believe that sedation should be given. If it is given, short-term medication only should be used until further evalution can be accomplished.

Long-term medication

The use of long-term psychotropic medication must be determined in follow-up evaluations.

Follow-up

1. Follow-up is very important both medically and, as discussed above, psychologically. Appointments should be scheduled for two to three weeks, six weeks and at three and six months for further evaluation.
2. Further laboratory evaluation for transmission of STDs and pregnancy should occur as detailed in Table 25.1.
3. Through a thorough understanding and continuing relationship and therapy the rape victim will be able to cope better with her trauma.

Conclusions

Sexual assault is serious and induces a life crisis, which inflicts major psychological and physiological trauma upon the victim. Sensitive physician involvement is important. Specific treatment and testing for pregnancy and infectious STDs is required.

REFERENCES

1. Zonana HV, Norko MA. Forensic psychiatry: Sexual predators. *Psychiatr Clin North Am* 1999;**22**:1–18.
2. Koss M. Rape: Scope, interventions and public policy responses. *Am Psychol* 1993;**48**:1062–9.
3. Tyra P. Older women: Victims of rape. *J Gerontol Nurs* 1993;**19**:7–12.

4. Holmstrom LL, Burgess AW. Sexual behavior of assailants during reported rapes. *Arch Sex Behav* 1980;**9**:427–39.

5. Dupre AR, Hampton HL, Morrison H, Meeks GR. Sexual assault. *Obstet Gynecol Surv* 1993;**48**:640–8.

6. US Bureau of Justice. *Statistics Data Report.* Department of Justice, Bureau of Justice Statistics, Washington DC, 1996.

7. Holmes MM, Resnick HS, Frampton D. Follow-up of sexual assault victims. *Am J Obstet Gynecol* 1998;**179**:336–42.

8. Dietz P, Hazelwood R, Warren J. The sexually sadistic criminal and his offenses. *Bull Am Acad Psychiatry Law* 1990;**18**:163–78.

9. Groth AN. Psychodynamics of rape. In Groth AN, ed., *Men Who Rape.* Plenum Press, New York, 1979, pp. 12–83.

10. Burgess AW, Fehder WP, Hartman CR. Delayed reporting of the rape victim. *J Psychosoc Nurs* 1995;**33**:21–9.

11. Schwartz RH, Weaver AB. Rohypnol, the date rape drug. *Clin Pediatr* 1998;**37**:321.

12. Anglin D, Spears KL, Hutson R. Flunitrazepam and its involvement in date or acquaintance rape. *Acad Emerg Med* 1997;**4**:323–6.

13. Dunn SF, Gilchrist VJ. Sexual assault. *Primary Care* 1993;**20**:359–73.

14. Silverman DC, Kalick SM, Bowie SI, Edbril SD. Blitz rape and confidence rape: A typology applied to 1,000 consecutive cases. *Am J Psychiatry* 1988;**145**:1438–41.

15. Sanday PR. *Fraternity Gang Rape.* New York University Press, New York, 1990.

16. Ullman SE. A comparison of gang and individual rape incidents. *Violence Vict* 1999;**14**:123–33.

17. Kilpatrick DG, Best CL, Saunders BE, Veronen LJ. Rape in marriage and in dating relationships: How bad is it for mental health? *Ann NY Acad Sci* 1988;**528**:335–44.

18. Burgess AW, Holmstrom LL. Adaptive strategies and recovery from rape. *Am J Psychiatry* 1979;**136**:1278–82.

19. Davis R, Taylor B, Bench S. Impact of sexual and nonsexual assault on secondary victims. *Violence Vict* 1995;**10**:73–84.

20. Moscarello R. Psychological management of victims of sexual assault. *Can J Psychiatr* 1990;**35**:25–30.

21. Gruber AJ, Pope HG. Compulsive weight lifting and anabolic drug abuse among women rape victims. *Comp Psychiatr* 1999;**40**:273–7.

22. van der Kolk BA. The body keeps score: memory and the evolving psychobiology of posttraumatic stress. *Harvard Rev Psychiatry* 1994;**1**:253–5.

23. Kope S. Sexuality. In Ranson SB, McNeeley SG, eds., *Gynecology for the Primary Care Provider.* WB Saunders Co., Philadelphia, 1997, pp. 82–7.

24. Regehr C, Regehr G, Bradford J. A model for predicting depression in victims of rape. *J Am Acad Psychiatry Law* 1998;**26**:595–605.

25. Muram D, Hostetler BR, Jones CE, Speck PM. Adolescent victims of sexual assault. *J Adolesc Health* 1995;**17**:372–5.

26. Cartwright PS, Moore RA. The elderly victim of rape. *South Med J* 1989;**82**:988–9.

27. Harrison A. Primary care of lesbian and gay patients: Educating ourselves and our students. *Fam Med* 1996;**28**:10–23.

28. Erickson CA. Rape and the family. In Figley CR, ed., *Treating Stress in Families,* Brunner Mazel, New York, 1989, pp. 257–89.

29. Ullman SE. Do social reactions to sexual assault victims vary by support provider? *Violence Vict* 1996;**11**:143–57.

30. Kimerling R, Calhoun KS. Somatic symptoms, social support and treatment seeking among sexual assault victims. *J Consult Clin Psychol* 1994;**62**:333–40.

31. Koss MP, Woodruff WJ, Koss PG. Criminal victimization among primary care medical patients: prevalence, incidence and physician usage. *Behav Sci Law* 1991;**9**:85–96.

32. Golding JM, Cooper ML, George LK. Sexual assault history and health perceptions: Seven general population studies. *Health Psychol* 1997;**16**:417–25.

33. Boisset-Pioro MH, Esdaile JM, Fitzcharles MA. Sexual and physical abuse in women with fibromyalgia syndrome. *Arthritis Rheum* 1995;**38**:235–41.

34. Smith ES, Biet M. Case management and legal considerations. Presentation at University of Nevada LV School of Dentistry, Las Vegas, NV, 1999.

35. Glaser JB, Hammerschlag MR, McCormack WM. Current concepts: Sexually transmitted diseases in victims of sexual assault. *N Engl J Med* 1986;**315**:625–7.

36. Ruckman LM. Victims of rape. The physician's role in treatment. *Curr Opin Obstet Gynecol* 1993;**5**:721–5.

26 Depression and premenstrual syndrome

Jo Ann Rosenfeld, MD

《Depression is a common problem that has been reported in greater frequency in women than in men. Diagnosis and treatment requires the understanding of medical, social, and psychological factors and interactions. Effective treatments are available and are important because suicide is a major cause of death for younger women.《

Epidemiology

1. Depression is very common.
   a. Five to 8 percent of all outpatients seen by primary care physicians have the diagnosis of depression.[1] Ten percent of individuals may have a depression during any year. The lifetime prevalence is 17 percent,[2] although up to 45 percent of those individuals who can be considered "high utilizers" of primary care services may have depression.[3]
   b. Approximately 60 percent of those individuals with anxiety and mood disorders are seen first in a primary care setting. Only approximately 20 percent of these are referred to a mental health specialist.[3]
   c. The incidence of depression does not seem to vary by race. In a large observational study of 900 young women, 21 percent of white, 28 percent of African-Americans, and 29 percent of Hispanic women reported severe depressive symptoms. Both white and African-American women with depression were likely to report being sexually assaulted, and unemployed.[4] Studies of older women vary. In one study of more than 2500 women in Detroit, African-American older women reported a higher level of depressive symptoms and unemployment was again related significantly to depression.[5]
2. The detection rate in primary care settings is 60 to 64 percent.[2]
   a. Detection is important because depression leads to greater impairment

and disability than diabetes, lung disease, back problems, and hypertension.

b. Major depressive disorders are associated with a 15 percent suicide rate.[2]

c. Only two-thirds of those who suffer depression seek treatment and only 10 percent receive adequate doses of antidepressants.[2]

3. Depression is more common in women.

a. The National Comorbidity Survey found a lifetime prevalence of depression for women of 21.3 percent and 12.7 percent for men.[6]

b. Depression occurs earlier in women and has occurred in progressively younger women with each decade since World War II.

c. Depression in women is more likely to be longer and recurrent, with greater seasonal effects on mood.[7]

> Depression is more common in women.

Reasons for gender disparity

This gender difference starts as early as adolescence. The cause of this disparity is disputed; differences in endocrine, social, sociological, psychological, and environmental causes and stresses have all been suggested. There are gender differences in the function of some neurotransmitters, but whether this is the cause is uncertain. Sociological factors such as the differing way adults react to male and female children have been proposed as etiologies. Introspective behaviors may be more encouraged in girls and these may worsen or intensify depression. The increased childhood sexual abuse in women may lead to an increased incidence of depression. Increased stressors in women in family and careers, pregnancy, infertility, and single parenthood coupled with greater social isolation have also been proposed as causes for the gender disparity. Differences in health care provider diagnosis and sensitivity and differences in patient presentation have also been suggested as causes.

Risk factors (Table 26.1)

1. The risk factors for all individuals for depression and those specifically for women are listed in Table 26.1.

2. Other medical illnesses and psychiatric diagnoses place women at higher risk of developing depression. Psychiatric problems are more common in patients

Table 26.1. Risk factors for depression in women and men

For men or all individuals
- Past history
  - Family history of depression
  - Personal history of depression
- Medical history
  - Serious medical illness
  - Antisocial personality disorder
  - Sexual dysfunction
- Social history
  - Life stress
  - Lack of social supports
  - History of substance abuse
  - Cigarette smoking
  - Alcohol use

Specifically women
- Past history
  - Loss of parent before age 10 years
  - Childhood history of physical or sexual abuse
- Medical history
  - History of mood disorders after pregnancy
- Social history
  - Marijuana use
  - Use of high-progesterone oral contraceptive pill
  - Use of gonadotropin stimulants for infertility evaluation
  - Single parenthood
  - Unhappy or abusive marriage
  - Presence of young children in home

Data from Brody DS, Thompson TL, Larson DB et al. Recognizing and managing depression in primary care. *Gen Hosp Psychiatry* 1995;**17**:93–107. Boswell EB, Stoudemire A. Major depression in the primary care setting. *Am J Med* 1996;**101**:6A-3S to 9S.

with medical illness and psychiatric disorders may affect the clinical outcome of medical disorders. Depressive symptoms are present in 24 to 46 percent of hospitalized medically ill patients with diseases such as cancer, myocardial infarction, Parkinson's disease and stroke (see below).[3]

Clinical symptoms

1. Vegetative symptoms include changes in appetite and libido. Sleep disturbances are common and include difficulty in falling asleep, staying asleep, and

early morning awakening. Unlike men, women can either become anorexic or eat too much or go on binges of eating. Loss of libido is another common symptom.

2.   Changes in mood – sadness, weeping, crying, irritability. Women may be more frustrated and angry than depressed.

3.   Changes in motivation – anhedonia ("Everything's an effort"), loss of interest or pleasure in usual activity, difficulty concentrating.

4.   Changes in behavior – social withdrawal, psychomotor retardation or agitation. Women may become nearly agoraphobic, stay in the house, and interact very little.

5.   Cognitive symptoms – low self-esteem, guilt, delusions, especially somatic hopelessness, helplessness, and thoughts of suicide and death.

6.   The "typical" symptoms of depression may be more difficult to detect in the elderly.

7.   The presentation may be different in women. Women may be more likely to have a seasonal component and atypical depressive symptoms such as hypersomnia, hyperphagia, carbohydrate craving, weight gain, "heavy feelings" in arms and legs, and evening mood worsening.

8.   Women are more likely to have depressive symptoms associated with eating disorders and headaches and less likely to have associated antisocial behavior, obsessive–compulsive disorders and alcoholism than men.[7]

> Women may be more likely to have a seasonal component and atypical depressive symptoms such as hypersomnia, hyperphagia, carbohydrate craving, weight gain, "heavy feelings" in arms and legs, and evening mood worsening.

Diagnosis

Differential

There are various medical and psychiatric conditions that can mimic or obscure the diagnosis of depression. The woman should be examined for the following:

1.   Comorbid medical conditions that can cause depression (Table 26.2).

2.   Medications that can cause or exacerbate depression (Table 26.3).

3.   Coexisting nonmood psychiatric disorders such as anxiety and anxiety disorders including obsessive–compulsive disorder and panic disorder with and without agoraphobia, substance abuse and schizoaffective disorder, especially if the depression has psychotic elements.[8]

4.   Dementia, especially in the elderly.

Table 26.2. Illnesses causing depressive-like mood syndromes

- Endocrine
  - Hypothyroidism
  - Apathetic hyperthyroidism
  - Cushing's disease
  - Hyperparathyroidism
- Nutritional
  - Vitamin B12 deficiency
  - Alcohol or substance abuse
- Treatment
  - Medications
- Other chronic diseases
- Connective tissue
  - Lupus
  - Cancer
  - Stroke
  - Heart disease
  - CNS disease – Parkinson's disease and multiple sclerosis, Alzheimer's disease

CNS, central nervous system.

5. Family factors.
6. Stressful life events.
7. Alcohol or substance abuse.
8. Level of social isolation.
9. Each patient with depressive symptoms should be assessed for suicidal risk (see below).

Diagnostic criteria

The diagnosis criteria for major depression is taken from the *Diagnostic and Statistical Manual of Mental Disorders* (DSM) *IV* (Table 26.4). Various good screening tools exist including the Beck Inventory (13 questions), the General Health Questionnaire, and the Geriatric Depression Scale.

Treatment

1. Treatment is counselling, cognitive-behavioral therapy and/or antidepressant medications.
2. There is some evidence that exercise can be beneficial. In a cross-sectional study of more than 3400 men and women, there was a consistent association between enhanced psychological well-being and regular physical exercise.[9]

Table 26.3. Medications that can cause depression

- Antihypertensives
  - Clonidine
  - Hydralazine
  - Hydrochlorothiazole
  - Methyldopa
  - Propranolol (all beta-blockers)
  - Reserpine
  - Spironolactone
  - Guanethidine
- Analgesics
  - Ibuprofen
  - Indomethicin
  - Opiates
- Antiepileptics
  - Phenytoin
  - Phenobarbital
  - Carbamazepine
- Antihistamines
- Antineoplastic agents
- Antibiotics
  - Ampicillin
  - Griseofulvin
  - Isoniazid HCl
  - Metronidazole
  - Nitrofuradantoin
  - Penicillin
  - Tetracycline
- Cardiovascular drugs
  - Digoxin
  - Lidocaine
  - Procainamide
- Hormones
  - Steroids
  - ACTH
  - ?OCPs
- Sedatives
  - Barbiturates
  - Benzodiazepines
  - Chloral hydrate
- Stimulants
  - Amphetamines
- Other CNS drugs
  - Amantidine
  - Butyrophenones
  - Phenothiazines

ACTH, adrenocorticotropic hormone; OCP, oral contraceptive pill; CNS, central nervous system.

Table 26.4. DSM-IV Diagnostic criteria for a major depressive episode

Patients must have more than five symptoms on a daily basis for at least 2 weeks.

- Essential symptoms
  - Depressed mood
  - Anhedonia
- Psychological symptoms
  - Recurrent thoughts of death and/or suicide plans or attempts
  - Difficulty in thinking or concentrating
  - Feelings of guilt or worthlessness
- Physical symptoms
  - Changes in sleep
  - Changes in appetite or weight
  - Change in psychomotor activity

From *Diagnostic and Statistical Manual of mental disorders*, 4th edn. American Psychiatric Association, Washington, DC, 1994.

Another randomized study that examined older patients found that 156 women and men responded as well at 16 weeks to exercise or antidepressants. However, those on antidepressants responded more quickly to therapy.[10]

3. Psychotherapeutic counselling is indicated as an integral part of the treatment of depression. Studies have shown that women with depression do better with counselling and pharmacological treatment than with medication alone,[11] especially patients with more severe depressions.[12]

4. Psychopharmacological treatment is standard in most cases of depression. Eighty percent of patients respond to medication.[6]

   Treatment is indicated in individuals with the following problems:

   a. Major depressive or manic-depressive disorders.
   b. Depressive symptoms causing suicidal thoughts, considerable distress, or impacting on ability to perform usual activities.
   c. Symptoms lasting more than two to three weeks, especially if the patient is isolated.
   d. An inability to cope.
   e. Mild symptoms and a history of depression.
   f. A request for treatment.

5. Use of antidepressants in women may be different because of differing pharmacokinetics. Women show greater absorption and plasma concentrations at similar doses. They may need lower doses because they develop increased side effects. Especially, in women, there may be a need to treat comorbid anxiety, panic, phobias, and eating disorders.

Table 26.5. Antidepressant medications

Name	Dose (mg)	FDA pregnancy category	Drowsiness	Insomnia	CV problems	GI effect
Tricyclics						
Amitryptyline (Elavil)	75–300	D	+ + + +	0	+ + +	0
Desimpramine(Norpramin)	50–300	C	+	+	+ +	0
Doxepin (Sinequan)	75–300	C[a]	+ + + +	0	+ +	0
Nortriptyline (Pamelor)	50–200	D	+	0	+ +	0
Nontricyclics						
Bupropion (Wellbutrin)	225–450	B	0	+	+	+
Trazodone (Desyrel)	150–600	C	+	+	+	+
Vanlafaxine (Effexor)	75–225	C	+	+	0	+ + + +
Nefazodone (Serzone)	300–600	C	+ +	+	+	0
SSRIs						SD
Fluoxetine (Prozac)[b]	10–40	C[c]	0	+ +	0	+ + +
Paroxetine (Paxil)	20–50	C	0	+ +	0	+ + +
Sertraline (Zoloft)	50–200	C	0	+ +	0	+ + +
Lithium	900–1200	D[d]				

CV, cardiovascular; GI, gastrointestinal; SSRI, selective serotonin reuptake inhibitor; SD, also associated with sexual dysfunction as side effect; + signs indicate degree of effect.

[a]Associated with apnea in breast-fed infants.

[b]May be drug of choice in pregnant or fertile women.

[c]Associated with GI effects and insomnia in breast-fed infants.

[d]Lithium toxicity in breast-fed infants.

6. Women may respond to some psychotherapeutic agents better, at a dose similar to that for men, perhaps because they have higher levels of the agents in their blood. The selective serotonin reuptake inhibitor (SSRI) sertraline worked better in women than in men, particularly in women with recurrent depression and those women with a first episode of depression.[13]

7. Medications include tricyclic antidepressants, SSRIs and a few other medications (see Table 26.5). Women with major manic-depressive disorders are also treated with lithium, and those with psychosis, schizophrenic elements or thought disorders often with phenothiazines or butypherones.

8. Choice of antidepressant: Unless there is a concern about cost, an SSRI is most likely the first choice for antidepressant. Sertaline may be more favored by many experts than fluoxetine. The patient should see an effect with SSRIs within seven to ten days.

    Tricyclic antidepressants work well, but have substantial side effects such as sedation, dry mouth, cardiovascular effects, and blurred vision. They take longer to work, usually 10 to 14 days before an effect is seen and the dose needs to be titrated up over weeks. Doxepin (Sinequan) has often been used in the elderly, because it may have fewer cardiovascular interactions. Desyrel, a quadricyclic antidepressant, works more quickly than tricyclic antidepressants and works well in returning rapid eye movement (REM) sleep to normal.

9. Any antidepressants must be started in low or standard doses.
    a. A single drug, often an SSRI, should be started. With tricyclic antidepressants, the dose is often increased slowly week by week, or twice a week, until an improvement is seen and as long as side effects are tolerable. An adequate trial of one medication should take six to eight weeks, before another drug is added or substituted.
    b. Individuals should be warned about side effects and urged to call if these are bothersome.
    c. Although some improvement in symptoms may be seen as early as one week, usually 10 to 14 days of treatment are needed to see progress.
    d. Patients who fail to respond within one to two months or worsen may need psychiatric referral.
    e. Only a small number of antidepressant tablets should be prescribed at one time, because of the risk of suicide. Antidepressants can cause serious cardiac arrhythmias in high or overdoses.

Psychopharmacological treatment is standard in most cases of depression. Eighty percent of patients respond to medication.

f. Women should be seen very often at first – at least every two weeks. Once an adequate dose is determined, once a month may be sufficient, if the patient is receiving additional counselling.

g. The medications should be continued four to eight months before tapering off.

h. SSRIs have become the agents of choice for depression, but only fluoxetine has data suggesting any safety during pregnancy. A surveillance study of more than 230 000 pregnancies showed that mothers who took fluoxetine during pregnancy had a major birth defect rate of only 1.8 percent (less than normal 2.8 to 3 percent).[14] Prospective studies have shown no increased fetal loss in mothers taking fluoxetine.[15]

i. Women who are pregnant or breast feeding should not be placed on lithium valproate, or carbamazepine.[16]

10. Other psychotropic drugs are also being investigated for use in depression. Gabapentin, an antiepileptic medication, has shown some promise in reducing depression symptoms, especially in patients who have not or only partially responded to other antidepressants[17] or those with chronic pain[18].

Usually 10 to 14 days of treatment are needed to see progress.

Risk of suicide

Risk factors

1. Women, especially those under age 30 years, are more likely to attempt suicide but are successful less often than men. They are more likely to have guilt feelings.[7]

2. Women choose less lethal methods.

3. Women at higher risk for suicide attempts include those with major depressive disorders, age younger than 30 years, who live alone, and those who have substance abuse problems, psychosocial stressors, and personality disorders.

4. Women who are at an increase risk for completed suicides include women with psychotic depression, substance abuse, previous suicide attempts, active ideation, divorced or widowed marital status, chronic medical illness, and those with panic or severe anxiety disorders.

Women, especially those under age 30 years, are more likely to attempt suicide but are successful less often than men.

Assessment for suicide risk

1. In all patients, their potential for suicide must be assessed. Patients must be asked about suicidal thoughts and plans. If they have suicide plans or active suicidal thoughts, they need emergency evaluation.

2. Other indications for immediate referral include psychotic ideation, such as hallucinations, and thought disorders.

3. The more precise, immediate and lethal the plan, the higher is the short-term risk. Rating of lethality is an estimate of potential fatality of suicide plan, method, and means, including means of rescue.[19]

4. The more socially isolated the woman is, with fewer resources and less social support, the higher is the risk of her suicide. Women who are socially isolated, live alone, have few contacts and are depressed may be at a higher risk of suicide and stronger or quicker treatment may be necessary.

> If they have suicide plans or active suicidal thoughts, they need emergency evaluation.

Ways to decrease risk of suicide

1. Safe environment: This may take hospitalization, close supervision and/or medications. Women are more likely to need hospitalization if they have poor impulse control, chemical dependency or alcoholism, a major depression or other psychiatric disorder.

2. Immediate or quick symptom relief, especially relief of pain, may decrease suicide risk.

3. Making a "no suicide contract" with the patient may decrease her risk of a suicide attempt. Creating methods of easily contacting physicians or health care advisors will help. (No voice mail or email contacts.)

4. Maximizing and identifying family and community resources and social support is important.

> Women are more likely to need hospitalization if they have poor impulse control, chemical dependency or alcoholism, a major depression, or other psychiatric disorder.

Special situations

Caregivers

Women often become the caregivers for their parents and/or their spouse. Twenty five percent of working women are caring for a disabled individual. By virtue of having more stress, caregivers are more likely to become depressed.

Table 26.6. Symptoms that occur in patients with cancer and depression

- Sense of failure
- Loss of social interest
- Feeling of being punished
- Dissatisfaction
- Suicidal ideation
- Indecision
- Loss of interest and crying indicated severe depression

Depression in caregivers is more likely if the patient being cared for had a psychiatric disorder or dementia (as high as 47 percent).[20]

Cancer patients

1. Cancer patients are more prone to depression. In an observational study, 47 percent of cancer patients had psychiatric problems, either adjustment disorders, depression (13 percent) or anxiety.[21] In another study, 25 percent of cancer patients had symptoms of depression.[19]

2. Untreated depression can cause more frequent clinic visits, increased cost, extended hospitalization, and reduced adherence to therapeutic protocols and worse quality of life.

3. Depression with cancer is more likely in women, in patients with advanced stages of cancer, or a history of preexisting mood disorders, and those with uncontrolled pain. In one study of breast cancer patients, 38 percent experienced a major depressive disorder, while 95 percent had dysphoria and/or insomnia, most within the first six months of treatment.[22]

4. Depression is harder to diagnose in a cancer patient because vegetative symptoms, such as weight loss, insomnia, fatigue, thoughts of death, and anergy may be caused by cancer, depression, or both.

5. Seven important symptoms in patients with depression and cancer are listed in Table 26.6.[23]

6. Depression can be treated successfully with antidepressants in cancer patients. However, practitioners are less likely to treat depression in a cancer patient, partially because they expect depression as a normal response. Depression does not automatically resolve when the cancer improves or is surgically removed.

7. Death from suicide occurs in only 2 to 6 percent of terminally ill patients. However, cancer patients are twice as likely to commit suicide as other patients with depression. Risk factors for suicide in depressed cancer patients are listed in Table 26.7.[24]

Table 26.7. Risk factors for suicide in cancer patients

- Poor prognosis
- Advanced stage of illness
- Mild delirium with poor impulse control
- Inadequately treated pain
- Major depression
- Premorbid psychiatric or personality disorders
- Alcohol abuse
- Prior suicide attempts
- Poor social supports
- Physical and emotional exhaustion

Chronic disease

Although many individuals with chronic disease develop depression, they should not be placed on antidepressants prophylactically. Antidepressant medications have too many side effects and interactions to be used prophylactically, without a diagnosis of depression. However, close observation, clinical suspicion and follow-up are essential. Depression worsens recovery or rehabilitation of many chronic diseases.

1. Cardiac disease: Although women develop cardiac disease later than men, almost one-half of all deaths in women are caused by heart disease. A 10-year prospective study reported that 8 to 44 percent of cardiac patients experience a major depression.[25] Depression usually occurs in the six months after a myocardial infarction or diagnosis of cardiac disease and can worsen rehabilitation or impede proper treatment. Confusion and lethargy can be signs of a myocardial infarction, congestive heart failure or depression in the elderly.

2. Stroke:
   a. There is a higher frequency of depression in patients with stroke, and depression may be difficult to diagnose, especially if the woman has an expressive or receptive aphasia.
   b. Major depressions occur in 1 to 25 percent and minor depressions in 10 to 30 percent of patients after a stroke.[26] The depression may be observed as primarily vegetative signs and mood disturbances. The patient may withdraw and refuse to cooperate with rehabilitation or therapy.
   c. Some stroke patients are at higher risk for depression (Table 26.8).
   d. Most stroke patients with depression show improvement within the first year, and only a small percentage suffer chronic and persistent depression lasting more than three years. Active treatment with antidepressant medications improves most patients' symptoms of depression.
   e. The stroke causes the depression and the depression worsens the recovery

Table 26.8. Risk factors for depression and severity of depression after stroke

- Younger age
- Greater impairment of activities of daily living
- Social impairment
- Prior personal or family history of psychiatric problems
- Nonfluent aphasia
- Cognitive impairment
- Enlarged ventricle to brain ratio
- Lesions close to left frontal pole in patients with subacute stroke
  Left cortical and left basal ganglia lesions were associated with an increased frequency of major depression

from stroke. Patients with depression showed significantly less recovery in activities of daily living after two years than nondepressed controls.[26] Stroke patients who had a depression were more likely to die; they were three and half times more likely to die in the first two to three years after a stroke than those who did not have a depression. However, these studies did not take into account treatment for depression, including medications. Antidepressant treatment may improve this increased risk of mortality.

Elderly

1. Major depressive illness is no more common in the general population of elderly than it is in young people – about 1 percent in community-dwelling elderly, up to 3 percent, if dysthymic patients are included.[27]

2. Major depression occurs in 17 percent of primary care patients over age 65 years, and is more likely in nursing home residents. The incidence of depression is higher in all patients in long-term care settings; in women in long-term care settings, up to 12 percent are depressed.

3. Depression in the elderly is more difficult to diagnose. Symptoms of depression such as loss of interest, fatigue, and decreased energy and appetite are sometimes mistakenly attributed to the normal aging process.[27]

4. Serious suicide attempts were more than twice as common in elderly depressed with somatic complaints than those without and increased in elderly men, especially those living alone.

5. The predisposition to depression in women continues into the older ages. Elderly women are no more likely than younger women to develop depression, but more of the elderly are women.

6. Treatment in the elderly is the same as in younger individuals, except that the elderly may be more sensitive to side effects and may develop adverse effects

Table 26.9. Research criteria for premenstrual dysphoric disorder

Presence of 5/11 symptoms with at least one-quarter occurring with menstrual cycle a week before menses and ceasing with onset of menses

These must interfere with social, occupational, sexual, or school functioning

These must be related to menstrual cycle and be confirmed by daily ratings of at least two cycles. One symptom must be present for at least one year related to menstrual cycles

- Physical symptoms
  - Breast tenderness or swelling, headaches, weight gain, bloated feelings, or joint or muscle pain
- Depressive symptoms
  - Changes in sleep
  - Lethargy, fatigue, lack of energy
  - Feeling sad or tearful
  - Markedly depressed mood, with hopelessness and self-deprecation
  - Anhedonia or decreased interest in activities
- Cognitive symptoms
  - Difficulty concentrating
- Anxiety symptoms
  - Feeling overwhelmed or out of control
  - Persistent marked irritability, anger, increased interpersonal conflicts, marked anxiety, tension, feeling of being on edge

when using relatively low doses of medications. Psychotherapy also works. Tricyclic antidepressant medications can create arrhythmias and depress cardiac function, negatively affect balance, memory and orthostatic pressure, increase falls, and increase urinary retention. SSRIs may be better in the elderly.

7. Electroconvulsive therapy (ECT) use has increased in the 1990s. The rate of ECT use per 10 000 Medicare beneficiaries also increased from 4.2 to 5.1 from 1987 to 1992.[28] There was a greater increase in use in older women, whites, and the disabled population (under age 65 years).

Depression in the elderly is more difficult to diagnose.

Premenstrual dysphoric disorder (Table 26.9)

1. Incidence: Between 3 and 5 percent of women meet the criteria for this disorder (Table 26.9). However, premenstrual syndrome (PMS) symptoms may affect 30 to 50 percent of women. The symptoms include affective lability, persistent irritability, intense anxiety, depressed mood, concentration difficulties, fatigue, changes in sleep and appetite, and physical symptoms.

2. Diagnosis is difficult because of lack of consensus regarding pathophysiology and its relation to other systems, including hormonal systems.

3. Treatment: The best treatment is unclear. Suggested treatment includes exercise, changes in diet – caffeine restriction, carbohydrate consumption, decreased alcohol, and treatment with progesterone, gonadotropin-releasing hormone antagonists, antidepressants and/or antianxiety drugs. Serotonin antidepressants (SSRIs) are effective in approximately half the patients,[29] and can be given in all or half of the menstrual cycle.

4. A RCT of 120 women compared four medications – fluoxetine (10 mg/day), alprazolam (0.75 mg/day), propranolol (20 to 40 mg/day) and pyridoxine (300 mg/day) for treatment of severe PMS over six months. Fluoxetine had a 65 percent improvement in PMS symptoms compared with propranolol 58.7 percent, alprazolam 55.6 percent, pyridoxine 45 percent and placebo 39 to 46 percent.[30] A metaanalysis of the use of vitamin B6 (pyridoxine 100 mg daily) that combined nine studies and 940 patients found that use of pyridoxine gave an OR to placebo of 1.69 in improvement of depressive symptoms and an OR of 2.32 of improvement of PMS symptoms.[31]

Depression during pregnancy

1. Incidence: Women are not more likely to become depressed in pregnancy. Depression rates are the same in pregnant and nonpregnant women. Having a depression in pregnancy is related to a previous history of depression.[7]

2. Treatment: Treatment during pregnancy is complicated. Most antidepressants, except buproprion (which is category B), are FDA category C or D, while lithium should not be used at all. Several large prospective studies showed no causal relationship between in utero exposure to tricyclic antidepressants, fluoxetine, or other SSRIs and teratogenicity.

Depression rates are the same in pregnant and nonpregnant women.

Postpartum depression

1. Postpartum depression can have significant sequelae for the mother, family, and child, with depressed maternal–infant bonding.

2. Incidence: There is a wide range of mood reactions reported after delivery. From 30 to 75 percent of women, depending on the study, have mild "postpartum blues" consisting of fatigue and lack of sleep, irritability, tearfulness and anxiety, lasting less than two weeks.[32]

3. Eight to ten percent of women have a major depression within six months of delivery. At six months postpartum, the same percentages of women have had

Table 26.10. Risk factors for postpartum depression

- Lack of spousal support
- Preterm infants
- Twins
- Less positive social adjustment
- Lower marital satisfaction
- Less gratification in parental role
- Poorer physical health
- Personal history of depression
- Family history of depression
- Stressful life events
- Difficulties in marital relationship
- Being an adolescent mother

a depression as control women. However there was a threefold higher rate of depression within five weeks of childbirth.[33] Approximately one to two per 1000 women have a postpartum depressive psychosis.

4. Symptoms of major depression include energy loss, guilt, fatigue, agitation, and psychomotor retardation, and these symptoms may occur more frequently than usual in major depression. Symptoms also include difficulty in taking care of the infant, disrupted family interactions, and excessive maternal anxiety about the infant. Fatigue is often a serious symptom and may extend for months, delaying resumption of normal activities.[34] A woman with postpartum depressive psychosis would show thought changes such as hallucinations and delusions and psychomotor retardation.

5. Risk factors (Table 26.10): Postpartum depression is related to lack of spousal support, preterm infants, twins, personal or family history of depression, stressful life events, and difficulties in marital relationship. Childbearing adolescents are more likely to be depressed than nonchildbearing peers. These symptoms are not associated with any social class, marital status, or parity.

6. Fatigue may instead be caused by medical problems. Other symptoms may include pallor, fever, and exertional dyspnea. Causes of fatigue can include:

   a. Anemia – iron or folate deficiency, or occasionally hemolysis from toxemia.

   b. Infections – postpartum endometritis, UTIs or mastitis.

   c. Hypothyroidism – postpartum autoimmune thyroiditis with asymptomatic thyrotoxic phase and symptomatic hypothyroidism can develop 4 to 12 weeks postpartum.

   d. Cardiomyopathy – postpartum cardiomyopathy may present as a life-threatening emergency or insidiously as fatigue and dyspnea.

Symptoms of major depression include energy loss, guilt, fatigue, agitation, and psychomotor retardation.

7. Diagnosis is difficult, often because many women may have feelings of inadequacy in the maternal role, sleeplessness, loss of appetite, and lack of energy.

8. Diagnosis would include a complete history of previous mood disorders, family and social situation, physical examination, complete blood count, sedimentation rate, and thyroid-stimulating hormone level.

9. A small prospective study of first-time mothers found that 38 percent developed late depressive symptoms. Late or longer-term depression was associated with chronic stresses such as maternal health problems, infant difficulties, or poverty and poor social support.[35]

10. Treatment: Major postpartum depression resolves within one year in two out of three patients but requires antidepressants.[36] If the mother is breast feeding, no medication is safe, but fluoxetine and sertraline (50 mg daily) are transferred in only insignificant amounts into breast milk.

   A prospective UK study in two large hospitals questioned women six to eight weeks postpartum to assess for mood disorders. Eighty-seven women were assigned to fluoxetine or placebo plus one or six sessions of counselling by a nurse. Those who responded to fluoxetine did so within one week. All groups had significant improvement. Adding counselling did not increase the rate of improvement.[37]

   Other studies suggest that there is great improvement within one week of entering counselling, and that eight sessions in three months proved significantly effective.[30] Counselling may be adequate in breast-feeding women and women who do not want to take medications.

11. Whether postpartum depression is maternal or parental is disputed. Twenty-two percent of first-time fathers reported a dysphoric mood and 30 percent of first-time fathers reported depressive symptoms.[38] There was a significant correlation between maternal and paternal depressive symptoms.

12. Increased spousal support and emotional support from the husband with infant care and housework related positively to maternal well-being.[39]

Counselling may be adequate treatment for depression in breast-feeding women and women who do not want to take medications.

Menopause

There is no good evidence that menopause causes or is related to depression.[8] A review of literature from 1966 to 1996 found only 43 studies addressing this and cumulative evidence failed to support decisions that menopause causes depression.[40]

Conclusions

For unknown reasons, depression is more common in women. However, it can be treated with medication, exercise and/or counselling. PMS is a diffuse diagnostic syndrome whose treatment is not well defined, but for which a variety of treatments may help in different women.

REFERENCES

1. Brody DS, Thompson TL, Larson DB et al. Recognizing and managing depression in primary care. *Gen Hosp Psychiatr* 1995;**17**:93–107.
2. Ferty JP. Barriers to the diagnosis of depression in primary care. *J Clin Psychiatry* 1997;**58**:5–10.
3. Boswell EB, Stoudemire A. Major depression in the primary care setting. *Am J Med* 1996;**101**:6A-3S to 9S.
4. Rickert VI, Wiemann CM, Berenson AB. Ethnic differences in depressive symptomatology among young women. *Obstet Gynecol* 2000;**95**:55–60.
5. Cochran DL, Brown DR, McGregor KC. Racial differences in the multiple social roles of older women: Implications for depressive symptoms. *Gerontologist* 1999;**39**:465–72.
6. Blazer DG, Kessler RC, McGonagle KA, Swarz MS. The prevalence and distribution of major depression in a national community sample: The national comorbidity survey. *Am J Psychol* 1994;**151**:979–86.
7. Bhatia SC, Bhatia SK. Depression in women: Diagnostic and treatment considerations. *Am Fam Physician* 1999;**60**:225–31.
8. Stotland NL, Stotland NE. Depression in women. *Obstet Gynecol Surv* 1999;**54**:519–24.
9. Hassmane P, Kiovula N, Uutela A. Physical exercise and psychological well-being: A population study in Finland. *Prev Med* 2000;**30**:17–25.
10. Blumenthal JA, Babyak MA, Moore KA et al. Effects of exercise training on older patients with major depression. *Arch Intern Med* 1999;**159**:2349–56.
11. Frank E, Grochocinski VJ, Spanier CA et al. Interpersonal psychotherapy and antidepressant medication: Evaluation of a sequential treatment strategy in women with recurrent major depression. *J Clin Psychiatry* 2000;**61**:51–7.
12. Thase ME, Greenhouse JB, Frank E et al. Treatment of major depression with psychotherapy or psychotherapy–pharmacotherapy combinations. *Arch Gen Psychiatry* 1997;**54**:1009–15.
13. Malt UF, Roback OH, Madsbu HP, Bakke O, Loeb M. The Norwegian naturalistic treatment study of depression in general practice: Randomised double blind study. *BMJ* 1999;**318**:1180–4.
14. Briggs GG, Freeman RK, Yaffe SJ, eds., *Drugs in Pregnancy and Lactation*, 4th edn. Williams & Wilkins, Baltimore, MD, 1994.

15. Chambers CD, Johnson KA, Dick LM et al. Birth outcomes in pregnant women taking fluoxetine. *N Engl J Med* 1996;**335**:1010–15.

16. Chaudron LH, Jefferson JW. Mood stabilizers during breastfeeding: A review. *J Clin Psychiatry* 2000;**61**:79–90.

17. Sokolski KN, Green C, Maris DE, DeMet EM. Gabapentin as an adjunct to standard mood stabilizers in outpatients with mixed bipolar symptomatology. *Ann Clin Psychiatry* 1999;**11**:217–22.

18. Maurer I, Volz HP, Sauer H. Gabapentin leads to remission of somatoform pain disorder with major depression. *Pharmacopsychiatry* 1999;**32**:255–7.

19. Valente SM, Saunders JM. Diagnosis and treatment of major depression among people with cancer. *Cancer Nurs* 1997;**20**:168–77.

20. Livingston G, Manela M, Katona C. Depression and other psychiatric morbidity in carers of elderly people living at home. *BMJ* 1996;**312**:153–6.

21. Derogatis LF, Morrow GR, Getting J et al. The prevalence of psychiatric disorders among cancer patients. *JAMA* 1983;**249**:751–7.

22. Duff LS, Greenberg DB, Younger J, Ferraro MG. Iatrogenic acute estrogen deficiency and psychiatric syndromes in breast cancer patients. *Psychosomatics* 1999;**40**:304–9.

23. Cavanaugh S, Clard DC, Gibbons RD. Diagnosing depression in the hospitalized medically ill. *Psychosomatics* 1983;**4**:809–15.

24. Massie MH, Gagnon P, Holland JC. Depression and suicide in patients with cancer. *J Pain Symptom Manage* 1994;**55**:325–40.

25. Cohen-Cole SA, Kaufman KG. Major depression in physical illness: Diagnosis, prevalence and antidepressant treatment a ten year review, 1982–1992. *Depression* 1993;**1**:181–204.

26. Robinson RG. Neuropsychiatric consequences of stroke. *Annu Rev Med* 1997;**48**:217–29.

27. Rasking MA. Depression in the elderly. *Can J Psychol* 1992;**37**:4–6.

28. Rosenbach ML, Hermann RC, Dorwart RA. Use of electroconvulsive therapy in the Medicare population between 1987 and 1992. *Psychiatr Serv* 1997;**48**:1537–42.

29. Freeman EW, Rickels K, Arrendondo F et al. Full or half cycle treatment of severe premenstrual syndrome with a serotonergic antidepressant. *J Clin Psychopharmacol* 1999;**19**:3–8.

30. Diegoli MSC, da Fonseca AM, Diegoli CA, Pinotti JA. A double blind trial of four medications to treat severe premenstrual syndrome. *Int J Gynecol Obstet* 1998;**62**:63–7.

31. Wyatt KM, Dimmock PW, Jones PW, Shaugh O'Brien PM. Efficacy of vitamin B-6 in the treatment of premenstrual syndrome: Systematic review. *BMJ* 1999;**18**:1375–81.

32. O'Hara MW, Schlechte JA, Lewis DA, Wright EJ. Prospective study of postpartum blues. Biological and psychosocial factors. *Arch Gen Psychol* 1991;**48**:801–6.

33. Wisner KL, Peindl DS, Gigliotti T, Hanusa BH. Obsessions and compulsions in women with postpartum depression. *J Clin Psychiatry* 1999;**60**:176–81.

34. Atkinson LS, Baxley EG. Postpartum fatigue. *Am Fam Physician* 1994;**50**:1231–44.

35. Sequin L, Potvin L, St-Denis M, Loiselle J. Depressive symptoms in the late postpartum among low socioeconomic status women. *Birth* 1999;**26**:157–63.

36. Bright D. Postpartum mental disorders. *Am Fam Physician* 1994;**50**:889–94.

37. Appelby L, Warner R, Whitton A, Faugher B. A controlled study of fluoxetine and cognitive-behavioral counselling in the treatment of postnatal depression. *BMJ* 1997;**314**:932–6.

38. Soliday E, McCluskey-Faucett K. O'Brien M. Postpartum affect and depressive symptom in mothers and fathers. *Am J Orthopsychiatry* 1999;**69**:30–7.

39. Gjerdingen DK, Froberg DG, Fontaine P. The effects of social support on women's health during pregnancy, labor and delivery, and the postpartum period. *Fam Med* 1991;**23**:370–5.
40. Nicol-Smith L. Causality, menopause and depression: A critical review of the literature. *BMJ* 1996;**313**:1229–32.

27 Addiction

Jo Ann Rosenfeld, MD

Definition

1. Addiction is a compulsive obligatory use of a substance or medication, characterized usually by dependence, tolerance, and a withdrawal syndrome, if stopped, and often by disruption to medical, social, and family life. Addiction usually includes periods of chronic intoxication or periodic craving.[1]
2. Alcoholism is a chronic disease, occasionally fatal and usually progressive, in which there is preoccupation with the use of alcohol, to the detriment of family, health, and social life. Drug abuse, similarly, is the chronic compulsion for a particular drug.
3. Addiction is a personal, medical, family, social, and societal problem that affects more than just the patient. The family physician plays an important role as counsellor, advocate, therapeutic agent, and coordinator of care for the individual with an alcohol or drug abuse problem.

> Addiction is a personal, medical, family, social and societal problem that affects more than just the patient.

Alcoholism

Definitions

There are four levels of alcohol use:

1. Social drinkers: Ten percent of all individuals abstain totally from alcohol use; therefore 90 percent of individuals are social drinkers or drink more.
2. Individuals with "at risk" consumption: These individuals have a level of alcohol intake that, if maintained, may be a risk to their health. Twenty-eight percent of men and 11 percent of women are at risk.
3. Problem drinkers: At this level of consumption, drinking or addiction causes serious problems to the drinker's family, social network, work, and society.

This occurs in 1 to 2 percent of the population.

4. Alcoholism: Addiction to alcohol.[1]

Impact

1. In 1997 there were approximately 200 000 individuals with alcohol addiction in the UK. Approximately 4.6 million individuals in the USA are alcoholic and approximately one-third of these are women.[2]
2. Medical impact: Alcohol abuse increases the risk of death in heavy drinkers, older individuals and former drinkers. In 1997, this led to 3000 premature deaths in the UK. Alcoholism accounted for 80 percent of suicides, 40 percent of the motor vehicle accidents, 50 percent of murders, and 25 percent of drownings in the UK.[1]
3. Social impact: Alcohol abuse can be linked to one-third of the divorces, one-third of the episodes of child abuse, one-fifth of hospital admissions, and one-third of all homelessness.[1] The cost of alcohol abuse is higher than $100 billion dollars in the USA.[3]
4. Women who abuse alcohol are more likely to be homeless, have dependent children that need help, be single, divorced or separated, abused, and have a history of sexual abuse as children.[4]

Impact on women

1. More men than women have problems with alcoholism. However, the gap is narrowing. More men than women become alcoholic; this difference is not genetic but may be caused by variations in environmental pressures to drink or not drink heavily.
2. Four percent of all excessive deaths among women, and 9 percent decreased life expectancy can be related to alcoholism.[5]
3. The greatest incidence of heavy drinking in women was in women aged 34 to 49 years (9 percent) followed by women aged 21 to 34 years (6 percent).[6]
4. Twenty-three percent of men and 4.7 percent of women had an alcoholic disorder over their lifetime.[7] For alcohol dependence, the lifetime prevalence in men is 20.1 percent and in women 8.2 percent.[8]
5. At the same level of alcohol use/abuse, women are more likely to feel significant effects and more likely to become medically ill. Women who drink have higher blood alcohol levels at lesser intakes than men, as do the elderly,

---

Women who abuse alcohol are more likely to be homeless, have dependent children that need help, be single, divorced or separated, abused and have a history of sexual abuse as a child.

because both groups have lower total body water. Women have half the amount of the enzyme gastric alcohol dehyrogenase that metabolizes alcohol. Thus women achieve, with similar alcohol intakes to men, higher blood alcohol levels, a higher level of liver pathology with half the consumption, and, once it develops, progression of liver disease at faster rates with lower survival rates. Both women and the elderly have more complications from alcohol abuse and a higher risk of alcohol–drug interactions.[4]

6. Native American women are 36 times more likely to develop alcoholic cirrhosis and six times more likely to die from it than other women.[9]

> Women achieve, with similar alcohol intakes to men, higher blood alcohol levels, a higher level of liver pathology with half the consumption, and, once it develops, progression of liver disease at faster rates with lower survival rates.

Medical effects

1. Heart disease:
   a. Alcohol use has a dose dependent U-shaped curve effect on cardiovascular (CV) mortality. Moderate amounts of alcohol use decrease CV mortality as compared with abstinent individuals. However, alcohol abuse increases the CV mortality. This may be caused by alcohol's effects on platelets and HDL cholesterol levels.
   b. In an observational study of more than 85 000 women, those who consumed light to moderate amounts of alcohol (one to three drinks per week) had a lower risk of death from CV disease, especially those older than age 50 years.[10]
   c. All mortality: Alcohol increases the rate of death from suicide, cancers, and cirrhosis.[11] However, women with the heaviest alcohol consumption (more than 30 g) daily had the highest rate of mortality caused by increased risk of death from non-CV disease including breast cancer and cirrhosis.[12]
   d. Individuals who drink heavily are more likely to smoke cigarettes. Alcohol abuse is associated with increased rates of death from cancer of the mouth, esophagus, pharynx, larynx, and liver. Heavy drinking men (more than six drinks per day) had an RR of 1.6 for non-CV death. Women with similar levels of alcohol abuse had an increased relative risk of death of 2.2 compared with men.[13]

2. Hypertension: Alcohol abuse increases blood pressure levels. An observational study of more than 9000 individuals across Europe (4800 of whom were women) found that women as well as men who drank more than 300 mL/week had higher blood pressure readings.[14]

3. Other problems: Alcoholics, especially older alcoholics, were more likely to have diabetes and hip fractures.[15]
4. Endocrine changes:
    a. Heavy alcohol use is associated with menstrual irregularities including anovulation, menorrhagia, oligomenorrhea, premenstrual syndrome and luteal phase dysfunction, recurrent amenorrhea, and early menopause.[16]
    b. Alcoholism also increases the risk of spontaneous abortion and breast cancer.
    c. Sexual relations are less important to women alcoholics, but after a year's abstinence sexual function and pleasure returns to normal.[17]
    d. Alcohol abuse decreases fertility even at less than five drinks per week. In a fertility clinic, women who drank one to five drinks per week had an OR of 0.61 of conceiving as compared with abstinent women. Women who drank more than 10 drinks weekly had an OR of 0.34 of conceiving.[18]

> Women with similar levels of alcohol abuse had an increased relative risk of death of 2.2 compared with men.

Pregnancy

1. Alcoholism in pregnant women can lead to medical complications and fetal effects. Pregnant alcoholic women have a greater incidence of intrauterine growth retardation.[9]
2. Twenty percent of pregnant women continue to use alcohol. Three percent of women binge drink and 2 to 9 percent are heavy drinkers during pregnancy.[19]
3. Alcohol is a teratogen. Although it is known that binge or heavy drinking is related to fetal alcohol syndrome (FAS) and fetal alcohol effects (FAE), the "safe" amount of alcohol in pregnancy is not known. Pregnant women are therefore urged not to drink. Alcohol abuse is the most preventable cause of mental retardation. FAS occurs in 1.9/1000 births worldwide and 2.2/1000 births in North America. In alcohol-abusing women, the incidence rises to 25/1000.[9]
4. FAS is a syndrome of prenatal and postnatal growth retardation, mental retardation and particular morphology affecting face, hands and stature, including micrognathia, small hands, ears, fingers, toes and feet, antimongolian slant of eyes, wide bridged nose, midface hypoplasia, single palmar crease and short stature. FAE is growth and mental retardation without the facial dysmorphology.

The elderly and alcohol abuse

1. Alcoholism is less prevalent in the elderly. Fifteen percent of men and 12 percent of women older than age 60 years in community clinics drank alcohol excessively.[20]

2. However, alcohol abuse in the elderly is associated with an increased incidence of depression, drug interactions, accidents, and emergency room and hospital visits. Elderly individuals with alcohol abuse are more likely to have cognitive impairment, heart arrhythmias, vascular effects, and social problems.

3. Approximately half of the elderly use some alcohol and 60 to 80 percent use medications for which there may be a risk of interactions, including NSAIDs, aspirin, sedatives, narcotics, antidepressants, antihypertensive medication, H2 blockers, warfarin, heart failure, gout and diabetes medications. Thirty-eight percent of the elderly, in an observational study, used both alcohol and high risk medication.[10]

4. Detecting alcoholism in the elderly may be more difficult. Those older individuals who are retired were more likely, in an observational study, to be heavy drinkers than those employed. The CAGE screening test (see below) worked less well and identified only half of the elderly drinkers. Physicians who are concerned about alcoholism in the elderly should also ask about quantity and frequency of alcohol consumption.[14]

> Alcohol abuse in the elderly is associated with an increased incidence of depression, drug interactions, accidents, and emergency room and hospital visits.

Diagnosis

1. Screening tests:
   a. A part of addiction often is denial of the problem. This is a major difficulty in treatment. Various screening tests have therefore been developed to help the physician determine whether the individual has an alcohol problem. Validated on men, some of these tests are not quite as accurate in women and the elderly.
   b. One of the best-studied screening tests is the CAGE or CAGE for drugs. Two positive answers is 60 to 90 percent sensitive and 40 to 60 percent specific for alcohol or drug abuse (Table 27.1).[20] The CAGE does not focus on current use, but on lifetime use, and it will not detect those individuals early in the course of the disease.
   c. An additional question on tolerance has been validated for pregnant women (Table 27.1). The question on tolerance may provoke a positive

Table 27.1. T-CAGE questions adapted to include drugs

T – How many drinks does it take to make you feel high?

- Have you felt you ought to **C**ut down on your drinking or drug use?
- Have people **A**nnoyed you by criticizing your drinking or drug use?
- Have you felt **G**uilty about your drinking or drug use?
- Have you ever had a drink, or used drugs first thing in the morning to steady your nerves or to get rid of a hangover or to get the day started? (**E**ye-opener)

Two or more "yes" answers indicate a need for a more in-depth assessment. Even one positive response should raise a red flag about problem drinking or drug use

Adapted from Schulz JE, Parran T Jr. Principles of identification and intervention. In Graham AW, Shultz TK, eds., *Principles of Addiction Medicine*, 2nd edn. American Society of Addiction Medicine, Chevy Chase, MD, 1998, pp. 249–52.

Table 27.2. Additional questions for women

- Has alcohol ever affected your relationship with husband or children?
- Do you use any medications for nerves?
- Do you carry alcohol in your purse or other secret place?
- Do you drink alone?
- Has your appearance changed or have you neglected it?

From Beebe D. Addictive behaviors. In Rosenfeld JA, ed., *Women's Health in Primary Care*. Williams & Wilkins, Baltimore, MD, 1997, pp. 227–40.

answer and less denial. With pregnant women, the physician may want to ask additional questions. Even one positive answer on the CAGE for a pregnant woman is significant.[21]

d. The CAGE, also, is not as sensitive for women because women are more likely to drink at home and less likely to be identified. Additional questions to detect alcohol disease in women are important (Table 27.2).

2. The social history may provide clues to alcoholism. Signs of family stress, domestic abuse, divorce, separation, difficulty keeping appointments, trouble at home and work or losing jobs, financial problems and frequent motor vehicle accidents are associated with alcohol abuse. An arrest for driving while intoxicated is 75 percent associated with alcoholism; two arrests for driving while intoxicated is 95 percent sensitive for alcoholism.

3. The medical history may give evidence of alcohol abuse. Depression, hepatitis or any liver disease, pancreatitis, unexplained intermittent seizures, myocardial infarctions at a young age, sleep or sexual dysfunction, cancer of the mouth or esophagus, anxiety, personality changes, menstrual disorders,

infertility, blackouts, gout and/or drug addiction or benzodiazepine use can be associated with alcoholism.

4. Physical signs of hyperestrogen states such as telangictasias may give evidence of alcohol abuse.

5. Laboratory tests may be used but are not sensitive or specific. The best test is the glutamyl galactose tolerance (GGT), liver function test that is often elevated when the individual has alcoholic liver disease. Serum levels of glutamyl oxaloacetate transferase and glutamyl pyruvate transferase may also be elevated.

> The CAGE questionnaire is not as sensitive for women because women are more likely to drink at home and less likely to be identified.

Treatment

1. Approximately one-third recover without any professional help.[1]

2. The individual often does not seek treatment until the medical and social consequences are calamitous and urgent. However, women are more likely to notice and recognize a problem with alcohol abuse and seek help earlier. Women and the elderly do as well as men in treatment.

3. Many treatment options – inpatient, outpatient, structured many ways – have been used. Abstinence is recommended. Physicians can make a difference in their office and through appropriate referrals.

4. Treatment for women alcoholics may be more difficult because the woman may be divorced or separated, and un- or underemployed and separated, thus, from any medical insurance. Women may have dependents and child care problems (Table 27.3).

> Women are more likely to notice and recognize a problem with alcohol abuse and seek help earlier.

5. Treatment options:

   a. Brief interventions: A metaanalysis found that very brief interventions were not successful in decreasing alcohol use in women or men, but repeated extended brief interventions in physician's office over several minutes did decrease alcohol abuse among women. The women had an average decrease of 51 g or four drinks per week.[22] Brief interventions are based on the stages of change described by J. O. Prochaska and C. C. DiClemente.[23]

   Another clinical trial of brief physician advice for older alcoholics found that intervention in the family physician's office caused significant reduction in seven-day alcohol use, with decrease in episodes of binge drinking

Table 27.3. Special needs of woman alcoholic or drug abuser

- Home and income: May be single, with dependent children or homeless – do they have adequate housing?
- Social Services: Help with children, foster-care, public assistance, etc.
- Marital counselling: Marriage often troubled, spousal abuse, divorce, separation
- Insurance: Partially, under- or unemployed – may not have insurance or means of obtaining health care?
- Multiply addicted: May be dependent on alcohol, illicit and prescription drugs
- Vocational training: Partially, under- or unemployed
- Medical care: Coexistent medical problems or pregnancy
- Child care: Help while she gets help

(74 percent) and frequency of excessive drinking (62 percent) at 3, 6, and 12 months.[19]

b. Group programs: Alcoholics Anonymous (AA) has been the traditional outpatient alcohol treatment program, and approximately 6 to 10 percent of all individuals, and 12 to 20 percent of those with alcohol problems have attended an AA meeting. Thirty percent of AA members are women.[9]

AA and other 12-step recovery programs are effective. Of half of those who stay for a year, 67 percent remain sober and of those who remain for two years 85 percent remain sober.[24] Studies of more than 8000 patients including adolescents found that those in AA were 50 percent more likely to be sober.[25]

c. There are traditional consultant addiction specialists whose approach has positive results in 80 percent of cases.[26]

6. Pharmacotherapy:

a. Disulfiram can be useful early in recovery. It causes a severe, sometimes fatal, toxic reaction if alcohol is used. The alcoholic must therefore be prepared to remain abstinent.

b. Naltrexone is a long acting opioid that blocks the euphoric effect of opiates. It has been promoted as adjunctive treatment for alcohol dependence. In a controlled study, those on naltrexone had reduced craving and increased rate of abstinence for 12 weeks.[27]

Physicians can make a difference in their office and through appropriate referrals.

Drug addiction

Impact

1. Six percent of the US population have a drug use disorder. Thirty percent of adults in the UK have used illicit drugs at some time, but the prevalence of misuse of prescription drugs is greater.[1]
2. The most commonly abused illicit drug in the USA is marijuana, with 10 million users. At least 13 million Americans use at least one illicit substance in any month. Two million use cocaine, 600 000 weekly. The greatest use is in the age group 18 to 25 years, and leads to 20 000 deaths per year in the USA.[28]
3. Drug abuse disorders are more common in men (7 percent) as compared with women (5 percent).[29] However, drug abuse is the second most common psychiatric disorder in women.[30] Women are more likely to abuse prescription drugs such as benzodiazepines, anxiolytics and psychotropic medication.
4. Lifetime use of cocaine is greater in poor, minority, and adolescent women, who have small children vulnerable to neglect. The complications for cocaine abuse are the same as for men. However, women, the elderly, and patients with liver disease have greater susceptibility to cocaine's effects, especially the cardiotoxic effects including cardiomyopathy, myocarditis, left ventricular hypertrophy, pulmonary embolism, tachycardia, myocardial infarctions, and sudden death.

> Drug abuse is the second most common psychiatric disorder in women.

Clinical presentation

1. Medical history: Clues to addiction and drug abuse problems include social and medical problems. Depression, divorce, job loss, unemployment and abuse are all associated with addiction. Medical complications include infection, bacteremia, cellulitis, endocarditis, and HIV infection. Complications from addiction lifestyle include poor nutrition, cigarette smoking, alcoholism, and homelessness.[31]
2. During pregnancy:
   a. All these problems impact on pregnancy. Eleven to 24 percent of pregnant women in the USA use illicit drugs during pregnancy.[31]
   b. Fetal effects include prematurity, low birth weight, abruptio placentae, preterm birth, increased incidence of spontaneous abortion, mental retardation, neonatal abstinence syndrome, neonatal infections, sudden infant death syndrome, neurobehavioral abnormalities, and poorer outcomes.

Table 27.4. Screening for drug misuse

Give the patient a list of illicit drugs

- Have you misused one of the substances more than five times in your life?
- Have you ever found you needed to increase your use of substance in order to get the same effect?
- Have you ever had emotional or psychological problems from using drugs – like feeling crazy or paranoid or uninterested in things?

Adapted from Rose K, Vurnam MA, Smith GR. Development of screeners for depressive disorders and substance disorder history: *Med Care* 1993;**31**:189–200.

c. Intensive prenatal substance abuse care and counselling can improve outcomes, although facilities for pregnant addicts are often difficult to fine.

d. Heroin use was associated with small babies, by an average of almost 500 g. Methadone use in pregnant women produced smaller babies but larger than for those women who used heroin.[32]

e. In an observational study, 2.3 percent of more than 7400 women used cocaine during pregnancy or tested positive, although only one in 10 admitted to using it. Eleven percent of women admitted to marijuana or tested positive. Cocaine was not associated with low birth weight or increased preterm babies, although it was associated with increased incidence of abruption.[33]

Diagnosis

The CAGE or CAGE for drugs or Rose Questionnaire (Table 27.4)[34] can be used to screen for drug addiction. Those medical and social clues for alcoholism, including alcohol abuse itself, are also clues to drug addiction. Family can often add information to the diagnosis.

Treatment

Treatment can be outpatient, inpatient or a combination, and include pharmacotherapy. The family physician has a part in the treatment program.

1. Recovery is a "process of adaption and growth in a previously addicted patient now committed to a lifestyle excluding use of psychoactive substances." Recovery is medical, psychological and social. The patient must be committed to abstinence.[27]

2. The family physician will be needed, although the patient may not want any medication. She may be cautious, embarrassed or rejecting the physician. The physician should be careful not to prescribe narcotics, benzodiazepines or

antitussives containing alcohol. Medical problems such as gastritis, hepatitis, HIV, and withdrawal symptoms may need treatment.

3. Family members should be involved.

4. Pharmacotherapy: Three drugs have been used in drug addiction – methadone, LAAM (L-alpha-acetylmethadol) a long-acting methadone opiate agonist that can be given only three times a week, and naltrexone. Methadone daily doses greater than 60 mg are more effective in retaining patients in treatment. Naltrexone blocks opiate receptors, preventing the euphoric rush.

   Heroin-addicted women can be treated with methadone. Methadone-treated pregnant women attended twice as many treatment days for outpatient addiction treatment as those not receiving methadone.[35]

Conclusions

Addiction, alcohol, and substance abuse occur in women and affect women differently, often more seriously with less substance abuse. All addictions, but especially alcohol, cause many serious health consequences and worsen other medical conditions. Screening tests are available, and treatment opportunities exist, so physicians should be sensitive to the possibility of addiction in their women patients.

REFERENCES

1. Ashworth M, Gerada C. ABC of mental health: Addiction and dependence: II. Alcohol. *BMJ* 1997;**315**:358–60.

2. Wilsnack SC, Wilsnack RW. Epidemiology of women's drinking. *J Subst Abuse* 1991;**3**:133–57.

3. National Institute on Alcohol Abuse and Alcoholism. *Ninth Special Report to the US Congress on Alcohol and Health.* Publication no. 97-4017. National Institutes of Health, Bethesda, MD, 1997.

4. Beebe D. Addictive behaviors. In Rosenfeld JA, ed., *Women's Health in Primary Care.* Williams & Wilkins, Baltimore, MD, 1997, pp. 227–40.

5. Makela P, Valkonene T, Martelin T. Contribution of deaths related to alcohol use to socioeconomic variation in mortality: Register based follow up study. *BMJ* 1997;**315**:211–16.

6. Wilsnack RW, Wilsnack SC, Klassen AD. Women's drinking and drinking problems: Patterns from a 1981 survey. *Am J Public Health* 1984;**74**:1231–8.

7. Helzer JE, Burnam A, McEvoy LT. Alcohol abuse and dependence. In Robins LN, Regier DA, eds., *Psychiatric Disorders in America: The Epidemiologic Catchment Area Study.* The Free Press, Macmillan, Inc., New York, 1991, pp. 81–115.

8. Kessler RC, Crum RM, Warner LA. Lifetime co-occurence of DSM-IIIR alcohol abuse and

dependence with other psychiatric disorders in the National Comorbidity Survey. *Arch Gen Psychiatry* 1997;**54**:313–21.

9. Quinby PM, Graham AV. Substance abuse among women. *Primary Care* 1993;**20**:131–41.

10. Fuchs CS, Stampfer MJ, Colditz GA et al. Alcohol consumption and mortality among women. *N Engl J Med* 1995;**332**;1245–50.

11. Tun MJ. Alcohol consumption and mortality among middle-aged and elderly US adults. *N Engl J Med* 1997;**337**:2705–14.

12. Hanna E, Dufour MC, Elliott S, Stinson F, Harford TC. Dying to be equal: Women, alcohol, and cardiovascular disease. *Br J Addict* 1992;**87**:1593–7.

13. Marmot MG, Elliott P, Shipley MJ et al. Alcohol and blood pressure: the INTERSALT study. *BMJ* 1994;**308**:1263–7.

14. Adams WL, Barry KL, Flemin MF et al. Screening for problem drinking in older primary care patients. *JAMA* 1996;**276**:1964–7.

15. Sarkola T, Makisalo H, Fukunaga T, Eriksson CJ. Acute effect on estradiol, estrone, progesterone, prolactin, cortisol and luteinizing hormone in premenopausal women. *Alcoholism* 1999;**23**:976–81.

16. Gavler JS, Rizzo A, Roassaro L et al. Sexuality of alcoholic postmenopausal women: Effects of duration of alcohol abstinence. *Alcoholism* 1994;**18**:269–71.

17. Jense TK, Hjollund NH, Henriksen TB et al. Does moderated alcohol consumption affect fertility? Follow-up study among couples planning first pregnancy. *BMJ* 1998;**317**:505–10.

18. Day NL, Cottreau CM, Richardson GA. The epidemiology of alcohol, marijuana, and cocaine use among women of childbearing age and pregnant women. *Clin Obstet Gynecol* 1993;**36**:232–45.

19. Fleming MF, Manswell LB, Barry KL, Adams W, Staffacher EA. Brief physician advice for alcohol problems in older adults. *J Fam Pract* 1999;**48**:378–84.

20. Schulz JE, Parran T Jr. Principles of identification and intervention. In Graham AW, Shultz TK, eds., *Principles of Addiction Medicine*, 2nd edn. American Society of Addiction Medicine, Chevy Chase, MD, 1998, pp. 249–52.

21. Cullen TA, Moriah KA. Screening for alcohol abuse in pregnancy. *Am Fam Physician* 1995;**51**:1137–41.

22. Poiolainen K. Effectiveness of brief interventions to reduce alcohol intake in primary care populations: A meta-analysis. *Prev Med* 1999;**28**:503–9.

23. Prochaska JO, DiClemente CC. Stages and processes of self-change of smoking: Toward an integrative model of change. *J Consult Psychol* 1983;**51**:390–5.

24. Makela K. Rates of attrition among the members of Alcoholics Anonymous in Finland. *J Stud Alcohol* 1994;**55**:91–5.

25. Hoffman NG, Miller NS. Treatment outcomes for abstinence-based programs. *Psychiatr Ann* 1992;**22**:312–27.

26. Johnson, V. *I'll Quit Tomorrow*. Harper & Row, New York, 1980.

27. Del Toro IM, Thom DJ, Beam HP, Horst T. Chemically dependent patients in recovery: Roles for the family physician. *Am Fam Physician* 1996;**53**:1667–81.

28. Haverkos HW, Stein MD. Identifying substance abuse in primary care. *Am Fam Physician* 1995;**52**:2029–35.

29. Anthony JC, Helzer JE. Syndromes of drug abuse and dependence. In Robins LN, Regier DA, eds., *Psychiatric Disorders in America*. The Free Press, Macmillan, New York, 1991, pp. 116–54.

30. Maroney JT, Allen MH. Cocaine and alcohol use in pregnancy. *Adv Neurol* 1994;**18**:231–42.

31. Jannson LM, Sivikis D, Lee J et al. Pregnancy and addiction. *J Subst Abuse* 1996;**13**:321–6.

32. Hulse GK, Milkne E, English DR, Holman CD. The relationship between maternal use of heroin and methadone and infant birth weight. *Addiction* 1997;**92**:1571–9.

33. Shiono PH, Klebanoff MA, Nugent RP et al. The impact of cocaine and marijuana use on low birth rate. *Am J Obstet Gynecol* 1995;**172**:19–24.

34. Rose K, Vurnam MA, Smith GR. Development of screeners for depressive disorders and substance disorder history. *Med Care* 1993;**31**:189–200.

35. Svikis DS, Lee JH, Haug NA, Stitzer ML. Attendance incentives for outpatient treatment effects in methadone and non-methadone maintained drug-dependent women. *Drug Alcohol Depend* 1997;**48**:33–41.

28 Eating disorders

Janet Lair, MD

Eating disorders and disordered eating patterns are problems that disproportionately affect women of all ages.

Epidemiology

Impact

Women account for 90 to 95 percent of all cases of eating disorders diagnosed. Anorexia is seen in 1 percent and bulimia in 4 to 5 percent of the female population. In a prospective study of adolescents in Australia, 3.3 percent of adolescent girls and 0.3 percent of boys had a partial eating disorder. Girls who dieted at a severe level were 18 more times as likely to develop an eating disorder.[1]

Anorexia nervosa

This disease has the highest mortality of any psychiatric disorder.[2]

Incidence

The incidence of eating disorders has two peaks in adolescence corresponding to the onset of puberty (11 to 13 years) and late adolescence (18 to 20 years). Eating disorders can be seen at any age and in men as well as in women. Disordered eating patterns (without a specific diagnosis) may occur in 20 to 40 percent of adult women.[3]

Risk factors

In certain populations, the incidence is much higher. Groups of women at increased risk include adolescents, athletes, dancers and models.[4] Once thought to affect mostly young, white and relatively affluent women, recent surveys have shown that they equally affect women in all ethnic groups and income categories. In one telephone survey of more than 7300 women, African-American women were as likely as white women to report binge eating or vomiting, and more likely to report fasting and laxative or diuretic abuse within the previous three months.[5]

> Eating disorders equally affect women in all ethnic groups and income categories.

Associated medical problems

1. Women with eating disorders are more likely to have a history of sexual abuse. Women with bulimia were more likely than those with anorexia to report unwanted sexual experiences.[6]
2. Women with disabilities are more likely to have altered or disordered eating patterns.[7]
3. Women with psychiatric morbidity – obsessive-compulsive personality disorders, dysthymia, panic attacks, and depression disorders – may be more likely to have altered eating patterns and disorders.[1,8]

> Women with psychiatric morbidity may be more likely to have altered eating patterns and disorders.

Definitions (see Table 28.1)

Etiology

As more is learned about the increasing problem of eating disorders in society, it becomes clear that this condition fits a disease model that represents a complex set of biological, psychological, sociological, and spiritual factors. There are features of eating disorders that suggest a biological tendency or predetermination. Other psychological, spiritual and social features suggest these as etiological factors (Table 28.2).[9]

Clinical presentation (see Table 28.3)

Diagnosis and evaluation

1. Diagnosis is important, although presentation is often subtle. A few questionnaires for diagnosis exist, including the Eating Disorders Inventory, but these

Table 28.1. Definitions

Anorexia nervosa

Anorexia nervosa occurs in individuals who have:
- A body weight of 15 percent or more below normal weight for height or body mass index less than 17.5
- Restricted their caloric intake
- A fear of weight gain
- A distorted perception of body size, shape or weight
- Amenorrhea for 3 months after menarche or primary amenorrhea

Bulimia nervosa

Individuals have bulimia nervosa if they have:
- Recurrent binge eating (2 episodes/week for 3 months)
- Recurrent purging (2 times/week for 3 months)
- Recurrent emesis
- Laxative/enema abuse
- Excessive exercise
- Fasting/restricting between binge episodes
- Excessive concern over body image/weight/shape

Binge eating is defined by the consumption of large quantities of food in a short time period.

Binge eating disorder

is defined as:
- Recurrent overeating without purging behaviors
- Distress over abnormal eating
- Perceived lack of control over eating
- Feelings of guilt or shame
- Eating disorder, not otherwise specified
- Disordered eating that does not fall into the other three categories or has mixed features

are not screening tools. A five-question screening test called SCOFF (Table 28.4) has been suggested recently. With two or more questions positive, the SCOFF test is 100 percent sensitive for anorexia and bulimia, with a specificity of 87.5 percent.[10]

2. A multidisciplinary approach is often best for the woman with an eating disorder. This includes nutritional assessment and counselling by a nutritionist experienced in eating disorders, psychological support and treatment for the individual and family, and medical evaluation and follow-up for complications.

3. In young women (prepuberty and young adolescence), a failure to follow the normal growth curve or experiencing a gain in height without a commensurate gain in weight should be suspicious for early onset eating disorder. This is

Table 28.2. Features of eating disorders suggesting etiologies

Biological features
- Gender-specific pattern
- Women: men ratio of 15 : 1
- Age predominance
- Adolescence
- Serotonin research
- Appetite/behavior regulation
- Response to selective serotonic reuptake inhibitors
- Increased incidence in twins and families

Psychological features
- High incidence of comorbid illness
- Depression
- Anxiety, panic disorder
- Obsessive-compulsive disorder
- Personality disorder
- Substance abuse (bulimia)
- Distorted body image
- Personality traits
- Low self-esteem
- Perfectionism (anorexia)
- Drive for thinness (anorexia)
- Somatization (bulimia)

Sociological features
- Cultural high regard for extreme thinness
- Beliefs that thinner is healthier, sexier, more appealing
- Fat phobia
- Media messages to diet/lose weight

Spiritual
- Difficulty with self acceptance/love
- Social isolation/secrecy
- Obsession with food/weight/body

of great concern as this is the period most critical for accrual of adequate bone mass to last a woman's lifetime. Early onset of eating disorder carries a higher risk of development of osteoporosis.[11]

4. History:

a. The history should include onset and duration of illness, precipitating factors – diets and recent stresses.

Since the etiology of eating disorders is complex, a multidisciplinary approach to treatment works best.

Table 28.3. Symptoms of eating disorders

Anorexia
- Syncope/dizziness
- Dehydration/hypotension
- Hypoglycemia
- Amenorrhea/oligomenorrhea
- Referral from friends/family for weight loss
- Suicide attempts

Bulimia
- Somatic complaints – often gastrointestinal
- Dental referral
- Dehydration
- Self-referral with request for diet/weight concerns

Binge eating disorder
- Self-referral with weight concern or lack of control
- Overeating behavior

Table 28.4. The SCOFF questionnaire

1. Do you make yourself **S**ick because you feel uncomfortably full?
2. Do you worry you have lost **C**ontrol over how much you eat?
3. Have you recently lost more than **O**ne stone (14 lbs, 6.4 kg) in a 3-month period?
4. Do you believe yourself to be **F**at when others say you are too thin?
5. Would you say that **F**ood dominates your life?

From Morgan JF, Reid F, Lacey JH. The SCOFF questionnaire: Assessment of a new screening tool for eating disorders. *Br Med J* 1999;**319**:1467–8.

    b. The woman's highest and lowest weights, usual diet, dieting efforts, eating patterns, and exercise behaviors should be determined.

    c. She should be asked if she exhibits purging behaviors. Questions about body image perceptions and menstrual history are important.

    d. Finally, the woman should be screened for coexistent psychiatric disorders, substance and alcohol abuse, and sexual and physical abuse. Use of medication, herbal/natural products, and nonprescription drugs should be established.

5. Physical examination:

    a. The physical examination should include, at least, a height and weight measurement (use the same scale for each visit), vital signs, and orthostatic blood pressure and pulse.

    b. Noting the woman's general body habitus, and skin, the presence of gooseflesh, lanugo, and acrocyanosis, and her skin color and turgor is important.

c. Hypercarotenemia can occur from binge eating.

d. Russell's sign–dorsal hand lesions (calluses from inducing vomiting), edema, teeth erosions, and periodontal inflammation can occur.

e. Examination of the head and neck may also show parotid and thyroid gland enlargement.

f. The cardiovascular examination might show irregular heartbeats, tachycardia, or bradycardia.

g. Examination of the abdomen may show distension, increased bowel sounds, epigastric tenderness, or hepatosplenomegaly.

h. The woman may have musculoskeletal atrophy and poor muscle tone, abnormal tendon reflexes, a tremor, an abnormal gait, a different affect, and even confusion and coma.[12]

6. Laboratory evaluation: A minimal evalution includes the following:

a. A complete blood count to look for signs of malnutrition, such as anemia, leukopenia, or thrombocytopenia.

b. Electrolytes to eliminate diabetes or metabolic disturbances as causes for these symptoms, or a result from the disorder and vomiting.

c. Level of thyroid-stimulating hormone to evaluate for possible thyroid disease. Hyperthyroidism can have similar symptoms.

d. Consider performing an electrocardiogram when the woman's weight is 20–25 percent below ideal body weight, she has used ipecac or has symptoms of syncope, excessive vomiting, diarrhea, or evidence of hemodynamic compromise. Women with anorexia were found to have lower heart rates, lower R wave values in lead V6 and a longer QRS interval than other young women, but whether these were related to electrolyte disturbance was not known.[13]

> Women with anorexia were found to have lower heart rates, lower R wave values in lead V6 and a longer QRS interval than other young women.

Complications of eating disorders

1. Complications occur in proportion to the severity of the eating disorder and the duration. The clinician is more likely to see significant complications with weights less than 75 to 80 percent of ideal body weight, and with frequent vomiting and/or the use of laxatives and diuretics to achieve weight loss. A

Table 28.5. Complications of eating disorders

- Osteoporosis
- Dental erosions/caries
- Cardiac arrhythmias
- Cardiomyopathy
- Hypotension/hypovolemia
- Constipation/decreased gastrointestinal motility
- Abnormal liver function tests
- Esophagitis, esophageal tears
- Hypoglycemia
- Electrolyte disturbance
- Hypokalemia, hypomagnesemia, hyponatremia
- Metabolic alkalosis
- Hyperphosphatemia
- Euthyroid sick syndrome
- Delayed growth and/or puberty
- Amenorrhea, oligomenorrhea
- Infertility
- Increased pregnancy loss, low birth weight infants
- Stress fractures
- Hair loss, dry skin
- Anemia, thrombocytopenia, leukopenia
- Suicide risk

longer duration and more severe illness increases the risk of other complications (Table 28.5).

2. Morbidity/mortality:
   a. Significant short-term and long-term morbidity occur in women with eating disorders. Mortality is about 0.5 percent per year in women with anorexia and generally infrequent in women with bulimia.
   b. Suicide, cardiovascular compromise, and starvation in the most severe cases account for most of these deaths.
   c. A retrospective study of 246 women with anorexia, followed for 11 years, found a crude mortality rate of 5.1 percent, with a higher than normal suicide rate.[14] Another review suggests that suicide is not more common in women with anorexia.[15]

Significant short-term and long-term morbidity occur in women with eating disorders.

LIVERPOOL JOHN MOORES UNIVERSITY
LEARNING SERVICES

Table 28.6. Indications for immediate hospitalization for treatment of eating disorders

- Weight more that 25 percent below ideal body weight
- Rapid weight loss
- Significant medical complications
  - Electrolyte/metabolic abnormalities
  - Cardiac abnormalities
  - Gastrointestinal bleeding, esophageal rupture
- Significant psychological complications
  - Worsening depression
  - Risk of suicide
- Failure of outpatient treatment after 3 to 6 months

Treatment

1. For most women, outpatient treatment is possible. Ideally all three components – nutritional therapy, psychological counselling, and medical support – should be included in the treatment plan. If the professionals involved in treatment have the individual's consent to discuss and coordinate the care plan, the treatment works most efficiently.
2. Treatment tends to be lengthy and costly for most eating-disordered patients.
3. Occasionally women will require an inpatient admission for treatment. Indications for hospitalization are listed in Table 28.6.
4. Treatment goals include reversal of abnormal eating patterns. Some experts believe that until refeeding produces a certain weight gain, the woman cannot benefit from psychological and nutritional therapy.
5. Treatment includes reversal of malnutrition, psychological intervention, treatment of comorbid conditions, individual therapy, family therapy (adolescents/young adults), group therapy (bulimia), cognitive-behavioral interventions, and monitoring for medical complications. Some studies, including a RCT of 220 women with bulimia followed for one year, have found that cognitive-behavioral therapy was superior to interpersonal therapy in terms of number of women recovered and eating in normal patterns.[16]
6. Pharmacological treatment:
   a. Antidepressant therapy, especially use of selective serotonin reuptake inhibitors (SSRIs), has been shown to decrease binge/purge episodes in women bulimia and binge eating disorder and, after refeeding, help with

Nutritional therapy, psychological counselling, and medical support should be included in the treatment plan.

weight gain in women with anorexia. Their use also decreases obsessional thinking and prevents relapses.[17]

b. If the woman has coexisting depression, SSRIs and tricyclic antidepressants can be used. Bupropion is generally avoided in eating disorders because of concern about the possibility of seizures.

c. Women with these conditions also need hormonal supplementation. Treatment with estrogen/progesterone may prevent bone mass loss and osteoporosis. Often OCPs are used. If osteoporosis has already occurred, treatment with bone remineralization agents such as alendronate or calcitonin may be needed as well. Recovery from anorexia does not always mean recovery of lost bone mineral density, although there is not an increased incidence of fractures after recovery.[18]

Treatment with estrogen/progesterone may prevent bone mass loss and osteoporosis.

Course of illness/prognosis

1. Recovery: Outcome studies of more severely ill individuals from specialized treatment centers have shown that 50 percent of the women experience full recovery.[14] Thirty percent improve but continue to struggle with eating/body image issues and 20 percent have chronic eating disorders without substantial improvement. Populations with less severe illness have not been as intensively followed long term. Spontaneous remission and full recovery may be more common in milder forms of disordered eating.

2. Another important feature of eating disorders is that they change over time in many cases. A woman with anorexia may become bulimic eventually. Bulimic individuals may begin to restrict and later become anorexic.

3. Relapse often occurs in response to stressful events.

Conclusion

Eating disorders represent an increasingly common challenge to the clinician who treats women of all ages. Identification of the individual at risk is often difficult as the symptoms are frequently hidden from the health care provider and the woman may deny that a problem exists. Once the individual is identified, locating experienced providers of nutritional, psychological, and medical care can be a challenge. Given the current insurance climate, obtaining coverage for the recommended services and intensity of care may place effective treatment out of reach financially for many women.

Despite the many challenging aspects of caring for the woman with disordered eating or an eating disorder, assisting her in the process of recovery and return to a healthful, balanced life can be immensely rewarding.

REFERENCES

1. Patton GC, Selzer R, Coffer C, Carlin JB, Wolfe R. Onset of adolescent eating disorders: Population based cohort study over 3 years. *BMJ* 1999;**318**:765–8.
2. Vitiello B, Lederhendler I. Research on eating disorders: Current status and future prospects. *Biol Psychiatry* 2000;**47**:777–86.
3. American Psychiatric Association. Practice guidelines for eating disorders. *Am J Psychiatry* 1993;**150**:2.
4. Santonastaso P, Frederici S, Farrar A. Full and partial syndromes in eating disorders: A 1-year prospective study of risk factors among female students. *Psychopathology* 1999;**32**;50–6.
5. Striegel-Moore RH, Wilfrey DE, Pike KM, Dohm FA, Fairburn CG. Recurrent binge eating in black American women. *Arch Fam Med* 2000;**9**:83–7.
6. Waller G. Sexual abuse as a factor in eating disorders. *Br J Psychiatry* 1991;**159**:664–71.
7. Gross SM, Ireys HT, Kinsman SL. Young women with physical disabilities: Risk factors for symptoms of eating disorders. *J Dev Behav Pediatr* 2000;**21**:87–96.
8. Zaider TI, Johnson JG, Cockell SJ. Psychiatric comorbidity associated with eating disorder symptomatology among adolescents in the community. *Int J Eat Disord* 2000;**28**:58–67.
9. Becker AE, Greenspoon SK, Klibanski A, Herzog DB. Eating disorders. *New Engl J Med* 1999;**340**:1092–8.
10. Morgan JF, Reid F, Lacey JH. The SCOFF questionnaire: Assessment of a new screening tool for eating disorders. *BMJ* 1999;**319**:1467–8.
11. Putukian M. The female athlete triad. *Clin Sports Med* 1998;**17**:675–96.
12. Casper R. Recognizing eating disorders in women. *Psychopharmacol Bull* 1998;**34**:267–9.
13. Panagiotopoulos C, McCrindle BW, Hick K, Katzman DK. Electrocardiographic findings in adolescents with eating disorders. *Pediatrics* 2000;**105**:1100–5.
14. Herzog DB, Greenwood DN, Dorer DJ et al. Mortality in eating disorders: A descriptive study. *Int J Eat Disord* 2000;**28**:20–6.
15. Coren S, Hewitt PL. Is anorexia nervosa associated with elevated rates of suicide. *Am J Public Health* 1998;**88**:1206–7.
16. Agras WS, Walsh T, Fairburn CB, Wilson GT, Kraemer HC. Outcome predictors for the cognitive behavior treatment of bulimia nervosa. Data from a multisite study. *Arch Gen Psychiatry* 2000;**57**:459–66.
17. Kaye WH, Gendall K, Strober M. Serotonin: Implications for the etiology and treatment of eating disorders. *Eating Disord Rev* 1999;**10**:1–3.
18. Harman D, Crisp A, Rooney B et al. Bone density of women who have recovered from anorexia nervosa. *Int J Eat Disord* 2000;**28**:107–12.

Common medical problems

29 Coronary heart disease

Valerie Ulstad, MD

In recent years, the clinical understanding of coronary heart disease (CHD) in women has been greatly enhanced. There are important differences between men and women concerning CHD.

Introduction

1. The similarities between men and women with respect to CHD outweigh the differences. CHD does not discriminate on the basis of gender. CHD remains the number one killer of women and men. Since 1984, CHD has annually globally killed more women than men.[1]
2. Prevention of CHD is a major health issue for women.
   a. Women often do not believe they are at risk for CHD.
   b. Common misperceptions are that CHD is a man's disease and that the most likely threat to a woman's life is breast cancer. Over a lifetime, a woman is 10 times more likely to develop CHD than she is breast cancer.[2]
   c. Coronary bypass surgery or angioplasty with stent placement does not prevent future heart attacks.[3] These procedures only relieve ischemia in the distribution of established stenoses. Future heart attacks are prevented by the prevention of plaque formation in the coronary arteries and by stabilization and regression of existing plaque through lifestyle modification.
3. Efforts must continue to empower all women to take personal preventative action to prevent CHD.

Coronary heart disease remains the number one killer of women and men.

Primary prevention: Reducing the incidence of CHD in women

Research

Two important studies have been the foundation of our understanding of CHD risk factors in women.

1. The Framingham Heart Study is an important longitudinal cohort study of cardiovascular disease and was the first to systematically study this process in women. The study started in 1948 and included women from the beginning. The initial rationale for inclusion of women was to understand why, compared with young men, young women seemed to be protected from CHD.

    The Framingham study's most important contributions to the understanding of CHD in women include:

    a. That women develop CHD manifestations 10 years later than men.
    b. That women tend to present with angina as their initial manifestation of CHD, whereas men tend to present with myocardial infarction (MI).
    c. That silent or clinically unrecognized MI is more common in women than in men.
    d. That the case fatality rate for acute MI is higher in women.[4]

    The Framingham study established the concept of the cardiovascular risk factor and showed that risk factors for CHD are similar in women and men.

2. The Nurses' Health Study (NHS) begun in 1976, has been the foundation of specifically characterizing CHD risk in women. Initial enrollment included 120 000 women between ages 30 and 55 years with participants now aged 50 to 75 years. Every two years, this cohort fills out extensive questionnaires about their health and lifestyles and the questions are periodically changed, allowing examination of the relationship between different lifestyle factors and medical outcomes.[5]

3. The fundamentals of reducing the incidence of CHD in women suggested by these two landmark studies include smoking cessation, control of lipids, control of systolic and diastolic hypertension, regular physical activity of moderate intensity, a healthy diet, and weight control.

Women develop coronary heart disease manifestations 10 years later than men.

Nonmodifiable risk factors for CHD (Table 29.1)

1. Incidence: The incidence of CHD in women aged 35 to 44 years is 1 per 1000, increasing to 4 per 1000 in women aged 45 to 54 years. In the fifth decade, the incidence of CHD is half that of men. By the sixth decade, the incidence of

Table 29.1. Risk factors in coronary heart disease in women

Nonmodifiable risk factors for CHD
- Age
- Race
- Family history
- Low socioeconomic status

Major modifiable risk factors
- Cigarette smoking
- Hypertension
- Lipid abnormalities
  - An elevated serum cholesterol level greater than 260 mg/dL
  - LDL cholesterol elevation
  - Low HDL cholesterol
  - Elevated triglyceride
- Diabetes mellitus
- Obesity
- Sedentary lifestyle

LDL, low density lipoprotein; HDL, high density lipoprotein.

CHD is equal in women and men. One in four women older than age 65 years has CHD.[6]

2. Race: CHD is a particularly important threat to African-American women, who have a higher incidence of CHD and an earlier mortality from CHD than both African-American men and white women and men. The decline in CHD morbidity and mortality over the last 20 years has also been less dramatic in black women compared to white women. [7] Data from other racial groups is sparse. However, the risk factors for myocardial infarction in an urban area of Japan are the same as in Western countries. The most significant risk factor is diabetes.[8] Those individuals with risk factors are at high risk for heart disease.[9]

3. Family history: Family history is a risk factor for CHD. If an individual's first-degree male relative younger than age 55 years or first-degree female relative younger than 65 years developed clinically manifest CHD or experienced unexplained death, her risk of CHD is increased. A family history of early heart disease in female relatives is a strong predictor for CHD.[10]

4. Socioeconomic status: Low socioeconomic status is significantly associated with the development of CHD in women, because of the likelihood of the presence of more CHD risk factors, including higher BMI, physical inactivity, cigarette smoking, and elevated LDL cholesterol.[11]

5. Family-related variables in women such as cultural habits, socioeconomic status, education, and insurance coverage may play a role in the modification

of atherosclerotic development and progression, the recognition of adaptation to disease, and recovery from serious illness.[12]

One in four women older than age 65 years has coronary heart disease.

Major modifiable risk factors (Table 29.1)

1. Cigarette smoking:
   a. Twenty-three percent of US women are currently cigarette smokers.[13] Smoking is the major cause of CHD in young and middle-aged women, accounting for up to half of all coronary deaths.[14]
   b. There is a dose–response effect associated with smoking in women. A woman who smokes one to four cigarettes per day is at twice the risk of an acute MI as a nonsmoker, while a woman who smokes more than 45 cigarettes per day has a risk that is 11 times higher than that of a nonsmoker.[14] Women who smoke have their first MI 19 years earlier than women who do not smoke.[15]
   c. After smoking cessation, the risk falls back to the level of a nonsmoking woman within three to five years (the risk of lung cancer takes much longer to drop back to baseline). This is independent of the amount smoked, the age of quitting or the duration of the smoking habit.[16]
   d. Other disadvantageous effects of smoking include lower HDL cholesterol levels, lower serum estrogen levels, increase in serum fibrinogen levels, and earlier onset of menopause. Complete cessation of nicotine use and avoidance of passive nicotine inhalation should be the goal.

Smoking is the major cause of coronary heart disease in young and middle-aged women, accounting for up to half of all coronary deaths.

2. Hypertension:
   a. Systolic and diastolic hypertension, defined as a blood pressure of more than 140/90 mmHg and the use of antihypertensive medication, strongly and independently increases the risk of CHD in women.[17] Reducing blood pressure with medication decreases cardiovascular morbidity and mortality in women to the same extent as it does in men.[18]
   b. More women than men develop hypertension as they get older. In women older than age 45 years, 60 percent of white women are hypertensive and 79 percent of African-American women are hypertensive and the majority of women with hypertension are under poor control.[7]
   c. Isolated systolic hypertension (ISH) is predominantly a disease of older

Reducing blood pressure with medication decreases cardiovascular morbidity and mortality in women to the same extent as it does in men.

women, affecting approximately 30 percent of women over 65 years.[19] Control of ISH is associated with a marked decrease in stroke and fatal and nonfatal MI.

d. Weight loss, avoidance of alcohol, cessation of the use of NSAIDs, smoking cessation, sodium restriction, adequate potassium, calcium and magnesium intake and regular exercise are important elements in a strategy to control hypertension. Nonpharmacological treatment of hypertension is important to consider because it can be extremely effective and often allows avoidance of the expense and side effects of medication.[20]

Nonpharmacological treatment of hypertension is important.

3. Lipid abnormalities:
    a. Lipid abnormalities are important predictors of CHD risk in women. Recently data on the effects of lipid lowering in women have increased dramatically. An elevated serum cholesterol level in women is as predictive of later CHD events as it is in men.[21] A woman with a serum cholesterol level of greater than 260 mg/dL has a relative risk for CHD mortality of 1.4 compared to a woman with a cholesterol < 200 mg/dL.[22]
    b. Recent RCTs have demonstrated that cholesterol lowering reduces CHD endpoints in subjects with CHD and high cholesterol levels (20 percent of subjects were women),[23] those with CHD and average cholesterol levels (14 to 17 percent of subjects were women),[24] and those without CHD with average cholesterol levels (17 percent of subjects were women).[25] In these studies, lowering cholesterol levels significantly reduced CHD deaths, the risk of stroke, and total mortality without an increase in noncardiovascular deaths.
    c. LDL cholesterol: LDL cholesterol is the major atherogenic lipoprotein in women. The higher the levels, the higher the CHD risk.[10] LDL levels do not predict CHD risk as strongly in women as they do in men.[21]
    d. HDL cholesterol: HDL cholesterol, a stronger predictor of CHD risk in women than LDL, is second only to age as a predictor of death from cardiovascular disease among women.[26] Women with an HDL less than 50 mg/dL have an increased mortality (RR = 1.7) compared to women with

An elevated serum cholesterol level in women is as predictive of later coronary heart disease events as it is in men.

High density lipoprotein cholesterol, a stronger predictor of coronary heart disease risk in women than low density lipoprotein cholesterol, is second only to age as a predictor of death from cardiovascular disease among women.

HDL over 50 mg/dL. An HDL level of greater than 60 mg/dL is considered protective against CHD.[10]

e. Triglycerides: Elevated triglyceride levels have been shown to be an independent risk factor for CHD in women.[27] Whether the elevated risk associated with elevated triglycerides is related to the triglycerides themselves, or whether they are a marker for the metabolic syndrome that includes low levels of HDL cholesterol, small dense LDL particles and nonlipid factors, such as hypertension, insulin resistance, and a prothrombotic state, is not presently clear.[28]

f. Therapy: Diet and exercise should be the cornerstones of lipid-lowering therapy. Dietary therapy should be tailored to reduce dietary cholesterol and saturated fats, replacing them with monounsaturated and polyunsaturated fats. Calorie restriction should be recommended if weight loss is indicated. Frequent and consistent encouragement about dietary compliance and weight control by the clinician will maximize success. If diet, weight reduction, and exercise have not reduced LDL cholesterol to desired levels in three to six months, drug therapy should be considered.

g. Lifestyle changes that increase HDL include weight loss, smoking cessation, and regular physical activity. The first steps in treatment of hypertriglyceridemia are nonpharmacological, including weight loss, reduced calories from saturated fat, reduced simple carbohydrates, abstinence from alcohol, and increased physical activity.[10]

h. In women, as in men, treatment decisions are based on the LDL levels, although consideration of all the lipid parameters are important in counselling patients regarding life style modification. A fasting total cholesterol, HDL and triglyceride level are obtained and the LDL level is calculated from these levels (see Table 29.2). There is, unfortunately, ample evidence that these guidelines are not implemented successfully in women or men.[29] Of the 2763 women with vascular disease recruited for the Heart and Estrogen/Progestin Replacement Study (HERS) trial, only 9 percent met the National Cholesterol Education Program (NCEP) (Table 29.2) goals of LDL cholesterol less than 100 mg/dL.

i. Lipid management is a rapidly changing area of CHD prevention. The Air

Diet and exercise should be the cornerstones of lipid-lowering therapy.

Table 29.2. National Cholesterol Education Program guidelines for target lipid levels in the treatment of hyperlipidemia

LDL cholesterol	100 mg/dL	Women with established vascular disease
	130 mg/dL	Women with no atherosclerosis and two or greater risk factors
		Women ⩾ 55 years
		Premature menopause without estrogen replacement
		Family history of premature CHD
		Smoking
		Hypertension
		HDL < 35 mg/dL
		Diabetes
	160 mg/dL	Women with fewer than 2 risk factors
	100 mg/dL	Women with diabetes
Triglyceride levels	200 mg/dL	
HDL cholesterol	> 60 mg/dL	

LDL, low density lipoprotein; HDL, high density lipoprotein; CHD, coronary heart disease. Data from Walden CE, Retzlaff BM, Buck BL, McCann BS, Knopp RH. Lipoprotein lipid response to the National Cholesterol Education Program Step II diet by hypercholesterolemic and combined hyperlipidemic women and men. *Arterioscler Thromb Vasc Biol* 1997;**17**:375–82.

Force/Texas Coronary Atherosclerosis Prevention Study (AFCAPS/Tex-CAPS) examined the effect of lovastatin therapy in women and men who were healthy (without CHD) with low levels of HDL cholesterol (< 50 mg/dL in women), LDL cholesterol levels of 130 to 190 mg/dL and triglyceride levels less than 400 mg/dL. Therapy with lovastatin reduced the risk of first major coronary event by 36 percent in the study population in general, by 54 percent in women, and by 34 percent in men.[25] Only 17 percent of the group that attained treatment benefit would have qualified for treatment under the current NCEP guidelines. New treatment goals are likely as the clinical trial evidence mounts that in men and in women lower cholesterol levels should be the goal.

4. Diabetes mellitus:
   a. Diabetes is a more potent risk factor for CHD in women than in men and negates the gender differential in the age of CHD onset.[30] Diabetes

Diet and exercise should be the cornerstones of lipid-lowering therapy.

eliminates the protective effect of estrogen on CHD in women. Mortality rates from CHD are three to seven times higher among diabetic women than among nondiabetic women as compared with rates that are two to four times higher among diabetic men compared with men without diabetes.[31]

b. Optimal control of diabetes is important for a variety of reasons, but the increased risk of subsequent cardiovascular events probably persists compared to the nondiabetic.[32] Diabetics must vigorously modify other cardiovascular risk factors to avoid compounding the CHD risk.

> Diabetes eliminates the protective effect of estrogen on coronary heart disease in women.

5. Obesity:
   a. There is a direct positive association between obesity and the risk of CHD in women. Although obesity is associated with diabetes mellitus, lipid abnormalities and hypertension in women, an independent effect of obesity persists even after adjustment for known cardiovascular risk factors.[33] In the NHS, the risk of CHD was over three times higher among women with a BMI of 29 or higher than among lean women.
   b. Even women who were mildly to moderately overweight (BMI 25 to 28.9) had nearly twice the risk of CHD compared with lean women.[34]
   c. Direct evidence that weight loss reduces CHD risk is lacking. These data are difficult to obtain, in part caused by the difficulties in maintaining weight loss.[30]
   d. Excess abdominal and upper body adiposity is associated with a particularly high risk of CHD in women.[34] The risk of CHD rises steeply among women whose waist to hip ratio is higher than 0.8.[35] Whether the risk associated with body fat distribution can be modified is uncertain.

> There is a direct positive association between obesity and the risk of coronary heart disease in women.

6. Sedentary lifestyle:
   a. Physically active women have a significant graded reduction in CHD risk as compared with sedentary women.[36]
   b. All-cause mortality is lower in physically fit women and higher levels of fitness have been shown to offer a greater mortality benefit for women than for men.[37]
   c. Women can improve their risk factor profiles, particularly by raising HDL levels, by increasing their level of physical activity.[38]
   d. Older women are at higher risk for cardiac events and are least likely to

engage in regular physical activity. Every woman in the USA should accumulate 30 minutes or more of moderate-intensity physical activity (equivalent of walking briskly at 3 to 4 miles/hour (4 to 6.8 km/hour)) on most days of the week.[39]

Every woman should accumulate 30 minutes or more of moderate-intensity physical activity (equivalent of walking briskly at 3 to 4 miles/hour (4 to 6.8 km/hour)) on most days of the week.

Other issues in CHD risk reduction: Drugs for primary and secondary prevention

Hormone replacement therapy

1. Until recently, the only data available about the potential magnitude of the cardioprotective effect of estrogen were from case control and observational studies. Although these studies consistently suggested a 50 percent reduction in CHD in women taking estrogen,[40] the studies, by the nature of their design, are subject to bias caused by known and unknown factors that may be overrepresented in the treatment or control group. The most ardent skeptics of these studies have postulated that intrinsically healthier women were more likely to have taken estrogen, leading to an apparent beneficial effect of estrogen on cardiovascular health.[41]

2. Estrogen has been shown to reduce LDL cholesterol levels and increase HDL levels by 10 to 15 percent.[42] The lipid benefits may account for as much as half of the apparent protective effect seen with estrogen.[43]

3. Estrogen has also been shown to have direct beneficial effects on the vasculature and endothelial function.[44]

4. The Postmenopausal Estrogen/Progestin Interventions Trial (PEPI) was a three-year multicenter, placebo-controlled RCT, designed to assess the effects of unopposed estrogen and three combination estrogen-plus-progestin (HRT) regimens on CHD risk factors in 875 healthy postmenopausal women aged 45 to 64 years.[45] This study showed that estrogen alone or in combination with a progestin significantly improved the lipid profile in healthy women. The beneficial lipid effects were somewhat attenuated by progestin. All four hormonal regimens increased triglyceride levels. This study looked only at effects on risk factors and did not examine clinical CHD endpoints. Thus it simply advanced the biological plausibility that hormones may protect the heart.

5. HERS, the first randomized double blind placebo controlled trial of HRT (conjugated estrogen 0.625 mg + MPA 2.5 mg daily) for CHD prevention in

women, was designed to assess whether HRT alters the cardiac risk in post-menopausal women with established CHD.[46] The primary outcome evaluated was CHD death or nonfatal MI. After an average follow-up of 4.1 years, no statistically significant difference was found between HRT and placebo.

6. In the first year of HERS, HRT increased the risk of cardiac events (RR = 1.52), but after two years there appeared to be benefit of HRT. The relative risk of using HRT as compared to placebo for mortality in years four and five was 0.67. The hypothesis that HRT is beneficial in women with CHD was not refuted by this study, but it was not as strongly supported as many had expected. The study was underpowered because the CHD event rate was expected to be 5 percent per year but it was only 3.3 percent per year in the placebo group. The follow-up period was also shorter than expected because most of the participants joined the study in the last six months of the 18-month recruitment period. Other confounders in the study were that many women were on "statin" drugs and angiotensin-converting enzyme inhibitors. This study raised more questions than it answered. Does progesterone attenuate the benefits of estrogen? Were the CHD events within the first year of HRT events thrombotic in nature? Are there women prone to thrombotic events who should not take HRT? A two-year follow up is planned and new studies are being developed to address these questions.

7. The Women's Health Initiative (WHI) is a large-scale multicenter randomized trial evaluating preventative therapies including HRT in healthy post-menopausal women.[47] This study should help to determine the effect of hormone supplementation on heart disease, osteoporosis, and breast cancer in healthy postmenopausal women. The results of the WHI trial cannot be expected until approximately 2006.

8. Until the results of this trial are available, health care providers will need to make individual decisions with patients based on available data. A discussion of risks and benefits of HRT should be offered to each patient. A uniform recommendation for HRT for every postmenopausal woman cannot yet be made. The potential effect on the overall health of the woman is important to consider. Estrogen may significantly decrease the risk of CHD, the risk of fractures caused by osteoporosis and the frequency of disabling peri-menopausal symptoms; however, it is a well-recognized cause of endometrial cancer and gall bladder disease. The possible influence of estrogen replacement therapy on the development of breast cancer is not yet clear,

---

The relative risk of using hormone replacement therapy as compared with placebo for mortality in years four and five was 0.67.

although the increased risk is likely to be small.[48] Until the results of randomized trials are available, the observational study evidence supporting the use of estrogen to prevent CHD has to be considered on its inferential merit.

A uniform recommendation for hormone replacement therapy for every postmenopausal woman cannot yet be made.

Aspirin

1. A recent Consensus Statement by the American College of Chest Physicians recommends aspirin 80 to 325 mg daily for all individuals older than age 50 years with one or more of the major cardiovascular risk factors.[49] This recommendation is based largely on the impressive 44 percent reduction in risk of acute MI seen in the Physicians' Health Study among male physicians aged 40 to 90 years taking aspirin daily.[50]

2. The NHS showed a reduction in MI risk in women who took one to six aspirin per week.[51] The soon to be published Women's Health Study is a randomized trial of low dose aspirin (100 mg on alternate days) in over 40 000 healthy female health professionals, aged 45 years or older.[7] Aspirin may reduce the risk of CHD but it may increase the risk of hemorrhagic stroke in women.[52]

Studies showed a reduction in myocardial infarction risk in women who took one to six aspirin per week.

3. Aspirin reduces the incidence of subsequent MI, stroke, and death from cardiovascular causes by 25 percent in women and men with established vascular disease.[53] Aspirin has been shown to have benefit in women and men with evolving MI.[54]

4. The recommended dose of aspirin for secondary prevention is 100 to 325 mg daily continued indefinitely.

The recommended dose of aspirin for secondary prevention is 100 to 325 mg daily continued indefinitely.

Vitamin E

The NHS examining the relationship between vitamin E consumption and the risk of CHD in women found that the use of vitamin E supplements was associated with a small but reduced risk of CHD.[55] Any potential benefit of antioxidant vitamins in the prevention of CHD is likely to be small; thus, reliable data can come only from large-scale randomized trials in women. The usual dose of vitamin recommended for primary prevention is 400 to 800 IU/day, since the minimum dose to prevent LDL oxidation is 400 IU.[56]

Homocysteine

Mild elevations of homocysteine (> 15 mmol/L) are associated with increased risks of CHD, peripheral vascular disease, stroke, and venous thromboembolism.[57] There is observational trial evidence that folic acid and vitamin B6 supplementation may be important in CHD prevention in women.[58] Supplementation of the diet with folic acid and vitamins B6 and B12 reduces homocysteine levels and prevents masking of vitamin B12 deficiency that can result from folic acid supplementation alone.

Increasing women's self-advocacy

1. Chest pain is the most common initial manifestation of CHD in women.[4]
2. Encouraging women patients to promptly seek medical evaluation of chest pain and educating providers regarding the evaluation of chest pain in women remain important challenges. The way in which women experience and interpret their symptoms is probably related to the likelihood that they will seek medical attention promptly when they develop symptoms.
3. Women dramatically underestimate their own risk of CHD, despite the fact that they seek chronic medical care more often than men.[59] Women and elderly patients tend to delay longer than men and younger individuals in seeking medical care after the onset of acute coronary symptoms.[60] This may be caused by denial, poor self-advocacy, attribution of symptoms to other processes, and/or failure to recognize symptoms of acute coronary disease.

> Women dramatically underestimate their own risk of coronary heart disease, despite the fact that they seek chronic medical care more often than men.

Chest pain in women

History

1. The clinical evaluation of chest discomfort begins with a good history, including an assessment of location, quality and duration of the discomfort, and precipitating and palliating factors. Angina is the clinical manifestation of myocardial ischemia caused by an imbalance between myocardial oxygen supply and demand. Any activity that increases the workload of the heart can precipitate angina in a person with a significant (⩾ 70 percent) stenosis in a coronary artery.

2. Classic situations that provoke angina are exertion, emotional stress, cold, sexual activity, and after a meal. Angina is more common in the first hours after awakening. Anginal discomfort typically lasts from two to five minutes and the abnormal chest sensation completely disappears between episodes. Chest discomfort that has been constant for days to weeks is not angina. Classic ischemic pain is relieved by cessation of activity (decreases oxygen demand) or nitroglycerin (promotes coronary vasodilation therefore increasing blood supply).

> Angina is more common in the first hours after awakening.

3. Angina pectoris is characterized by substernal discomfort that may radiate to the neck or left arm, but it can be perceived anywhere between the xyphoid process and the ears. Angina is a disagreeable pressure-like sensation, not stabbing or sharp in nature. Discomfort that is pleuritic or positional is not angina.
4. Community education programs have traditionally focused on men as being susceptible to CHD and have focused on chest pain as the presenting symptom of heart disease. Clinical features that suggest angina are the same in women and men.[61]
5. A woman's risk factors should be considered in the evaluation of chest discomfort, but atherosclerosis can exist in women without recognized risk factors. The absence of risk factors does not rule out the clinical diagnosis of myocardial ischemia. If symptoms of angina begin suddenly in a woman with no previous symptoms, if such symptoms occur at rest in a woman with previously known CHD, or if low level exertion provokes chest discomfort that seems to be ischemic, the woman should be promptly evaluated.
6. Nonchest symptoms are common in women with MI. Although most women have chest pain as part of their initial presentation with MI, they are significantly more likely than men to present with nausea, upper abdominal pain, neck and shoulder pain, dyspnea, and fatigue.[62]
7. Patients (especially women) have been shown to delay seeking medical care when their cardiac symptoms do not match their expectations.[63] Delay in seeking care may adversely affect outcomes in women with acute coronary syndromes.

> Nonchest symptoms are common in women with myocardial infarction.

Differential diagnosis

1. Chest pain in women is a diagnostic dilemma. Chest pain is the most

common presenting symptom for women with CHD but when compared with men, women have more chest pain that is not caused by CHD.

2. While women with CHD are just as likely to have exertional angina as men, such women are more likely to experience angina at rest, during sleep, or with mental stress.[64]

3. Women have a higher prevalence than men of vasospastic angina and microvascular angina, both of which are associated with atypical chest pain patterns, are often treated differently, and have a more favorable prognosis than epicardial coronary disease.[65]

4. Just as in men, acute chest discomfort in women should be systematically and consistently evaluated and triage decisions made promptly, with adequate follow-up. Stratifying women with chest pain into categories of low, intermediate, and high probability of CHD based on existence of minor and major determinants of disease is possible and will aid in decision-making.[66]

> Women have a higher prevalence than men of vasospastic angina and microvascular angina.

5. The clinical history helps to determine which woman has a high likelihood of a significant coronary stenosis as the cause of the symptoms. Classification of the symptoms into the categories of typical angina, atypical angina, or nonspecific chest pain is an important first step. In the Coronary Artery Surgery Study (CASS), 20 000 patients with chest pain (19 percent women, aged 30 to 70 years) were prospectively enrolled and underwent coronary angiography to determine CHD prevalence in the various chest discomfort syndromes.[67] The definitions of these classes of chest pain come from this study.

   a. Typical angina was defined as substernal discomfort that was precipitated by exertion, relieved by rest or nitroglycerin in less than 10 minutes, and radiated to the shoulders, jaw or ulnar aspect of the left arm.

   b. Atypical chest pain or atypical angina was defined as having most of the features of angina yet the discomfort was unusual in some aspect such as unusual pattern of radiation, nitroglycerin not always being effective, or that the pain went away only after 15 to 20 minutes of rest.

   c. Nonspecific pain has none of the features of typical angina.

   Significant CHD, defined as an epicardial stenosis of $\geqslant 70$ percent or left main coronary stenosis of $\geqslant 50$ percent, was found in 72 percent of women and 93 percent of men with typical angina, in 36 percent of women and 66 percent of men with atypical chest pain, and in 6 percent of women and 14 percent of men with nonspecific chest pain.[68] Thus women and men with typical angina and men with atypical chest pain are three subgroups with a relatively high prevalence of significant CHD. Women with atypical chest pain

Table 29.3. Stress test sensitivity and indications for type of stress test for women with chest pain

	Typical chest pain	Atypical chest pain	Nontypical chest pain
Percentage likelihood of significant CAD (epicardial stenosis of $\geqslant 70$ percent or left main coronary stenosis of $\geqslant 50$ percent)	72	36	6
"Regular" stress test	Postmenopausal with normal ECG	Maybe, but if this is positive, continue with imaging stress test	No
Imaging stress test	Premenopausal with normal ECG, or abnormal ECG	Yes, or after regular stress test, or abnormal ECG	No

CAD, coronary artery disease; ECG, electrocardiogram.

are at an intermediate prevalence. Women and men with nonspecific chest pain have a low prevalence of significant CHD.

Women and men with typical angina and men with atypical chest pain are three subgroups with a relatively high prevalence of significant CHD.

Stress testing

1. The clinical assessment of the likelihood of CHD is important because it dictates the next step in the clinical evaluation and affects the interpretation of stress test results. The stress electrocardiogram (ECG) or graded exercise test is a relatively inexpensive test that is widely available and often used as the next step in the evaluation of chest pain. Unfortunately, the specificity for stress testing for significant CHD is much less in women (Table 29.3). For example, women are 5 to 20 times more likely to have a false positive stress test than men.[69]

2. In the postmenopausal woman with typical angina, if the baseline ECG is normal, a regular treadmill is probably the test of choice. Since the pretest probability of an important obstruction is fairly high (72 percent), a positive test will further increase the likelihood that the woman has an important coronary lesion.

3. In premenopausal women with typical angina, the approach should probably be more like that in women with atypical angina (see below) because there is a lower prevalence of disease in this subset of women.

4. In the woman with atypical angina with a normal baseline ECG, there is a 36 percent pretest probability of an important coronary lesion. A positive regular treadmill test enhances the posttest probability to only 40 to 50 percent. Most of the positive stress tests in this category will be false positive. A repeat stress test using another imaging modality such as echocardiogram or nuclear imaging should be done before referring the patient for angiography. An alternative and potentially more cost-effective strategy in the woman with atypical chest pain would be to begin with an imaging stress test.[70] In this situation, a negative exercise test (regular or with imaging) is powerful in excluding significant CHD because the low pretest probability is lowered further by the negative test.[71]

5. In a woman with nonspecific chest pain who has no features of angina pectoris, exercise testing should not be done for the diagnosis of CHD. The rate of false positives is high when the test is applied to a population with a low prevalence of disease.

6. If the baseline ECG is abnormal, an imaging modality should be used with stress testing. Causes of resting ECG abnormalities include intraventricular conduction abnormalities (left bundle branch block (LBBB) and right bundle branch block), left ventricular hypertrophy and use of digoxin.

7. Even if the resting ECG is normal, the ST segment depression during exercise is not interpretable if the woman is on digoxin. Absence of ST-segment depression, during an exercise test in a woman receiving digoxin, is considered a valid negative response.[72]

8. Pharmacological nuclear studies should be used in women with LBBB (to avoid artifactual perfusion defects that occur with exercise testing with or without imaging) or who cannot exercise secondary to other medical problems such as orthopedic, neurological, or peripheral vascular disease. Agents such as dipyridamole, dobutamine or adenosine can be used to induce pharmacological stress.

9. The low sensitivity (70 percent) and specificity (60 percent) of regular treadmill testing in women has led to a marked increase in studies involving exercise testing with echocardiographic or nuclear imaging. The increasing availability of prognostic as well as diagnostic information from these studies continues to refine noninvasive testing in women.[73] For example, in both men

The specificity for stress testing for significant CHD is much less in women.

and women, cardiac events were extremely rare in those with normal techne-tium-99^m sestamibi exercise nuclear scans (0.6 percent of women and 1.4 percent of men). Patients with abnormal scans had significantly higher rates of cardiac events (6.9 percent in women and 10.9 percent in men).[74] In another study, although abnormal sestamibi scans were equally predictive of adverse events in women and men, the types of event differed. Women with abnormal scans were more likely to develop unstable angina and heart failure and men were more likely to develop MI and death.[75]

10. A stress test is not simply positive or negative. A "nondiagnostic" stress test is not the same as a negative stress test. This usually means that the test was inconclusive often because of the patient's inability to reach 85 percent of her age-predicted maximal heart rate. This type of stress test can give the clinician useful information but should not be interpreted as a negative test.

   a. Predictors of subsequent cardiac events based on a routine Bruce stress test are chest pain during maximal exercise, duration of exercise less than six minutes, failure to attain 90 percent of age-predicted maximal heart rate, and ischemic ST-segment depression, particularly if it lasts more than four minutes into recovery.

   b. A woman with reproduction of her anginal symptoms at a low level of exercise with significant ST-segment depression would have a high probability of having severe three-vessel CHD or significant left main disease and should probably be referred for catheterization to assess her revascularization options.

   c. A woman with angina and excellent exercise tolerance with symptoms of angina occurring at eight minutes on the Bruce protocol with 1 mm of ST depression developing at that time probably does not have severe disease and probably does not need a catheterization. She does require aggressive risk factor modification and antianginal therapy.

   d. If a stress test is truly negative, the patient can be followed. The assumption should not be, however, that the woman does not have CHD, but rather that the woman has a low likelihood of a significant coronary obstruction. Preventive recommendations to inhibit the formation of atherosclerotic plaque should be made in any woman with chest discomfort. Other causes of chest discomfort should be pursued according to the clinical characteristics of the discomfort.

In the woman with atypical angina with a normal baseline electrocardiogram, there is a 36 percent pretest probability of an important coronary lesion. A positive regular treadmill test enhances the posttest probability to only 40 to 50 percent.

11. Contraindications to stress testing include severe aortic stenosis, unstable angina, severe anemia, electrolyte disturbances, and decompensated heart failure.[71]

Contraindications to stress testing include severe aortic stenosis, unstable angina, severe anemia, electrolyte disturbances, and decompensated heart failure.

Treatment of CHD in women

1. Female gender has been shown to be a risk factor for delayed presentation and for delayed treatment in acute MI.[76] During the evaluation of chest pain, women are likely to be treated differently from men, especially when there is no prior diagnosis of CHD. For example, women presenting to the hospital with signs and symptoms of acute coronary disease are less likely than men with similar symptoms to be admitted for evaluation.[77]

2. A large clinical trial that included large numbers of men and women with acute MI showed that women have angina before MI as frequently and with more debilitating effect than men. Prior to the MI, physicians took a less aggressive approach to women. This difference could not be explained by differences in coronary risk factors or cardiac medications. Women underwent cardiac catheterization only half as often after their MI as men did but women were revascularized similarly to men after their coronary anatomy was known.[78] This has been called the Yentl syndrome (after the 19th-century heroine of Isaac Bashevis Singer's short story) because once a woman showed she is just like a man (she has a proven MI), she was treated like a man.[79]

3. Although women with MI have more serious presentations, with greater prevalence of tachycardia, rales, heart block, and congestive heart failure on presentation,[60] women are less likely to receive thrombolytics (even after controlling for eligibility) and receive it later than men do. This delay in presentation reduces the potential benefit from thrombolytic therapy.[58]

4. Although older age is the most important prognostic factor after acute MI, patients older than age 75 years are six times less likely to receive thrombolytic therapy than younger patients. The elderly have potentially the most to gain from reperfusion strategies because of their high absolute mortality rate.[80] This may disproportionately affect women because they have their MIs, on average, 10 years later than men.

5. Mortality reduction rates with thrombolytic therapy are similar in men and women.[59] Women do not differ significantly from men with regard to either

early infarct-related artery patency or reocclusion after thrombolytic therapy or ventricular functional response to injury/reperfusion.[81] Female sex is not a risk factor for intracranial hemorrhage if the patient's age, blood pressure, and body weight are taken into account.[82]

> Patients older than age 75 years are six times less likely to receive thrombolytic therapy than younger patients.

Acute myocardial infarction

1. Women tend to have their MIs at older ages than men, with a higher case fatality rate.[83]

2. They are more likely than men with MI to have a history of hypertension, diabetes, congestive heart failure, cerebrovascular disease, and elevated total cholesterol levels.

3. The increased morbidity and mortality in older females with MI can be accounted for by their advanced age and coexisting, age-related conditions. Among patients under age 50 years with MI, the mortality rate during hospitalization was more than twice as high among women as among men. The difference in rates diminished with increasing age and was no longer significant after age 74 years.

4. The clinical presentation and outcomes of 3662 women and 8480 men with acute coronary syndromes were recently compared.[84] Outcomes varied by sex depending upon the type of acute coronary syndrome. Women were more likely than men to have unstable angina rather than acute myocardial infarction. Women with unstable angina had a better prognosis than their male counterparts. Women with acute MI with ST-segment elevation had a poorer prognosis and those without ST-elevation had similar outcomes to men. Among patients with MI, a smaller percentage of women than men presented with ST-segment elevation. Coronary angiography was performed in 53 percent of the women vs. 59 percent of the men and showed that more women had clinically insignificant coronary disease compared with men.

5. Treatment of women with MI by direct angioplasty may result in a lower mortality and hemorrhagic stroke rate than treatment with thrombolytic therapy, whereas these therapies yield similar outcomes in men.[85]

> Among patients under age 50 years with myocardial infarction, the mortality rate during hospitalization was more than twice as high among women as among men.

6. Women with acute infarction are more likely to be treated with nitrates, digoxin, and diuretics than are men and are less likely to receive thrombolytics, antiarrhythmics, antiplatelet agent, and beta-blockers.[86] Beta-blockers provide a significant improvement in postinfarction survival in women that is at least equal to if not greater than that for men.

7. Women are less likely to be referred for cardiac rehabilitation and more likely to drop out of rehabilitation programs if they actually enroll.

8. After infarction, women have more anxiety and depression. They also have less psychosocial support, since they are more likely to be widows and to have low incomes. Women with greater sources of emotional support have better survival after an MI compared to women with fewer resources for support.[87]

> Women with acute infarction are more likely to be treated with nitrates, digoxin, and diuretics than are men and are less likely to receive thrombolytics, antiarrhythmics, antiplatelet agents, and beta-blockers.

Revascularization therapy

The Bypass Angioplasty Revascularization Investigation (BARI) was the largest RCT comparing coronary artery bypass graft (CABG) and angioplasty in men and women with multivessel CHD. The study included 27 percent women, thereby becoming one of the largest studies of women undergoing revascularization. The extent of CHD was similar in women and men and CABG and angioplasty were equally effective in both groups. There were similar in-hospital and long-term survival rates in men and women.[88] Previous studies had reflected as much as a twofold increase in in-hospital mortality in women as compared with men.[7] The more recent results of the BARI trial and others are felt to reflect improvements in technology and procedures.

Conclusions

Prevention of CHD is a major health issue for women. Thanks to huge educational and advocacy efforts, awareness of CHD among women is increasing. Risk factor modification is the cornerstone of prevention. Early symptom recognition by the patient and complete evaluation by health care providers are crucial to provide women with proven beneficial therapies.

REFERENCES

1. American Heart Association. *2000 Heart and Stroke Facts: Statistical Update.* American Heart Association, Dallas, TX, 1999.

2. Grady D, Rubin SM, Petitti DB et al. Hormone replacement therapy to prevent disease and prolong life in postmenopausal women. *Ann Intern Med* 1992;**117**:1016–37.

3. Forrester JS, Shah PK. Lipid lowering versus revascularization: An idea whose time (for testing) has come. *Circulation* 1997;**96**:1360–2.

4. Lerner DJ, Kannel WB. Patterns of coronary heart disease morbidity and mortality in the sexes: A 26-year follow-up of the Framingham population. *Am Heart J* 1986;**111**:383–90.

5. Rich-Edwards JW, Manson JE, Hennekens CH, Buring JE. The primary prevention of coronary heart disease in women. *N Engl J Med* 1995;**332**:1758–66.

6. Bush TL. The epidemiology of cardiovascular disease in postmenopausal women. *Ann NY Acad Sci* 1990;**592**:263–71.

7. Mosca L, Manson JE, Sutherland SE et al. Cardiovascular disease in women. A statement for healthcare professionals from the American Heart Association. *Circulation* 1997;**96**:2468–82.

8. Kashihara H, Ohno H, Tamura M, Kawakubo K, Gunji A. Risk factors for ischemic heart disease in an urban area of Japan. A case-control study in AMHTS. *Methods Inf Med* 2000;**39**:223–8.

9. Mannami T, Baba S, Ogata J. Strong and significant relationships between aggregation of major coronary risk factors and the acceleration of carotid atherosclerosis in the general population of a Japanese city: The Suita Study. *Arch Intern Med* 2000;**160**:2297–303.

10. NCEP Summary of Second Report of the National Cholesterol Education Program (NCEP) Expert Panel on Detection, Evaluation, and Treatment of High Blood Cholesterol in Adults (Adult Treatment Panel II). *JAMA* 1993;**269**:3015–23.

11. Winkelby MA, Kraemer HC, Ahn DK, Varady AN. Ethnic and socioeconomic differences in cardiovascular disease risk factors. *JAMA* 1998;**280**:356–62.

12. Judelson DR. Coronary heart disease in women: Risk factors and prevention. *J Am Womens Assoc* 1994;**49**:186–97.

13. Pierce JP, Fiore MC, Novotny TE, Hatziandreu EJ, Davis RM. Trends in cigarette smoking in the United States: Projections to the year 2000. *JAMA* 1989;**261**:61–5.

14. Willett WC, Green A, Stampfer MJ et al. Relative and absolute excess risk of coronary heart disease among women who smoke cigarettes. *N Engl J Med* 1987;**317**:1303–9.

15. Hansen EF, Andersen LT, Von Eyben FE. Cigarette smoking and age at first acute myocardial infarction, and influence of gender and extent of smoking. *Am J Cardiol* 1993;**71**:1439–42.

16. Rosenberg L, Palmer JR, Shapiro S. Decline in the risk of myocardial infarction among women who stop smoking. *N Engl J Med* 1990;**322**:213–17.

17. Joint National Committee on the Detection, Evaluation, and Treatment of Blood Pressure. The Fifth Report of the Joint National Committee on Detection, Evaluation, and Treatment of Blood Pressure (JNC-V). *Arch Intern Med* 1993;**153**:154–83.

18. Gueyffier F, Boutitie F, Boissel JP et al. Effect of antihypertensive drug treatment on cardiovascular outcomes in women and men: A meta-analysis of individual patient data from randomized controlled trials. *Ann Intern Med* 1997;**126**:761–7.

19. SHEP Cooperative Research Group. Prevention of stroke by anti-hypertensive drug treatment in older persons with isolated systolic hypertension: Final results of the Systolic Hypertension in the Elderly Program (SHEP). *JAMA* 1991;**265**:3255–64.

20. Whelton PK, Appel LJ, Espeland MA et al. Sodium reduction and weight loss in the treatment of hypertension in older persons: A randomized controlled trial of nonpharmacologic interventions in the elderly (TONE). TONE Collaborative Research Group. *JAMA*;**279**:839–46.

21. Manolio TA, Pearson TA, Wenger NK et al. Cholesterol and heart disease in older persons and women. *Ann Epidemiol* 1992;**2**:161–76.

22. Bass KM, Newschaffer CH, Klag MJ, Bush TL. Plasma lipoprotein levels as predictors of cardiovascular death in women. *Arch Intern Med* 1993;**153**:2209–16.

23. Scandinavian Simvastatin Survival Study Group. Randomised trial of cholesterol lowering in 4444 patients with coronary heart disease: The Scandinavian simvastatin survival study (4S). *Lancet* 1994;**344**:1383–9.

24. Lewis SJ, Sacks FM, Mitchell JS et al. for the CARE investigators. Effect of pravastatin on cardiovascular events in women after myocardial infarction: the cholesterol and recurrent events (CARE) trial. *J Am Coll Cardiol* 1998;**32**:140–6.

25. Downs JR, Clearfield M, Weis S et al. Primary prevention of acute coronary events with lovastatin in men and women with average cholesterol levels: Results of AFCAPS/TexCAPS. *JAMA* 1998;**279**:1615–22.

26. Jacobs DR Jr., Meban IL, Bangdiwala SI, Criqui MH, Tyroler HA. High-density lipoprotein cholesterol as a predictor of cardiovascular disease mortality in men and women: The follow-up study of the Lipid Research Clinic Prevalence Study. *Am J Epidemiol* 1990;**131**:32–47.

27. Castelli WP. The triglyceride issue: A view from Framingham. *Am Heart J* 1986;**112**:432–7.

28. Grundy SM. Hypertriglyceridemia, atherogenic dyslipidemia, and the metabolic syndrome. *Am J Cardiol* 1998;**81**:18B–25B.

29. Schrott HG, Bittner V, Vittinghoff E, Herrington DM, Hulley S, for the HERS Research Group. Adherence to National Cholesterol Education Program treatment goals in postmenopausal women with heart disease: The Heart and Estrogen/Progestin Replacement Study (HERS). *JAMA* 1997;**277**:1281–6.

30. Rich-Edwards JW, Manson JE, Hennekens CH, Buring JE. The primary prevention of coronary heart disease in women. *N Engl J Med* 1995;**332**:1758–66.

31. Barrett-Connor E, Wingard DL. Sex differential in ischemic heart disease mortality. I. Diabetics: A prospective population-based study. *Am J Epidemiol* 1983;**118**:489–96.

32. The Diabetes Control and Complications Trial Research group. The effect of intensive treatment of diabetes on the development and progression of long term complications in insulin-dependent diabetes mellitus. *N Engl J Med* 1993;**329**:977–86.

33. Manson JE, Stampfer MJ, Colditz GA et al. A prospective study of obesity and the risk of coronary heart disease in women. *N Engl J Med* 1990;**322**:882–9.

34. Kaplan NM. The deadly quartet: Upper body obesity, glucose intolerance, hypertriglyceridemia, and hypertension. *Arch Intern Med* 1989;**149**:1514–20.

35. Bjorntorp P. Regional patterns of fat distribution. *Ann Intern Med* 1985;**103**:994–5.

36. Kushi LH, Fee RM, Folsom AR, Mink PJ, Anderson KE, Sellers TA. Physical activity and mortality in postmenopausal women. *JAMA* 1997;**277**:1287–92.

37. Blair SN, Kohl HW III, Paffenbarger RS Jr., Clark DG, Cooper KH, Gibbons LW. Physical fitness and all-cause mortality: A prospective study of healthy men and women. *JAMA* 1989;**262**:2395–401.

38. Greendale GA, Bodin-Dunn L, Ingles S. Leisure, home and occupational physical activity and cardiovascular risk factors in postmenopausal women. The Postmenopausal Estrogen/

Progestin Intervention (PEPI) Study. *Arch Intern Med* 1996;**156**:418–24.

39. Pate RR, Pratt M, Blair SN et al. Physical activity and public health. A recommendation from Centers for Disease Control and Prevention and the American College of Sports Medicine. *JAMA* 1995;**273**:402–7.

40. Stampfer MJ, Colditz GA. Estrogen replacement therapy and coronary heart disease in women: A quantitative assessment of the epidemiologic evidence. *Prev Med* 1991;**20**:47–63.

41. Barrett-Connor E. Postmenopausal estrogen and prevention bias. *Ann Intern Med* 1991;**115**:455–6.

42. Nabulsi AA, Folsom AR, White A et al. for the Atherosclerosis Risk in Communities Study Investigators. Association of hormone replacement therapy with various cardiovascular risks factors in postmenopausal women. *N Engl J Med* 1993;**328**:1069–75.

43. Bush TL, Barrett-Connor E, Cowan LD et al. Cardiovascular mortality and noncontraceptive use of estrogen in women: Results from the Lipid Research Clinics Program Follow-up Study. *Circulation* 1987;**75**:1102–9.

44. Williams JK, Adams MR, Herrington DM, Clarkson TB. Short-term administration of estrogen and vascular responses of atherosclerotic coronary arteries. *J Am Coll Cardiol* 1992;**20**:452–7.

45. Writing Group for the PEPI Trial. Effects of estrogen or estrogen/progestin regimens on heart disease risk factors in postmenopausal women. The Postmenopausal Estrogen/Progestin Interventions (PEPI) trial. *JAMA* 1995;**273**:199–208.

46. Hulley S, Grady D, Bush T et al. for the Heart and Estrogen/Progestin Replacement Study (HERS) Research Group. Randomized trial of estrogen plus progestin for secondary prevention of coronary heart disease in postmenopausal women. *JAMA* 1998;**280**:605–13.

47. Rossouw JE, Finnegan LP, Harlan WR et al. The evolution of the Women's Health Initiative: Perspectives from the NIH. *J Am Med Women Assoc* 1995;**50**:50–5.

48. Collaborative Group on Hormonal Factors in Breast Cancer. Breast cancer and hormone replacement therapy: Collaborative reanalysis of data from 51 epidemiological studies of 52,705 women with breast cancer and 108,411 women without breast cancer. *Lancet* 1997;**350**:1047–59.

49. American College of Chest Physicians. Fifth consensus on antithrombotic therapy. *Chest* 1998;**114**(5 Suppl):439S–769S.

50. The Steering Committee of the Physicians' Health Study Research Group. Final report from the aspirin component of the ongoing Physicians' Health Study. *N Engl J Med* 1989;**321**:129–35.

51. Manson JE, Stampfer MJ, Colditz GA et al. A prospective study of aspirin use and primary prevention of cardiovascular disease in women. *JAMA* 1991;**266**:521–7.

52. He J, Whelton PK, Vu B, Klag MJ. Aspirin and risk of hemorrhagic stroke: A meta-analysis of randomized controlled trials. *JAMA* 1998;**280**:1930–5.

53. Antiplatelet Trialist' Collaboration. Collaborative overview of randomised trials of anti-platelet therapy. I. Prevention of death, myocardial infarction, and stroke by prolonged antiplatelet therapy in various categories of patients. *BMJ* 1994;**308**:81–106.

54. ISIS-2 (Second International Study of Infarct Survival). Randomised trial of intravenous streptokinase, oral aspirin, both or neither among 17,187 cases of suspected myocardial infarction: ISIS-2. *Lancet* 1988;**2**:329–60.

55. Stampfer MJ, Hennekens CH, Manson JE et al. Vitamin E consumption and the risk of coronary disease in women. *N Engl J Med* 1993;**328**:1444–9.

56. Faggiotto A, Poli A, Catapano AL. Antioxidants and coronary artery disease. *Curr Opin Lipidol*

1998;**9**:541–9.

57. Boushey CJ, Beresford SAA, Omenn GS, Motulsky AG. A quantitative assessment of plasma homocysteine as a risk factor for vascular disease: Probable benefits of increasing folic acid intakes. *JAMA* 1995;**274**:1049–57.

58. Rimm EB, Willett WC, Hu FB. Folate and vitamin B6 from diet and supplements in relation to risk of coronary heart disease in women. *JAMA* 1998;**297**:359–64.

59. Douglas PS. Coronary artery disease in women. In Braunwald E, ed., *Heart Disease.* WB Saunders Co., Philadelphia, pp. 1704–14.

60. Newby LK, Rutsch WR, Califf RM et al. Time from symptom onset to treatment and outcomes after thrombolytic therapy. *J Am Coll Cardiol* 1996;**27**:1646–55.

61. Cunningham MA, Lee TH, Cook EF et al. The effect of gender on the probability of myocardial infarction among emergency department patients with acute chest pain: A report from the Multicenter Chest Pain Study Group. *J Gen Intern Med* 1989;**4**:392–8.

62. Yarzebski J, Bigelow C, Savageau J, Gore JM. Sex differences in symptom presentation associated with acute myocardial infarction: A population-based perspective. *Am Heart J* 1998;**136**:189–95.

63. Johnson JA, King KB. Influence of expectations about symptoms on delay in seeking treatment during myocardial infarction. *Am J Crit Care* 1995;**4**:29–35.

64. Pepine CJ. Angina pectoris in a contemporary population: Characteristics and therapeutic implications. TIDES Investigators. *Cardiovasc Drugs Ther* 1998;**12** (Suppl 3):211–16.

65. Sullivan AK, Holdright DR, Wright CA et al. Chest pain in women: Clinical, investigative, and prognostic features. *BMJ* 1994;**308**:883–6.

66. Douglas PS, Ginsburg G. The evaluation of chest pain in women. *N Engl J Med* 1996;**334**:1311–15.

67. Espinola-Klein C, Rupprecht HJ, Erbel R, Nafe B, Brennecke R, Meyer J. Ten-year outcome after coronary angioplasty in patients with single-vessel coronary artery disease and the results of the Coronary Artery Surgery Study. *Am J Cardiol* 2000;**85**:321–6.

68. Chaitman BR, Bourassa MG, Davis K et al. Angiographic prevalence of high-risk coronary artery disease in patient subsets (CASS). *Circulation* 1981;**64**:360–7.

69. Miller DD. Noninvasive diagnosis of CAD in women. *J Myocard Ischem* 1995;**7**:263–8.

70. Marwick TH, Anderson T, Williams MJ et al. Exercise echocardiography is an accurate and cost-effective technique for detection of coronary artery disease in women. *J Am Coll Cardiol* 1995;**26**:335–41.

71. Pratt CM, Francis MJ, Divine GW, Young JB. Exercise testing in women with chest pain. Are there additional exercise characteristics that predict true positive test results? *Chest* 1989;**95**:139–44.

72. Chaitman BR. Exercise testing. In Braunwald E, ed., *Heart Disease.* WB Saunders Co., Philadelphia, 1997, pp. 153–76.

73. Heupler S, Mehta R, Lobo A et al. Prognostic implications of exercise echocardiography in women with known or suspected coronary artery disease. *J Am Coll Cardiol* 1997;**30**:414–20.

74. Miller D. Prognostic impact of stress myocardial perfusion imaging in women. *J Myocard Ischem* 1995;**7**:269–73.

75. Duca MD, Travin MI, Herman SD et al. Abnormal stress Tc-99m sestamibi SPECT imaging in women vs. men: Same management, same prognosis, different events. *J Am Coll Cardiol* 1996;**27**(Suppl):381A.

76. Behar S, Gottlieb S, Hod H et al. Influence of gender in the therapeutic management of

patients with acute myocardial infarction in Israel. *Am J Cardiol* 1994;**73**:438–43.

77. Silbergleit R, McNamara RM. Effect of sex on the emergency department evaluation of patients with chest pain. *Acad Emerg Med* 1995;**2**:115–19.

78. Steingart RM, Packer M, Hamm P et al. Sex differences in the management of coronary artery disease. *N Engl J Med* 1991;**325**:226–30.

79. Healy B. The Yentl syndrome. *N Engl J Med* 1991;**325**:274–6.

80. White HD, Van de Werf FJJ. Thrombolysis for acute myocardial infarction. *Circulation* 1998;**97**:1632–46.

81. Woodfield SL, Lundergan CF, Reiner JS et al. Gender and acute myocardial infarction: Is there a different response to thrombolysis? *J Am Coll Card* 1997;**29**:35–42.

82. Gore JM, Granger CB, Simoons ML et al. Stroke after thrombolysis. Mortality and functional outcomes in the GUSTO-I trial. Global use of strategies to open occluded coronary arteries. *Circulation* 1995;**92**:2811–18.

83. Vaccarino V, Parsons L, Every NR, Barron HV, Krumholz HM. Sex-based differences in early mortality after myocardial infarction. *N Engl J Med* 1999;**341**:217–25.

84. Hochman JS, Tamis JE, Thompson TD et al. Sex, clinical presentation and outcome in patients with acute coronary syndromes. *N Engl J Med* 1999;**341**:226–32.

85. Stone GW, Grines CL, Browne KF et al. Comparison of in-hospital outcome in men versus women treated by either thrombolytic therapy or primary angioplasty for acute myocardial infarction. *Am J Cardiol* 1995;**75**:987–92.

86. Clarke KW, Gray D, Keating NA, Hampton JR. Do women with acute myocardial infarction receive the same treatment as men? *BMJ* 1994;**309**:563–6.

87. Eaker ED. Social and psychologic aspects of coronary heart disease in women. *Cardiol Rev* 1998;**6**:182–90.

88. Jacobs AK, Kelsey SF, Brooks MM et al. Better outcome for women compared to men undergoing coronary revascularization. *Circulation* 1998;**98**:1279–85.

30 Diabetes mellitus type II

Ann Brown, MD

Introduction

1. Living with diabetes is a full time job. Affected individuals live with it every moment of their lives, continuously and relentlessly making decisions and choices that take the fact of their carbohydrate metabolism into account. Thus diabetes weaves itself into the fabric of a life, and does so whether the affected person wills it or not. It is a condition greatly affected by lifestyle, diet, stress, exercise, and access to care and supplies. Its course is determined in large part by these factors.

2. Coaching a person about self-management strategies must take into account the social context of the disorder. Providers must be as vigilant for denial, guilt, depression, overwork and diabetes burn-out as for other complications of the disease.[1]

3. This is what often makes management strategies different for men and women. The disease itself is not significantly different, but coping strategies may be. Understanding individual responses to living with their chronic condition, and helping to build effective management strategies, is critical for a successful provider–patient partnership.

4. New strategies for effective diabetes care are desperately needed. The majority of people with diabetes in this country have suboptimal glucose control; one survey showed mean fasting glucose values of 180 mg/dL.[2] Yet, recent studies have clearly shown that even modest glucose reduction improves long-term outcomes, driving the search for innovative ways to help people achieve the best possible glucose control. Strategies that emphasize participation and the incorporation of body, mind, and spirit may be effective and mutually rewarding.

5. This chapter discusses clinical aspects of diabetes management, with emphasis on gender when it is relevant. It reviews epidemiology and natural history,

pathophysiology and diagnostic criteria. It then discusses available evidence regarding cardiovascular risk management, HRT, and exercise. The chapter emphasizes the importance of attention to mental health in every management plan, and advocates the concept of self-management as a replacement for "compliance" or "adherence". In keeping with the style of this text, a medical management protocol is presented in algorithm form (see Table 30.5), accompanied by a table summarizing each medication (see Table 30.4). This chapter does not address the important issue of management of gestational diabetes. For an excellent review of this subject, the reader is referred to a recent report,[3] and updates provided regularly by the American Diabetes Association.

> Understanding individual responses to living with their chronic condition, and helping to build effective management strategies, is critical for a successful provider–patient partnership.

Epidemiology and natural history

1. Data from the CDC indicate that more women than men are affected by diabetes.[4] The difference in self-reported prevalence rates is small, but appears to be most pronounced among those aged 75 years and older. Because women live longer, there are more women than men with diabetes.

2. Larger differences in prevalence are found when racial and ethnic groups are compared. The National Health and Nutrition Examination Survey (NHANES) III conducted between 1988 and 1994 showed that whereas 7.2 percent of whites aged 40 to 74 years have type II diabetes, almost twice as many African-Americans (12.5 percent) and Mexican Americans (13.7) have the diagnosis (Figure 30.1).

3. According to the NHANES III survey, 8 million people in the USA know they have diabetes mellitus, and another 8 million have diabetes but are unaware of it.[5] Considering only those with a known diagnosis, the National Center for Health Statistics reports that the prevalence of diabetes increased from 0.93 percent in 1958 to 3.1 percent in 1993.[2] The growth of the epidemic, and the poor record of diagnosing hyperglycemia early, together pose an enormous challenge to the health care system, and to individual providers.

> Because women live longer, there are more women than men with diabetes.

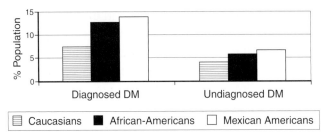

Figure 30.1.   Prevalence of type II diabetes by race. DM, diabetes mellitus. (From Harris MI, *Diabetes in America*: Epidemiology and scope of the problem. *Diabetes Care* 1998;**21**:C11–C14.)

Pathophysiology

Three major metabolic problems occur in type II diabetes. New therapeutic agents (see below), with their prescribing guidelines, target each of these important defects.

1. Insulin resistance: In normal physiological functioning, glucose enters cells under the direction of insulin. Insulin interacts with cell surface receptors to trigger a series of intracellular events that lead to the translocation of GLUT-4 transport molecules to the cell surface. Glucose enters cells through these transporters by a process of facilitated diffusion. Once inside, glucose is converted to energy. The term insulin resistance describes a condition in which this process is impaired.

   The precise derangement in insulin action in type II diabetes is not known. In fact, insulin resistance may develop as a result of different metabolic defects in different individuals. The common end result is a compensatory hypersecretion of insulin by the pancreatic beta cells, resulting in hyper-insulinemia. Many tissues, such as skeletal and cardiac muscle and adipose tissue, rely on insulin for optimum glucose uptake. Skeletal muscle comprises the largest mass of insulin-responsive tissue, and its metabolism contributes disproportionately to the degree of insulin resistance seen clinically.

2. Increased hepatic glucose output: In the fed state, insulin levels rise in response to increasing blood glucose levels, and act to suppress hepatic glucose output. Through this mechanism, the liver can serve as a source of glucose in the fasting state (low insulin levels) but ceases this function in the fed state. However, in type II diabetes, insulin resistance at the liver results in excessive hepatic glucose output, thus contributing to overall hyperglycemia.

3. Impaired beta cell function: Defects in beta cell function include impaired first phase (stored) insulin release, and insufficient insulin production to

compensate fully for insulin resistance. Some investigators believe that at least two defects must occur for type II diabetes to develop: insulin resistance and impaired beta cell function. This theory helps to explain why some people with insulin resistance do not progress to type II diabetes.

4. Diabetes progresses with time. Insulin sensitivity and beta cell function decline with aging. As a result, insulin resistance can progress to impaired glucose tolerance. With time, this advances to postprandial hyperglycemia with normal fasting glucose, and then to hyperglycemia both in the fasting state and postprandially. At some point in this progression, insulin production ceases to compensate adequately for glycemic surges and begins to decline. Late in the disease process, very little insulin may actually be produced. The practical consequence of this disease progression is that therapy may require intensification over time.

Diagnostic criteria[6]

1. Individuals with normal glucose tolerance will maintain fasting plasma glucose levels below 110 mg/dL (6.1 mmol/L). During an oral glucose tolerance test (OGTT) using a 75 g glucose load, the two-hour plasma glucose will not rise above 140 mg/dL (7.8 mmol/L). The diagnostic criteria for impaired fasting glucose, impaired glucose tolerance, type II diabetes and gestational diabetes are summarized in Table 30.1.

2. Though the line dividing diabetes from normal glucose tolerance is somewhat arbitrary, the diagnostic criteria are based on studies that show a steep rise in the prevalence of retinopathy in individuals with glucose levels above these values.

3. The American Diabetes Association (ADA) recommends screening high risk individuals every three years. Identified risk factors are listed in Table 30.2.

4. The diagnostic standards are based on plasma glucose measured in the laboratory using enzymatic methods. Results from capillary blood glucose monitoring devices should not be used to make the diagnosis. They are less accurate than laboratory testing, may not be regularly standardized, and may give confusing results, since some are calibrated to report plasma blood values, and others whole blood. Plasma glucose values will be 10 to 15 percent higher than whole blood glucose values.

The American Diabetes Association recommends screening high risk individuals every three years.

Table 30.1. Diagnostic criteria for type II diabetes

Normal	FPG < 110 mg/dL and 2 hour OGTT value < 140 mg/dL	Based on OGTT using 75 g oral glucose solution
Impaired fasting glucose	FPG ⩾ 110 mg/dL and < 126 mg/dL	
Impaired glucose tolerance	2 hours OGTT BG < 200 mg/dL and ⩾ 140 mg/dL	
Diabetes	FPG ⩾ 126 mg/dL (7.0 mmol/L), random BG ⩾ 200 mg/dL (11.1 mmol/L) with symptoms of polyuria, polydipsia, and/or unexplained weight loss, or 2-hour post 75 g glucose challenge BG ⩾ 200 mg/dL (11.1 mmol/L)	
Gestational diabetes	A plasma glucose at 1 hour after a 50 g oral glucose challenge of ⩾ 140 mg/dL necessitates a diagnostic challenge with 100 g oral glucose, with plasma glucose determined at 1, 2, 3, and 4 hours. If two of four of the following values are exceeded, gestational diabetes is diagnosed: fasting 105 mg/dL, 1 hour 190 mg/dL, 2 hours 165 mg/dL, 3 hours 145 mg/dL	Screening can be done in the nonfasting state with a 50 g oral glucose load

FPG, fasting plasma glucose; OGTT, oral glucose tolerance test; BG, blood glucose.

Rationale for tight glucose control

1. The Diabetes Control and Complications Trial (DCCT), completed in 1993, clearly documented significant reductions in microvascular complications in patients with type I diabetes with tight blood glucose control (average glucose 155 mg/dL) when compared with usual care (average glucose 231 mg/dL).[7] No threshold hemoglobin A1c values were found. This means that any reduction in average glucose can improve microvascular outcomes in these patients. These results have been extrapolated to apply to patients with type II diabetes, and recent evidence supporting this translation has been provided by the United Kingdom Prospective Diabetes Study (UKPDS).

Table 30.2. Risk factors for type II diabetes mellitus

- Family history of diabetes (parents or siblings)
- Obesity with BMI $\geqslant 27\,kg/m^2$
- Race/ethnicity (African-American, Hispanic, Native Americans, and Pacific Islanders)
- Previously identified impaired fasting glucose or impaired glucose tolerance
- Hypertension
- Low HDL cholesterol and/or high total glucose
- History of gestational diabetes or delivery of babies over 9 lbs (> 4 kg)

BMI, body mass index; HDL, high density lipoprotein.

The UKPDS demonstrated similar benefit to good glycemic control in people with type II diabetes. This important and complicated study is succinctly summarized in an ADA Position Statement.[8] Briefly, microvascular events were reduced by 25 percent in individuals with aggressive management (average glucose of 150 mg/dL) compared with those with usual management (average glucose of 200 mg/dL).

2. The investigators also monitored macrovascular events such as stroke and myocardial infarction to determine whether these important events could be prevented with tight blood glucose control. Though the difference was not significant, there was a trend toward a reduced risk of macrovascular events for those patients with better glucose control.

3. The UKPDS also demonstrated the critical importance of blood pressure control in individuals with diabetes. Event rates for cardiovascular outcomes decreased by 24 to 54 percent with intensive blood pressure management.

4. Further, beta-blockers and angiotensin-converting enzyme inhibitors appeared to be equally effective. The myocardial infarction rate decreased by 21 percent, but this was not statistically significant ($p = 0.13$). Based on the study results, UKPDS investigators recommend aggressive blood pressure control for all people with diabetes, with a goal of achieving blood pressures of less than 135/85.

There was a trend toward a reduced risk of macrovascular events for those patients with better glucose control.

Management strategies

Long-term goals

The goals of long-term diabetes care are the maintenance of health, and the prevention and treatment of complications. Achieving these goals requires glycemic control, cardiovascular risk factor management, and a productive therapeutic alliance between the individual with diabetes and the health care team. These are each discussed below. Additional and continually updated information can be found in "Clinical Practice Recommendations", an annual January supplement to the journal *Diabetes Care*.[9]

Self-management

The goal of diabetes education is to provide individuals with tools to make good decisions about managing their disease. General information about diabetes is also important, but specific strategies for managing day to day challenges require special focus and ask that the patient assume a central role in determining which interventions are possible and which are not. Within this framework, concepts such as compliance and adherence lose some of their meaning.[10] Instead, the issues of barriers to self-care, disease-related stresses, and social support become central. These challenges create the context for educational efforts, and guide the development of plans that are meaningful and realistic.

Team work

The ongoing process of diabetes education is ideally accomplished with a team of providers, each addressing different aspects of self-care, and reinforcing a common goal. The physician plays an important role in the team, but time-intensive work with a diabetes educator, nutritionist, and mental health professional provides the tools to manage the enormous number and variety of diabetes-related decisions that a patient encounters daily.

Cardiovascular risk management

Aggressive management of cardiovascular risk factors is a fundamental priority in diabetes care. All individuals with diabetes should be considered very high risk, whether or not a documented event has occurred (see Chapter 29).

1. Cholesterol: Diabetes mellitus eliminates the protective effect of female sex on cardiovascular disease risk. Practically, this means that women with diabetes, like men with diabetes, have at least two risk factors for CHD (sex and diabetes). Thus the goal LDL cholesterol for all women with diabetes is at least less than 130 mg/dL for those without known CHD, and less than 100 mg/dL for those with CHD. Some authorities, including the National Cholesterol

Aggressive management of cardiovascular risk factors is a fundamental priority in diabetes care.

Education Project (NCEP) Adult Treatment Panel II and the ADA suggest a goal LDL cholesterol of $< 100\,\text{mg/dL}$ for all individuals with diabetes, whether or not a documented event has occurred.[11,12] This suggestion arises from expert opinion (rather than primary prevention data) that most adults with diabetes have vascular disease and that waiting for an event delays important treatment. Further, they argue that aggressive cholesterol management might help to reduce the disturbing 50 percent fatality rate seen in the first year following a CHD event.

2. Secondary prevention data come principally from two large trials. The Scandinavian Simvastatin Survival Study (4S) and Cholesterol and Recurrent Events (CARE) study both included participants with type II diabetes and have recently published subgroup analyses.[13,14] Both studies showed a significant reduction in event rate with statin therapy. In the 4S study, LDL cholesterol reduction with simvastatin resulted in a 55 percent decrease in event rate among men and women with diabetes and hyperlipidemia. The CARE trial evaluated a subgroup of 586 participants with diabetes and average cholesterol levels and found that pravastatin decreased the relative risk for a recurrent coronary event by 25 percent.

3. Aspirin: Aspirin therapy has been shown to reduce cardiovascular events and mortality in individuals with diabetes.[15] The strongest evidence exists for secondary prevention, with event rate reduction (20 to 25 percent) similar to those seen in individuals without diabetes. Primary prevention data come from the US Physicians' Health Study in which male physicians with diabetes experienced a reduction in myocardial infarction from 10.1 to 4.0 percent using aspirin 325 mg every other day.[16] Evidence of efficacy in women with diabetes is not available. The ADA recommends that all individuals over age 30 years with diabetes take enteric-coated aspirin at doses of 75 to 325 mg daily, unless contraindicated.[17] The presence of retinopathy is not considered a contraindication to aspirin therapy.

4. Smoking cessation: Smoking and diabetes each deliver toxic insult to the vasculature. Because of an already profound risk for cardiovascular disease, smokers with diabetes should be counselled to quit, and assisted in their efforts with appropriate pharmacological and behavioral support at every opportunity. Some authorities suggest that providers treat smoking like a vital sign, a basic parameter to be evaluated and addressed at each visit.[18] For many individuals, particularly women, the potential for weight gain after smoking cessation may pose a significant barrier to quitting. Acknowledging

Diabetes mellitus eliminates the protective effect of female sex on cardiovascular disease risk.

the possibility of weight gain, and planning preventive strategies, should be part of the counselling process.

5. Angiotensin-converting enzyme (ACE) inhibitor therapy with ramipril has recently been shown to reduce several important cardiovascular endpoints in patients at high risk for heart diseases, including patients with diabetes.[19] The measured reductions were myocardial infarction (22 percent), stroke (33 percent), cardiovascular death (37 percent) and total mortality (24 percent). These results were verified for patients with diabetes in a subgroup analysis of 3577 out of 9500 total participants in the Heart Outcomes Prevention Evaluation (HOPE) study.

> The American Diabetes Association recommends that all individuals over age 30 years with diabetes take enteric-coated aspirin at doses of 75 to 325 mg daily, unless contraindicated.

Postmenopausal hormone replacement therapy

Many observational and physiological studies support the use of estrogen for both primary and secondary prevention of cardiovascular disease.[20] The only RCT to date that has evaluated the effect of HRT on cardiovascular disease outcomes, the Heart Estrogen/Progestin Replacement (HERS) did not provide the expected support for these studies.[21] At the end of five years, the HRT and placebo groups had similar event rates, with higher event rates in the first year among HRT users. Though the study excluded women with poorly controlled diabetes (fasting blood glucose > 300 mg/dL), almost 20% of the participants had diabetes. The investigators concluded that HRT does not prevent recurrent events in women with existing CHD. However, because a downward trend in event rates was seen over the course of the study, those already on HRT do not need to stop taking it. The study did not address women without known coronary disease, so recommendations for primary prevention still rely on data from observational studies (see Chapter 29).

1. Postmenopausal HRT is well tolerated in women with diabetes. In particular, it does not adversely affect glucose control.[22]

2. However, HRT has potentially important effects on lipid metabolism. For instance, oral estrogen can significantly increase serum triglycerides, exacerbating a significant underlying problem in diabetes. Transdermal estrogen offers the advantage of direct absorption into the systemic circulation. By circumventing the gastrointestinal tract and the associated "first pass" metabolism by the liver, transdermal delivery minimizes the stimulatory effect of estrogen on hepatic triglyceride synthesis.[23]

3. Women with hypertriglyceridemia should undergo triglyceride lowering treatment prior to initiation of HRT. Frequently, this will simply entail aggressive blood glucose lowering. However, if that fails, medical therapy with a fibrate (e.g., gemfibrozil or fenfibrate), or fish oil may be necessary. Nicotinic acid effectively reduces triglycerides, but, because it induces significant hyperglycemia, it should be used with caution in women with diabetes.

4. Estrogen also has significant effects on LDL and HDL cholesterol concentrations. Both oral and transdermal estrogen can induce significant reductions in LDL cholesterol,[24] while only oral estrogens appear to raise HDL cholesterol.

5. Different progestins also have varying effects on lipids. MPA attenuates the beneficial rise in HDL cholesterol seen with estrogen.[25] However, micronized progesterone does not share this metabolic effect, and may thus provide an advantage, especially for women with low HDL cholesterol values.

6. Despite the evidence that HRT can exert a strong and beneficial effect on plasma lipids, cardiovascular outcome data for HRT in women with diabetes are few. One case control study documented no increased risk of myocardial infarction in diabetic women using HRT, and suggested a possible benefit.[26] However, statins have been more extensively studied, and the strength of data favors statin therapy for cardiovascular risk reduction. Thus, when lipid lowering is the primary objective, statins should be first-line therapy.

Postmenopausal hormone replacement therapy is well tolerated in women with diabetes.

Dietary therapy

ADA guidelines suggest that 30 percent or fewer calories come from fat, and that no more than one-third of these should come from saturated fat.[12] Ten to 15 percent of calories can come from protein, leaving the majority of calories (60 percent) to come from carbohydrates.

1. Dietary preferences develop early in life, under the influence of culture and tradition. Food choices that have become habit over a lifetime are difficult to change. Thus many patients will find it difficult to make major and sustainable changes in their dietary habits, even if they understand the reasons behind the recommended modifications. Dietary prescriptions are important, but by themselves they rarely result in meaningful alterations in ingrained habits.

2. Individualized nutritional counselling that takes culture, tradition, and the emotional nuances of eating behaviors into account is an invaluable adjunct to medical therapy. Providers can contribute greatly to the work of nutritionists by reinforcing behavioral nutritional principles during regular visits.

Table 30.3. Some suggested recommendations for providers to offer regarding healthy eating behavior. (Add more of your own)

- Eat regularly and avoid the temptation to skip meals. If your schedule is too hectic to eat reliably, we should consider a more flexible regimen with more frequent dosing of short acting agents
- Try to combine carbohydrates with fats, proteins or fiber to slow absorption and prevent rapid rises in blood glucose. This may be especially important at breakfast, a meal that is frequently high in carbohydrates
- Limit saturated fats – these are the fats that tend to be solid at room temperature
- Use more mono- and polyunsaturated fats such as canola oil or olive oil
- Nothing is off limits, even sugar (sucrose). Everything can be eaten in moderation
- Eat a variety of foods
- Portion sizes often tend to be larger than they need to be. Try smaller portions
- Bedtime snacks, if you need them, should have some protein or fat. A snack with only carbohydrates is metabolized more quickly and may not last overnight
- A "diabetic diet" is a healthy diet, and is appropriate for the whole family

Table 30.3 lists examples of the types of suggestion that may prove valuable to patients, and that can be incorporated into medical visits.

Exercise

1. Exercise and diet remain the mainstays of all therapeutic interventions for type II diabetes and prevention of cardiovascular disease. Evidence supporting the utility of physical activity in preventing type II diabetes and generally improving insulin sensitivity comes from a variety of sources.

2. Epidemiological studies have documented a strong protective effect of physical activity on the development of type II diabetes. In the Nurses' Health Study, women who self-reported vigorous exercise at least once a week, had a lower risk of developing type II diabetes over an eight-year follow up period than sedentary women.[27] A follow-up, prospective observational study found that fewer coronary events occurred in women aged 40 to 65 years who engaged in either brisk walking or vigorous exercise over an eight-year period.[28] In a controlled prospective trial, another study recently reported that, among Chinese patients with impaired glucose tolerance, greater daily activity level was associated with lower risk of type II diabetes over a six-year period.[29] The incidence of myocardial infarction did not change significantly over the course of the study.

3. Exercise modulates insulin resistance by increasing glucose uptake in active muscles during and following physical activity.[30] Muscle contraction and insulin each acutely increase the mobilization of GLUT-4 transporters to the

cell surface, with a resultant increase in facilitated diffusion of glucose into skeletal muscle cells. The exercise effect on skeletal muscle GLUT-4 transporters has been shown both in nondiabetic individuals, and those with type II diabetes.[31]

4. Human exercise studies suggest that low and moderate physical activity can induce significant improvements in whole body insulin sensitivity. One study that used a glucose clamp to study the acute effects of low intensity bicycling in obese patients with type II diabetes, found that glucose uptake nearly doubled during exercise.[32] In a study of insulin-resistant, nonobese first-degree relatives of patients with type II diabetes, participants had a 40 percent increase in insulin sensitivity after a six-week regimen of moderate exercise.[33] Interestingly, this was a larger effect than has been seen with either metformin (16 to 25 percent) or troglitazone (20 percent).

5. Because of the magnitude of its effect, and because of the associated cardiovascular benefits, physical activity is a critical component of diabetes self-management. A recent US Surgeon General's report recommends 30 minutes of moderate physical activity most days of the week.[34]

6. Before beginning a new exercise regimen, individuals with diabetes should be evaluated for factors that might influence recommendations. Such factors include cardiovascular disease status, with a careful history to detect clues to the presence of silent ischemia, the presence of peripheral neuropathy, and the existence of untreated retinopathy.

Mental health

Depression

1. Depression occurs more commonly in women who have a chronic illness, including diabetes. Depression and diabetes have many symptoms in common, including fatigue and changes in weight or appetite, so evaluating symptoms carefully is important. Clinical studies evaluating women with diabetes have shown that cognitive-behavioral therapy and use of tricyclic antidepressants both improve depression scores.[35,36]

2. Tricyclic antidepressants, such as amitriptyline and nortriptyline, may have unwanted appetite stimulant effects, potentially complicating therapy. Second-generation antidepressants such as the selective serotonin reuptake inhibitors (SSRIs) do not stimulate the appetite and may even improve insulin sensitivity.[37] Their effectiveness in treating depression has not been specifically tested in women with diabetes, but they are commonly used, and used successfully.

Depression and diabetes have many symptoms in common, including fatigue and changes in weight or appetite.

Therapeutic options and suggested algorithm

Table 30.4 lists currently available medications, their doses, and mechanisms of action. The accompanying algorithm in Table 30.5 provides a suggested approach to their use. This algorithm is modified from several recently published papers[38–40] and incorporates several overarching principles.

1. Metformin and sulfonylureas are currently considered first-line therapy, after diet and exercise have failed to bring glucose into the goal range. Metformin is preferred in obese individuals, since it does not promote weight gain. Sulfonylureas are generally less expensive, but in addition to weight gain, they can cause hypoglycemia. This is particularly true if blood glucose control is (appropriately) tight.

2. Only brief intervals are needed to determine whether a particular therapy is working. For diet and exercise, this could be two weeks. For metformin and the thiazolidinediones, which take longer to reach maximal effect, six to eight weeks should be enough to determine whether blood sugars are likely to reach goal values.

3. Combination oral therapy produces excellent results, allowing many individuals to reach near-normal blood glucose levels.

4. Bedtime insulin is often a good way to introduce injections into a regimen. Physiologically, it decreases hepatic glucose output overnight, resulting in a lower fasting glucose. Psychologically, it does not seem as daunting as changing to insulin entirely.

Special populations

Reproductive age women

1. Pregnancy: Ideally, all pregnancies in women with diabetes should be planned, and normal glucose levels achieved before conception.[41] There is increased intrauterine death and congenital malformation in the fetuses of women who conceive while hyperglycemic. All sexually active reproductive age women should receive contraceptive counselling.

2. The low dose OCPs available today do not cause deterioration in blood glucose control in women with prior gestational diabetes[42] or in those with

type I diabetes.[43] These pills generally contain 20–50 μg of ethinylestradiol (5 mg of ethinylestradiol is roughly equivalent to 0.625 mg of conjugated equine estrogens). Extrapolating these findings, women with type II diabetes can safely take OCPs, provided that they do not smoke, have hypertension, or have other contraindications to OCP therapy. Blood pressure should be monitored after initiation, since an idiosyncratic rise occurs in some women.

3. In the absence of contraindications, oral contraceptives can be used until the menopausal transition, at which time postmenopausal HRT can be initiated. Because postmenopausal HRT does not provide contraception, alternative methods of birth control should be used during the perimenopausal transition.

4. In young women and men, the presence of diabetic ketoacidosis usually indicates the absence of insulin, and a diagnosis of type I diabetes. However, patients with type II diabetes can occasionally present with significant ketonuria and even ketoacidosis. This can occur when long standing hyperglycemic stress results in temporary pancreatic beta-cell exhaustion, and insulin deficiency. In this situation C-peptide, a marker of pancreatic insulin production, may be undetectable. The distinction between types I and II diabetes can thus be difficult, especially if the individual falls into the age group typical of type I diabetes. Clues to the presence of type II diabetes include obesity and a family history of type II diabetes. In these individuals, insulin can be used initially, followed by a measurement of C-peptide after at least six weeks of aggressive blood glucose-lowering therapy. If C-peptide is now present, oral agents can be introduced and an attempt made to wean onto insulin.

5. Polycystic ovary syndrome:
    a. PCOS affects an estimated 5 to 8 percent of reproductive age women and is frequently associated with abnormal carbohydrate metabolism.[44] Oligo-amenorrhea and hirsutism, with or without obesity, acne, or acanthosis nigricans characterize PCOS.
    b. Recent studies have documented significant insulin resistance in these women, with one study showing a staggering 20 percent prevalence of previously undiagnosed type II diabetes among obese women with PCOS.[45] Thus women with irregular menses and male-pattern hair growth comprise a group of women at potentially high risk for developing diabetes at a young age.
    c. Because of the opportunity for early intervention, obese women with PCOS

All pregnancies in women with diabetes should be planned.

Table 30.4. Medications for the treatment of type II diabetes

Generic name	Brand name	Dosing range	Comments[a]
Glipizide	Glucotrol	5 mg q.a.m. to 20 mg b.i.d. a.c.	Take 30 minutes before meals
Glipizide	Glucotrol XL	5–20 mg q.d.	Pills release drug slowly through laser-drilled hole in capsule. Therefore, capsules should not be broken. Long duration of action may decrease fasting hyperglycemia more effectively than non-XL formulation
Glyburide	Micronase	2.5 mg q.d.–10 mg b.i.d. a.c.	Take 30 minutes before meals
Glyburide	Diabeta	Same as Micronase	Take 30 minutes before meals
Glyburide	Glynase	3–6 mg b.i.d. a.c.	Micronized glyburide
Glimepiride	Amaryl	1–4 mg q.d. max. dose 8 mg/day	Sulfonylurea. Stimulates pancreatic insulin release
Repaglinide	Prandin	0.5–2.0 mg t.i.d. a.c.	Nonsulfonylurea stimulates pancreatic insulin release. Very short acting, allows more flexible timing because it is taken when meal available
Acarbose	Precose	50 mg t.i.d. a.c. is maximum dose, though can go up to 100 mg t.i.d. a.c. in large people	Delays carbohydrate absorption in small intestine by inhibiting alpha-glucosidases. Start low (e.g., 25 mg p.o. q.d.) and increase dose slowly, e.g., by 25 mg every 2 weeks. This minimizes side effects of loose stools and flatulence. Take pill with first bite of meal for best effect
Miglitol	Glyset	25–100 mg t.i.d. a.c.	Alpha-glucosidase inhibitor. No significant differences from acarbose
Metformin	Glucophage	500–1000 mg b.i.d. a.c. usual dose Maximum dose 2500 mg/day	Decreases hepatic glucose production Do not use if Cr > 1.6 in men or 1.4 in women, if LFTs elevated, or in chronically hypoxic conditions such as COPD, CHF Side effects of intestinal gas and loose stools usually resolve in 2–4 weeks Discontinue before procedures requiring i.v. contrast and during hospitalizations (conditions predisposing to dehydrated state), but $t_{1/2}$ short so do not withhold necessary emergency procedures

Table 30.4. (*cont.*)

Generic name	Brand name	Dosing range	Comments[a]
Rosiglitazone	Avandia	2 mg q.d.–4 m.g. b.i.d.	Insulin sensitizer Thiazolidinedione class Monitor LFTs (ALT) every 2 months for first year, then periodically thereafter May exacerbate CHF, cause edema Not contraindicated in renal insufficiency Approved as monotherapy, in combination with sulfonylureas and metformin
Pioglitazone	Actos	15–45 mg q.d.	Insulin sensitizer Thiazolidinedione class Monitor LFTs (ALT) every 2 months for first year, then periodically thereafter May exacerbate CHF, cause edema Not contraindicated in renal insufficiency Approved as monotherapy, and combine with sulfonylurea, metformin, and insulin
Human insulin		Duration: Peak:	
	Regular	6–8 hours 4 hours	
	NPH	8–12 hours 6–8 hours	Take Reg insulin 30 min a.c. meals for best effect
	Lente	8–12 hours	Can pre-draw insulin: mixtures of Reg + NPH are stable for a week when refrigerated.
	70/30	8–12 hours 70% NPH, 30% Reg	Mixtures of Reg + L are not stable and must be used immediately
Lispro insulin	Humalog	Duration: Peak: 4 hours 30–60 min	Take lispro insulin immediately before eating

q.a.m., every morning; Cr, creatinine; LFT, liver function test; ALT, alanine transferase; COPD, chronic obstructive pulmonary disease; CHF, congestive heart failure; Reg, regular insulin; NPH, neutral protamine Hageman; L, lispro insulin.

[a]FDA approved indications may differ somewhat from these suggested uses.

Table 30.5. Suggested strategies for management of type II diabetes

FBG < 200 or random BG < 250, or in early phases of diabetes with good pancreatic reserve	FBG 200–300 or random BG > 250, or in mid-phase of diabetes	FBG > 300 or random BG > 450, or in late stages of diabetes with failing pancreatic reserve
↓	↓	↓
Emphasize meal plan and exercise	Start oral agent: metformin (first choice for obese individuals) OR SFU or repaglinide Alternatives: Rosiglitazone or pioglitazone (TZDs) Acarbose/miglitol (alpha-glucosidase inhibitors) Insulin Continue to emphasize meal plan and exercise	Start insulin therapy[a] 0.3–0.7 U/kg per day in divided doses: Reg + NPH a.m. and Reg + NPH a.c. supper Give 2/3 a.c. breakfast and 1/3 a.c. supper Divide a.m. shot into 1/3 Reg and 2/3 NPH and p.m. shot into 1/2 Reg and 1/2 NPH, e.g., 36 U/day = 8 Reg/16 N a.m. and 6 Reg/6 NPH p.m.
↓		↓
If BGs not in target range in 1 month, add oral agent (See next column) ↗	If BGs not in target range after 2 weeks on maximum dose, use combination therapy with: SFU + metformin or alpha glucosidase inhibitor or TZD OR Add bedtime NPH insulin to oral agent	If persistent a.m. hyperglycemia and/or nocturnal hypoglycemia consider: Reg + NPH a.m., Reg a.c. supper, NPH at h.s. (e.g., split evening shot)
	↓	↓
	If BGs not in target range after 2 weeks on maximum doses add third agent, or add h.s. NPH, or change to insulin-only regimen (See next column) ↗	If BGs erratic with frequent lows, consider: Reg before each meal and NPH at h.s. (4 shots per day for more flexibility with each dose)

FBG, fasting blood glucose; BG, blood glucose; Reg, regular insulin; NPH, neutral protamine Hageman; TZDs, thiazolidinediones; SFU, sulfonylurea; a.c., before meals; b.s., before sleep.

[a]For type I diabetes management, start at lower end of scale (0.3 U/kg per day). All insulin regimens may be used in type I patients.

should be carefully monitored for diabetes and insulin resistance. This can be accomplished through glucose tolerance testing, or assessment of insulin resistance.

d. One recent study found that a fasting glucose to insulin ratio of < 4.5 correlated with insulin resistance when measured with the gold standard clamp technique.[46]

The low dose oral contraceptive pills available today do not cause deterioration in blood glucose control in women with prior gestational diabetes or in those with type I diabetes.

Elderly

Elderly individuals with diabetes may require special equipment to accommodate handicaps such as visual impairment or poor motor coordination due to arthritis or stroke. The ADA, in their patient-oriented publication *Diabetes Forecast*, provides a resource guide summarizing products for a variety of special needs.[47]

Conclusions

Diabetes is very common in women and in the elderly, who are most often women. Rigorous diagnosis and treatment will help to prevent the serious microscopic side effects and important macroscopic worsening of heart, kidney, and great vessel disease that increases mortality. Lifestyle changes, diet, exercise, and medication will all help to reduce the consequences of this disease.

REFERENCES

1. Welch GW, Jacobson AM, Polonsky WH. The problem areas in diabetes scale. An evaluation of its clinical utility. *Diabetes Care* 1997;**20**:760–6.
2. Harris MI. Diabetes in America: Epidemiology and scope of the problem. *Diabetes Care* 1998;**21**:C11–C14.
3. Jovanovic L. American Diabetes Association's Fourth International Workshop–Conference on Gestational Diabetes Mellitus: summary and discussion. Therapeutic interventions. *Diabetes Care* 1998;**21**(Suppl 2):B131–B317.
4. Website: www.cdc.gov/hchs/fastats/pdf/10199t58.pdf
5. Harris M. Classification, diagnostic criteria, and screening for diabetes. In *Diabetes in America*, 2nd edn. NIH Publication no.95-1468. NIH/NIDDK, Bethesda, MD, 1995.

6. The Expert Committee on the Diagnosis and Classification of Diabetes Mellitus. Report of the Expert Committee on the Diagnosis and Classification of Diabetes Mellitus. *Diabetes Care* 1997;**20**:1183–97.

7. The Diabetes Control and Complications Trial Research Group. The effect of intensive treatment of diabetes on the development and progression of long-term complications in insulin-dependent diabetes mellitus. *N Engl J Med* 1993;**329**:977–86.

8. American Diabetes Association. Implications of the United Kingdom Prospective Diabetes Study. *Diabetes Care* 1998;**21**:2180–4.

9. American Diabetes Association. Clinical practice recommendations 2000. *Diabetes Care* 2000;**23**(suppl 1):S1–S116.

10. Luftey KE, Wishner WJ. Beyond "Compliance" is "Adherence": Improving the prospect of diabetes care. *Diabetes Care* 1999;**22**:635–9.

11. Haffner S. Management of dyslipidemia in adults with diabetes (technical review). *Diabetes Care* 1998;**21**:160–78.

12. American Diabetes Association. Management of dyslipidemia in adults with diabetes. *Diabetes Care* 2000;**23**:S57–S60.

13. Pyorala K, Pederson TR, Kjekshus J et al. Cholesterol lowering with simvastatin improves prognosis of diabetic patients with coronary heart disease. A subgroup analysis of the Scandinavian Simvastatin Survival Study (4S). *Diabetes Care* 1997;**20**:614–20.

14. Goldberg RB, Mellies MJ, Sacks FM et al. Cardiovascular events and their reduction with pravastatin in diabetic and glucose-intolerant myocardial infarction survivors with average cholesterol levels: Subgroup analyses in the Cholesterol and Recurrent Events (CARE) trial. *Circulation* 1998;**98**:2513–19.

15. ETDRS Investigators. Aspirin effects on mortality and morbidity inpatients with diabetes mellitus. Early Treatment Diabetic Retinopathy study report 14. *JAMA* 1992;**268**:1292–300.

16. Colwell JA. Aspirin therapy in diabetes (technical review). *Diabetes Care* 1997;**20**:1767–71.

17. American Diabetes Association. Aspirin therapy in diabetes. *Diabetes Care* 2000;**23**:S61–S62.

18. Haire-Joshu D, Glasgow RE, Tibbs TL. Smoking and diabetes (technical review). *Diabetes Care* 1999;**22**:1887–98.

19. The Hope Study Investigators. Effects of ramipril on cardiovascular and microvascular outcomes in people with diabetes mellitus: Results of the HOPE study and MICRO-HOPE substudy. *Lancet* 2000;**355**:253–9.

20. Grady D, Rubin SM, Petitti DB et al. Hormone therapy to prevent disease and prolong life in postmenopausal women. *Ann Intern Med* 1992;**117**:1016–37.

21. Hulley S, Grady D, Bush T et al. Randomized trial of estrogen plus progestin for secondary prevention of coronary heart disease in postmenopausal women. Heart and Estrogen/Progestin Study (HERS) Research Group. *JAMA* 1998;**280**:605–13.

22. Samaras K, Hayward CS, Sullivan D et al. Effects of postmenopausal hormone replacement therapy on central abdominal fat, glycemic control, lipid metabolism, and vascular factors in type II diabetes: A prospective study. *Diabetes Care* 1999;**22**:1401–7.

23. Bhathena RK, Anklesaria BS, Ganatra AM et al. The influence of transdermal oestradiol replacement therapy and medroxyprogesterone acetate on serum lipids and lipoproteins. *Br J Clin Pharmacol* 1998;**45**:170–2.

24. Meschia M, Bruschi F, Soma M et al. Effects of oral and transdermal hormone replacement therapy on lipoprotein (A) and lipids: A randomized controlled trial. *Menopause* 1998;**5**:157–62.

25. Writing Group for the PEPI Trial. Effects of estrogen or estrogen/progestin regimens on heart disease risk factors in postmenopausal women. The Postmenopausal Estrogen/Progestin Interventions (PEPI) trial. *JAMA* 1995;**273**:199–208.

26. Kaplan RC, Heckbert SR, Weiss NS et al. Postmenopausal estrogens and risk of myocardial infarction in diabetic women. *Diabetes Care* 1998;**21**:1117–21.

27. Manson JE. Physical activity and incidence of non-insulin-dependent diabetes mellitus in women. *Lancet* 1991;**338**:774–8.

28. Manson JE, Hu FB, Rich-Edwards JW et al. A prospective study of walking as compared to vigorous exercise in the prevention of coronary heart disease in women. *N Engl J Med* 1999;**341**:650–8.

29. Pan X, Li G, Hu Y et al. Effect of diet and exercise in preventing NIDDM in people with impaired glucose tolerance. The Da Qing impaired glucose tolerance and diabetes study. *Diabetes Care* 1997;**20**:537–44.

30. Annuzzi G, Riccardi G, Capaldo B et al. Increased insulin-stimulated glucose uptake by exercised human muscles one day after prolonged exercise. *Eur J Clin Invest* 1991;**21**:6–12.

31. Goodyear LJ, Kahn BB. Exercise, glucose transport, and insulin sensitivity. *Annu Rev Med* 1998;**49**:235–61.

32. Usui K, Yamanouchi K, Asai K et al. The effect of low intensity bicycle exercise on the insulin-induced glucose uptake in obese patients with type 2 diabetes. *Diabetes Res Clin Pract* 1998;**41**:57–61.

33. Perseghin G, Price T, Petersen KF et al. Increased glucose transport – phosphorylation and muscle glycogen synthesis after exercise training in insulin resistant subjects. *N Engl J Med* 1996;**335**:1357–62.

34. US Department of Health and Human Services. *Physical Activity and Health: A Report of the Surgeon General.* Centers of Disease Control and Prevention, National Center for Chronic Disease Prevention and Health Promotion. US Government Printing Office, Washington, DC, 1996.

35. Lustman PJ, Griffith LS, Freedland KE et. al. Cognitive behavior therapy for depression in type 2 diabetes mellitus. A randomized, controlled trial. *Ann Intern Med* 1998;**129**:613–21.

36. Lustman PJ, Griffith LS, Clouse RE et al. Effects of nortriptyline on depression and glycemic control in diabetes: Results of a double-blind, placebo-controlled trial. *Psychosom Med* 1997;**59**:241–50.

37. Maheux P, Ducros F, Bourque J et al. Fluoxetine improves insulin sensitivity in obese patients with non-insulin-dependent diabetes mellitus. *Int J Obes Relat Metab Disord* 1999; **21**:97–102.

38. DeFronzo RA. Pharmacologic therapy for type 2 diabetes mellitus. *Ann Intern Med* 1999;**131**:281–303.

39. Mazze RS, Etzwiler DD, Strock E et al. Staged diabetes management. Toward an integrated model of diabetes care. *Diabetes Care* 1994;**17**(Suppl 1):56–66.

40. Feinglos M, Bether AM. Treatment of type 2 diabetes mellitus. *Med Clin North Am* 1998;**82**:757–90.

41. Kjos SL, Buchanan TA. Gestational diabetes mellitus. *N Engl J Med* 1999;**23**:1749–56.

42. Kjos SL, Peters RK, Xiang A et al. Contraception and the risk of type 2 diabetes mellitus in Latino women with prior gestational diabetes mellitus. *JAMA* 1998;**280**:533–8.

43. Petersen KR, Skouby SO, Jespersen J. Contraception guidance in women with pre-existing disturbances in carbohydrate metabolism. *Eur J Contracept Reprod Health Care* 1996;**1**:53–9.

44. Dunaif A, Graf M, Mandeli J et al. Characterization of groups of hyperandrogenic women with

acanthosis nigricans, impaired glucose tolerance, and/or hyperinsulinemia. *J Clin Endocrinol Metab* 1987;**65**:499–507.

45. Legro RS, Kunselman AR, Dodson WC et al. Prevalence and predictors of risk for type 2 diabetes and impaired glucose tolerance in polycystic ovary syndrome: A prospective, controlled study in 254 affected women. *J Clin Endocrinol Metab* 1999;**84**:165–9.

46. Legro RS, Finegood D, Dunaif A. A fasting glucose to insulin ratio is a useful measure of insulin sensitivity in women with polycystic ovary syndrome. *J Clin Endocrinol Metab* 1998;**83**:2694–8.

47. American Diabetes Association Resources Guide 2000. *Diabetes Forecast*, January 2000:1–72.

Thyroid disorders

William Hueston, MD

Thyroid disorders comprise a wide range of problems that affect the normal functioning of the thyroid gland. These conditions can be grouped into several large categories that include inflammatory diseases of the thyroid (i.e., thyroiditis), autoimmune stimulation of the thyroid (Graves' disease), benign thyroid nodular diseases, and thyroid cancers. While the manifestations of thyroid disease are usually obvious if the presentation is classic, subtle changes in thyroid function, especially in the elderly, can lead to confusion about the diagnosis and treatment for complications of the thyroid condition rather than the underlying thyroid problem. Since thyroid disorders are the second most common endocrine disorder after diabetes, primary care physicians will encounter many individuals with these problems.

Epidemiology

Occurrence

Thyroid disease affects 1 out of 200 adults (0.5 percent), but is more commonly seen in the elderly and in women.[1,2] By the time adults reach older ages, about 5 percent have a thyroid abnormality, most commonly hypothyroidism.

Sex risk

The risk of thyroid disease in women is 10 times higher than that in men. For example, about 2 percent of the female adult population has been hyperthyroid during their lifetime compared to 0.2 percent of men.[1]

The risk of thyroid disease in women is 10 times higher than that in men.

529

Relative frequency

Hypothyroidism is much more common than hyperthyroidism, nodular disease, or thyroid cancer. Thyroid nodules occur in between 4 percent and 8 percent of all individuals and, like other thyroid problems, increase in incidence with age. While nodules are more common in women, thyroid carcinoma is more common in women than in men.[3] However, thyroid cancer represents a higher percentage of cancer deaths in men (0.24%) than in women (0.16%).[4]

Clinical presentation

Hypothyroidism

1. Patients with hypothyroidism generally present with a constellation of symptoms that include lethargy, weight gain, hair loss, dry skin, slowed mentation or forgetfulness, and a depressed affect.
2. In older patients, hypothyroidism can be confused with Alzheimer's or other conditions that cause dementia.
3. In women, hypothyroidism is often confused with depression.
4. Physical findings that can occur with hypothyroidism include a low blood pressure and bradycardia, nonpitting edema, generalized hair thinning along with hair loss in the outer third of the eyebrows, skin drying, and a diminished relaxation phase of reflexes. The challenge in early hypothyroidism is to differentiate the generalized symptoms that characterize hypothyroidism from the many other conditions that can cause similar symptoms of tiredness and dysthymia.
5. Amenorrhea or oligomenorrhea may be a symptom of hypothyroidism.

> In older patients, hypothyroidism can be confused with Alzheimer's or other conditions that cause dementia.

Hyperthyroidism

1. Hyperthyroidism usually presents with progressing nervousness, tremor, palpitations or an irregular heart rate when atrial fibrillation is present, weight loss, dyspnea on exertion, and difficulty concentrating.
2. Physical findings include a rapid pulse and elevated blood pressure with the systolic increasing to a greater extent than diastolic, creating a wide pulse-pressure hypertension. Additionally, cardiac dysrhythmias such as atrial fibrillation may be evident on examination. A resting tremor may be noted on physical examination.

3. Oligomenorrhea or hypermenorrhea can be symptoms of hyperthyroidism.

Thyroid storm (thyroid crisis)

1. Thyroid storm represents an acute hypermetabolic state associated with sudden release of large amounts of thyroid hormone. This occurs more often in Graves' disease, but can occur in acute thyroiditis conditions.
2. Individuals with thyroid storm present with confusion, fever, restlessness, and sometimes with acute psychotic-like symptoms.
3. Physical examination shows tachycardia, elevated blood pressure, and sometimes fever. Cardiac dysrhythmias may be present or develop. They will have other signs of high output heart failure (dyspnea on exertion, peripheral vasoconstriction) and may exhibit signs of cardiac or cerebral ischemia.
4. Thyroid storm is a medical crisis requiring prompt attention and reversal of the metabolic demands from the acute hyperthyroidism.

Thyroid nodules

1. Most thyroid nodules are asymptomatic and found on routine health examinations of women. In rare cases, the nodule may be very large and compressing nearby structures, but most benign nodules grow slowly.
2. Nodules under 4 cm in size are rarely malignant.
3. Nodules usually do not produce symptoms of hypo- or hyperthyroidism, but autonomously functioning adenomas may cause hyperthyroidism. In this situation, the adenoma is not under the control of thyroid-stimulating hormone (TSH) and continues to produce thyroid hormones despite inappropriately high levels.

Most thyroid nodules are asymptomatic and found on routine health examinations of women.

Laboratory and radiological evaluation

Blood levels of circulating thyroid hormones

1. Both T4 and T3 are highly protein bound. These hormones bind to a number of serum proteins including thyroid-binding globulin (TBG), which has a special affinity for T4 and T3. Under normal circumstances, 99 percent of T4 and 97 percent of T3 are protein bound.

2. Congenital absences of TBG occur, appearing in genetic patterns. In these patients, both total T4 and T3 levels are extremely low, although patients are usually euthyroid.

3. Other physiological conditions that alter serum proteins can influence total thyroid hormone levels while total free thyroid remains normal. The high ratio of bound to free thyroid hormones means that measurements of total T4 and T3 may not reflect levels of free thyroid hormone.

4. Radioimmunoassays (RIA) that measure free T3 are available that can avoid confusion over bound and free hormone levels. In addition, total T4 measurements can be paired with a test that measures bound levels of T4, called the T3 resin uptake test (T3RU). The combination of these two tests, often termed the free thyroid index or sometimes referred to as a T7, can offer better indications of thyroid status in patients.

Thyroid stimulating hormone levels

1. Measuring the amount of TSH in the blood can assess thyroid function in most hypo- or hyperthyroid individuals. Since, in normal individuals, TSH rises with low free thyroid levels and falls when free thyroid is elevated, it is an alternative measure for actual circulating levels of the free thyroid hormones.

2. However, when the cause of the thyroid dysfunction is abnormal production of TSH, the test may be misleading. In the case of secondary hypothyroidism, i.e., thyroid deficiency due to low levels of TSH production, both TSH and thyroid hormones levels will be low.

3. In most circumstances it is not necessary to measure both TSH and thyroid hormones. Only when the TSH level appears to contradict the clinical appearance of the patient, such as a low TSH in a patient suspected of hypothyroidism, should thyroid hormones testing be done.

Measuring the amount of thyroid-stimulating hormone in the blood can assess thyroid function in most hypo- or hyperthyroid individuals.

Thyrotropin-releasing hormone stimulation testing

If pituitary dysfunction is suspected, further evaluation of the anterior pituitary function can be performed using a thyrotropin-releasing hormone (TRH) stimulation test. In this test, TSH levels are determined before and after administration of intravenous TRH. In normal circumstances, infusion of TRH results in a modest rise in TSH. With pituitary dysfunction, the TSH response is absent or blunted. If an exaggerated rise in TSH is noted, this indicates that the pituitary is normal and that the lack of production of TSH reflects an abnormality in TRH production in the hypothalamus.

Other blood tests

Other diagnostic tests for the thyroid include measurement of thyroid antibodies. These antibodies are found in Graves' disease and usually cause stimulation of the thyroid gland resulting in hyperthyroidism.

Radionucleotide thyroid scanning

1. Radionucleotide scanning of the thyroid provides both a direct image of the thyroid and an indication of thyroid functioning. Imaging is performed using either an isotope of technetium (^{99m}Tc) or iodine (^{123}I). These radionucleotides are taken up by the active thyroid and, in the case of ^{123}I, incorporated into thyroid hormones.

2. ^{99m}Tc is preferred over radiolabelled iodine for scanning for a couple of reasons. First, the radiation dose from ^{99m}Tc is much lower than that delivered by ^{123}I. Secondly, uptake of radioactive iodine is altered by the use of thyroid-suppressing medications. This means that patients who have had their hyperthyroidism controlled by thyroid-suppressing drugs must have their medications withdrawn before an adequate scan can be completed. Use of ^{99m}Tc is not affected by thyroid-suppressing medications, avoiding any risk to the patient from the temporary discontinuation of her medications.[5]

3. Imaging of the thyroid after the administration of one of these agents allows visualization of active and inactive areas of the thyroid as well as an indication of the level of activity in that area of the thyroid gland. Similarly, thyroid nodules can be localized and determined to be thyroid hormone-producing ("hot" nodules) or nonthyroid hormone-producing ("cold" nodules).

> Radionucleotide scanning of the thyroid provides both a direct image of the thyroid and an indication of thyroid functioning.

Ultrasound

Ultrasound scans are used primarily as a confirmatory test following the visualization of a nonfunctioning nodule on thyroid scans. In the presence of a cold nodule, ultrasound can be used to differentiate a hypoechoic nodule, which raises suspicion of a thyroid cancer from a solid nonfunctioning nodule, which is usually a "burned out" adenoma, and a thyroid cyst, which is rarely malignant.

Magnetic resonance imaging

1. When a thyroid mass is suspected, but cannot be differentiated from other possible neck masses, MRI is the test of choice. MRI provides excellent resolution among neck structures such as the thyroid, muscle, and lymphoid tissue.

2. An MRI scan can be used to determine what structures are involved and, if a thyroid cancer is suspected, evaluate the extent of involvement of adjacent structures.

3. In contrast to MRI, CT provides poor differentiation among the soft tissues of the neck and has little advantage over ultrasound despite considerable differences in the cost.

Thyroid disorders

Thyroiditis

Thyroiditis encompasses a number of unrelated clinical conditions that involve either autoimmune, infectious, or unknown insults to the thyroid. Symptoms may include painless or tender enlargement of the thyroid, hyper- or hypothyroid symptoms, and even fever and other stigmata of invasive bacterial infections.

1. Chronic lymphocytic (Hashimoto's) thyroiditis:
   a. Hashimoto's thyroiditis is the most common type of thyroiditis and is seen most often in middle-aged women. The prevalence of Hashimoto's has increased dramatically in the USA in the last 50 years.
   b. It presents with nonpainful enlargement of the thyroid.
   c. About 20 percent of patients presenting with Hashimoto's will already be hypothyroid either clinically or on measurement of TSH. Patients with Hashimoto's often go on to develop hypothyroidism, but progression is generally slow.
   d. Hashimoto's is caused by an autoimmune disease; 95 percent of patients will have antithyroid perixodase (formerly known as antimicrosomal) antibodies in their serum.

2. Subacute lymphocytic (painless or silent) thyroiditis:
   a. Subacute lymphocytic thyroiditis is also autoimmune mediated, but the immune insult is usually more transient.
   b. Patients with subacute lymphocytic thyroiditis often have fairly acute enlargement of the thyroid without tenderness (hence, the label "painless").

    c. Autoimmune inflammation of the thyroid may result in the release of preformed thyroid hormone resulting in a period of hyperthyroidism. Following this hyperthyroid phase, patients may become hypothyroid as the injured thyroid undergoes repair.

    d. Fewer than 10 percent of patients will have permanent hypothyroidism.

3. Subacute granulomatous (giant cell thyroiditis or de Quervain's) thyroiditis:

    a. Subacute lymphocytic thyroiditis is similar to subacute lymphocytic thyroiditis, except it is not autoimmune mediated but is believed to arise from a viral infection. In subacute granulomatous thyroiditis, patients usually have a viral illness preceding their symptoms and the thyroid enlargement is mildly painful.

    b. The clinical presentation of subacute granulomatous thyroiditis is similar to subacute lymphocytic with a hyperthyroid stage followed by euthyroid or a hypothyroid periods.

    c. Acute inflammation in the thyroid may be treated with aspirin or other NSAIDs or, in severe cases, with prednisone. Usually steroids administered at 40 mg/day results in a rapid reduction in thyroid pain and after a week the steroids can be tapered over two to four weeks. However, prednisone withdrawal may result in a rebound in thyroid swelling and tenderness in approximately 20 percent of patients. Antiinflammatory drugs may provide symptomatic benefit, but there is little evidence that antiinflammatory treatment reduces the duration of the inflammatory process or changes the long-term likelihood of hypothyroidism.[6]

    d. Approximately 10 percent of patients will require permanent thyroid replacement.

4. Suppurative thyroiditis:

    a. Suppurative thyroiditis is an acute bacterial infection of the thyroid gland usually with *Staphylococcus aureus*, *Streptococcus pyogenes* (Group A strep), or *Streptococcus pneumoniae*. It is a rare condition, with only 224 cases reported between 1900 and 1980.[6] However, thyroid infection with opportunistic organisms such as cytomegalovirus, *Mycobacterium avium-intercellulare* complex, and *Pneumocystis carinii* has become more common in patients with HIV and other immunosuppressive disorders.[6]

    b. Patients have a tender, swollen thyroid, fever, elevated white blood cell count and other manifestations of an acute bacterial illness. Occasionally thyroid abscesses can develop.

    c. Suppurative thyroiditis is treated like any other acute, serious bacterial infection. Parenteral administration of antibiotics to cover the likely organisms (*Staph. aureus* and streptococcal species) is indicated.

    d. Fluctuence may signal abscess formation. Abscesses can be confirmed by ultrasound (if large) or by thyroid scanning (if small). These should be surgically drained.

  e. Unless extensive damage to the thyroid has occurred, patients usually have normal thyroid function following clearance of the acute infection.

5. Invasive fibrous (Reidel's) thyroiditis:
  a. This condition presents with a gradually enlarging, firm but nontender thyroid. In this condition, thyroid tissue is infiltrated with dense fibrous tissue that causes a hard, woody goiter.
  b. Patients are usually euthyroid, although a small minority can develop hypothyroidism over time.
  c. Occasionally, because the large, firm thyroid may be uncomfortable or compress nearby structures, surgical removal of the thyroid is warranted. Otherwise, monitoring for symptoms of hypothyroidism is all that is needed.

6. Treatment of hypothyroidism: Treatment is simple and inexpensive. Treatment should start with 50 μg (0.050 mg) of thyroid replacement daily. After one month's use, a repeat TSH is performed. If it is still elevated, the dosage is titrated up slowly. Usually 100 to 125 μg is the daily dose needed.

> Hashimoto's thyroiditis is the most common type of thyroiditis and is seen most often in middle-aged women.

Graves' disease

1. Graves' disease is the most common cause of hyperthyroidism.
2. Graves' disease is an autoimmune disorder caused by immunoglobulin G antibodies that bind to TSH receptors and initiate the production and release of thyroid hormone. Like most of the autoimmune conditions noted in thyroiditis, Graves' disease is more common in women.
3. In addition to the hyperthyroid symptoms noted above, approximately 50 percent of patients with Graves' disease also exhibit exophthalmos.
4. Thyroid hormones will be elevated, with a corresponding low TSH.
5. On thyroid scan, diffuse increased uptake of radiolabelled iodine will be found; this distinguishes Graves' disease from thyroid hormone-producing nodules.
6. The single diagnostic test that differentiates Graves' disease from other causes of hyperthyroidism is the detection of thyroid-receptor antibodies, specific for Graves'.

> Graves' disease is the most common cause of hyperthyroidism.

7.   There are three approaches available to treat Graves' disease (Table 31.1):

  a.   Radioactive iodine is the treatment of choice for Graves' disease in adult patients who are not pregnant. Radioactive iodine should not be used in children or breast-feeding mothers. There is also concern that the administration of radioactive iodine in patients with active ophthalmopathy may accelerate progression of eye disease. For this reason, some experts initially treat Graves' disease with oral suppressive therapy until the eye disease is stabilized.

  b.   Antithyroid drugs are well tolerated and successful at blocking the production and release of thyroid hormones in patients with Graves' disease. These drugs work by blocking the organification of iodine. Propylthiouracil (PTU) also prevents peripheral conversion of T4 to the more active T3. PTU must given in divided doses (two or three times per day), whereas methimazole and carbimazole can be administered once a day. The most serious side effect of these drugs is agranulocytosis that occurs in 3 per 10 000 patients per year. All of these drugs are relatively safe in pregnancy, but associations of carbimazole with aplasia cutis and the decreased release of PTU in breast milk make PTU the favored treatment in pregnant or potentially pregnant women. Antithyroid drugs are especially useful in adolescents where Graves' disease may go into spontaneous remission after 6 to 18 months of therapy.

  c.   Surgery is reserved for women where medication and radioactive iodine ablation are not acceptable treatment strategies or where a large goiter is present that compresses nearby structures or is disfiguring. Surgical results for Graves' disease after one year show that approximately 80 percent of patients will be euthyroid, 20 percent may be hypothyroid, and 1 percent remain hyperthyroid. Recurrence of hyperthyroid occurs at a rate of 1 percent to 3 percent per year. Complications of surgery include damage to the superior laryngeal nerve (1 to 2 percent of cases) and possible hypocalcemia from inadvertent removal of parathyroid tissue.

The single diagnostic test that differentiates Graves' disease from other causes of hyperthyroidism is the detection of thyroid-receptor antibodies.

Thyroid storm

1.   Thyroid storm is an acute event related to the release of large amounts of thyroid hormone in a short period of time. This condition is usually seen with acute onset of Graves' disease, but also may be encountered with abrupt onset

Table 31.1. Treatment of hyperthyroidism

Treatment	Best in which patients	Dose	Comments
Radioactive iodine	Adult patients who are not pregnant Radioactive iodine should not be used in children or breast-feeding mothers		Some experts initially treat Graves' disease with oral suppressive therapy until eye disease is stabilized
Antithyroid medication	Pregnant women Women in whom there is a concern that the administration of radioactive iodine in patients with active ophthalmopathy may accelerate progression of eye disease Adolescents where Graves' disease may go into spontaneous remission after 6 to 18 months of therapy	PTU must be given in divided doses (two or three times a day) Methimazole and carbimazole can be administered once a day	Antithyroid drugs are well tolerated and successful The most serious side effect of these drugs is agranulocytosis that occurs in 3 per 10 000 patients per year PTU is the favored treatment in pregnant or potentially pregnant women
Surgery	Women in whom medication and radioactive iodine ablation are not acceptable treatment strategies OR Patients with a large goiter that compresses nearby structures or is disfiguring		After 1 year shows that approximately 80 percent of patients will be euthyroid, 20 percent may be hypothyroid, and 1 percent remain hyperthyroid Recurrence of hyperthyroid occurs at a rate of 1 to 3 percent per year Complications of surgery include damage to the superior laryngeal nerve (1 to 2 percent of cases) and possible hypocalcemia from inadvertent removal of parathyroid tissue

PTU, propylthiouracil.

of thyroiditis or in stable patients who are under physiological stress such as with severe infections, surgery, or trauma.

2. The *urgent* treatment of thyroid storm is essential to prevent ischemia complications. Administration of high doses of PTU (100 mg every six hours) to quickly block thyroid release and reduce peripheral conversion of T4 to T3 and high doses of beta-blockers (propranalol 1 to 5 mg i.v. or 20 to 80 mg orally every four hours) are the optimal strategy to control symptoms of thyrotoxicosis and prevent complications. Hydrocortisone (200 to 300 mg/day) also is used to prevent possible adrenal crisis.

The *urgent* treatment of thyroid storm is essential to prevent complications of ischemia.

Thyroid nodules

1. Solitary thyroid nodules are usually asymptomatic and are discovered primarily during routine medical examination.

2. An exception to this is an autonomous nodule that produces thyroid hormones without TSH control and in which symptoms of hyperthyroidism are frequently present.

3. The most common type of nodule (about 40 percent) is a simple colloid cyst. Other types of nodule include adenomas, carcinomas (see below), metastatic disease from breast kidney or prostate tumors, lymphomas, or a benign neoplasm such as a neurofibroma, hamartoma, or teratoma.

4. On examination, most benign nodules are soft and cystic or may be tender. Cervical lymph nodes should not be enlarged.

5. Further evaluation with radionucleotide scanning should reveal a functioning nodule or, in the case of an autonomous adenoma, may reveal a "hot" nodule, with suppression of the remainder of the thyroid. In some instances, an adenoma may "burn out" and appear "cold".

6. Cold nodules: Since nonfunctioning nodules may represent thyroid cancers, further evaluation with fine needle biopsy is recommended. Ultrasound also may be useful to determine whether the nodule is cystic (and likely to be benign) as opposed to solid. In cystic nodules, no further treatment is necessary.

7. Functioning nodules: For functional nodules, an attempt at suppression with exogenous thyroid is indicated to determine whether the nodule is under the control of TSH. Functioning adenomas that respond to TSH will suppress after administration of exogenous thyroid hormone. In women with these types of nodule, the disease can be controlled with small doses of thyroid hormones.

8. Autonomously functioning nodules: Autonomous nodules do not suppress and may cause symptoms of hyperthyroidism. These nodules may need to be treated with antithyroid medications or radioactive iodine. For large nodules, surgical excision may be considered.

> Since nonfunctioning nodules may represent thyroid cancers, further evaluation with fine needle biopsy is recommended.

Thyroid cancers

1. Thyroid cancers are more common in women than in men. Thyroid cancer is more common in patients with familial colonic polyposis and hamartomas (Cowden's syndrome). Previous breast, renal, or central nervous system malignancy also increases the risk for a primary thyroid cancer.
2. Two classes of primary thyroid cancer exist: medullary cancer (10 percent of all cancers) and adenocarcinomas.
   a. Nodules suggestive of thyroid cancer are often hard and fixed and may involve adjacent cervical tissue. Nodules larger than 4 cm should also be suspected of being malignant.
   b. Paralysis of the vocal cords and/or cervical lymphadenopathy are other concerning signs.
   c. Definitive diagnosis should be made with thyroid biopsy. Most often this can be achieved through a fine needle aspiration biopsy.
   d. Adenocarcinomas are the most common type of thyroid cancer and can be subcategorized into five different groups: papillary (60 percent of all cancers), follicular (25 percent), medullary, Hürthle cell, and anaplastic carcinomas (< 5 percent).
      i. Papillary carcinoma is the most common but least aggressive form of thyroid cancer. Follicular cancers with some papillary components also behave like papillary carcinomas. These tumors tend to remain in the thyroid gland and, if they do spread, metastasize only to local lymph nodes.
      ii. Follicular cancer, on the other hand, metastasizes to lung and bone. These two kinds of cancer combined have a 97 percent cure rate when treated with surgery, radioactive iodine and thyroid suppression.
      iii. Medullary carcinoma is also aggressive and often part of the multiple endocrine neoplasia (MEN) syndrome. Surgical resection may initially control symptoms, but is not curative. Other chemotherapeutic agents can help to slow the spread of disease.
      iv. One subtype of follicular carcinoma, the Hürthle cell tumor, tends to metastasize to bone frequently and be more invasive and have a poor prognosis.

v. Anaplastic thyroid tumors have a very bad prognosis. This is a very aggressive tumor that rapidly invades adjacent tissue. Surgery, chemotherapy, and iodine radiation are usually ineffective at preventing metastases. Patients rarely survive for more than six months from diagnosis.

e. Non-Hodgkin's lymphoma (NHL) of the thyroid is increasing in incidence. There is a relationship between chronic lymphocytic (Hashimoto's) thyroiditis and NHL, so as the prevalence of chronic lymphocytic thyroid disease increases, NHL should increase as well. This type of tumor should be suspected when patients with chronic lymphocytic thyroiditis develop superimposed thyroid nodules. Surgery is the primary therapeutic option with supplemental radiation and chemotherapy.

Thyroid cancers are more common in women than in men.

Special populations

Pregnancy

1. Pregnant women often have a goiter and have elevated T4 levels with normal TSH levels. Thyroid levels may be difficult to diagnose during pregnancy.
2. Mild hyperthyroidism in pregnancy can mimic hyperemesis gravidarum and women with intractable vomiting may need TSH levels checked.
3. Women with any question of hypothyroidism in pregnancy must be treated with adequate to high levels of thyroid replacement to prevent cretinism in the infant. Two to three months postpartum, the woman can then be assessed to determine thyroid levels.
4. Pregnant women with hyperthyroidism should be treated with PTU (Table 31.1).

Mild hyperthyroidism in pregnancy can mimic hyperemesis gravidarum.

Women on oral contraceptive pills

Women on OCPs often have both a slightly enlarged thyroid or goiter, and, although euthyroid, an elevated T4 with normal TSH, as in pregnancy.

Postpartum thyroiditis

1. Postpartum thyroiditis occurs in between 2 percent and 17 percent of all women in the first six months after delivery.

2. The symptoms of hypothyroidism may mimic those of normal new mother-hood (tiredness, weight gain, lethargy) or postpartum depression.
3. The etiology of the thyroiditis is believed to be autoimmune and the clinical features are similar to chronic lymphocytic (Hashimoto's) thyroiditis.
4. In contrast to Hashimoto's, a large percentage of women (40 percent) remain hypothyroid after the onset postpartum.

Adolescents and children

1. A goiter can be found in 1 percent to 3 percent of healthy teenage girls on routine health examinations. Many of these represent subclinical Graves' disease or chronic lymphocytic thyroiditis.
2. As noted earlier, Graves' disease in adolescent girls tends to resolve sponta-neously. Symptomatic treatment with antithyroid medications for 6 to 18 months may provide time for remission to occur. Most remissions are perma-nent.
3. Chronic lymphocytic thyroiditis is more common than Graves' disease in adolescents, but rarely causes hyper- or hypothyroidism. Antiperoxidase anti-bodies usually disappear after about two years, signalling a resolution of the thyroiditis.

Elderly women

1. The incidence of thyroid disease increases with age. Between 8 percent and 12 percent of older women have hypothyroidism.
2. The symptoms of hypothyroidism in older women can easily be confused with or complicate other disorders such as depression, dementia, and conges-tive heart failure.
3. To confuse matters further, individuals with hyperthyroidism in older age groups can behave as if they are hypothyroid, with lethargy and confusion. The only clue to the hyperthyroid state may be the development of new onset atrial fibrillation.
4. TSH may not be a good screening tool for thyroid disease in older individuals. Approximately 1 percent of older women have chronic mild to moderate elevations in their TSH levels, with no evidence of disease. Treatment of these individuals with "subclinical hypothyroidism" is controversial.

The symptoms of hypothyroidism in older women can easily be confused with or complicate other disorders such as depression, dementia, and congestive heart failure.

Thyroid medications and drug interactions

Several potential drug interactions complicate the use of thyroid replacement in individuals with comorbid conditions. These include interactions with the following:

1. Coumadin: Coumadin effect is enhanced with increases in thyroid hormone doses.
2. Oral hypoglycemics: Effect of these agents blunted by increases in thyroid hormone dose.
3. Estrogens: Administration of hormone replacement with estrogens increases thyroid hormone binding and may require higher doses of thyroid hormone.
4. Clofibrate (may reduce thyroid hormone absorption).

Screening for thyroid abnormalities

The US Preventive Services Task Force does not recommend screening for thyroid disease.[7] If screening is being considered, older women, who comprise the population with the greatest risk of asymptomatic disease, should be targeted.

The US Preventive Services Task Force does not recommend screening for thyroid disease.

Conclusions

Although hypothyroid disease is much more common than hyperthyroidism, both affect women to a great degree. Early detection and close follow-up of treatment will avoid serious complications.

REFERENCES

1. Turnbridge WM, Evered DC, Hall R et al. The spectrum of thyroid disease in a community: The Wickham survey. *Clin Endocrinol* [Oxford] 1977;**7**:481–93.
2. Sawin CR, Castelli WP, Hershman JP, McNamara P, Bacharach P. The aging thyroid. Thyroid deficiency in the Framingham study. *Arch Intern Med* 1985;**145**:1386–8.
3. dos Santos Silva I, Swerdlow AJ. Sex differences in the risks of hormone-dependent cancers. *Am J Epidemiol* 1993;**138**:10–28.
4. Boring CC, Squires TS, Tong T. Cancer statistics, 1993. *CA Cancer J Clin* 1993;**43**:7–26.

5. Shamma FN, Abrahams JJ. Imaging in endocrine disorders. *J Reprod Med* 1995;**37**:39–45.

6. Farwell AP, Braverman LE. Inflammatory thyroid disorders. *Otolaryngol Clin North Am* 1996;**29**:541–56.

7. Report of the US Preventive Services Task Force. *Guide to Clinical Preventive Services*, 2nd edn. Williams & Wilkins, Baltimore, MD, 1996.

32 Hypertension and stroke

Jo Ann Rosenfeld, MD

HYPERTENSION

Hypertension is the most important risk factor in the development of CHD, myocardial infarction (MI) and stroke. Hypertensive women are four times more likely than age-matched controls to develop CHD.[1] The treatment of hypertension has led to a remarkable decrease in the incidence of MI and stroke.

Epidemiology and natural history

1. Unfortunately, not all individuals with hypertension are diagnosed. Fewer individuals receive treatment and fewer are in good control, although this has improved in the past years. Approximately 70 percent of individuals who have hypertension are aware of it, approximately 54 percent receive treatment, but only 27 percent are in good control. However, this has increased from 10 percent over the past 25 years.[2]
2. More women than men have hypertension. Although similar percentages of men and women develop hypertension, the incidence of hypertension increases with age and more elderly people are women.
3. Because of more effective treatment of hypertension, the mortality and morbidity from stroke and MI have declined. Age-adjusted rates of death from stroke declined by 60 percent and rates of death from CHD declined by 53 percent in women and men, whites, and African-Americans.
4. In women older than age 50 years, there has been a real reduction in stroke mortality. One-half of the benefit of stroke reduction in white women and two-thirds of the benefit of stroke reduction in African-American women can

Table 32.1. Stage of hypertension

Stage	BP readings	Evaluation
Severe or stage 3	> 110/ > 180	Evaluate or treat immediately but at least within 1 week
Stage 2	160–179/100–109	Evaluate or treat within 1 month
Stage 1	140–159/90–99	Confirm within 2 months
High normal	130–139/85–89?	Recheck in one year

BP, blood pressure.

be attributed to improvement in hypertensive control.

5. Untreated hypertension worsens a woman's quality of life. Surveys of untreated hypertensive women found that cognitive and sleep functions and sense of well-being were inversely related to diagnosis, degree, and duration of hypertension.[3] Women who were hypertensive reported poorer social activity and physical health status. However, having hypertension was not related to the incidence of anxiety or depression.[3]

More women than men have hypertension.

Diagnosis (Table 32.1)

1. Measurement of blood pressure should occur on two separate occasions, in an individual who has sat upright for at least five minutes and has not smoked or had coffee in the past half-hour. Both arms should be measured, at least for the first few times.
2. The cuff should be of adequate size for the patient – approximately two-thirds of the height of the arm.
3. The diagnosis is made by the recording of two elevated blood pressure readings.
4. White coat hypertension: Episodic elevation of blood pressure, primarily when taken by a health professional. This occurs in approximately 10 percent of those with hypertension. It is more common in men than women, but is not totally benign. White coat hypertension is associated with an increase in left ventricular mass and left ventricular hypertrophy.[4]

Table 32.2. Minimal laboratory evaluation for new patients with hypertension

After a history and physical

- Blood
  - Electrolytes
  - Complete blood count
  - BUN and creatinine
  - Glucose[a]
  - Cholesterol and triglycerides[a]
- Urine analysis
- Electrocardiogram

BUN, blood urea nitrogen.

[a]These are best done fasting. If they are taken at random levels, if elevated, they should be repeated fasting before a diagnosis is suggested.

Table 32.3. Causes of secondary hypertension

- Alcohol abuse
- Renal parenchymal disease
- Renovascular disease
- Endocrinopathies
  - Pheochromocytoma
  - Cushing's syndrome
  - Primary aldosteronism

Evaluation

1. The evaluation for the hypertension patient is minimal, because most individuals have primary or essential hypertension (Table 32.2).[5]
2. Treatable causes of hypertension, although rare, are listed in Table 32.3.
3. Signs that might indicate a more complete evaluation are listed in Table 32.4.
4. These abnormalities might indicate a more intensive evaluation, including creatinine clearance and 24-hour urine for protein and uric acid, glycosylated hemoglobin levels, echocardiography, and specific tests for endocrinopathies.

Treatment

Gender disparity in research concerning treatment

Most trials of treatment have primarily or exclusively studied men. However, with the evidence that the treatment of hypertension improved men's

Table 32.4. Indications for more intensive evaluation for secondary hypertension

- Hypertension that is difficult to control
- Early onset of hypertension, especially in a woman younger than age 30 years
- Rapid progression or sudden worsening of hypertension
- Weight loss or truncal obesity
- A rapid rise in BUN or creatinine while on an ACEI
- Hypokalemia, suggesting an endocrine cause
- Abnormal urine analysis, proteinuria, creatinine or BUN suggesting renal disease
- Hyperglycemia

BUN, blood urea nitrogen; ACEI, angiotensin-converting enzyme inhibitor.

morbidity and mortality, a similar analysis was accomplished for women. The INDANA (Individual Data Analysis of Antihypertensive Intervention Trials) analysis examined the results of more than 20 000 women and men in seven drug RCTs, some double, some single blinded.[6] Treatment significantly and statistically improved the risk for all major coronary events, fatal coronary events, and stroke for men, but not for coronary events or total mortality in women, perhaps because the rates of these events were lower in women. However, treatment of hypertension did reduce incidence of stroke, fatal stroke, and cardiovascular events in women.

Risk stratification

The Joint National Commission[2] suggests that evaluation, follow-up and treatment be based on level of hypertension and risk of cardiovascular disease, using both lifestyle modifications and drug therapy (Table 32.5).

Lifestyle modification

1. Diet: A low salt, low cholesterol diet can improve blood pressure and decrease cardiovascular morbidity and mortality.
2. The change in sodium intake does not have to be large. Removing extra salt from the table, and reducing consumption of high salt foods can reduce the average salt intake from 15 g to 5 to 7 g daily. In one placebo-controlled RCT, changing regular salt to low sodium, high potassium, high magnesium mineral salt reduced systolic blood pressure (SBP) by an average of 7.6 mm and diastolic blood pressure (DBP) by an average of 3.3 mm in 100 men and women aged 55 to 75 years.[7]
3. Weight modification:
   a. There is a definite independent association between hypertension and

Table 32.5. Risk stratification and treatment

| | Blood pressure | | |
Risk group	High normal	Stage 1	Stages 2 to 3
No risk factors	Lifestyle mod.	Lifestyle mod.[a]	Drug therapy
At least one risk factor No target organ damage	Lifestyle mod.	Lifestyle mod.	Drug therapy
More than one risk factor Diabetes or target organ damage	Drug therapy	Drug therapy	Drug therapy

mod., modification.

[a]Try for 12 months.

Taken from *The Sixth Report of the Joint National Committee on Prevention, Detection, Evaluation and Treatment of High Blood Pressure.* NIH publication no. 98-4080. National Institutes of Health, Bethesda, MD, 1997.

obesity. The Nurses' Health Study (NHS) showed that those women with BMI greater than 31 had an RR of 6.31 of developing high blood pressure. In addition, an increase in weight of 1 kg (2.2 lbs) was associated with a 12 percent increased risk of developing hypertension.[8]

b. As well, losing weight will lower blood pressure. Even a short-term, small weight loss will reduce blood pressure. The risk of hypertension was reduced by 15 percent by a weight loss of 5 to 10 kg. A weight loss of more than 10 kg (22 lbs) will reduce the individual's risk of hypertension 26 percent.[7]

A low salt, low cholesterol diet can improve blood pressure and decrease cardiovascular morbidity and mortality.

4. Exercise: An active lifestyle may reduce blood pressure in hypertensive individuals. A metaanalysis examining studies in which aerobic exercise was used in hypertensive patients found that those patients that exercised without drug therapy had a small reduction (1 to 2 percent) in resting SBP and DBP.[9]

Losing weight, as little as 10 percent, will lower blood pressure.

Drug therapy

1. Not all trials of medication included women, or if the trials did, they may not have analyzed the data by sex. However, basically, women can use any

Table 32.6. Some common drugs used to treat hypertension

Agent	Dose (daily)
Diuretics	
Thiazide type (usually once daily)	
Chlorothiazide	125–500 mg
Hydrochlorothiazide	12.5–50 mg
Chlorthalidone	12.5–50 mg
Indapamide	1.25–5 mg
Metolazone – Zaroxolyn	1.25–5 mg
Loop	
Bumetanide	0.5–5 mg in 2 or 3 doses
Furosemide	20–320 mg in 2 or 3 doses
Potassium sparing	
Amiloride	5–10 mg in 1 or 2 doses
Spironolactone	12.5–100 mg in 1 or 2 doses
Triamterene – Dyrenium	50–150 mg in 1 or 2 doses
Beta-blockers	
Acebutolol – Sectral	200–1200 mg in 1 or 2 doses
Atenolol – Tenormin	25–100 mg in 1 or 2 doses
Bisoprolol – Zebeta	5–20 mg in 1 dose
Metoprolol – Lopressor	50–200 mg in 1 or 2 doses
Nadolol – Corgard	20–240 mg in 1 dose
Penbutolol – Levatol	20 mg in 1 dose
Pindolol	10–60 mg in 2 doses
Propranolol – Inderal	40–240 mg in 2 doses
Timolol – Blocadren	10–40 mg in 2 doses
Angiotensin-converting enzyme inhibitors	
Captopril	12.5–150 mg in 2 or 3 doses
Enalapril – Vasotec	2.5–40 mg in 1–2 doses
Fosinopril – Monopril	10–40 mg in 1 or 2 doses
Lisinopril – Prinivil	5–40 mg in 1 dose
Moexipril	7.5–30 mg in 1 or 2 doses
Quinapril – Accupril	5–80 mg in 1 or 2 doses
Ramipril – Altace	1.25–20 mg in 1 or 2 doses
Angiotensin receptor antagonists	
Candesartan cilexetil – Atacand	8–32 mg in 1 dose
Losartan – Cozaar	25–100 mg in 1 or 2 doses
Valsartan – Diovan	80–320 mg in 1 dose
Alpha-beta-blockers	
Carvedilol – Coreg	12.5–50 mg in 2 doses
Labetalol	200–1200 mg in 2 doses

Table 32.6. (*cont.*)

Agent	Dose (daily)
Calcium-channel blockers	
Diltiazem	120–360 mg in 2 doses
Verapamil	120–480 mg in 2 or 3 doses
Dihydropyridines	
Amlodipine	2.5–10 mg in 1 dose
Felodipine –Plendil	2.5–10 mg in 1 dose
Isradipine – DynaCirc	5–10 mg in 2 doses
Nicardipine	60–120 mg in 3 doses
Nifedipine – extended release	30–90 mg in 1 dose
Alpha-adrenergic blockers	
Prazosin	First day: 1 mg at bedtime; maintenance: 1–20 mg in 2 or 3 doses
Terazosin – Hytrin	First day: 1 mg at bedtime; maintenance: 1–20 mg in 1 dose
Doxazosin – Cardura	First day: 1 mg at bedtime; maintenance: 1–16 mg in 1 dose
Central alpha-adrenergic agonists	
Clonidine	0.1–0.6 mg in 2 or 3 doses
Transdermal – Catapres TTS	One patch weekly (0.1 to 0.3 mg/day)
Guanabenz	4–64 mg in 2 doses
Methyldopa	250 mg to 2 g in 2 doses
Direct vasodilators	
Hydralazine	40–200 mg in 2 to 4 doses
Minoxidil	2.5–40 mg in 1 or 2 doses

medication used for treatment of hypertension by men. However, there may be differences in side effects and effectiveness.

2. One medication should be started and its effect observed. Usually, the dose of the first medication should be increased until side effects occur, before a second drug is started (Table 32.6).

3. The Joint National Commission suggests that, although the choice of the medication should be individualized, both men and women should be started on a diuretic or a beta-blocker first.[2]

4. There is no one perfect antihypertensive drug for all women (Table 32.6). Three studies, for example, suggest that many drugs can work equally well in women.

   a. One double blind multicentered RCT that included 309 women aged 60 to

80 years examined the effects of atenolol (50 to 100 mg daily), enalapril (5 to 20 mg daily), and isradipine (1.25 to 5.0 mg twice daily) on hypertensive control and the quality of life. Hydrochlorothiazide (HCTZ) was added, if needed. The three groups did not differ in degree of reduction of DBP or in supplementation of HCTZ. However, women on enalapril were more likely to have a cough and women on atenolol were more likely to have had a dry mouth.[10]

b. In the Systolic Hypertension in the Elderly Program (SHEP) trial, a community based multicentered double blind placebo-controlled RCT of treatment of isolated systolic hypertension (ISH) in men and women older than age 60 years, chlorthalidone (12.5 to 25 mg daily) or atenolol (25 to 50 mg daily) was compared to placebo. The treatment groups did respond with lower blood pressures. Neither therapy affected triglycerides, cholesterol, glucose, potassium or uric acid levels.[11]

c. A third, more recent, European RCT of two new drugs examined the response of 93 postmenopausal women with essential hypertension. It compared the new angiotensin-converting enzyme inhibitor (ACEI) moexipril (15 mg daily) to calcium channel antagonist nitrendipine (20 mg daily) in women aged 44 to 70 years over eight weeks. Both medicines were equally effective in lowering blood pressure, but more women on moexipril had a cough (9 percent) and more women (> 20 percent) on nitrendipine had headaches and flushing.[12]

Women can use any medication used for treatment of hypertension in men.

5. Specific drugs:
   a. Although a beta-blocker or a diuretic should be considered as first choice, the choice of therapy in women, as in men, should be individualized.
   b. The side effects of beta-blockers have not been as extensively examined in women as in men. The incidence of beta-blocker-induced depression may be more frequent in women. Sexual dysfunction induced by beta-blockers has been extensively examined in men but not in women.
   c. Women may respond less well on ACEIs than men and they are more likely to develop a cough. ACEIs are suggested for women with diabetes or congestive heart failure. Those on the second-generation ACEIs experience cough less often.[13] Women of childbearing years who are at risk for pregnancy should not use ACEIs, unless they use an effective method of contraception. ACEIs are contraindicated in pregnancy.

There is no one perfect antihypertensive drug for all women.

d. In retrospective studies, use of calcium channel blockers in elderly women had a reported and unexplained increased association with cancer, especially breast cancer. In a retrospective analysis of more than 3200 women older than age 65 years, women who use calcium channel antagonists had an RR of 2.57 of developing cancer. This risk was not explained and was not associated with any other group of antihypertensive medications.[14] More recent studies have not supported this correlation.

> Although a beta-blocker or a diuretic should be considered as first choice, the choice of therapy in women, as in men, should be individualized.

Special populations

Elderly

1. Importance: A higher percentage of elderly individuals than younger individuals have high blood pressure. Treating hypertension in the elderly is important and treatment does decrease their risk of morbidity and mortality. In a metaanalysis of studies of elderly hypertensive individuals, treatment reduced blood pressure by an average of 15/6 and reduced nonfatal and fatal major coronary events, fatal and nonfatal strokes and death of any cause in the elderly.[15]

2. In older individuals, SBP is a better predictor of events – CHD, stroke, and renal disease – than DBP.

3. Treatment: As with younger individuals, treatment should begin with lifestyle modifications. Even older individuals will respond to modest salt reduction and weight loss.

4. Pharmacological treatment: If the blood pressure goal is not achieved with lifestyle modifications, pharmacological therapy is indicated. In the elderly woman, the starting dose of medication should be lower, about half that in the younger woman.

5. Thiazides and/or beta-blockers have been shown to decrease mortality and morbidity. Combined diuretics are a better choice for the elderly because they reduce the incidence of hypokalemia and the need for potassium replacement.

6. Elderly women who used the calcium-channel antagonist nitrendipine had a 42 percent reduction in coronary events and congestive heart failure but this is not available in the USA. Other dihydropyridine calcium channel antagonists can be used.[2]

Treating hypertension in the elderly is important and treatment does decrease their risk of morbidity and mortality.

Oral contraceptive pills

1. Women on combination estrogen-containing OCPs usually demonstrate a slight increase in SBP and DBP.
2. Hypertension is more common in women on OCPs, especially if they are obese and older. Smokers who are older than age 35 years should not take OCPS.[2]
3. If women on OCPs develop hypertension, the OCPs should be stopped until the hypertension is under control. Once blood pressure is controlled, OCPs, especially low dose estrogen or progesterone-only OCPs, may be used, especially if the risks for pregnancy are higher than the risks for hypertension.

If women on oral contraceptive pills develop hypertension, the pills should be stopped until the hypertension is under control.

Chronic hypertension in pregnancy

The complete discussion of hypertension in pregnancy is beyond the scope of this chapter.

1. Diagnosis: Some women who have not had regular blood pressure measurements before pregnancy may not know they have chronic hypertension. If discovered, hypertension should be treated before pregnancy or as early in pregnancy as possible.
2. Medication: Women who are pregnant should not use diuretics and ACEIs. Alpha-methyldopa and hydralazine have been used in pregnant women with hypertension problems. Calcium channel antagonists, especially nifedipine, have been used in some situations. Beta-blockers have been used but are associated with growth retardation of the fetus.

Preeclampsia

1. The etiology of preeclampsia (PE) and eclampsia are still not known.
2. They are a major cause of maternal mortality in the USA and UK.[15]
3. Incidence: PE occurs in 8 to 24 percent of women and is more likely in women whose mother had PE.
4. Definition: Pregnancy-induced hypertension is the occurrence of blood

pressure readings of 140/90 or more on at least two occasions four hours apart after the 20th week of pregnancy in a woman who was known to be normotensive before. In these women, blood pressure returns to normal by the sixth week postpartum. If proteinuria (> 500 mg/dL per day) occurs with this, the woman has PE.

5. Eclampsia is unpredictable. More than one-third of eclamptic seizures occur before classic symptoms of proteinuria or hypertension appear and 44 percent occur postpartum.[16]

6. Research into the cause and treatment of PE is plagued by lack of consistency in diagnosis.

7. Long-term consequences:
   a. Hypertension that occurs close to term or after 37 weeks is not associated with an adverse outcome and has been associated with larger babies.
   b. Multiparous women who develop pregnancy-induced hypertension or PE are six to seven times more likely to become hypertensive in later life.

> Multiparous women who develop pregnancy-induced hypertension or preeclampsia are six to seven times more likely to become hypertensive in later life.

Menopause

1. Incidence: After menopause, the incidence of hypertension increases in women until there is equal incidence in both sexes.

2. HRT does not cause hypertension and hypertension is not a contraindication to HRT. Use of estradiol in a small prospective study actually lowered arterial blood pressure. Use of HRT may reduce other cardiovascular risk factors.

STROKE

Stroke occurs equally in men and women, but occurs more often in the elderly and more women are elderly. A stroke is a clinical cerebrovascular event caused by ischemia, thrombosis, or hemorrhage. It is a personal catastrophe that can cause death, disability or loss of independence. A stroke has a tremendous cost to the individual and strokes cause incredible cost to society in rehabilitation and long-term care. Because treatment is seldom possible, primary and secondary prevention are essential.

> Stroke occurs equally in men and women, but occurs more often in the elderly and more women are elderly.

Epidemiology

1. Strokes are the third leading cause of death in the USA, causing more deaths in men and women than chronic lung disease, accidents, pneumonia, diabetes, and HIV infection.[17] Approximately half a million individuals yearly have a first stroke.

2. Stroke mortality and incidence increases with age. The frequency of stroke doubles with every 10 years of age over age 55 years.[18] Three-quarters of all strokes occur in those older than age 65 years.

3. As women get older than age 65 years, they are more likely than men to have strokes.[19]

4. African-American men and women are more likely to die from a stroke than white men and women in the USA and Europe.[20]

Natural history of stroke

1. Strokes have become less lethal, although the first stroke is fatal in 30 percent. Between 1965 and 1985, there was a rapid and accelerating decline in the mortality of strokes in all areas of the USA and most industrialized countries.[21]

   A retrospective study in Finland found that the changes in cardiovascular risk factors can explain the observed changes in mortality in stroke (60 percent in women, 66 percent in men). In women, the changes in DBP and decreased incidence of smoking predicted half of the 60 percent decrease in mortality.[22]

2. More women than men die from strokes; strokes account for 16 percent of all deaths in women, as compared with 8 percent in men.[23]

3. Because of increased treatment of hypertension, the incidence of stroke has decreased in past years in both men and women.[24]

Primary prevention

The US National Stroke Association has identified six major and four lifestyle risk factors, which, if treated or modified, may prevent strokes.[25] These six factors include hypertension, myocardial infarction, atrial fibrillation (AF), diabetes mellitus, hyperlipidemia, and asymptomatic carotid artery stenosis. There are four modifiable lifestyle risk factors, including smoking, alcohol use,

Table 32.7. Risk factors for stroke

Major factors
- Hypertension
- Myocardial infarction
- Atrial fibrillation
- Diabetes mellitus
- Hyperlipidemia
- Asymptomatic carotid artery stenosis

Modifiable lifestyle risk factors
- Smoking
- Alcohol use
- Physical inactivity
- Poor diet

physical inactivity, and poor diet (Table 32.7).

Other risk factors include older age, male gender, history of prior strokes or transient ischemic attacks (TIAs), impaired cardiac function, African-American race, and a family history of strokes.

Educational level, the presence of coronary artery disease, angina and physical functioning level were not risk factors for stroke.

Hypertension

1. Hypertension is the most important risk factor for stroke in women.[25]
2. RCTs have shown that treatment of hypertension definitely decreases the risk of stroke. Treatment that reduces DBP by an average of 5 mm reduces the risk of stroke by 42 percent.[25] In the elderly, the SHEP trial found that the treatment of ISH decreased the risk for stroke by 36 percent.[26]
3. Individuals with hypertension should try to have their blood pressure in good control. Blood pressure levels should be lower than 140/90 and even 135/85.

Atrial fibrillation

1. AF is a common arrhythmia and, if the individual with AF is anticoagulated with warfarin, risk of stroke is decreased. About 16 percent of all individuals and one-third of those older than age 75 years who suffer an ischemic stroke have AF (Figure 32.1).[27]
2. AF can be asymptomatic and discovered by chance on physical examination or the patient can complain of irregular heartbeat, "skipping" beats, congestive heart failure, exercise intolerance, shortness of breath, dyspnea on exertion, or signs of heart failure and respiratory distress.

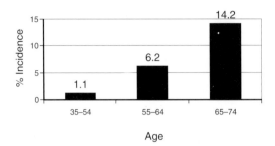

Figure 32.1.   Incidence of atrial fibrillation in women, by age.

3. Treatment for AF is cardioversion, electrically or chemically. Cardioversion is most effective when delivered as soon after AF starts as possible. Elderly individuals have as much chance at successful cardioversion as younger individuals. Although often used, drugs such as digoxin, quinidine, and other antiarhythmic drugs used to maintain cardioversion have not been proven as effective as electrical conversion.

4. The incidence of atrial fibrillation increases with age (Figure 32.1). Approximately 1 percent of the US population or 1.8 million individuals has AF.[28]

5. Correlation between AF and stroke: Although the Framingham study did not find a correlation,[29] several RCTs have shown that AF is an independent risk factor for stroke. AF increases the risk of ischemic stroke fivefold.[26] The Oxfordshire Community Stroke Project found that individuals with AF who have a stroke have an increased early mortality.[30]

6. Prevention therapy (Table 32.8):

   a. Several RCTs have found that anticoagulation reduces the risk of stroke by 70 percent in patients with AF.[31]

   b. Anticoagulation is difficult to maintain, requires frequent visits and blood tests and serious risks, including gastrointestinal and cardiovascular hemorrhage. The elderly on anticoagulation have an increased risk of severe hemorrhage.

   c. Further studies continue as to the most effective method of anticoagulation with the fewest side effects.[32]

      Three large placebo-controlled, double blind RCTs – the Stroke Prevention in Atrial Fibrillation Study (SPAF I) in the USA following 1330 patients,[33] the European Atrial Fibrillation Trial (EAFT),[34] and the Atrial Fibrillation, Aspirin and Anticoagulation Study (AFASAK) investigating 1007 patients[35] for more than one year – showed that warfarin use halved the rate of stroke and death as compared with placebo.

      However, when patients on warfarin were compared with those on aspirin in a continuation of the SPAF I, certain groups had a lower rate of

Table 32.8. Prevention of stroke in patients with atrial fibrillation

Age	Definitely	Consider
Primary prevention		
< 65 – no risk factors	Aspirin 325 mg/day	Warfarin INR 1.6–3.0
> 65 – no risk factors	Aspirin or warfarin	
65–75 – diabetes, HBP	Warfarin	INR 2.0–3.0
> 75 – diabetes, HBP	Warfarin	INR 1.6–2.5
Secondary prevention		
(After a TIA or stroke)		
All ages	Warfarin	INR 1.6–3.0

HBP, high blood pressure; INR, international normalized ratio; TIA, transient ischemic attacks.

strokes on aspirin than those on warfarin.[36] Warfarin was more effective than aspirin in preventing ischemic stroke but there was an increased incidence in intracranial hemorrhage in the patients treated with warfarin, especially in older patients. Warfarin caused a higher total number of strokes, including hemorraghic strokes, than aspirin in patients older than age 75 years. The risk of bleeding is a serious concern.

d. Contraindications (Table 32.9) to anticoagulation with warfarin include a history of bleeding from any source, such as gastrointestinal or genitourinary, or liver disease. Those women who cannot return frequently to monitor their levels of anticoagulation with monthly to weekly prothrombin times should not be placed on warfarin. Those with alcoholism, seizures or a history of falls or gait disturbances may not be good candidates. Women on anticonvulsants, OCPs, or other medications that affect the liver's cytochrome P-450 system should be prescribed warfarin only with great caution (Table 32.10).

e. Bleeding can be minimized if warfarin is used only to produce an international normalized ratio of 2.0 to 3.0 rather than greater than 3.0. Elderly patients showed an increased rate of bleeding with INRs > 3.0, and younger patients with INRs > 4.0.

Anticoagulation reduces the risk of stroke by 70 percent in patients with AF.

Myocardial infarction

A woman's risk of stroke is increased 30 percent in the first month after MI, and then 1 to 2 percent yearly after MI. Anticoagulation can prevent a stroke

Table 32.9. Contraindications to warfarin use to prevent strokes in women with atrial fibrillation

Medical history
- History of bleeding
- Liver disease
- Gait disturbances
- History of falls
- Seizure disorder
- Medications[a]

Social history
- Unable to cooperate with frequent monitoring
- Alcoholism

[a]See Table 32.10.

Table 32.10. Drugs that interfere with Warfarin's action

Increases its levels	Decreases its levels
Allopurinol	Antithyroid hormone drugs
Androgens	Carbamazepine
Cimetadine	Cholestyramine
Clofibrate	Griseofulvin
Disulfiram	Rifampin
Erythromycin	Spironolactone
Glucagon	Thiazide diuretics
Metronidazole	
Omeprazole	
Ranitidine	
Salicylates (high dose)	
Tamoxifen	
Thyroid hormone	
Trimethoprim/sulfa	

after a MI, particularly in women with AF. INRs of 2.0 to 3.0 should be the recommended range. Aspirin use may reduce the risk, although it has not yet been proven to prevent a first stroke.

Hyperlipidemia

RCTs have shown that treatment of hyperlipidemia prevents stroke in men. The simvastatin studies investigating patients with coronary heart disease and hyperlipidemia found that treatment reduced the incidence of stroke and TIA (RR = 0.7 in the treated group).[37] In hyperlipidemic MI patients, pravastatin reduced the risk of stroke.

Diabetes

More women than men have diabetes, and diabetes increases the risk of stroke 1.4 to 1.7 times. Although "good control" of hyperglycemia has not been proven to decrease the risk of stroke, care of diabetes will help to decrease other cardiovascular and renal risk factors and end-organ damage.

Carotid artery stenosis

1. Importance: The risk of stroke is increased in women with carotid artery stenosis, although treatment, which is angioplasty or surgical endarectomy, in asymptomatic patients (primary prevention) has not been shown to improve mortality or reduce the risk of stroke.

   One RCT, the CASANOVA (carotid artery stenosis asymptomatic narrowing: operation versus aspirin) study, in 1982–8 compared immediate endarterectomy with medical treatment (aspirin and/or dipyradamole) and possible later endarterectomy. No difference in mortality or stroke rate was found between medical and surgical therapy.[38] There was no placebo group.

2. Secondary prevention, treatment of symptomatic carotid stenosis after a stroke or TIA, improves mortality and reduces the risk of future events.

3. Clinical symptoms: Carotid artery stenosis can be silent, or it can sometimes be inferred by detection of carotid arterial bruits on physical examination. It may be found by radiological or doppler study after a TIA.

4. In a metaanalysis of hypertensive elderly women, those who had endarectomies had an increased risk of contralateral stroke and death compared with men.[39]

> Treatment of symptomatic carotid stenosis after a stroke or transitory ischemic event improves mortality and reduces the risk of future events.

Lifestyle factors

1. Smoking: The increased risk of stroke correlates with the number of cigarettes a woman smokes. The NHS found that smokers had two times the risk of stroke and the risk of stroke was dose related. In addition, stopping smoking decreased the risk of stroke.[40]

2. Alcohol Use: Regular alcohol use increases the risk of hypertension and

stroke.[41] No RCTs have proved that reducing alcohol consumption decreases stroke risk.

3. Exercise: Encouraging an active lifestyle may have beneficial effects through a variety of mechanisms.

4. Low fat diet: Eating a healthy low cholesterol, low sodium diet has been linked to a decreased risk of stroke.

Secondary prevention of strokes: after a TIA or first stroke

Definition

TIAs are focal ischemic neurological deficits that resolve within 24 hours. They can present with slurred speech, aphasia, visual problems, amaurosis fugax ("a curtain came down over vision"), paresis or hemiparesis, numbness, ataxia. Most TIAs last less than 15 minutes and 60 to 70 percent resolve within one hour.[42]

Importance

TIAs predict stroke occurrence. Only one out of five strokes are preceded by a TIA. However, one out of three women who have a TIA will have a stroke within five years, one out of five within one month.

Diagnosis

1. Differential diagnosis: Other diseases can present like TIAs, including drug toxicity, metabolic disturbances, seizures and syncope, labyrinthine disorders, tumors, subdural hematomas, small hemorrhages, and transient migraines.

2. Diagnostic evaluation: For a woman with a TIA, this includes an electrocardiogram and 24-hour Holter monitoring, and echocardiography to detect valvular and cardiac wall disease. A CT of the head is suggested because it may show signs of infarction in up to 40 percent of patients with TIAs. An MRI scan is superior to CT in detecting abnormalities and previous strokes, particularly in brainstem, subcortical, or lacunar infarcts, and may be indicated.

3. Carotid evaluation: Evaluation for possible significant carotid stenosis is essential. Angiography is the gold standard, but it is invasive and has mortality and morbidity, including renal failure in 2.5 percent, TIAs in 4.5 percent, strokes in 0 to 5.5 percent of patients and cardiovascular problems in 0.2 to 2

percent of procedures.[43] An ultrasound of the carotids is a better screening test for detection and characterization of carotid stenosis.

Treatment and secondary prevention

1. The primary treatment for TIAs is to modify the risk factors for TIAs and stroke. The patient should be urged to quit smoking, exercise, and eat a low fat diet. Hypertension should be detected and adequately treated.

2. All patients should be started on aspirin, ticlopidine, or other anticoagulant, if not contraindicated.

3. Surgical treatment of non-symptomatic carotid stenosis, if present, is essential for prevention of strokes. The use of endarectomy prevents further stroke in patients with 60 to less than 100 percent stenosis of the carotid arteries.[18]

   Several RCTs showed beneficial effect of surgery. The North American Symptomatic Carotid Endarectomy Trial (NASCET) examined patients who had a disabling stroke within 120 days and the patients were randomized to medical therapy (aspirin and control of lipid, hypertension, and diabetes as needed) or surgical therapy. There was only a 9 percent incidence of stroke or death in surgically treated patients compared with 26 percent in the medically treated group.[44] The European Carotid Surgery Trial, a multicentered prospective RCT, found that, for those patients with severe stenosis, the occurrence of stroke or death was 21.9 percent in the medically treated group and 12.3 percent in surgical group.[45]

4. Choice of anticoagulant:

   a. Aspirin: Use of aspirin after a TIA has been proven to reduce TIAs and stroke in men. Two RCTs found that an aspirin dose as low as 30 mg/day (but definitely 75 mg/day) could prevent strokes in men.[46,47] Whether aspirin prevents further strokes in women, especially elderly women, is under investigation.

   b. Aspirin-intolerant patients – use of ticlopidine or clopidogrel: Ticlopidine has been shown to reduce stroke incidence by 20 to 30 percent after a TIA in men and women. In one placebo-controlled RCT of more than 3000 patients up to age 94 years, use of ticlopidine was effective in reducing the risk of stroke. However, ticlopidine had increasingly more severe and serious side effects than aspirin. Twenty percent of the patients who took ticlopidine experienced diarrhea, 10 percent a skin rash, and 1 percent neutropenia, although there was less peptic ulceration than in aspirin users.[42]

   Ticlopidine should therefore be reserved for patients with intolerance or allergy to aspirin, or those who have further symptoms or strokes while on aspirin, because of its expense, its increased monitoring needs and risks. Because of the risk of neutropenia, white blood counts and differentials are required every two weeks for the first three months.

Clopidogrel bisulfate (75 mg/day) and other new ADP-receptor antagonists may be easier to use than ticlopidine. Clopidogrel does not cause leukopenia, and, thus, it requires no recurrent blood testing. An international RCT comparing clopidogrel to aspirin in more than 19 000 patients found clopidogrel more effective in reducing risk of ischemic stroke, MI or vascular death than aspirin.[48]

c. Recommendations in women: Since the ticlopidine studies included women, use of the drug was suggested as more effective and the drug of choice for women rather than aspirin. Recent studies suggest that aspirin's benefit for preventing TIAs in men extends to women. More recent studies suggest that clopidogrel may be used instead of ticlopidine.

5. Anticoagulation for patients with a TIA or stroke with AF: More women than men who have a stroke have AF. Anticoagulation is important for a woman who has had a TIA or a stroke and has AF. The European Atrial Fibrillation RCT showed that the rate of stroke was significantly reduced by aspirin (by 15 percent) or by the use of warfarin (by 66 percent).[28] Warfarin use should be considered in patients who have had a TIA or stroke and have AF. In patients in whom bleeding is a concern, use of aspirin or clopidogrel may be sufficient.

All patients should be started on aspirin, ticlopidine, or other anticoagulant, if not contraindicated.

Oral contraceptive pills

1. Risk of stroke: Although the risk of stroke is very low in women of childbearing age, OCP use does increase the risk, especially if the woman has coexistent hypertension, is older than age 35 years and/or smokes. Early studies suggest an increased risk if the woman used pills with an estrogen dose far higher than those presently used (Figure 32.2).

A case-controlled retrospective study in 2242 women in 17 countries, found that the OR for developing an ischemic stroke in women who used OCPs was

Although the risk of stroke is very low in women of childbearing age, use of oral contraceptive pills does increase the risk, especially if the woman has coexistent hypertension, is older than age 35 years and/or smokes.

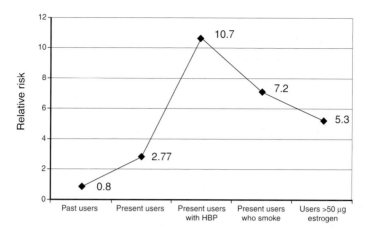

Figure 32.2.   Relative risk of ischemic stroke by OCP users. HBP, high blood pressure.

3.0 but these women were much more likely to have coexistent hypertension or smoking or be using high estrogen OCPs.[49]

2. Dose of estrogen and risk of stroke: Women taking OCPs with greater than 50 μg ethinylestradiol have an increased risk of ischemic stroke (RR = 2.9[50] to 5.3[51]). Women who use OCPs with 35 μg ethinylestradiol have a 2.7 relative risk of ischemic stroke. However, women who are on OCPs, are younger than age 35 years, and do not have hypertension have no increased risk of stroke.

3. Duration of use: Once stopped, the relative risk of stroke returns to that of women who did not use OCPs (RR = 0.5 to 0.8).[52] There is no relation between length of use and risk of stroke.[51]

> Women who are on oral contraceptive pills, are younger than age 35 years, and do not have hypertension have no increased risk of stroke.

Conclusions

Most patients who have hypertension are women and this is the most common risk factor for stroke. Hypertension is often silent, and careful and accurate measurement of blood pressure will help to diagnose and follow this disease. Treatment includes lifestyle changes, diet, exercise, and medication, many of which work effectively. Good control will prevent serious complications of heart disease, stroke and mortality.

REFERENCES

1. Mercuro G, Zonco S, Pilia I et al. Effects of acute administration of transdermal estrogen on postmenopausal women with systemic hypertension. *Am J Cardiol* 1997;**80**:652–7.

2. Joint National Committee on Prevention, Detection, Evaluation and Treatment of High Blood Pressure. *The Sixth Report of the Joint National Committee on Prevention, Detection, Evaluation and Treatment of High Blood Pressure.* NIH publication no. 98-4080. National Institutes of Health, Bethesda, MD, 1997.

3. Robbins MA, Elias MF, Croog SH, Colton T. Unmediated blood pressure levels and quality of life in elderly hypertensive women. *Psychosom Med* 1994;**56**:251–9.

4. Muschooll MW, Hense HW, Brockel U et al. Changes in left ventricular structure and function in patients with white coat hypertension. Cross-sectional survey. *BMJ* 1998;**317**:565–70.

5. Kaplan NM. Renal parenchymal hypertension. In Kaplan NM, *Clinical Hypertension*, 7th edn. Williams & Wilkins, Baltimore, MD, 1997, pp. 281–99.

6. Gueyffier F, Boutitie F, Boissel JP et al. Effect of antihypertensive drug treatment on cardiovascular outcomes in women and men. *Ann Intern Med* 1997;**126**:761–7.

7. Geleijnse JM, Wetteeman JC, Bak AA, Breijen JH, Grobee DE. Reduction in blood pressure with a low sodium, high potassium, high magnesium salt in older subjects with mild to moderated hypertension. *BMJ* 1994;**309**:436–40.

8. Huang Z, Willett WC, Mason JE et al. Body weight, weight change and risk for hypertension in women. *Ann Intern Med* 1998;**128**:81–8.

9. Kelley GA. Aerobic exercise and resting blood pressure among women: A meta-analysis. *Prev Med* 1999;**28**:264–75.

10. Croog SH, Elias MF, Coilton T. Effects of antihypertensive medications on quality of life in elderly hypertensive women. *Am J Hyperten* 1994;**7**:329–39.

11. Savage PJ, Pressel SL, Curb JD et al. Influence of long-term, low-dose, diuretic-based antihypertensive therapy on glucose, lipid, uric acid and potassium levels in older men and women with isolated systolic hypertension. *Arch Intern Med* 1998;**158**:741–51.

12. Agabiti-Rosei E, Ambrosinione E, Pireeli A, Stimpel M, Zanchetti A. Efficacy and tolerability of moexipril and nitrendipine in postmenopausal women with hypertension. MADAM study group. *Eur J Clin Pharmacol* 1999;**55**:185–9.

13. Papdemetriou V, Prisant LM, Neutel JM, Weir MR. Efficacy of low-dose combination of bisoprolol/hydrochlorothiazide compared with amlodipine and enalapril in men and women with essential hypertension. *Am J Cardiol* 1998;**81**:1363–6.

14. Fitzpatrick AL, Daling JR, Furberg CD, Kronmal RA, Weissfeld JL. Use of calcium channel blockers and breast carcinoma risk in postmenopausal women. *Cancer* 1997;**80**:1438–47.

15. Pearce KA, Furberg CD, Rushing J. Does anithypertensive treatment of the elderly prevent cardiovascular events or prolong life? A meta-analysis of hypertension treatment trials. *Arch Fam Med* 1995;**4**:943–50.

16. Rosenfeld JA. Hypertension occurring postpartum for the first time: Was it pre-eclampsia? *Tenn Med J* 1992;**85**:465–6.

17. Landis SH, Murray T, Bolden S, Wingo PA. Cancer statistics, 1999. *CA Cancer J Clin* 1999;**49**:8–31.

18. McCann RL. Surgical management of carotid artery atherosclerotic disease. *South Med J* 1993;**86**:2S-23 to 28.

19. Kaarisalo MM, Immonen-Raiha P, Martilla RJ et al. Atrial fibrillation and stroke: Mortality and causes of death after first acute ischemic stroke. *Stroke* 1997;**28**:311–15.

20. Agency for Health Care Policy and Research Clinical Practice Guideline: Post stroke rehabilitation: Assessment, referral and patient management. *Am Fam Physician* 1995;**52**:461–70.

21. Barker WH, Mulllooly JP. Stroke in a defined elderly population 1967–1985. *Stroke* 1997;**28**:283–90.

22. Vartianen E, Sarti C, Tuomilehto J, Kuulasmaa K. Do changes in cardiovascular risk factors explain changes in mortality from stroke in Finland? *BMJ* 1995;**310**:901–4.

23. Bouser MG. Stroke in women. *Circulation* 1999;**99**:463–7.

24. Shuaib A, Boyle C. Stroke in the elderly. *Curr Opin Neurol* 1994;**7**:41–7.

25. Morey SS. National Stroke Association develops consensus statement on prevention of stroke. *Am Fam Physician* 1999;**60**:314–15.

26. SHEP Cooperative Research Group. Prevention of stroke by antihypertensive drug treatment in older persons with isolated systolic hypertension: Final results of the Systolic Hypertension in the Elderly Program (SHEP). *JAMA* 1991;**265**:3255–64.

27. English KM, Channer KS. Managing atrial fibrillation in elderly people. *BMJ* 1999;**318**:1088–9.

28. Hart RG, Sherman DG, Easton JD, Cairns JA. Prevention of stroke in patients with nonvalvular atrial fibrillation. *Neurology* 1998;**51**:674–81.

29. Wolf PA, Kannel WB, McGee DL et al. Duration of atrial fibrillation and imminence of stroke: The Framingham Study. *Stroke* 1983;**14**:664–7.

30. Sanderock P, Bamford J, Dennis M et al. Atrial fibrillation and stroke: Prevalence in different types of stroke and influence on early and long term prognosis (Oxfordshire Community Stroke Project). *BMJ* 1992;**305**:1460–5.

31. Albers G. Atrial fibrillation and stroke. Three new studies, three remaining questions. *Arch Intern Med* 1994;**154**:1443–57.

32. Nademanee K, Kosar EM. Long term antithrombotic treatment for atrial fibrillation. *Am J Cardiol* 1998;**82**:37N–41N.

33. The Stroke Prevention in Atrial Fibrillation Investigators. The Stroke Prevention in Atrial Fibrillation Study: final results. *Circulation* 1991;**84**:527–39.

34. The EAFT Study Group. Secondary prevention in non-rheumatic atrial fibrillation after transient ischemic attack or minor stroke. *Lancet* 1993;**342**:1255–62.

35. Petersen P, Godtfredsen J, Boysen G, Andersen ED, Andersen B. Placebo-controlled, randomized trial of warfarin and aspirin for prevention of thromboembolic complication in chronic atrial fibrillation. The Copenhagen AFASAK study. *Lancet* 1989;**I**:175–9.

36. The Stroke Prevention in Atrial Fibrillation Investigators. Warfarin versus aspirin for prevention of thromboembolism in atrial fibrillation: The Stroke Prevention in Atrial Fibrillation Study II. *Lancet* 1994;**343**:687–91.

37. Randomized trial of cholesterol lowering in 4444 patients with coronary heart disease: The Scandinavian Simvastatin Survival Study, 4S. *Lancet* 1994;**344**:1383–9.

38. McCann RL. Surgical management of carotid artery atherosclerotic disease. *South Med J* 1993;**86**:2s-23-28.

39. Rothwell PM, Slattery J, Warlow CP. Clinical and angiographic predictors of stroke and death from carotid endarectomy: Systemic reviews. *BMJ* 1997;**315**:1571–7.

40. Colditz GA, Bonita R, Stampfer MJ et al. Cigarette smoking and risk of stroke in middle aged women. *N Engl J Med 1988*;**318**:937–41.

41. Gorelick PB, Sacco RL, Smith DB et al. Prevention of a first stroke: A review of guidelines and a

multidisciplinary consensus statement from the National Stroke Association. *JAMA* 1999;**281**:1112–19.

42. Brass LM, Fayad PB, Levine S. Transient ischemic attacks in the elderly: Diagnosis and treatment. *Geriatrics* 1992;**47**:36–44.

43. Vrielink A, Eikelboom BC, Klop RBJ, Taks AC. Carotid surgery without angiography. *Ann Chirurg Gynaecol* 1992;**81**:155–7.

44. North American Symptomatic Carotid Endarterectomy Trial Collaborators. Beneficial effects of carotid endarterectomy in symptomatic patients with high grade carotid stenosis. *N Engl J Med* 1991;**325**:445–53.

45. European Carotid Surgery Trials Collaborative Group. MRC European Carotid Surgery Trial: Interim results for symptomatic patients with severe or with mild carotid stenosis. *Lancet* 1991;**337**:1235–43.

46. Hart RG, Harrison MJ. Aspirin wars:The optimal dose of aspirin to prevent stroke. *Stroke* 1996;**27**:585–7.

47. The Dutch TIA Trial Study Group. A comparison of two doses of aspirin (30 mg v 283 mg a day) in patients after a transient ischemic attack or minor ischemic stroke. *New Engl J Med* 1991;**325**:1261–6.

48. Paciaroni M, Bogousslavasky J. Clopidogrel for cerebrovascular prevention. *Cerebrovasc Dis* 1999;**9**:253–60.

49. WHO collaborative study of cardiovascular disease and steroid hormone contraception. Ischemic stroke and combined oral contraceptives: Results of an international multicenter case control study. *Lancet* 1996;**348**:498–505.

50. Lidegaard O. Oral contraception and risk of a cerebral thromboembolic attack: Results of a case-control study. *BMJ* 1993;**306**:956.

51. Haemorrhagic stroke, overall stroke risk, and combined oral contraceptives: results of an international, multicentre, case-control study. WHO collaborative study of cardiovascular disease and steroid hormone contraception. *Lancet* 1996;**348**:505–10.

52. Petitti DB, Sidney S, Bernstein A, Wolf S, Quesenberry C, Ziel HK. Stroke in users of low-dose oral contraceptives. *N Engl J Med* 1996;**335**:8–15.

33 Osteoporosis, osteoarthritis, and rheumatoid arthritis

Jo Ann Rosenfeld, MD

Osteoporosis, osteoarthritis, and rheumatoid arthritis are chronic common diseases that affect women predominantly and cause a significant disability.

Osteoporosis

Osteoporosis (OP) is a condition in which an individual develops a low bone mass or density (BMD), resulting in an increased risk of fractures. This occurs in women and men, but there is an increased rate of bone loss in post-menopausal women.

OP leads to an increased risk of fractures, resulting in health complications such as pneumonia and lung disease and chronic obstructive pulmonary disease, chronic pain, disability, and loss of independence.

Epidemiology

1. OP is common and its incidence increases with age. The prevalence of OP in women aged 50 to 54 years in the UK is between 2.0 and 3.5 percent. The prevalence rises to 14 to 20 percent in women aged 70 to 74 years.[1]
2. There is an increasing risk of fracture with decreasing bone density. A decrease of one standard deviation in bone density increases the risk of fractures 1.5 to 3 times.[1]
3. One in six white women will have an OP-related hip fracture in her lifetime. Fifty-four percent of 50-year-old women will have an OP related fracture during their lifetimes. The lifetime risk of a hip fracture for a 50-year-old British woman is 14 percent, a vertebral fracture 11 percent and radial fracture 13 percent.[1] This risk is as great as that of heart disease and six times higher than breast cancer.

4. OP causes more than 150 000 fractures in the UK yearly, including 60 000 hip fractures.[1]

5. Vertebral fractures occur in 25 percent of white women by age 65 years, and result in some institutionalization for more than half. There is a mortality rate of 5 to 20 percent within the first year after vertebral fracture.[2]

Risk factors

Case-controlled and prospective studies have found that the risk factors for OP-related hip fractures include being a woman, menopause, being of white or Asian race, cigarette smoking, low body weight, and inactivity (Table 33.1).

1. The more risk factors a woman has, the greater is her risk of hip fracture. The risk rises from a rate of 1.1 hip fractures per 1000 women-years for those women with two or fewer risk factors to a high of 9.4/1000 women-years with more than five risk factors.[3]

2. However, risk factors have a poor specificity and sensitivity in predicting either bone density or risk of fractures in individuals.[4]

3. Menopause: After menopause a woman's rate of bone turnover and loss of bone mass increase precipitously, and use of estrogen in HRT (see below) reduces the incidence of OP, improves bone mass and prevents fractures.

4. Low weight: Women who are underweight and those who lose weight are at higher risk for OP. A prospective study found that postmenopausal women who lose weight over two years had an increased risk of OP (RR = 1.32/10 lbs or 4.5 kg lost).[5]

5. Cigarette smoking: Whether smoking is a risk factor and how strong is disputed. Several studies correlate active cigarette smoking and OP. However, one study found that smoking was not a risk factor when the data were controlled for weight, health, and difficulty walking. Smokers were in poorer health, had more difficulty rising from a chair, spent fewer hours on their feet, were less likely to walk, and had faster heart rates.[3]

6. Alcohol use: Alcohol ingestion was associated with lower risk of hip fracture but not after adjustment for better self-reported health and ability to stand up from a chair.

7. Chance of falling: Fractures occur in 3 to 6 percent of individuals who fall. At least one fall occurs in 30 percent of individuals older than age 70. Individuals with balance and gait disturbances, tremors, difficulty walking or seeing, or on psychotropic medications are at higher risk of falling, and, if they have OP, fracturing a bone.

Table 33.1. Risk factors for fractures from osteoporosis

Family history and demographic factors
- Older age
- History of maternal hip fracture
- White or Asian race

Medical history
- Postmenopausal
- Poor self-rated health
- Previous hyperthyroidism
- Stroke
- Current use of medications
  - Long-acting benzodiazepines
  - Tricyclic antidepressants
  - Anticonvulsant medications
  - Steroids
- Any fracture since age 50 years

Social history
- Alcohol use
- Poor nutrition
- On feet less than 4 hours a day
- Limited ADLs and physical activity

Physical examination
- Resting pulse > 80 beats per minute
- Poor memory
- Confusion
- Disorientation
- Poor vision
- Low distant depth perception
- Poor strength
- Absent deep tendon reflexes
- Slow rising from sitting
- Inability to tandem walk

ADLs, activities of daily living.
Data from Cummings SF, Nevitt MC, Browner WS et al. Risk factors for hip fracture in white women. A prospective study. *N Engl J Med* 1995;**332**:767–71.

Primary prevention

Routine preventive care of women and older men, especially white and Asian women, should include assessment of OP risk. Counselling, including use of HRT, diet and physical activity and consideration of other concurrent medical conditions, is important.

1. Exercise in premenopausal women can increase their total BMD. Thus, when the woman is postmenopausal, she will start with a higher BMD and OP will be prevented for a longer period of time.

2. Similarly, dietary supplementation of calcium – 1500 mg daily for teenagers, 1000 mg daily for adult women, 1500 mg daily for postmenopausal women – can increase BMD and prevent OP. Additional use of vitamin D may be needed, if the woman cannot get enough from light exposure or drinking vitamin D-enriched milk.

3. HRT, in postmenopausal women: Use of HRT, either estrogen or estrogen and progesterone, in postmenopausal women is protective against development of OP, helps to reverse the bone loss, and prevents fractures. HRT is the cornerstone of preventive therapy for osteoporosis and fractures in women.

    a. Estrogen decreases bone resorption and increases cortical and trabecular bone density. Its greatest effect is in the first few years after menopause when the bone turnover would be at its highest.

    b. Current postmenopausal users of estrogen have a decreased risk for hip, wrist, and vertebral fractures. Women who use estrogen have a 25 percent decrease in the risk for hip fractures.[6]

    c. Rapid bone loss occurs when HRT is stopped.

    d. The optimal starting and duration of estrogen use is not yet determined, although starting as soon after menopause as possible is suggested.

        i. The magnitude of the effect of HRT was greater if HRT was started as early as possible in menopause. The effect of HRT was diminished, if it was initiated more than five years after menopause.

        ii. Women who are younger than age 75 years need at least seven years' (and perhaps as long as nine to ten years') use of estrogen to improve the BMD.

        iii. Whether estrogen use helps BMD if started after age 75 years is unknown. However, there is a demonstrated effect in women over age 70 years and with established OP.[2]

    e. Use of HRT has been proved to decrease the risk and occurrence of osteoporotic fractures (Table 33.2). Long-term use was associated with a 75 percent reduction in wrist fractures.[2] An International Consensus Development conference on osteoporosis concluded that estrogen therapy is the only well-established preventive measure that could decrease the number of osteoporotic fractures.[7]

Routine preventive care of women and older men, especially white and Asian women, should include assessment of osteoporosis risk.

Table 33.2. Relative risk of osteoporosis-related fracture with HRT use by duration of use

	Current user		Past user	
	< 10 years	> 10 years	< 10 years	> 10 years
Hip	0.8	0.27	0.97	1.67
Wrist	0.75	0.25	0.79	0.90
All nonspinal	0.67	0.60	0.92	1.00

Data from Cauley JA, Seeley DG, Enrud K et al. Estrogen replacement therapy and fractures in older women. *Ann Intern Med* 1995;**122**:9–16.

f. A dose of 0.625 mg daily conjugated estrogen is considered the minimal effective dose. However, even a daily dose of 0.3 mg conjugated estrogen can work to increase lumbar vertebral bone density. Doses of 1.0 mg estradiol or 50 to 100 µg of transdermal estradiol daily are equivalent.

g. Use of progestin or smoking does not diminish the beneficial effects of the estrogen.

h. There are considerable questions about estrogen's continued and long-term use. Fewer than 14 percent of women in the USA prescribed estrogen continue it for one year. Rates for continued use in Europe range from 8 to 25 percent.

   i. Women who exercise, have a healthy diet and low cardiovascular risk factors, and who are more likely to be closer to ideal body weight are more likely to continue estrogen.

   ii. Why women do not take estrogen or why they stop has not been well researched.

i. Side effects of estrogen use include increased coaguability, with increased risk of deep venous thrombosis, pulmonary embolism and stroke, endometrial hyperplasia and cancer, and breast cancer.

   i. Use of estrogen increases the rate of deep venous thromboses.

   ii. Use of estrogen alone is restricted to women who have had a hysterectomy. Women with an intact uterus must take a progestin in addition to prevent endometrial hyperplasia and increased risk of endometrial cancer.

   iii. There is an increased risk of breast cancer in long-time users of HRT. The Nurses' Health Study showed that the greatest risk was for women who used HRT for more than five years and were older than age 60 years. HRT is contraindicated in women with breast cancer.[2]

Women who are younger than age 75 years need at least seven years' use of estrogen to improve the BMD.

iv. Premenopausal women who develop amenorrhea related to anorexia, low weight, or excessive exercise are also at risk for OP, and may preserve bone mass by using OCPs. Low dose OCPs offer protection against OP. Whether depot-MPA offers this protection as well is uncertain.

v. Research studies do not yet suggest the routine prophylactic use of selective estrogen receptor modulator agents (SERMs) such as tamoxifen and raloxifene for primary prevention.

A dose of 0.625 mg daily conjugated estrogen is considered the minimal effective dose.

Secondary prevention

Secondary prevention is determination of individuals who have OP at a preclinical stage and institution of therapy to increase BMD and prevent fractures.

Diagnosis

The diagnosis of OP may be suggested by a new or pathological fracture or noticed incidentally on an X-ray.

1. Evaluation – history and physical: A history of bone fractures, thinness in an older woman, kyphoscoliosis or a loss of height may suggest OP. There are few physical findings. In some centers, any elderly person who fractures a bone is evaluated for OP.
2. Laboratory evaluation: There are metabolic bone diseases that can mimic OP. A minimal laboratory evaluation includes the following:
   a. Calcium and alkaline phosphatase. These levels are normal in OP, but abnormal in metabolic bone diseases such as hyperparathyroidism and vitamin D deficiency osteopenia.
   b. Thyroid-stimulating hormone: Hyperthyroidism or excessive use of exogenous thyroid in hypothyroid individuals can lead to excessive bone loss.
   c. Serum protein electrophoresis may be needed if other signs of multiple myeloma are present.
   d. There have been new assays of bone protein metabolites in blood and urine but their clinical significance and reliability are controversial.
3. X-rays: Standard X-rays do not determine early or mild bone loss.

A history of bone fractures, thinness in an older women, kyphoscoliosis or a loss of height may suggest osteoporosis.

4. Bone mineral densitometry is useful. Treatment is recommended when values are one to two or more standard deviations (SD) below peak bone mass (not corrected for age) (see below).

5. Absorptiometry of lumbar spine and hip provides the most precise measure.

6. Bone density measurement by dual energy X-ray absorptiometry (DEXA) scans is the most sensitive and suggested diagnostic modality. DEXA scans can assess bone mass both at axial and appendicular sites.

   a. Values are expressed as a "Z-score", representing the SD from the mean matched for age and sex.

   b. There is also a "T-score", which is the deviation from values for a young adult. A "T-score" below 2.5 SD defines osteoporosis, and 1.0 to 2.5 SD below average defines osteopenia.

   c. Osteopenia may be an indication for prophylaxis, depending on the age of the woman and risk factors. Osteoporosis is an absolute indication for treatment (secondary prevention).

7. Whether screening for OP is indicated is disputed. In the USA, without complete evidence, menopause alone is considered an indication for scanning and DEXA scans are covered biannually by Medicare.[8]

   In the UK, recent editorials and a metaanalysis of prospective studies of 11 populations (90 000 women-years) suggest that, although measurement of BMD can predict who is at greater risk for fractures, it cannot predict which individual will sustain a fracture. Thus screening menopausal women is not recommended.[9] Indications for densitometry are included in Table 33.3.

Whether screening for osteoporosis is indicated in all women is disputed.

Treatment

Treatment with drugs does not restore bone, but does prevent its further loss, and, thus, decreases the risk for fractures.

1. Lifestyle modifications:

   a. Exercise can increase BMD, especially with use of other methods, including diet, calcium, and estrogen. Estrogen and exercise actually increased bone density values in women with low BMDs who were followed for two years.[10] Good exercise includes weight-bearing exercise such as walking, jogging, rowing, and weight lifting.

   b. Moderation in use of caffeine and alcohol can decrease the bone mass loss rate.

   c. Dietary supplementation of calcium and vitamin D is inexpensive and may

Table 33.3. Indications for densitometry

Primary prevention
- In women with multiple risk factors
  - Smoking
  - White or Asian race
  - Hyperthyroidism
  - Chronic steroid use
  - Menopause
  - Secondary amenorrhea
    ? Prolonged use of depot-MPA
    Premature ovarian failure
    Anorexia nervosa

Secondary prevention
- In women > age 50 years with any fracture
- In woman with pathological fracture
- Radiological or clinical evidence of vertebral abnormality

Tertiary prevention
- Monitoring of therapy

Data from Compston JE, Cooper C, Kanis JA. Bone densitometry in clinical practice. *BMJ* 1995;**310**:1507–10.

increase BMD up to 1 percent over two years. Postmenopausal women need 1000 to 1500 mg elemental calcium daily. In elderly women, as little as 1000 mg daily may retard bone loss. The major side effect is constipation; it may be contraindicated in women with calcium renal stones.

One study of more than 3500 men and women who took 500 mg elemental calcium and 700 to 800 IU vitamin D daily found that there was one fracture less for every 45 woman (or man)-years of use. This was a risk reduction of 25 to 32 percent.[8]

d. Improvement of vision will not improve BMD, but will reduce the likelihood of falls.

e. Cessation of medications: Many medicines used for comorbid conditions can cause osteoporosis (Table 33.4). Also, medications that affect balance (psychotropic drugs, benzodiazepines, anticholinergic drugs, antihistamines) or cause postural hypotension (diuretics, antihypertensives) should be modified or stopped, to prevent fractures, if possible.

2. Pharmacological treatment:

a. Estrogen use or HRT is the treatment of choice for secondary prevention. However, HRT is contraindicated in some women and unacceptable in others (Table 33.5).

Table 33.4. Medications that can worsen osteoporosis

- Diuretics
  - Thiazides
  - Chlorthalidone
- Corticosteroids
- Antiseizure medications
- Cancer chemotherapeutic agents

Table 33.5. Contraindications to use of estrogen in postmenopausal women

- History of estrogen-dependent cancers
  - Breast
  - Endometrium
  - Cervical
  - Ovarian
- History of thrombosis
  - Deep venous thrombosis
  - Pulmonary embolism
  - Stroke
- Unexplained/undiagnosed breast lump
- Unexplained/undiagnosed vaginal bleeding

b. SERMS: Tamoxifen and raloxifene (Table 33.6):

   i. Tamoxifen: When tamoxifen was used for the treatment of breast cancer, it was noticed that its use increased BMD. However, although it also improves lipid profile, it increases the risk of thromboembolic disease and hepatic and endometrial tumors. It has not therefore been used specifically to improve BMD and prevent or treat OP.

   ii. Raloxifene has tissue-specific effect. Raloxifene is a SERM that has an antagonistic effect on breast tissue (against breast cancer) and an antagonistic effect on uterus (so no increase in endometrial tumors) and an agonistic effect on bone and cholesterol. This may make it an excellent drug for primary or secondary prevention of OP and improvement of lipids. More evidence is needed before it is recommended universally or prophylactically.

      1. Use of raloxifene in a three-year RCT trial of more than 6800 women decreased risk of vertebral fracture by half (RR = 0.5) at 60 or 120 mg/day. The risk of nonvertebral fractures was unchanged. Raloxifene increased BMD in femoral neck by 2.1 to 2.6 percent yearly. However, it increased the risk of deep venous thrombosis

Table 33.6. Pharmacological secondary prevention and treatment of osteoporosis

Treatment	Daily dose	Yearly cost $(US)
Exercise		Variable
Calcium	1000 mg	20–400
Vitamin D	700–800 IU	
Calcium/vitamin D		22
Alendronate	10 mg	> 600
Etridonate	400 mg	150
HRT	0.625 mg	200–300
Raloxifene	60 mg	700
Calcitonin	100 IU i.m.	400–700
	200 IU i.n.	

i.n., intranasally.

(RR = 3.3). Its use decreased the individual's risk of breast cancer and did not cause endometrial bleeding.[11]

2. Raloxifene lowers serum cholesterol levels. It may reduce cardiovascular risk in postmenopausal women. In one multicentered study of 300 nonobese menopausal women, raloxifene reduced LDL cholesterol, did not raise triglycerides, and increased HDL cholesterol, but not as much as HRT.[12]

iii. Other SERMS are rapidly being developed.

c. Biphosphonates: Etidronate (Didronel) and alendronate (Fosomax – 10 mg daily) are synthetic pyrophosphate analogs that decrease bone resorption.

i. When compared to placebo in a RCT, alendronate resulted in a BMD increase of 8.8 percent in vertebrae and 6.9 percent in the femoral neck and reduced all fractures from 18 to 13 percent.[2]

ii. These drugs are effective in decreasing rate of fractures. Another RCT compared women using calcium plus alendronate (5 or 10 mg daily for three years or 20 mg daily for two years) to those using just calcium and placebo. Use of alendronate was associated with a 48 percent decrease in new vertebral fractures, a decrease in progression of vertebral deformities and significant reduction in height loss.[13]

iii. These drugs also increase bone density. Another multicentered RCT of more than 2000 white women followed for three years found that alendronate increased average BMD, while decreasing by half the rate of vertebral fractures.[14]

iv. Gastrointestinal side effects are significant and include nausea, constipation, pain, and diarrhea. These drugs must be taken on an empty stomach with 8 oz (240 cm³) of water on awakening, at least half an hour before food, drink and other medications. They are expensive.

d. Calcitonin: Treatment with calcitonin causes a short-term decrease in bone resorption.

    i. The usual dose is 100 IU calcitonin salmon preparation or 0.5 mg recombinant form subcutaneously three times per week. This causes nausea.

    ii. Intranasal salmon calcitonin (200 IU) given once daily in alternating nostrils is also available.

e. Fluoride: Fluoride stimulates osteoblasts, but the bone growth it causes may be thin and the rate of fracture actually increased. It is therefore used in combination with calcium and vitamin D. The dose is 45 to 75 mg daily and gastrointestinal side effects are a problem.

f. Parathyroid hormone (PTH) use has been suggested. Intermittent low dose PTH can increase bone formation while high doses cause bone resorption. It is not generally used at present.

g. Growth hormone-releasing hormone and growth hormone use have been evaluated in small trials and have increased lumbar bone density.

> Dietary supplementation of calcium and vitamin D is inexpensive and may increase bone mass density up to 1 percent over two years.

Follow-up and further evaluation

A woman with a DEXA scan of 2 SD below nonage-controlled mean should be considered to have OP and started on treatment. Estrogen or HRT is the treatment of choice. Calcium and vitamin D supplementation is also suggested in all individuals who have or are at risk for OP. Dietary modification and exercise is also strongly suggested.

When HRT cannot or will not be used, SERMs, especially raloxifene would be the next treatment, with biphosphonates as the alternative.

This is a slowly progressive disease with long-term treatment necessary. The patient should be reevaluated in two years with a DEXA scan. Decreasing bone loss to less than 2 percent per year is an improvement and treatment should continue.

Arthritis

Arthritis is the most common chronic disease in women and causes more disability than any other disease.

1. In the USA by 2020 almost 60 million individuals will have arthritis.
2. Sixty to 85 percent of Americans over age 65 years have X-ray evidence of osteoarthritis (OA) and 35 to 50 percent have symptoms of pain, stiffness, and limitation of motion.
3. In the UK, 24 percent of all adults reported joint pain and 8 percent disability from arthritis.[15] In a typical UK general practice, 15 percent of the patients will have a connective tissue diagnosis and 3 to 4 percent will carry the diagnosis "osteoarthritis".[16]
4. Although perhaps not as immediately fatal as other diseases, nonetheless arthritis brings with it concerns about pain, deformity, isolation, loss of independence and privacy, fractures, and death. Yet, prevention of disability may be possible and treatment can improve complications of the disease.

> Arthritis brings with it concerns about pain, deformity, isolation, loss of independence and privacy, fractures, and death.

Osteoarthritis

Definition

Osteoarthritis is the degenerative disease of cartilage and joints; it has many etiologies and usually a slow, progressive nondeforming course. The joints most effected are usually the hands and large weight-bearing joints. Abnormalities in the cartilage can be associated with it.

Epidemiology

1. Osteoarthritis (OA) is very common (Figure 33.1). Twenty-four percent of women aged 64 to 75 years and more than half of women of more than age 75 years have symptomatic OA. An estimated 23 million women in the USA have OA,[17] and a British survey found that 8.7 percent of all individuals reported knee pain from OA.[18]
2. OA is a common cause of disability in the elderly, most of whom are women.
   a. This disability has social consequences, affecting work and employment.
   b. In women, arthritis can lead to disability that results in social isolation and

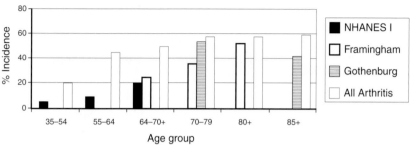

Figure 33.1.   Incidence of knee osteoarthritis and all arthritis in women (diagnosed by X-ray). (Data from: (1) NHANES I: Davis MA, Ettingher WH, Neuhaus JM. Obesity and osteoarthritis of the knee: Evidence from the National Health and Nutrition Examination Survey (NHANES I). *Semin Arthritis Rheum* 990;**20**:34–41. (2) Framingham: Felson DT. The epidemiology of knee osteoarthritis: Results from the Framingham Study. *Semin Arthritis Rheum* 1990;**20**:42–50. (3) Gothenburg: Bagge E, Bjelle A, Eden S, Svanborn A. Osteoarthritis in the elderly: Clinical and radiologic features in 79 and 85 years olds. *Ann Rheum Dis* 1991;**50**:535–9. (4) All arthritis: CDC. National Health Interview Survey 1989–1991. *MMWR Morb Mortal Wkly Rep* 1995;**44**:329–34.)

homeboundness, which, in turn, is a risk factor for nursing home placement.

3. OA of the knee, the most common joint affected, bothers more than half of older Americans and produces the greatest disability.

   a. Those individuals with OA of the knee are more than two times as likely to report difficulty walking and have a functional limitation.[17]

   b. It is the most common cause of difficulty with activities of daily living (ADLs) (Figure 33.2).

   c. Over half the women with OA of the knee report difficulty performing heavy chores and they are five times more likely to have trouble going up and down steps.

   d. Radiographic changes of the knee are present in one-third of individuals older than age 65 years.

4. However, 20 percent of those individuals with arthritis have never sought a physician's care.

Primary prevention:

Determining risk factors and altering these by behavior and lifestyle modifications, if possible, might avoid development of OA (Figure 33.3).

1. Framingham Study: Prospectively, 15.6 percent of elderly individuals developed knee arthritis in a 10-year period.[19] The Study identified three risk factors:

   a. Women had higher risk (RR = 1.8).

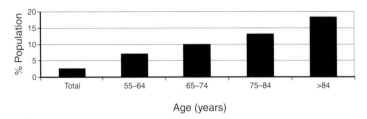

Figure 33.2.   Percentage of population with limitations caused by arthritis, by age. (Data from US Department of Health and Human Services. Arthritis prevalence and activity limitations – United States 1990. *MMWR Morb Mortal Wkly Rep* 1994;**43**:433–8.)

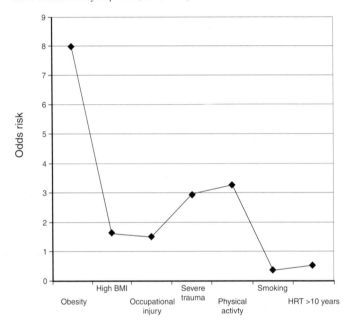

Figure 33.3.   Risk factors for osteoarthritis. BMI, body mass index; HRT, hormone replacement therapy.

   b. A higher baseline BMI (RR = 1.6) and weight change (RR = 1.4 per 10 lbs (4.5 kg) increase in weight) increased the risk of developing OA.
   c. Physical activity increased the risk of OA. Individuals with the highest quartile of activity had a relative risk of 3.3.
   d. Smokers had lower risk (RR = 0.4) of developing OA.
2.   Being a woman: OA has an increased incidence in women, with more rapid rise in the occurrence with age, particularly of small-joint hand arthritis.[20]
   a. An increase in symptoms with menopause has been documented for nearly 200 years.
   b. However, there is no relation between a woman's age of menarche or age at menopause or parity and development of OA.

    c. However, Heberden's nodes were three times more frequent in women whose age at menopause was above 50 years.

    d. The incidence of OA is increased in women who have had surgical menopause.[20]

    e. The course of OA in women may be different. Older women are more likely to report joint symptoms for the same level of radiographic severity of knee OA and OA of the hip progresses more rapidly in women than in men.[21]

> OA has an increased incidence in women, with more rapid rise in the occurrence with age.

3. OA and osteoporosis: Women with OA have less OP. There is an inverse relationship with OA and OP, probably linked first to obesity and increased BMI and secondly to the development of osteophytes. Obesity is linked to an increased incidence of OA and decreased incidence of OP. Osteophytes, bony overgrowths, occur in OA and increase the bone density. In addition, though, postmenopausal women with knee, hip, hand and multijoint OA have an increased BMD not explained by obesity and this increased BMD may predate menopause.[21]

4. OA and HRT and OCP use: Many studies show an inverse relationship between the use of HRT and development of OA, while a few show no difference.[21]

    a. In a cross-sectional study of more than 400 women of more than age 65 years, those who were currently using oral estrogen had a signficantly reduced risk of OA of the hip (RR = 0.57).[22]

    b. However, in a case-controlled study of more than 400 women, hip OA had no association with use of HRT, OCPs, parity, or hysterectomy.[23] Estrogen exposure and OA may be unrelated.

5. Obesity: Obesity increases the risk of knee, hip, and hand arthritis in women. However, whether this increased risk is caused by wear and tear or has a metabolic cause is undetermined. Women with a BMI of 27.3 or greater have a higher age-adjusted rate of arthritis.[24]

6. Physical activity: The effect of increased physical activity is complex.

    a. Increased activity has been linked to increased incidence of OA. Several studies including a Swedish case-controlled one found that the risk of hip OA leading to hip replacement was 2.3 times greater for individuals with high sports exposure and 1.5 times greater with medium sports exposure.[25]

    b. However, another case-controlled study that examined runners and community controls over eight years found that running protected against

> Obesity increases the risk of knee, hip, and hand arthritis in women.

disability and runners had less mortality. Older individuals who engage in vigorous running and aerobic activity had lower mortality and slower development of disability, fewer chronic joint pains but the same or more bone fractures. This effect was much more significant for women than for men. Women who did not run had much more disability than men or men and women runners.[26]

7. Occupational joint trauma: Long-term repetitive occupational use of joints is linked to an increased incidence of OA, especially bending and knee pain.

8. Primary prevention would include reducing risk factors. Some can be changed. Reducing weight can significantly affect the risk of development of OA of the knee in women. Weight reduction of 5.1 kg or 11.2 lbs over 10 years reduces the risk of symptomatic knee OA by 50 percent.[27] Also, reducing the physical demands of occupation can reduce the chance for OA.

> Weight reduction reduces the risk of symptomatic knee osteoarthritis by 50 percent.

Clinical presentation and diagnosis

1. Presentation:
   a. Women present with joint pain and stiffness.
   b. The disease waxes and wanes, and the course of the diseases varies among individuals.
   c. However, usually after months, the pain and disease "burn-out" in one joint.
   d. OA is a clinical diagnosis, established on the presence of joint stiffness, pain and the absence of systemic features (Table 33.7).

2. Examination: Examination shows large joints with crepitus with movement. Joint line tenderness and, later, decreased muscle strength, reduced range of motion and contractures may be found.

3. Radiological examination: X-ray findings do not correlate with severity of clinical disease or amount of pain. However, the presence of osteophytes is the radiographic feature that associated best with knee pain.[28] X-rays may show joint space narrowing and subchondral sclerosis.

4. Differential diagnosis includes several entities (Table 33.8).

> X-ray findings do not correlate with severity of clinical disease or amount of pain.

Treatment and secondary prevention

1. The goals of treatment are to maintain function, protect the joint, reduce pain and prevent complications and disability. Treatment must be individualized

Table 33.7. Criteria for diagnosis of osteoarthritis of hip and knees: American College of Rheumatology Classification Criteria

Hip
- Hip pain
- At least two of the following three items:
  - ESR < 20 mm/hour
  - Radiographic femoral or acetabular osteophytes
  OR
  - Radiographic joint pain narrowing

Knee
- Knee pain
- Radiographic osteophytes
- At least one of the following three items:
  - Age > 50 years
  - Morning stiffness ≤ 30 min every morning
  - Crepitus on motion

ESR, erythrocyte sedimentation rate.

Table 33.8. Differential diagnosis of osteoarthritis (OA)

- Crystalline arthritis
  - Calcium pyrophosphate disease (CPP): The incidence of CPP also increases with age. Ten to 15 percent of individuals aged 65 to 75 years and 30 to 60 percent of those over age 85 years have this. It occurs in areas affected by OA, but usually presents as acute monoarticular synovitis of knee, wrist, or shoulder. Structural changes are the same as in OA. Associated with hyperparathyroidism, hypothyroidism, gout, hypophosphatemia and hypermagnesemia. Treatment of primary cause does not affect chronic pyrophosphate arthropathy
  - Gout: Sudden onset of one red, warm, swollen joint or a chronic arthritis
- Connective tissue arthritides
  - Rheumatoid arthritis: Usually polyarthritis affecting small joints of hand, knees, shoulders, and hips and having systemic symptoms. Joints are often very swollen, hot, and tender
  - Psoriatic arthritis
- Infective arthritides
  - Septic arthritis: Usually a single, very swollen, tender, red hot joint in patient, with a fever, high white blood cell count, and systemic symptoms. May be caused by *Staphylococcus*, gonorrhea, or other organisms
  - Lyme arthritis: Usually starts as a single, warm, red joint, usually knees or elbows. Associated with tick bite (which may not be remembered) and sometimes with typical rash
- Traumatic arthritis

and includes exercise, education, and pain control.

Treatment must include:

a. Stabilization of coexisting disease.

b. Social and psychological support.

c. Physiotherapy and occupational therapy.

d. Pain control.

e. Exercise to keep up muscular conditioning.

f. Reduction of body weight to closer to ideal.

g. Use of assistive devices.

h. Self-management programs.

2. No screening tests to detect the disease before it is clinically obvious and, by treatment, change its course (secondary prevention) are available with OA.

3. Exercise:

a. Exercise can affect the course of disease and reduce the subsequent disability. However, few individuals receive an exercise prescription from their physician.

b. Individuals with arthritis often decondition and prolonged inactivity can lead to muscle weakness, decreased flexibility, poor endurance, osteoporosis, fatigue, depression, and low pain threshold.

c. A RCT found that individuals with OA who walked increased their walking distance and functional status and decreased their pain and their pain medication use.[29]

> Exercise can affect the course of the disease and reduce the subsequent disability.

4. Education: Patients need to be knowledgeable about their disease. A study of a self-management program that followed more than 100 women for 12 months found that using education and behavioral and cognitive modification techniques enhanced self-care management, improved physical and psychological health, and reduced pain.[30]

5. Pain control: Acetaminophen (up to 1000 mg every six hours) is the preferred analgesia. Only after this has been tried in maximal doses, should NSAIDs be used, and then in low dose pain dosages not high antiinflammatory doses to decrease the side effects of NSAIDs.

In the UK nearly 1.5 million person-years of NSAIDs are prescribed yearly. A practice guideline recommends that daily treatment should be acetaminophen (Tylenol, paracetamol). If NSAIDs are used, ibuprofen is the most appropriate alternative at a dose of 1.2 g daily.[16]

Side effects include upper gastrointestinal bleeding (gastric ulcers in 15 percent of those on chronic use), edema, hyponatremia, hyperkalemia, and renal and hepatic toxicity. A general policy of prescribing drugs to prevent gastrointestinal injury is not suggested.[16]

The role of topical NSAIDs is unclear.

6. Intraarticular steroid injections for single-joint arthritis can be used.
7. There is no use for systemic steroids or narcotics.
8. Surgery: Surgery is indicated in some patients with severe disease – either joint replacement or arthroscopy with debridement of cartilage and washout of joint space.
   a. The risks of surgery have decreased with new technology of prosthetic devices and new surgical techniques.
   b. Total hip replacement is an option for patients with disease of hip that cause:
      i. Chronic discomfort.
      ii. Considerable impairment.
      iii. Joint failure.
      iv. X-ray evidence of joint damage.
      v. Moderate to severe persistent pain.
      vi. Severe disability not relieved by extended course of nonsurgical management.

Acetaminophen (up to 1000 mg every six hours) is the preferred analgesia.

Rheumatoid arthritis

This is a systemic disease with multijoint arthritis that is usually progressive and often both disabling and deforming. Although primary and secondary prevention is not possible, use of effective disease-altering medications can affect the course of the disease.

Epidemiology

Rheumatoid arthritis (RA) is definitely a disease of women. There is some proof that estrogen use may affect its course.

1. Noticing that RA improved during pregnancy led to the discovery of steroid hormones.
2. OCP use may protect against RA or reduce the severity of the disease. A retrospective study found that women who used OCPs for more than five years had a RR of 0.1 of developing RA.[31]
3. Disease symptoms are less severe in the second half of the menstrual cycle.[32]

4. Women with RA had more children. In a retrospective study, it was found that having more than three children increased the risk of developing RA 4.8 times, and increased the risk of poorer prognosis.[31]

5. In the same retrospective study, women who breast fed their infants had twice the rate of RA.[31]

6. In one small RCT, however, use of postmenopausal estrogens caused no improvement in 33 women with RA followed for one year,[32] while in another small RCT of 107 women, more women (21 percent) given testosterone (50 i.m. every two weeks for one year) showed a significant improvement as compared with 4 percent of the placebo group.[33]

Clinical course

RA is a disabling disease that deforms and destroys joints, causes a loss of function and decreases the lifespan by an average of 13 to 18 years.[34]

1. RA occurs at any age but its peak incidence is at age 30 to 50 years, the ratio of women to men being 3 : 1.

2. Its course is variable.
   a. The disease waxes and wanes from weeks to years, with remissions and exacerbations occurring spontaneously.
   b. The disease ranges from mild to disabling and destructive. There is usually a remission in the first year.
   c. There is some evidence that individuals who develop the disease after age 60 years have a more severe course, greater burden in large and small joints, greater disease activity, and worse damage revealed on X-ray.
   d. Individuals with high rheumatoid factor titers and C-reactive protein titres often have a worse prognosis.
   e. Predictors of a more severe course, with earlier death, include being a man, younger age at onset, use of prednisone, being single, and having no occupation.

3. Any synovial-lined joint can be affected.
   a. Most commonly, RA starts as a bilateral symmetrical disease, although it can present asymmetrically.
   b. The joints most frequently affected are the small joints of hands and feet, wrists, knees, elbows, and geleno-humeral and acromioclavicular joints.

4. It is a systemic disease. It usually occurs in one of two forms – an acute arthritis involving single or multiple joints or a subacute form with multiple systemic manifestations. Systemic symptoms can include fatigue, fever, weight loss, anorexia, malaise, night sweats, parasthesias, and myalgias, and can precede the development of arthritis.

Table 33.9. 1987 criteria for rheumatoid arthritis

Four of seven of the following criteria are necessary for diagnosis:

1. Radiographic changes: Typical changes of posteroanterior hand and wrist X-rays – erosions or bony decalcifications

Clinical course

2. Morning stiffness lasting 1 hour
3. Arthritis of three or more joints at same time, seen by physician, consisting of swelling or joint effusions:

   Joints include proximal interphalangeal, metacarpophalangeal, wrist, elbow, knee, ankle, and metarsophalangeal joints

4. Rheumatoid nodules
5. Arthritis of hand joints
6. Symmetrical arthritis

Laboratory

7. Serum rheumatoid factor positive

Most commonly, rheumatoid arthritis starts as a bilateral symmetrical disease.

Diagnosis

1. Diagnosis of RA is clinical and usually gathered over a period of months to years (Table 33.9). The criteria in Table 33.9 have a 91 percent sensitivity and a 89 percent specificity for the diagnosis of RA.
2. Extraarticular manifestations:
   a. Fever.
   b. Rheumatoid nodules: These occur in 20 to 30 percent of individuals with RA, usually on extensor surfaces but they can occur anywhere.
   c. Muscle weakness and atrophy of skeletal muscles.
   d. Vasculitis: This can affect any system and is usually seen in individuals with high rheumatoid factor titers. This can cause polyneuropathy, gangrene, and visceral infarctions rarely.
   e. Lung and pleural symptoms: Fibrosis, nodules, pneumonitis, arteritis.
3. Radiological diagnosis:
   a. Early in the course of the disease the X-ray changes may not be symmetrical.
   b. There are usually both osseous and soft tissue manifestations. Findings include marginal erosions, uniform joint space loss, fusiform periarticular soft tissue swelling, and juxtaarticular osteoporosis.
   c. The MRI scan is becoming a good diagnostic test and can find early joint changes.

Findings include marginal erosions, uniform joint space loss, fusiform periarticular soft tissue swelling, and juxtaarticular osteoporosis.

4. Serological diagnosis:
   a. Anemia: This is usually a normocytic normochromic anemia, present in active RA.
   b. The erythrocyte sedimentation rate is usually elevated and C-reactive proteins are often present.
   c. Rheumatoid factor (RF): Rheumatoid factor comprises autoantibodies that occur in two-thirds of individuals with the disease. However, RF also occurs in 5 percent of normal individuals and in patients with lupus, Sjögren's syndrome, chronic liver disease, sarcoidosis, tuberculosis, and syphilis, and other diseases.
   d. Joint fluid analysis is not specific, but usually turbid, with decreased or normal glucose, increased protein and a white blood cell count of 5000 to 50 000, mostly polymorphonuclear lymphocytes.

Rheumatoid factor comprises autoantibodies that occur in two-thirds of individuals with the disease.

Treatment

The goals of therapy are relief of pain, reduction of inflammation, reduction of disability of joints and relief of systemic symptoms. Treatment includes behavioral and pharmacological therapy.

1. Life-altering therapy includes moderate exercise. Those individuals with RA who did exercise for more than five hours weekly for more than five years had less progression of joint damage, fewer hospitalizations, and less work disability.[35] Nonweight-bearing exercise such as swimming may help considerably.
2. Patient education and use of assistive devices are helpful.
3. Pharmacological treatment: There are four primary modes of treatment: (1) aspirin and NSAIDs, (2) oral steroids, (3) disease-modifying drugs (DMD), and (4) intraarticular steroid injections.
   a. When to go to DMDs is disputed. Traditionally, they are saved for patients who did not do well on NSAIDs and oral steroids or who had rapidly progressive disease. Recently, some experts suggested the use of DMDs earlier in the course, perhaps immediately.[34] Use of DMDs requires familiarity with their use (because of their potentially serious side effects) or consultation for continuing use.
   b. Aspirin and NSAIDs are used both for pain relief and control of inflamma-

tion. They work well but do not affect the progression of the disease. NSAIDs do have potentially serious gastrointestinal, hematological, and renal side effects and are some of the drugs most prescribed to women and elderly women.

c. Low dose systemic oral steroids will reduce pain and inflammation and may slow the progression of bone erosions. In a general practice in the UK, more than 1 percent of all patients were using chronic steroids and one-quarter of these were for RA.[36]

Oral steroids have been used as short-term medication, a bridge until DMDs work, and as chronic medication, but recently a RCT suggested that steroids work better short term than i.m. gold, although there was rebound in the group that used steroids.[37] In a metaanalysis of 34 studies, prednisolone, when compared to placebo or aspirin, chloroquine or deflazacort, did better at reducing the number of swollen joints short term, but the effect was not significant, and whether steroids reduce long-term joint deformation is unclear.[23]

Chronic steroid use has its own complications including OP, fractures, gastrointestinal side effects, and immunosuppression.

d. Disease-modifying drugs include gold compounds, methotrexate, D-penicillamine, and plaquinyl. These do not relieve pain and usually a NSAID must be given with them. They take weeks to show effect. However, they do produce significant improvement in approximately two-thirds of cases. The one most commonly used is methotrexate.

e. Intraarticular steroid injection for severe pain or inflammation of one joint can help.

f. Surgery plays a role in patients with severe intractable pain or disability.

Aspirin and nonsteroidal antiinflammatory drugs are used both for pain relief and control of inflammation.

Disability

More than half of women with RA become work disabled. Women who can modify their pace at work are less likely to become disabled. Women with the least autonomy over pace and schedule of work were 36 times more likely to be disabled than women with more autonomy.[38]

Conclusions

Arthritis most often occurs in women and is a major cause of disability.

Although prevention is difficult and screening does not change the course of the disease, treatment, palliation, and improvement are possible. Osteoporosis is a major cause of fractures in the elderly, especially women, and can thus cause disability, loss of independence, and death. Screening is possible and treatment is effective, but seeing improvement takes many years.

REFERENCES

1. Compston JE, Cooper C, Kanis JA. Bone densitometry in clinical practice. *BMJ* 1995;**310**:1507–10.
2. Bellatoni, ME. Osteoporosis and treatment. *Am Fam Physician* 1996;**54**:986–92, 995–6.
3. Cummings SF, Nevitt MC Browner WS et al. Risk factors for hip fracture in white women. *N Engl J Med* 1995;**332**:767–71.
4. Compston JE. Risk factors for osteoporosis. *Clin Endocrinol* 1992;**36**:223–4.
5. Ensrud KE, Cauley J, Lipschuts R, Cummings SR. Weight change and fractures in older women. *Arch Intern Med* 1997;**157**:857–61.
6. Cauley JA, Seeley DG, Enrud K et al. Estrogen replacement therapy and fractures in older women. *Ann Intern Med* 1995;**122**:9–16.
7. Consensus Conference. Osteoporosis. *JAMA* 1984;**252**:799–802.
8. Ullom-Minnich P. Osteoporosis. *Am Fam Physician* 1999;**60**:193–202.
9. Marshall D, Johnell O, Wedel H. Meta-analysis of how well measures of bone-mineral density predit occurrence of osteoporotic fractures. *BMJ* 1996;**312**:1254–9.
10. Prince RL, Smith M, Dick IM et al. Prevention of postmenopausal osteoporosis. A comparative study of exercise, calcium supplementation, and hormone-replacement therapy. *N Engl J Med* 1991;**325**:1189–95.
11. Ettinger B, Black DM, Mitlak BH et al. Reduction of vertebral fracture risk in postmenopausal women with osteoporosis treated with raloxifene: Results from a 3-year randomized clinical trial. *JAMA* 1999;**282**:637–742.
12. Walsh BW, Kuller LH, Wild RA et al. Effects of raloxifene on serum lipids and coagulation factors in healthy postmenopausal women. *JAMA* 1998;**279**:1445–51.
13. Lieberman UA, Weiss SR, Broll J et al. Effect of oral alendronate on bone mineral density and the incidence of fractures in postmenopausal osteoporosis. *N Engl J Med* 1995;**333**:1437–43.
14. Black DM, Cummings SR, Karpf DB et al. Randomized trial of effect of alendronate on risk of fracture in women with existing vertebral fractures. *Lancet* 1996;**348**:1535–41.
15. Litman K. A rational approach to the diagnosis of arthritis. *Am Fam Physician* 1996;**53**:1295–300, 1305–6.
16. Eccles M, Freemante N, Mason J. North of England Evidence Based Guideline Development Project: Summary guideline for non-steroidal anti-inflammatory drugs versus basic analgesia in treating the pain of degenerative arthritis. *BMJ* 1998;**317**:526–30.
17. Slemenda CW. The epidemiology of osteoarthritis of the knee. *Curr Opin Rheumatol* 1992;**4**:546–51.
18. O'Reilly SC, Muir KR, Doherty M. Knee pain and disability in the Nottingham community. *Br J Rheumatol* 1998;**37**:870–3.

19. Felson DT, Zhang Y, Hannan MT et al. Risk factors for incident radiographic knee osteoarthritis in the elderly: The Framingham study. *Arthritis Rheum* 1997;**40**:728–33.

20. Silman AJ, Newman J. Obstetric and gynecologic factors in susceptibility to peripheral joint osteoarthritis. *Ann Rheum Dis* 1996;**55**:671–3.

21. Nevitt MC, Felson DT. Sex hormones and the risk of osteoarthritis in women: Epidemiologic evidence. *Ann Rheum Dis* 1996;**55**:673–6.

22. Nevitt MC, Cumming NE, Hochberg MC et al. Association of estrogen replacement therapy with the risk of osteoarthritis of the hip in elderly white women. *Arch Intern Med* 1996;**156**:2073–81.

23. Dennison EM, Arden NK, Kellingray S et al. Hormone replacement therapy, other reproductive variables and symptomatic hip osteoarthritis in elderly white women: A case control study. *Br J Rheumatol* 1998;**37**:1198–202.

24. Callahan LF. Arthritis as a women's health issue. *Am J Rheumatol* 1965;**9**:159–62.

25. Vingard E, Alfredsson L, Malchau H. Osteoarthrosis of the hip in women and its relationship to physical load from sports activity. *Am J Sports Med* 1998;**26**:78–82.

26. Fries JF, Sing G, Morfeld D et al. Running and the developmentof disability with age. *Ann Intern Med* 1994;**121**:502–9.

27. Felson DT, Zhang Y, Anthony JM, Naimark A, Anderson JJ. Weight loss reduces the risk for symptomatic knee osteoarthritis in women: The Framingham Study. *Ann Intern Med* 1992;**116**:535–9.

28. Lanyon P, O'Reilly S, Jones A, Doherty M. Radiographic assessment of symptomatic knee osteoarthritis in the community definitions and normal joint space. *Am Rheum Dis* 1998;**57**:595–601.

29. Kovar P, Allegrante J, MacKenzie C et al. Supervised fitness walking in patients with osteoarthritis of the knees: A randomized controlled trial. *Ann Intern Med* 1992;**116**:529–34.

30. Barlow JH, Turner AP, Wrighty CC. Long-term outcomes of an arthritis self-management programme. *Br J Rheumatol* 1998;**37**:1315–19.

31. Jorgensen C, Picot MC, Bologna C, Sany J. Oral contraception, parity, breast feeding and severity of rheumatoid arthritis. *Ann Rheum Dis* 1996;**55**:94–8.

32. Van der Brink HR, van Everdingen AA, Van Wijk MJG, Jacobs JWG, Bijlsma JW. Adjuvant oestrogen therapy does not improve disease activity in postmenopausal patients with rheumatoid arthritis. *Am Rheum Dis* 1993;**52**:862–5.

33. Booij A, Biewenga-Booij CM, Huber-Bruning O et al. Androgens as adjuvant treatment in postmenopausal female patients with rheumatoid arthritis. *Am Rheum Dis* 1996;**55**:811–15.

34. Abyad A, Boyer JT. Arthritis and aging. *Curr Opin Rheumatol* 1992;**4**:153–6.

35. Nordermar R, Ekblom B, Zachrisson L, Lundquist K. Physical training in rheumatoid arthritis: A long term study. *Scan J Rheumatol* 1981;**10**:25–30.

36. Dennison EM, Cooper C. Corticosteroids in rheumatoid arthritis. *BMJ* 1998;**316**:789–90.

37. Van Gestel AM, Laan RF, Haagmsa CJ, Van de Putte LBA, Van Riel PC. Oral steroids as bridge therapy in rheumatoid arthritis patients starting with parental gold. *Br J Rheumatol* 1995;**34**:347–51.

38. Callahan LF, Rao J, Boutaugh M. Arthritis and women's health: Prevalence, impact and prevention. *Am J Prev Med* 1996;**12**:400–7.

Index

Note to index: where abbreviations are used to save space, they are explained at the relevant place in this Index